Congenital Diseases of the Heart

Congenital Diseases of the Heart

Clinical-Physiological Considerations

Abraham M. Rudolph, MD

University of California
San Francisco, CA, USA

Third Edition

WILEY-BLACKWELL

A John Wiley & Sons, Ltd., Publication

This edition first published 2009, © 2009 by Abraham Rudolph

Blackwell Publishing was acquired by John Wiley & Sons in February 2007. Blackwell's publishing program has been merged with Wiley's global Scientific, Technical and Medical business to form Wiley-Blackwell.

Registered office: John Wiley & Sons Ltd, The Atrium, Southern Gate, Chichester, West Sussex, PO19 8SQ, UK

Editorial offices: 9600 Garsington Road, Oxford, OX4 2DQ, UK
The Atrium, Southern Gate, Chichester, West Sussex, PO19 8SQ, UK
111 River Street, Hoboken, NJ 07030-5774, USA

For details of our global editorial offices, for customer services and for information about how to apply for permission to reuse the copyright material in this book please see our website at www.wiley.com/wiley-blackwell.

Library of Congress Cataloging-in-Publication Data
Rudolph, Abraham M., 1924–
Congenital diseases of the heart : clinical-physiological considerations / Abraham M. Rudolph. – 3rd ed.
p. ; cm.
Includes bibliographical references and index.
ISBN 978-1-4051-6245-6
1. Congenital heart disease. I. Title.
[DNLM: 1. Heart Defects, Congenital. WG 220 R917c 2009]
RC687.R73 2009
616.1′2043–dc22
ISBN 978-1-4051-6245-6 2008042565

A catalogue record for this book is available from the British Library.

Set in 9.5/12pt Minion by Graphicraft Limited, Hong Kong

1 2009

Contents List

Preface

The second edition of *Congenital Diseases of the Heart* was published in 2001. Since then, there have been remarkable advances in our understanding of many aspects of etiology, pathophysiology, clinical manifestations and management of congenital cardiovascular malformations.

Although the association of congenital cardiac lesions with many chromosomal anomalies had been recognized, specific gene defects responsible for cardiovascular anomalies have now been identified. One example is the NOTCH 1 gene mutation found in individuals with bicuspid aortic valve, as well as in those with hypoplastic left heat syndrome and aortic coarctation.

The extensive use of ultrasound examination for prenatal screening has facilitated diagnosis of congenital cardiovascular malformations in fetuses in utero. Previously it was thought that these lesions had little adverse effect during fetal life. However, the ultrasound studies are defining the influences of these anomalies on blood flow patterns and on development of the cardiac chambers and great vessels. This has stimulated efforts to relieve obstruction of the aortic valve to attempt to prevent the development of hypoplastic left ventricle. Furthermore, the effects of normal changes in the circulation during fetal development, on the hemodynamic changes associated with congenital cardiac lesions, are being defined.

Management of many congenital cardiovascular malformations has changed dramatically in recent years. Interventional cardiac catheterization techniques with percutaneous approach have largely replaced surgical thoracotomy to relieve obstructions and, in many instances, to close communications between the left and right sides of the heart. The low risk of these procedures and avoidance of thoracotomy has resulted in the temptation to close small defects and relieve minor obstructions, raising issues regarding the indications for these procedures.

These advances, as well as increasing knowledge of the hemodynamic changes associated with fetal and postnatal development, prompted me to embark on the preparation of this *Third Edition.* As in the previous editions, I have not attempted to provide a detailed discussion of all aspects of congenital cardiovascular disease, but have discussed the anomalies from the perspective of their impact at various stages of development – from fetus to neonate to child and adolescent. Because ultrasound examination and other techniques are largely replacing cardiac catheterization for diagnosis, I was tempted to drastically reduce the discussion of the procedure. However, at the urging of many of my colleagues I have retained these sections, because they felt they added to the understanding of the pathophysiology.

I am most grateful to Dr Norman Silverman, with whom I frequently have discussions about effects of congenital cardiac malformations on the fetus. His vast experience with echocardiography of fetuses has contributed enormously to assisting me to appreciate fetal hemodynamics. I also greatly appreciate the contributions of Dr. Charles Kleinman; he reviewed the manuscript and his comments, criticisms and suggestions have been most helpful.

I dedicate this edition to my wife, Rhona. She died soon after I embarked on this venture. She had always been most supportive and I sensed her enthusiastic encouragement throughout the preparation of this book.

CHAPTER 1

The fetal circulation

The circulation in the fetus differs from that in the adult. Knowledge of the course and distribution of the fetal circulation is important to our understanding of the manner in which various congenital heart lesions influence the normal circulation. The circulation undergoes continuous maturation during gestation, both morphologically and functionally, and these changes during development may be greatly influenced by congenital cardiac lesions. Furthermore, we now recognize that the clinical manifestations of congenital heart disease are intimately related to postnatal changes in the circulation. At birth, dramatic changes occur as the gas exchange function is transferred from the placenta to the lungs.

The presence of congenital heart lesions may profoundly affect the alterations in the circulation necessary for adaptation and postnatal survival. In this chapter I review current knowledge of the fetal circulation and its distribution and the changes that occur postnatally. The pulmonary circulation and the changes it undergoes after birth are described in Chapter 5 and fetal function and perinatal changes of the ductus arteriosus are discussed in Chapter 6.

Most of the information regarding the fetal circulation has been derived from the sheep, which has a gestational period of about 150 days as compared with the human of about 280 days. However, with the advent of ultrasound techniques, knowledge of the circulation of the normal fetus and of fetuses with congenital heart lesions has been increasing. It cannot be assumed that development in different species is the same at similar stages of gestation. This is not only because of inherent species differences but also because there are wide variations in the degree of maturity at the time of birth. The rat and the rabbit are relatively immature at birth, whereas the guinea pig is very mature at birth; the lamb is relatively mature and the human infant somewhat less mature. Furthermore, in considering distribution of the circulation, there are marked differences in body proportions. Whereas the brain in the mature lamb fetus is only about 3% of body weight, the human brain comprises about 12% of body weight in the term fetus. Despite these differences, observations we have made in previable human fetuses and ultrasound studies in the human fetus indicate that the course and distribution of the circulation are similar to those in the fetal lamb. However, as discussed below, the quantities of blood ejected by the ventricles and the volumes distributed to various organs differ considerably in human and lamb fetuses.

Because gestational period varies in different species, it is convenient, in making comparisons, to express gestation as a fraction of the normal period for the species. Thus, in the lamb with a 150-day gestation, 100 days is denoted as 0.66 gestation.

Postnatal circulation

Postnatally, respiratory gases enter and leave the body through the lungs, and energy sources are provided from the gastrointestinal tract, entering the portal venous system to be distributed to the liver. The adult circulation is characterized by serial flow of venous blood into the right atrium (Figure 1.1). It is ejected by the right ventricle into the pulmonary circulation to be oxygenated in the lungs and returns to the left atrium and ventricle to be ejected into the aorta for distribution to body organs. Carbon dioxide is removed and oxygen taken up in the lungs; a variable proportion of oxygen is extracted, and carbon dioxide and

Congenital Diseases of the Heart, 3rd edition. By A. Rudolph
© 2009 Blackwell Publishing, ISBN: 9781405162456

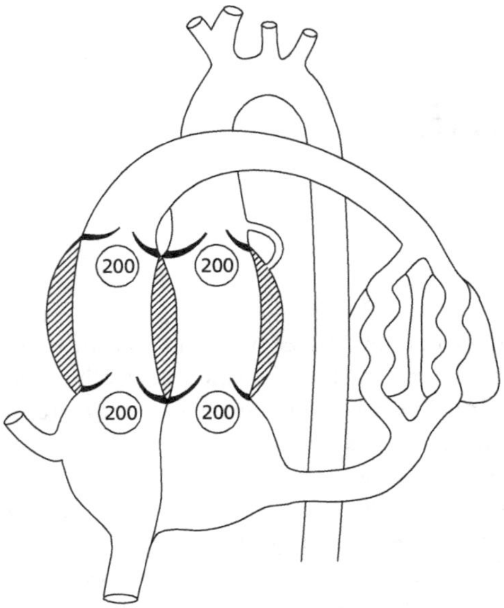

Figure 1.1 Course of blood flow in the adult circulation. The volumes of blood ejected by each ventricle and returning to each atrium are similar postnatally.

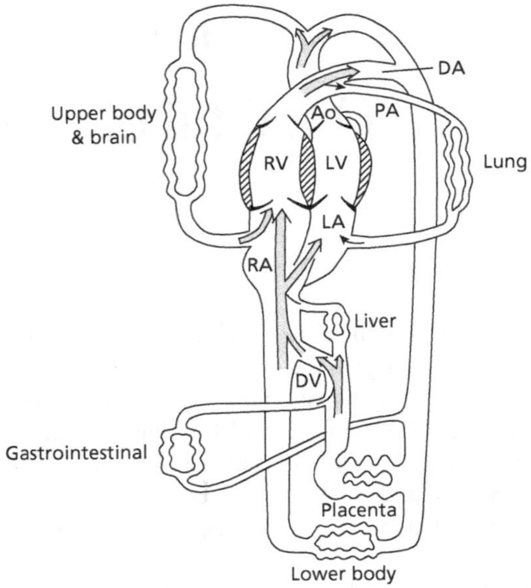

Figure 1.2 The general course of the mammalian fetal circulation. Ao, aorta; DA, ductus arteriosus; DV, ductus venosus; LA, left atrium; LV, left ventricle; PA, pulmonary artery; RA, right atrium; RV, right ventricle.

metabolites are added to blood by the tissues. Apart from minor amounts of bronchial venous blood that may enter the pulmonary vein and coronary venous blood that may empty directly into the left ventricular cavity, there is essentially no mixing of pulmonary venous and systemic arterial blood with poorly oxygenated systemic venous and pulmonary arterial blood. Postnatally, metabolic substrates, absorbed from the gastrointestinal tract into the portal venous system, are first delivered to the liver and then enter the systemic venous system and pass through the lungs before being delivered to tissues by the arterial circulation.

Circulation in the fetal lamb

Course of blood flow

The course of the circulation in the fetus is shown in Figures 1.2 and 1.3. Blood is oxygenated in the placenta and returns to the fetus through the umbilical veins, which enter the body through the umbilicus and join the portal vein. Umbilical venous blood has a Po_2 of about 32–35 mmHg when the mother is breathing ambient air and its oxygen saturation is about 80–85%. The umbilical vein

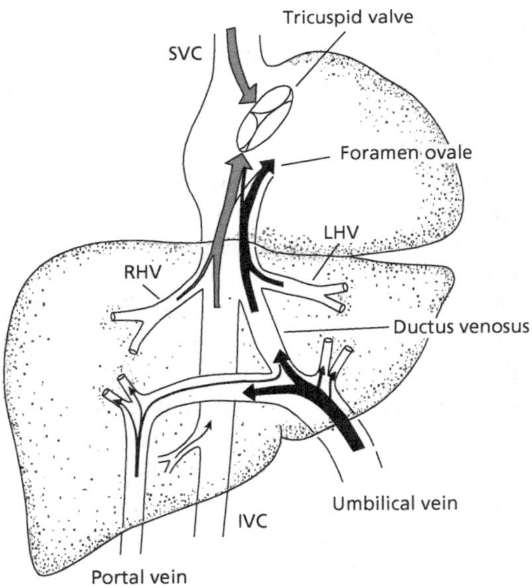

Figure 1.3 Course of blood flow in the region of the porta hepatis. Umbilical venous blood is distributed to the left lobe of the liver. The ductus venosus arises from the umbilical vein, which then arches to the right to join the portal vein. Portal venous blood is largely distributed to the right liver lobe and only a small proportion passes through the ductus venosus. IVC, inferior vena cava; LHV, left hepatic vein; RHV, right hepatic vein; SVC, superior vena cava.

passes from the umbilicus to the hilum of the liver; it provides branches to the left lobe of the liver and then divides into the ductus venosus and a large arcuate branch, which courses to the right in the hilum, where it is joined by the portal vein (Figure 1.3). Branches to the right lobe of the liver arise beyond this junction. The ductus venosus passes dorsally and cephalad through the liver parenchyma to join the inferior vena cava immediately beneath the diaphragm. The left hepatic vein joins the ductus venosus at its entry into the inferior vena cava, so there is a common entry orifice. In the sheep fetus this orifice is partly covered by a thin, valve-like membrane on its caudal edge [1]. The right hepatic vein enters the inferior vena cava separately, and the orifice is partly covered by a valve-like structure caudally. The function of these valve-like membranes is not known, but we have conjectured that they may facilitate directional flow of the various venous streams entering the inferior vena cava at this site. Previously, it was generally believed that umbilical and portal venous blood mixed in the porta hepatis and was then distributed to the left and right liver lobes and through the ductus venosus. However, Lind et al. [2] obtained umbilical venous angiograms in human fetuses immediately after delivery and suggested that umbilical venous blood passes preferentially to the left liver lobe and through the ductus venosus.

Using radionuclide-labeled microspheres, we were able to define not only the patterns of blood flow in the fetal liver but also the quantities of blood flowing through various channels in the fetal sheep [3]. Umbilical venous blood is distributed to the left lobe of the liver, through the ductus venosus, and via the arcuate branch, to the right liver lobe. Almost all portal venous blood is distributed to the right liver lobe. Only a small proportion, about 5–10% or less, passes through the ductus venosus and none is delivered to the left lobe. Thus the left lobe of the fetal liver receives well-oxygenated umbilical venous blood and a small supply from the hepatic artery. The right lobe receives a mixture of poorly oxygenated portal venous and umbilical venous blood, as well as a small amount from the hepatic artery. This accounts for the fact that the oxygen saturation of left hepatic venous blood is higher than that of right hepatic venous blood [4] (Figure 1.4).

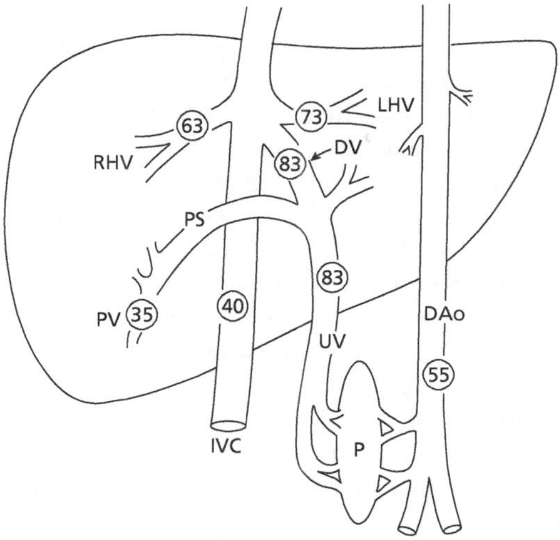

Figure 1.4 Blood oxygen saturations are shown in vessels in the region of the liver in the fetal lamb. DAo, descending aorta; DV, ductus venosus; IVC, inferior vena cava; LHV, left hepatic vein; P, placenta; PS, portal sinus; PV, portal vein; RHV, right hepatic vein; UV, umbilical vein.

The distributions of ductus venosus blood, blood from the distal inferior vena cava, and blood from the left and right hepatic veins have also been examined using radionuclide-labeled microspheres in fetal sheep [5]. Umbilical venous blood passing through the ductus venosus into the inferior vena cava is preferentially directed across the foramen ovale into the left atrium and left ventricle; only a small proportion passes into the right atrium and through the tricuspid valve. Abdominal inferior vena cava blood, in contrast, preferentially streams across the tricuspid valve into the right atrium and right ventricle and only a relatively small proportion crosses the foramen ovale to the left atrium. Blood from the left hepatic vein tends to follow the course of the ductus venosus stream, being preferentially distributed across the foramen ovale, whereas right hepatic venous blood preferentially streams across the tricuspid valve, following the course of abdominal inferior vena cava blood (see Figure 1.3). This preferential distribution of blood to the foramen ovale or the tricuspid valve suggests that there is streaming within the inferior vena cava between the liver and the heart. This can be observed directly in the fetal lamb when a right thoracotomy is performed. Observation of the thoracic portion of the inferior vena cava reveals well-oxygenated and poorly oxygenated blood streams. The anterior and right portion of the vessel is seen to have a poorly oxygenated stream, but blood flowing in the posterior and left portion is clearly well oxygenated. The streaming patterns in the inferior vena cava have also been observed by color flow Doppler studies. The ductus venosus stream has a velocity of about 55 cm/s and is directed largely through the foramen ovale, whereas distal inferior vena cava blood has a considerably lower velocity of about 15 cm/s and streams across the tricuspid valve. It is likely that the high velocity of the ductus venosus stream contributes to maintaining its preferential distribution across the foramen ovale. Ultrasound examination of human fetuses have also shown similar differences in ductus venosus and distal inferior vena cava velocities, and similar preferential streaming patterns.

The inferior margin of the atrial septum separates the entrance of the inferior vena cava from the left atrium, but the crescentic edge of the superior portion of the atrial septum, the crista dividens, overlies the inferior vena cava (see Figure 1.3). The posterior left portion of the inferior vena cava thus connects directly through the foramen ovale to the left atrium. During phases of the cardiac cycle, the eustachian valve and the lower portion of the atrial septum move in unison, either to the left to facilitate movement of blood through the foramen ovale, or to the right to enhance flow through the tricuspid valve [6]. The preferential streaming of ductus venosus and left hepatic venous blood through the foramen ovale distributes blood of higher oxygen saturation to the left atrium and ventricle and thus into the ascending aorta. Blood of lower oxygen saturation from the abdominal inferior vena cava and the right hepatic vein is preferentially distributed into the right ventricle and pulmonary artery.

The ductus venosus serves as a partial bypass of the hepatic microcirculation for umbilical venous blood. It may reduce the impedance to umbilical venous return by avoiding the need for all the blood to pass through the liver. Although it does facilitate passage of well-oxygenated blood to the left side of the heart, the proportion of umbilical venous blood that passes through the ductus varies greatly, both in the lamb and the human fetus, from about 20 to 90% [3,7]. In some species, such as the horse and the pig, the ductus venosus is not detectable in the latter part of gestation. The importance of the ductus venosus in the fetus is thus questionable, but it may be important in initiating some of the effects of aortopulmonary transposition on development of the pulmonary circulation (see Chapter 18).

Superior vena cava blood is largely directed by the tubercle of Lower to the tricuspid valve and is distributed into the right ventricle. Only about 5%, or less, flows through the foramen ovale into the left atrium in the normal fetus. Ultrasound examination of the fetal lamb indicates that the small amount of superior vena cava blood that enters the foramen ovale does so indirectly, by first flowing retrograde into the upper portion of the inferior vena cava and then entering the foramen. This phenomenon is markedly accentuated during fetal hypoxemia [6].

Right ventricular blood is ejected into the pulmonary trunk, and the larger proportion passes through the ductus arteriosus to the descending aorta, with the remainder entering the pulmonary circulation (Figure 1.5). Blood that passes from the pulmonary trunk through the ductus arteriosus is directed to the descending aorta; none passes retrogradely across the aortic isthmus to the ascending aorta and its branches. The left atrium receives blood from the foramen ovale and pulmonary veins, and then empties into the left ventricle, which ejects into the ascending aorta. Most ascending aortic blood is distributed to the coronary circulation, head and cerebral circulation, and upper extremities; only a small proportion passes across the aortic isthmus into the descending aorta. The major proportion of descending aortic blood is distributed to the umbilical–placental circulation and the remainder to the abdominal organs and the tissues of the lower trunk and lower extremities.

Admixture of oxygenated and systemic venous blood

In the adult circulation, there is essentially no mixing of oxygenated pulmonary venous and systemic venous blood. In the fetus, there are several sites of mixing. Portal and umbilical venous bloods enter the vessels in the porta hepatis. Blood from the ductus venosus, left and right hepatic veins, and abdominal inferior vena cava all enter the thoracic portion of the inferior vena cava. Admixture occurs

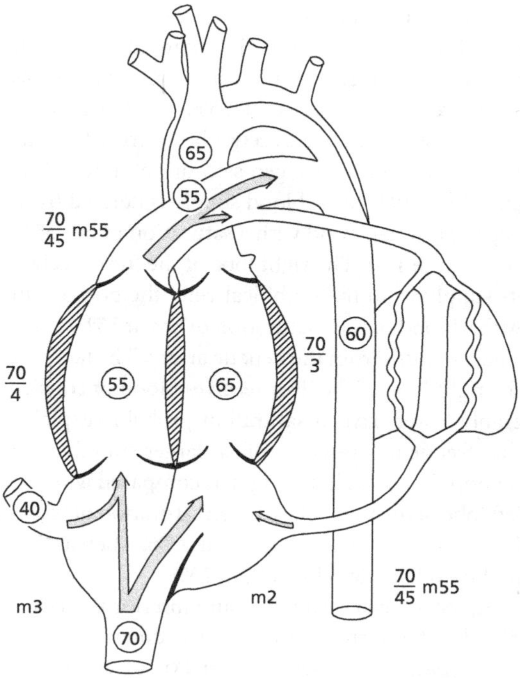

Figure 1.5 Course of the circulation in the heart and great vessels in the late-gestation fetus. The figures in circles within the chambers and vessels represent percent oxygen saturation levels. The figures alongside the chambers and vessels are pressures in mmHg related to amniotic pressure level as zero. m, mean pressure. The aortic arch and its branches are shown for both the human and the lamb. In the lamb, a single vessel, the brachiocephalic trunk, gives rise to carotid and subclavian arteries. In the human, the innominate and left carotid and subclavian arteries arise separately.

in the left atrium, where blood entering the foramen ovale from the inferior vena cava is joined by pulmonary venous blood. As mentioned above, the preferential streaming of blood partly separates the well-oxygenated and poorly oxygenated blood, favoring distribution of oxygenated blood into the left ventricle and ascending aorta and providing blood with a higher oxygen content to the heart, brain, and other upper body tissues. Systemic venous blood is preferentially directed into the right ventricle, pulmonary trunk, and ductus arteriosus to the descending aorta and its branches to the lower body, as well as to the placenta.

Because umbilical venous and vena cava blood is mixed, the blood delivered to the fetal body and the placenta contains varied proportions of oxygenated and systemic venous blood. Hence some umbilical venous blood is returned to the placenta after passing through the ductus venosus and foramen ovale or ductus arteriosus shunts without first being delivered to fetal tissues to permit oxygen uptake. This situation is equivalent to that occurring postnatally with some congenital heart lesions (e.g., atrial or ventricular septal defect), in which oxygenated blood passes from the left atrium or left ventricle into the right side of the heart to be recirculated to the lung. This, termed a *left-to-right shunt*, imposes an additional workload on the heart. Similarly, with congenital heart lesions in which systemic venous blood is shunted through an abnormal communication into the left side of the heart to be distributed back to the body tissues without passing through the lung, a *right-to-left shunt* occurs. The blood returning to the heart from the superior and inferior vena cava that is distributed to the fetal tissues without first being delivered to the placenta for oxygenation is effectively a right-to-left shunt. This effective right-to-left shunt contributes to inefficiency of the fetal circulation. In the sheep fetus under normal conditions, right-to-left shunt represents about 45% of superior vena cava and 53% of inferior vena cava blood [8]. Umbilical venous blood that passes through the ductus venosus and foramen ovale or ductus arteriosus and which is distributed back to the placenta is an effective left-to-right shunt. This represents about 22% of umbilical venous blood, and the combined left-to-right and right-to-left shunts constitute about 33% of the combined ventricular output of the fetal heart.

Intravascular pressures in the fetus

In the postnatal animal or human, it is customary to express pressures with reference to atmospheric pressure as the zero. However, the fetus is surrounded by amniotic fluid in the uterus within the abdomen, and all pressures are subjected to an increase from the environmental pressure. This changes if the intraabdominal pressure is increased by straining, distension with gas or feeding, and also by postural change; uterine contraction also produces an increase in all fetal intravascular pressures. It is therefore now customary to relate all fetal pressures to intraamniotic rather than to atmospheric pressure. The pressures shown in Figure 1.5 are expressed in relation to intraamniotic pressure. In the quietly standing ewe, intraamniotic pressure usually is about 8–10 mmHg above atmospheric pressure. When considering effective filling pressures of the cardiac ventricles, it is more appropriate to measure transmural pressure, or intraventricular minus pericardial pressure. Pericardial pressure is generally similar to intrapleural pressure, which is negative (i.e., lower than atmospheric pressure) postnatally. Mean pressure in the superior and inferior vena cava and the right atrium is about 2–3 mmHg. The *a* and *v* waves are about 4–5 mmHg, with the *a* wave only slightly higher. Left atrial pressures have a phasic contour similar to that of the right atrium, and the mean pressure is only 1–2 mmHg lower than right atrial pressure. Mean pressure in the portal sinus is 5–6 mmHg. Umbilical venous pressure is about 7–8 mmHg near the umbilical ring, and 2–3 mmHg higher near the placenta. Systemic arterial pressure increases with gestational age in the lamb fetus, from a mean level of 25–30 mmHg at about 60 days' gestation to 55–60 mmHg close to term. Figure 1.5 shows the pressures measured in various cardiac chambers in the late gestation fetal lamb *in utero*. The ductus arteriosus, connecting the pulmonary trunk with the descending aorta, has a diameter that, through most of gestation, is large enough to equilibrate pressures in the great arteries. The similarity of the systolic and diastolic pressures in the aorta and pulmonary artery has been observed in fetal lambs as young as about 60 days' gestation and to near term at about 145 days' gestation [9]. However, there is a tendency for systolic pressure in the pulmonary trunk to exceed that in the aorta by 5–8 mmHg during the last 10–14 days of gestation, presumably as a result of mild ductus arteriosus constriction. Left and right ventricular systolic pressures are similar to those in the ascending aorta and pulmonary trunk, and end-diastolic pressures are similar to the height of the *a* waves in the left and right atrium respectively.

Blood gases and oxygen saturation

Maternal arterial blood in the pregnant ewe has a Po_2 of 90–100 mmHg and a Pco_2 of about 35 mmHg. There is a large Po_2 gradient across the placenta, with a Po_2 of 32–35 mmHg in umbilical venous blood. Umbilical venous blood Pco_2 is about 40 mmHg and pH is 7.40. Because the P_{50} (the Po_2 at which hemoglobin is 50% saturated with oxygen) for fetal blood in the sheep is considerably lower (~19 mmHg) than that of adult blood (~31 mmHg), umbilical venous blood has an oxygen saturation of 80–85% (see Chapter 3). The left lobe of the liver receives blood from the umbilical vein with an oxygen saturation of 80–85%, and about 10% of its blood supply is derived from hepatic arterial blood with a saturation of 50–55% (see Figure 1.4). The right lobe of the liver receives its supply from the umbilical vein, the portal vein with a blood oxygen saturation of about 35%, and a small amount from the hepatic artery. The fact that the right lobe of the liver receives blood of considerably lower oxygen saturation probably explains the frequent presence of a larger number of hemopoietic cells in the right as compared with the left lobe of the liver. The oxygen saturation of blood in the right hepatic vein is about 65%, whereas that in the left hepatic vein is about 75%.

Superior vena cava blood and inferior vena cava blood distal to the entrance of the ductus venosus and hepatic veins both have a Po_2 of about 12–14 mmHg and an oxygen saturation of 35–40%. The Po_2 of right ventricular and pulmonary arterial blood is 18–20 mmHg and oxygen saturation is about 50%. Left ventricular and ascending aortic blood have a Po_2 of about 25–28 mmHg and an oxygen saturation of about 65%, whereas descending aortic blood has a Po_2 of 20–23 mmHg and an oxygen saturation of about 55%. Systemic arterial blood has a Pco_2 of 43–45 mmHg and a pH of about 7.38–7.39. The values for blood gases and oxygen saturations in the human fetus *in utero* are not well defined but are discussed below.

Effects of administering oxygen to the mother

Administering 100% oxygen to the ewe raises arterial oxygen saturation to 100% and the Po_2 to more than 400 mmHg. Fetal arterial Po_2 increases to only 30–35 mmHg with an oxygen saturation of about 80%. Umbilical venous blood Po_2 increases to 40–50 mmHg and oxygen saturation reaches 95–100% (see Chapter 3).

Cardiac output and its distribution

In the adult, the circulation passes in series through the right atrium, right ventricle and pulmonary artery, returning to the left heart and being ejected into the aorta and peripheral circulation. The cardiac output in the postnatal individual is expressed as the volume of blood flowing through the heart per unit time, and represents the volume of blood ejected by each ventricle. In the fetus, blood distributed to the various parts of the body and to the placenta is derived from the systemic venous return as well as the umbilical venous return, and the ventricles effectively act in parallel; blood to many organs is derived from both ventricles. Also, the outputs of the left and right ventricles are different in the fetus. It has therefore become customary to express the output of the heart as combined ventricular output (CVO), the sum of the volumes ejected by the two ventricles.

The CVO has been studied in human fetuses using ultrasound techniques, but measurements vary considerably (see below). Most reliable information is from studies in the sheep. In chronically instrumented fetal lambs during the latter months of gestation (term is about 145 days), CVO is about 450–500 mL/min per kg fetal body weight [9]. Umbilical–placental blood flow is about 200 mL/min per kg body weight, and blood flow to the fetal body is about 250–300 mL/min per kg. The right ventricle ejects about two-thirds and the left ventricle about one-third of CVO in the fetal lamb (Figures 1.6 and 1.7).

The umbilical–placental flow of about 200 mL/min per kg represents 40–45% of CVO. Umbilical venous blood entering the porta hepatis is distributed either to the liver or through the ductus venosus. Although the proportions vary, on average about 55% (range 20–90%) passes through the ductus venosus and 45% through the hepatic circulation. Thus about 110 mL/min per kg passes through the ductus venosus. The liver receives about 90 mL/min per kg fetal body weight of blood from the umbilical vein. Portal venous blood flow is about 30 mL/min per kg; most of this blood enters the right lobe of the liver. Inferior vena cava blood distal to the entrance of the hepatic veins and ductus venosus (abdominal inferior vena cava) is

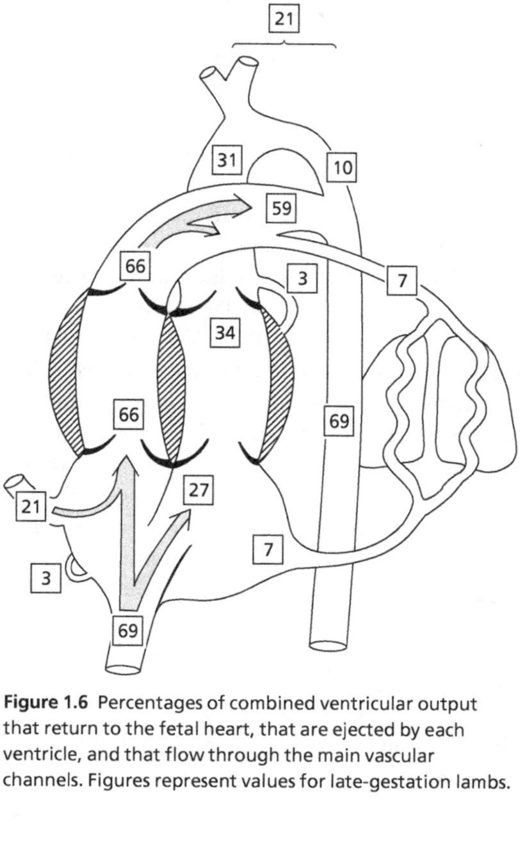

Figure 1.6 Percentages of combined ventricular output that return to the fetal heart, that are ejected by each ventricle, and that flow through the main vascular channels. Figures represent values for late-gestation lambs.

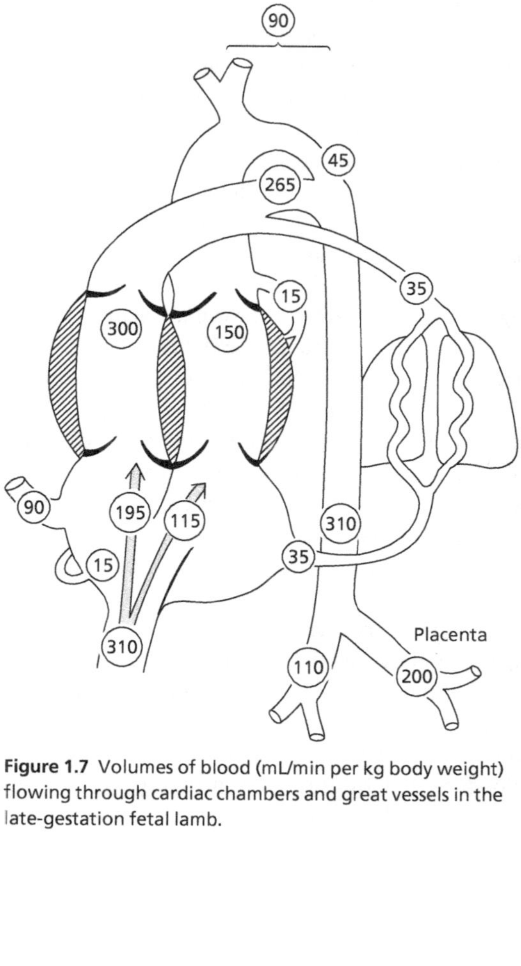

Figure 1.7 Volumes of blood (mL/min per kg body weight) flowing through cardiac chambers and great vessels in the late-gestation fetal lamb.

Table 1.1 Percent of combined ventricular output (%CVO) and actual blood flows distributed to organs in late-gestation lambs *in utero*.

Blood flow	*%CVO*[1]	*mL/100 g tissue*	*mL/kg fetal weight*
Brain	4.2	100	20
Heart	3.3	200	16
Liver	25.2	380	120
Kidney	2.9	190	14
Gut	5.2	55	25
Lung	5.2	95	25
Skin, muscle, bone	29.4	20	140
Placenta	39.4		180

1 Totals of %CVO are greater than 100 because a large proportion of liver blood flow is derived from umbilical–placental flow via the umbilical vein.

derived from the lower body organs and the lower extremities as well as the lower portion of the trunk. In the fetal lamb, this represents about 30% of CVO or about 140–150 mL/min per kg.

The blood entering the heart from the inferior vena cava includes ductus venosus, left and right hepatic venous, and abdominal inferior vena cava blood and constitutes about 70% of CVO, or about 315–350 mL/min per kg (Figures 1.6 and 1.7). About 115–125 mL/min per kg or about 25% of CVO passes through the foramen ovale to the left atrium; this blood is derived predominantly from the ductus venosus. Venous return from the superior vena cava is 90–95 mL/min per kg and represents about 21% of CVO. Most of this blood, as well as about 200 mL/min per kg of inferior vena cava blood passes through the tricuspid valve into the right ventricle. In addition, coronary venous blood enters the right ventricle. The right ventricle ejects about 300–325 mL/min per kg or about 66% of CVO. Only about 10–15% of the blood ejected by the right ventricle into the pulmonary trunk enters the pulmonary circulation; this constitutes about 8% of CVO or about 35–40 mL/min per kg fetal weight. The remainder, about 265–300 mL/min per kg, or about 60% CVO, passes through the ductus arteriosus.

The left ventricle receives about 115 mL/min per kg of blood passing through the foramen ovale and the 35 mL/min per kg from pulmonary venous return. It ejects about 150–170 mL/min per kg, or about 33% of CVO. Less than one-third of the blood ejected by the left ventricle passes across the aortic isthmus to the descending aorta. This represents about 10% of CVO or about 45 mL/min per kg. About 3% of CVO enters the coronary circulation and about 20% of CVO or about 90–100 mL/min per kg is distributed to the head, brain, upper extremities, and upper portion of the trunk. The proportions of CVO traversing the major arteries are reflected in the relative diameters of these vessels. The pulmonary trunk is very large, and the ascending aorta somewhat narrower; the descending aorta is also very wide, whereas the isthmus of the aorta is much narrower than the ascending or descending aorta and the ductus arteriosus. These features are discussed in Chapter 12. The blood flows to various fetal organs is shown in Table 1.1.

Hepatic flow is derived from the umbilical vein, portal vein and hepatic artery; flow to the left lobe is about 350 mL/min per 100 g tissue weight, whereas the right lobe receives about 450 mL/min per 100 g [4]. The proportions of the CVO distributed to the fetal organs and the placenta change with advancing gestation (Figure 1.8). There is a gradual reduction in the proportion of CVO directed to the placenta, from about 45% at 75–90 days (0.5–0.6 gestation) to 38–40% at term. The percentage of CVO distributed to the brain increases progressively, from about 2.2% at 0.5 gestation to 3% at term. The percentages of combined output to the lungs and gastrointestinal tract are fairly constant until about 120 days (0.8) gestation, but then increase rapidly [9]. The changes in actual blood flow per unit mass of tissue are shown in Figure 1.9. There are quite striking increases in flow per 100 g organ weight to the brain, gut and lungs, starting at

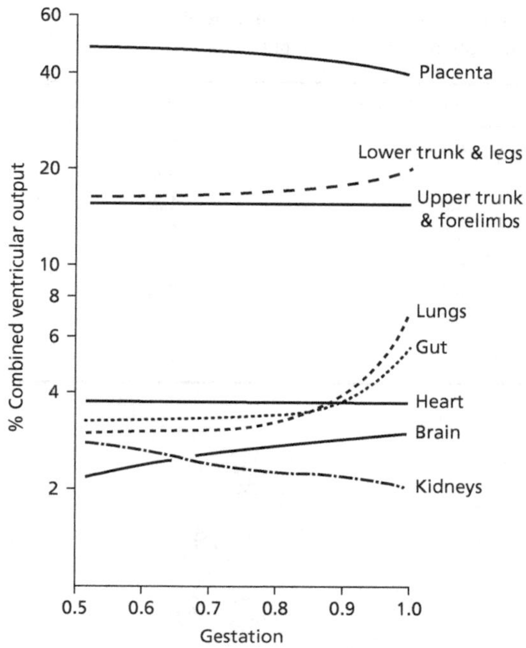

Figure 1.8 Changes in the percentage of fetal combined ventricular output distributed to various organs, body and limbs and the placenta at different gestational ages in the fetal lamb.

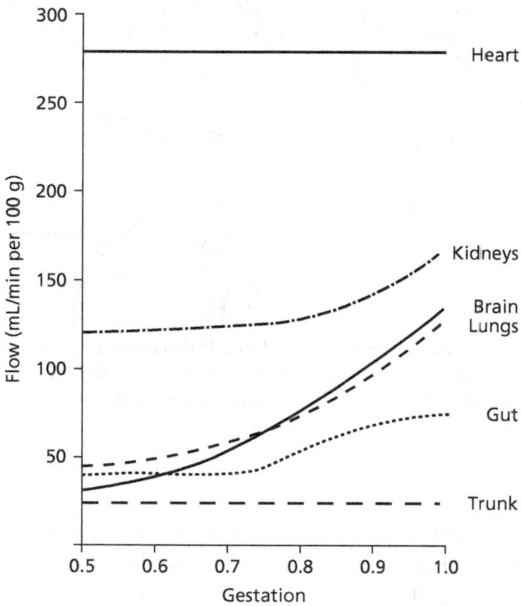

Figure 1.9 Changes in actual blood flow to various organs in the lamb during the latter half of gestation.

about 0.75 gestation (110 days). The cause of the increase in flow to these organs is not known; it could be related to increase in the size of the vascular bed, due to growth of new vessels, or to increased metabolic activity with vasodilatation, or a combination of these factors.

Oxygen delivery and oxygen consumption

One of the important functions of the circulation is to provide oxygen to the tissues. In the adult, oxygen delivery to the body is the product of arterial oxygen content and systemic blood flow, or cardiac output. In the fetus, calculation of oxygen delivery to the body is more complex. Umbilical–placental blood flow represents the volume of blood being presented to the site of oxygenation, whereas CVO minus umbilical–placental blood flow is the volume of blood delivered to the whole fetal body. Umbilical–placental blood flow determines oxygen uptake, and fetal body blood flow determines oxygen delivery to the fetus. However, the oxygen content of blood distributed to the organs supplied from the ascending aorta and to those supplied from the descending aorta are different. Oxygen delivery to an organ or tissue is determined by the oxygen content and the blood flow (see Chapter 3). In the fetus, pressures in the aortic and pulmonary arteries are almost identical, so blood flow to various fetal organs and to the umbilical–placental circulation is determined by local vascular resistance. This is influenced by the size, or cross-sectional area, of the vascular bed and by the degree of vascular constriction or dilatation. Oxygen delivery and oxygen consumption in various organs and tissues in the late-gestation lamb fetus are shown in Table 1.2.

Circulation in the human fetus

Studies in previable human fetuses have demonstrated that the general course of the circulation in the human fetus is similar to that in the lamb [7]. Figure 1.10 and Table 1.3 show average values for distribution of CVO and volumes of blood flow in the human fetal circulation, based on numerous studies [11–17].

Using ultrasound techniques, blood flow has been estimated in human fetuses based on measurement

Table 1.2 Oxygen consumption by tissues and organs in the late-gestation fetal lamb as a percentage of total consumption, as consumption per 100 g tissue weight, and as consumption per kg fetal weight.

Blood flow	*Percent of total*	*mL/100 g tissue*	*mL/kg fetal weight*
Brain	12	4.0	2.4
Heart	12	8.0	0.8
Liver	23	4.0	1.35
Kidney	4	2.6	0.5
Gut	5	0.4	0.4
Lung	4	0.6	0.25
Skin, muscle, bone	40	0.4	2.8
Total			8.5

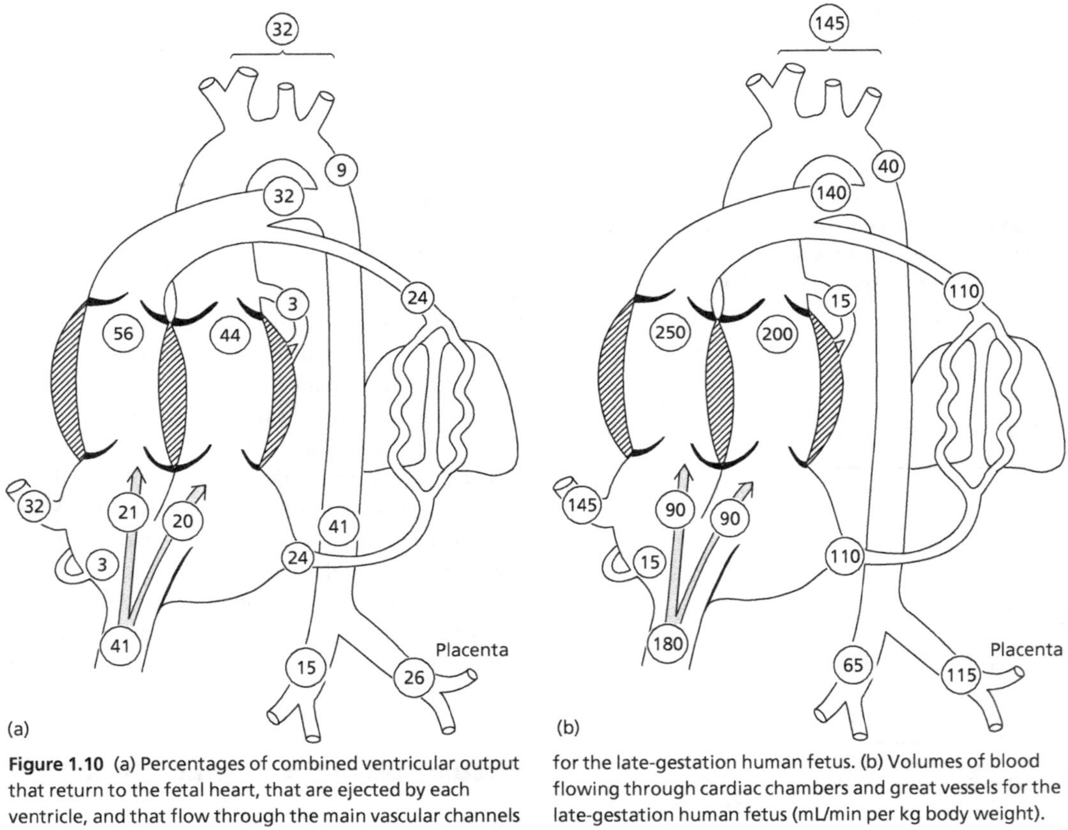

Figure 1.10 (a) Percentages of combined ventricular output that return to the fetal heart, that are ejected by each ventricle, and that flow through the main vascular channels for the late-gestation human fetus. (b) Volumes of blood flowing through cardiac chambers and great vessels for the late-gestation human fetus (mL/min per kg body weight).

of blood flow velocities and vessel diameter. There is considerable potential for error in these measurements and this may explain the variation in reported values for blood flows in published reports. Blood flows have been estimated at various sites; left and right ventricular outputs have been calculated from flow measurements across the mitral or tricuspid valves [10,11], or in the pulmonary trunk or ascending aorta [12–16]. Flows have also been measured through the ductus arteriosus and the

Table 1.3 Comparison of the distribution of blood flows in the sheep and human fetus as percent combined ventricular output (%CVO) and as actual blood flows (mL/min per kg fetal weight).

	Sheep[1]		*Human*[2]	
	%CVO	*mL/min/kg*	*%CVO*	*mL/min/kg*
Combined ventricular output	100	450	100	450
Left ventricular output	34	150	45	202
Aortic isthmus	10	45	8	36
Brain	3.5	16	24	107
Upper trunk, forelimbs	20.5	90	13	59
Right ventricular output	66	300	55	248
Ductus arteriosus	58	260	30	135
Pulmonary circulation	8	36	25	113
Descending aorta	68	305	38	171
Umbilical–placental circulation	40	180	26	112
Hepatic circulation	18	80	14	68
Ductus venosus	22	100	11	44
Lower body organs, hindlimbs	28	125	12	60
Superior vena cava	24	108	37	165
Inferior vena cava + umbilical flow	68	305	38	172
Foramen ovale	25	115	20	90

1 The values for sheep represent those obtained in fetuses in the latter part of gestation [9].

2 The values for human fetuses in the third trimester were obtained by ultrasound [10–17]; in view of the considerable variation in reported measurements, I have selected those I considered most appropriate.

common umbilical vein [17]. From these measurements it has been possible to calculate various other flows. Thus CVO is the sum of right ventricular output (RVO) and left ventricular output (LVO). Pulmonary blood flow is represented by RVO minus ductus arteriosus flow. Pulmonary blood flow has also been calculated from direct measurement of right and left branch pulmonary arteries in some studies [14,16]. Flow through the foramen ovale has been estimated from LVO minus pulmonary blood flow, because blood entering the left ventricles is derived from blood entering the left atrium through the foramen ovale and from pulmonary venous return.

Volume of blood flow ($\dot{Q}$) is determined from the product of average flow velocity (V_m) and cross-sectional area (πD^2). Because diameter (D) of the vessel is measured by ultrasound, the flow is calculated as:

$$\dot{Q} = V_m \times \pi D^2/4$$

It is apparent that, because the diameter is squared, small errors in measuring diameter could create major errors in calculation of flow. This would be a particular problem if vessel diameter is small. Also, in making these calculations, it is assumed that the diameter is constant throughout the cardiac cycle. An additional potential error is that the velocity should be recorded from the center of the vessel at an appropriate angle of insonation; this may be difficult to accomplish because of the position of the fetus in the maternal abdomen. When expressing blood flows in relation to fetal weight, it is necessary to use various formulae, based on age or various fetal measurements to estimate fetal weight and considerable error could be introduced into these calculations.

Table 1.3 shows a comparison of CVO and blood flow per kilogram of fetal weight, in the sheep and human fetus at about 0.8 gestation.

Left and right ventricular output

Estimates of CVO in the human fetus are similar to values measured in sheep fetuses. In the latter third of gestation CVO is about 400–450 mL/kg per min, whereas in earlier gestation it is somewhat higher. This compares with the fetal sheep levels of about 450–500 mL/kg per min. However, the proportions of combined output ejected by the left and right ventricles are quite different in the human. In the sheep, the ratio of right to left ventricular output is almost 2:1, whereas in the human, measurements vary from 1.2:1 to 1.5:1. The relatively higher proportion of blood ejected by the left ventricle appears to be related to the higher pulmonary blood flow in the human fetus and is important in providing the higher cerebral blood flow in the human fetus.

Cerebral blood flow

The relative weights of some organs are very different in the human compared with the lamb and thus the proportions of CVO distributed to body organs differ. Perhaps the most important factor is brain size; in the mature human fetus the brain constitutes 12% of body weight, as compared with 3% in the late-gestation lamb. It is reasonable to assume that the organ blood flow related to weight is similar in the two species. Near term, both human and sheep fetal body weights are about 3.5 kg, and brain weights are about 65 g in the sheep and 350 g in the human [18]. If it is assumed that blood flow to the brain is similar in relation to tissue weight (120 mL/min per 100 g), total brain flow would be about 80 mL/min in the sheep and about 420 mL/min in the human, or 22 and 120 mL/min per kg respectively in the term fetus (Table 1.4). Study of the proportions of CVO distributed to the brain in the primate versus the sheep show an enormous difference: 16% in the rhesus monkey versus 3–4% in the sheep fetus [19]. In the human fetus it is estimated that, in the third trimester, the brain receives about 24% of CVO. If LVO is 40–45% of CVO, about 25–30% of combined output is available for the peripheral circulation of the head and upper extremities and to traverse the ductus arteriosus to the descending aorta. Thus the proportion of combined output passing across the aortic isthmus is probably about 8%, similar to that in the lamb.

Table 1.4 Comparison of body weight, brain weight, and brain blood flow in the late-gestation lamb and human fetus.

	Lamb	*Human*
Body weight (g)	3500	3500
Brain weight (g)	65	350
Brain blood flow (mL/min per 100 g)	120	120
Total brain blood flow (mL/min)	78	420
Brain flow per kg body weight	22	120

Because cerebral blood flow is much higher in the human fetus, the volume of blood returning to the heart via the superior vena cava is proportionately considerably greater. In the lamb, about 24% of CVO returns via the superior vena cava, but in the human fetus superior vena cava flow probably represents about 37% of CVO ventricular output.

Umbilical–placental blood flow

In fetal lambs, umbilical–placental blood flow constitutes about 38–45% of CVO and is about 180–220 mL/min per kg fetal body weight The higher values are noted in younger fetuses at 0.5–0.75 gestation and the values decrease toward term [9]. A mean of about 55% of umbilical venous blood passes through the ductus venosus, but there is a wide range (20–90%) [3].

Umbilical–placental blood flow is much lower in the human than in the lamb fetus. In fetuses under 32 weeks' gestation it was reported to be about 32% of CVO, but after 32 weeks it fell to only about 21%. Flow was about 130–135 mL/min per kg estimated fetal weight before 32 weeks, but only about 90–100 mL/min per kg after 32 weeks [20]. In another report, umbilical blood flow was higher near term, about 117 mL/min per kg [21]. In the human fetus a mean of only 25–40% of umbilical venous blood passes through the ductus venosus, but there is also a wide range in the proportion [22].

Oxygen consumption in the human and lamb fetus is similar at about 7–9 mL/min per kg fetal weight. Umbilical venous oxygen saturations are about 80–85% in both the lamb and human fetus and umbilical arterial oxygen saturations are also similar at about 50%. The ability of the human fetus to maintain the same oxygen uptake per kilogram as the lamb when umbilical blood flow is about half as great is related to the much higher hemoglobin concentration and oxygen capacity in human fetal blood. Hemoglobin concentration in the human is about 16.5 g/dL with an oxygen capacity of 22.5 mL/dL near term compared with hemoglobin concentration of 8–9 g/dL and oxygen capacity of about 11–12 mL/dL in the sheep.

Pulmonary blood flow

In fetal lambs less than 0.8 gestation (120 days), only 3.5–4.0% of CVO is distributed to the lungs; after this there is a gradual increase to 7–9% at term (~145 days). Actual flow to the lungs is about 18–20 mL/min per kg fetal weight below 0.8 gestation and about 35–40 mL/min per kg at term. Reported values for pulmonary blood flow in human fetuses vary considerably. As mentioned above, in most reports pulmonary flow has been estimated as the difference between RVO and ductus arteriosus flow. Therefore possible errors in measurement of RVO or ductus arteriosus flow would tend to create variability in pulmonary flow. In those studies in which both left and right branch pulmonary artery flow was measured, errors in measurement in the two arteries could result in variability in estimation of total flow. It is thus not surprising that the magnitude of pulmonary blood flow in the human fetus has been reported to range from about 11% [15] to as much as 22–25% [12,14] of CVO. An increase in the proportion of CVO distributed to the lungs with advancing gestation has been reported [14]. In human fetuses less than 20 weeks' gestation, only about 13% entered the lungs, but after 32 weeks the lungs received 25% of CVO. Reported actual blood flow values would thus vary between 45 and about 120 mL/min per kg fetal weight.

Foramen ovale blood flow

Because of the complex velocity flow contour and the inability to define diameter of the foramen ovale, blood flow cannot be measured accurately by ultrasound in the human fetus. Foramen ovale flow, estimated from LVO minus pulmonary blood flow, constitutes about 30% of CVO in the fetal lamb [23]; it is slightly lower in younger fetuses and slightly higher in older fetuses. Reports in human fetuses vary considerably. In one study foramen ovale flow was about 30–33% of CVO in fetuses at all gestational ages [16]. However, in other reports it was about 18% of combined output before 20 weeks, but about 34% of combined output after 32 weeks' gestation [15].

Ductus arteriosus blood flow

In the lamb fetus about 90% of blood ejected by the right ventricle is directed through the pulmonary trunk and ductus arteriosus to the descending aorta. Thus more than half of CVO passes through the ductus. In the human, only about 55% of RVO passes through the ductus. RVO is also relatively lower than in the lamb so the proportion of CVO traversing the ductus is only about 30%.

Thus the major differences between the sheep and human fetus are more evident in the latter period of gestation and are characterized by the much greater cerebral and pulmonary blood flows and much lower umbilical–placental blood flow relative to fetal weight. The high cerebral flow accounts for the greater LVO in the human; because umbilical blood flow is derived largely from blood passing across the ductus arteriosus to the descending aorta, the low umbilical flow in the human accounts for the smaller flow across the ductus arteriosus and the lower RVO compared with the lamb.

Hepatic and ductus venosus blood flows

The pattern of flow in the liver region appears to be similar in the human and lamb fetus. Ultrasound examination of fetal lambs showed a blood flow velocity of 55–60 cm/s in the ductus venosus, whereas abdominal inferior vena cava velocity was only about 16 cm/s [6]. The ductus venosus stream was directed preferentially through the foramen ovale (see above). In the human fetus, blood flow velocity in the ductus venosus has been reported to be 65–75 cm/s, and the ductus venosus stream also flows preferentially through the foramen ovale [24].

Factors affecting perinatal cardiac output

Cardiac ventricular output is the product of heart rate and stroke volume. Stroke volume is determined by preload, afterload, and myocardial contractility. In isolated myocardial strips, the initial length of the myocyte, which determines sarcomere length, influences the force of muscle contraction. In the intact heart, ventricular volume at end diastole determines sarcomere length and the force of contraction and is the basis of the Frank–Starling mechanism. An increase in initial length or increase in end-diastolic ventricular volume increases the force of contraction of the muscle and, in the intact heart, increases stroke volume if other factors are unchanged. Afterload, or load on the muscle during development of active force, determines the degree of shortening. In the intact circulation, afterload is influenced by several factors (e.g., arterial pressure, compliance of the arterial system, and peripheral vascular resistance). In isolated myocardial strips, the greater the load on the muscle, the less the degree of muscle shortening. In the intact heart, an increase in afterload results in a reduction in stroke volume. Contractility is the intrinsic force of contraction of the muscle; with isolated muscle, increased contractility increases force developed and, in the intact heart, increases stroke volume, or developed pressure. In the cardiovascular system, a change in one factor influencing ventricular output may affect other parameters. It is therefore important to consider possible changes in these other parameters when assessing the effects of alteration of one regulatory factor.

Effects of heart rate

In the adult, cardiac output is relatively constant over a wide range of heart rates. Increasing heart rate to 150/min or decreasing it to 50/min from a resting rate of about 70/min does not alter output. Greater increases in heart rate may decrease cardiac output because the reduction in diastolic filling time does not permit adequate filling to maintain stroke volume. With very slow heart rates, stroke volume is increased to maintain cardiac output, but when maximal diastolic filling has been achieved, further slowing results in a decrease of ventricular output.

In studies in fetal sheep, spontaneous increases in heart rate above the resting level of about 160/min are associated with increases of ventricular output of up to 15–20%, and spontaneous decreases in heart rate results in a fall in output [25]. Because the cause of the spontaneous heart rate change was not known, it cannot be assumed that heart rate variation alone was responsible for the changes in ventricular output. For example, an increase in heart rate may be related to fetal activity or the onset of fetal respiratory movement. This may induce changes in sympathetic nervous activity that may affect myocardial contractility as well as heart rate. The effects of electrical pacing of the right or left atrium to increase rates to 240–300/min were studied in fetal lambs [25]. Pacing the atrium resulted in an increase in LVO of up to 15%, with only a small increase or no change in RVO. At rates above 300–320/min, ventricular output fell progressively with increasing rate, presumably because diastolic filling time is markedly reduced. RVO increased when the left atrium was paced, but LVO fell, often dramatically, by 50% or more. Normally the pressure pulses of the right and left atria are similar in the fetus, with a dominant *a* wave in both chambers; right atrial is slightly higher than left atrial pressure in all phases of the cardiac cycle. During pacing the left atrial pressure pulse is altered so left atrial pressure exceeds that in the right atrium during some phases of the cycle and interferes with flow through the foramen ovale into the left atrium, reducing left ventricular filling and output.

Vagal stimulation decreases both RVO and LVO; when heart rate falls from a resting level of 160/min to about 120/min, output decreases by 15–20%. Stroke volume increases slightly, but not adequately to maintain output as rate falls. Vagal stimulation results in an increase in systemic arterial pressure and a rise in intrapleural pressure in the fetus. The increase in arterial pressure causes an elevation of afterload and the increase in intrapleural pressure could reduce venous return to the heart. Thus the fall in ventricular output may not be the result of the bradycardia but of the associated changes.

Effect of preload and afterload

Preload and afterload are discussed together because there is usually an interaction between them in the intact circulation. If afterload is increased, the volume ejected by the ventricle during systole is reduced and residual ventricular volume increases. If ventricular filling is maintained, preload is greater with the next beat. *In utero* studies of fetal lambs have been performed to assess the role of preload on cardiac output. In most of these studies, ventricular end-diastolic or atrial pressures have been used as an index of preload. However, pressure measurements may not be a reliable indicator of volume, because ventricular compliance determines the volume at any particular pressure. Studies in isolated myocardium and intact hearts have shown that fetal myocardium is less compliant than that of the adult.

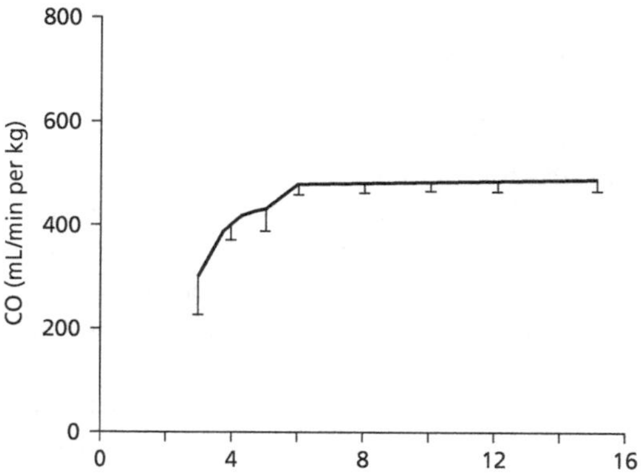

Figure 1.11 Changes in cardiac output (CO) associated with acute reduction of atrial pressure by blood removal and increase in atrial pressure by infusion of electrolyte solution in fetal lambs [26].

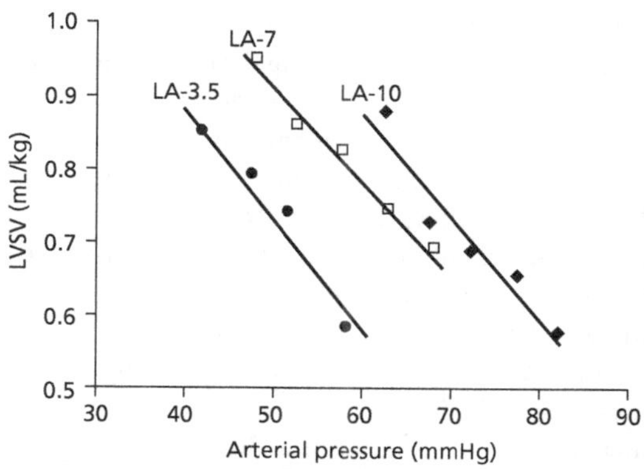

Figure 1.12 When systemic arterial pressure is regulated, an increase in pressure results in a decrease in left ventricular stroke volume (LVSV) at fixed left atrial pressure. At any level of arterial pressure, an increase in left atrial pressure increases left ventricular stroke volume.

Several investigators have studied the effects of decreasing or increasing preload in fetal lambs *in utero*. The preload was decreased by reducing fetal blood volume by removal of blood and increased by rapid intravenous infusion of electrolyte solution. A fall in right atrial and right ventricular end-diastolic pressure resulted in a marked decrease in ventricular output. Output rose when ventricular end-diastolic or atrial pressure increased by 2–4 mmHg above resting levels, but further increases in filling pressure did not result in greater output by the ventricle [26] (Figure 1.11).

This response is distinctly different from that of the adult heart, in which increases in atrial pressure to 15–20 mmHg are associated with a progressive increase in ventricular output. Based on these studies, it was proposed that the fetal heart is normally operating near the top of its ventricular function curve, so that a fall in preload results in a decrease in output. However, the rise in output associated with an increase in preload is limited because myocardial performance, or contractility, is relatively poor in the fetus.

In these studies, the effects of rapid infusion of electrolytes on arterial pressure were not considered. Associated with the infusion, fetal arterial pressure also increased and thus affected afterload. We examined the effects of changing preload at various constant levels of arterial pressure. Arterial pressure elevation dramatically reduced left ventricular stroke volume at all levels of mean atrial pressure [27] (Figure 1.12). At constant arterial pressure levels, progressive elevation of left atrial pressure increased left ventricular stroke volume even with atrial pressures as high as 10–15 mmHg. This study demonstrated that the fetal heart does respond to increases in preload by increasing its output. It did not, however, resolve whether performance of the fetal and adult myocardium are comparable.

Myocardial contractility

Studies of isolated myocardium from fetal and adult sheep have demonstrated that fetal myocardium develops less active tension than adult myocardium at similar muscle lengths. The maximal force that can be generated is considerably lower for fetal than for adult myocardium. Several differences in morphological and biochemical parameters of myocardium have been described that could account for the lesser contractility of fetal myocardium. Friedman [28] suggested that fetal myocardium contains fewer sarcomeres, or contractile units, in each myocyte. Also, as mentioned above, the parallel orientation of the myofibrils has not developed during early gestation.

Another factor that may be important is the development of the sarcoplasmic reticulum, which regulates movement of calcium ions essential for myocardial contraction. The fetal myocardial sarcoplasmic reticulum is well developed, but the T-tubular system, representing the extension of the sarcoplasmic reticulum to provide closer relations with the contractile elements, is either poorly developed or absent in immature myocardium. Not only are there structural differences in sarcoplasmic reticulum, but in studies with isolated sarcoplasmic reticulum vesicles calcium uptake was found to be impaired in fetal myocardium [29].

Local release of norepinephrine at sympathetic nerve endings is an important mechanism for increasing myocardial contractility. Morphological studies of fetal hearts using monoamine oxidase fluorescence have demonstrated absent or poor sympathetic innervation of the immature myocardium. The abundance of sympathetic nerve endings varies greatly at different periods of gestational and postnatal development among species. In the guinea pig, myocardial sympathetic innervation is almost fully developed at birth, whereas in the rabbit and rat there is almost no innervation at birth (it develops within 14–21 postnatal days). The sheep fetus has no detectable sympathetic innervation at 75 days (mid-gestation), but innervation begins to appear at 90–100 days and is abundant but not yet fully developed just before birth.

In addition to the difference in sympathetic innervation, possible differences in β-adrenergic receptor concentration in fetal and adult myocardium have been postulated. Although these differences in sympathetic innervation and β-adrenoceptor concentration may not be important in the resting fetal heart, they could influence the ability to respond to stress.

Circulatory regulation in the fetus

In the adult the systemic and pulmonary circulations are separate. Each ventricle is subjected to potentially different preload and afterload, and the stroke volume of each ventricle could vary greatly. The Frank–Starling mechanism is useful for adjusting the outputs of the two ventricles so that over a short period the ventricles eject similar volumes. A reduction in venous return to the right atrium reduces filling pressure and end-diastolic volume of the right ventricle, resulting in a decrease in stroke volume. Pulmonary blood flow and venous return to the left atrium and ventricle is reduced and stroke volume falls. An increase in systemic arterial pressure will restrict left ventricular stroke volume; end-diastolic volume will increase so that, with the next beat, greater force is generated to increase stroke volume.

In the fetus the presence of the foramen ovale tends to make right and left atrial pressures equal throughout the cardiac cycle. The ductus arteriosus provides a large communication between the aorta and pulmonary artery, which causes the pressures to be almost identical. In view of the similar atrial pressures and similar aortic and pulmonary arterial pressures, the differences in stroke volumes of the left and right ventricles in the fetal lamb are difficult to explain. Differences in afterload of the two ventricles could explain this. The aortic isthmus, which in the fetus is narrower than the ascending and descending aorta, might functionally separate the upper and lower body circulation to some extent. The left ventricle ejects into the ascending aorta and the vessels of the head and neck, a circulation that would be poorly compliant and have a relatively high vascular resistance. The right ventricle ejects into the pulmonary trunk and directly through the large ductus arteriosus into the descending aorta and its branches. This circulation would have a higher compliance and a lower resistance because it includes the umbilical–placental vasculature. This functional separation of the aorta at the isthmus has been demonstrated in fetal lambs. Rapid reduction in peripheral vascular resistance in the lower body circulation induced by a vasodilator causes a decrease in descending aortic pressure and an increase in right ventricular stroke volume for several beats, whereas ascending aortic pressure and LVO do not change. Similarly, injection of a vasodilator into the ascending aorta causes an evanescent decrease of ascending aortic pressure and increase in left ventricular stroke volume.

Baroreflex regulation

In the adult the arterial baroreflex modulates arterial pressure over a fairly narrow range. When arterial pressure is increased, the aortic and carotid baroreceptors respond, inducing reflex bradycardia, depression of myocardial contractility, and peripheral vasodilatation, all of which tend to decrease arterial pressure. When the aortic and carotid baroreflexes are abolished by bilateral section of the aortic and carotid afferent nerves, there is initially an increase in resting heart rate and arterial pressure, but within 1–2 days these parameters return to average levels present during the pre-denervation period. Wide swings of arterial pressure and heart rate occur around the average pressure and rate, in association with stimuli that produce small changes in the normal animal [30]. Arterial baroreceptors are functional in the fetus relatively early in gestation. In the fetal lamb, baroreflex sensitivity increases with gestational age from about 80 days' gestation; near term, it is as sensitive as in the neonate and adult in terms of the bradycardia induced by arterial pressure increase [31]. In fetal lambs, sinoaortic denervation results in the same wide variation in heart rate and blood pressure observed in adult animals. The variability is similar in fetal lambs and adult sheep, indicating that the baroreflex is fully operative in regulating arterial pressure in the late-gestation fetal lamb.

Chemoreflex regulation

Based on studies in acutely exteriorized lambs, it was proposed that the aortic and carotid chemoreceptors are relatively inactive in the fetus. However, more recent studies in fetal lambs have shown that they are active, at least in the latter third of gestation [32]. Responses to carotid chemoreceptor stimulation are much greater than to aortic receptor stimulation. The chemoreceptors are stimulated by hypoxemia and can be activated experimentally by intravascular injection of small doses of sodium cyanide. The cardiovascular response dominates, with bradycardia and immediate hypotension, but respiratory gasps are noted. The bradycardia can be abolished if the lambs are pretreated with atropine, indicating that the bradycardia is induced by vagus nerve stimulation. Confirmation that the cyanide response is the result of chemoreceptor stimulation was obtained by demonstrating the loss of the cardiovascular and respiratory responses in fetal lambs in which sinoaortic denervation had been accomplished [32].

In the adult, chemoreceptor stimulation may be associated with reflex peripheral vasoconstriction. This response has not been studied adequately in the fetus, but it can be inferred that the marked vasoconstriction induced in the peripheral circulation during hypoxia in fetal lambs (see below) is partly the result of chemoreceptor stimulation. It is apparent from studies in the fetal lamb that chemoreflex responses are different from those in the adult. The respiratory response in the adult animal dominates, whereas only minor and unsustained respiratory response results in the fetus. Whether it is due to a difference in chemoreceptor response or a difference in central response has not been resolved.

Fetal circulatory response to reduced oxygen delivery

The mechanisms responsible for decreased oxygen supply to the fetus and the effects on oxygen uptake and delivery are discussed in Chapter 3.

Heart rate and blood pressure response

In fetal lambs beyond about 110 days' gestation (term about 145 days), acute hypoxemia results in bradycardia and arterial hypertension. In one study a change of 4–5 mmHg in carotid arterial blood was necessary to produce bradycardia. Boekkooi *et al.* [33] have shown that the magnitude of the bradycardia is directly related to the degree of fall in oxygen saturation of carotid arterial blood. The bradycardia induced by hypoxemia can be abolished by atropine administration, indicating that it is induced reflexly through vagal stimulation. With extreme changes in Po_2 to levels below about 12 mmHg, the bradycardia cannot be completely prevented by atropine. It has been proposed that severe hypoxemia has a direct depressant effect on the heart that causes bradycardia. The hypothesis had been proposed that hypertension was the primary change, related to catecholamine-induced vasoconstriction, and that the bradycardia was a baroreflex response. However, as has been mentioned above, the bradycardia is the result of chemoreceptor stimulation. In chronic sinoaortic denervated fetal lambs, hypoxemia does not induce bradycardia even though it results in progressive hypertension.

With prolonged fetal hypoxemia, heart rate gradually increases although it does not usually achieve control values. The mechanism for this recovery is not defined, but it could be due to resetting of chemoreceptor sensitivity.

Cardiac failure in the fetus

Prior to the examination of fetuses *in utero* by ultrasound, it was thought that some stillborn fetuses with gross edema had cardiac malformations. With the advent of ultrasound it is now recognized that hydrops fetalis is frequently due to cardiovascular disturbances. Although decreased ventricular ejection, suggesting impaired cardiac function, can be recognized by ultrasound examination, the diagnosis of cardiac failure is usually made when the fetus is seen to have hydrops. Many conditions other than cardiovascular disturbances are associated with hydrops fetalis, including erythroblastosis fetalis due to Rh or other incompatibilities, severe anemia, hepatic dysfunction, and genetic conditions such as Turner syndrome. Cardiovascular factors associated with hydrops fetalis are listed in Table 1.5.

The hemodynamic feature common to all these causes of fetal hydrops is an increase in systemic venous pressure. We have shown experimentally in fetal lambs that acute constriction of the ductus arteriosus elevates right atrial and vena cava pressures. Increases in ventricular output associated with volume loading are also associated with an increase in right atrial pressure. Electrical pacing of the left or right atrium in fetal lambs alters the pressure contour and also raises right atrial and venous pressures. Bradycardia induced by stimulation of the vagus nerve is also associated with raised venous pressure.

It is of interest that, postnatally, the usual manifestation of cardiac failure is respiratory distress resulting from elevated pulmonary venous pressure and increased fluid transudation into the lungs. However, in the fetus, pulmonary edema is an unusual manifestation of cardiac failure. This can be accounted for by several factors.

- Pulmonary arterioles are markedly constricted and limit pulmonary blood flow as well as transmission of arterial pressure into the capillaries.
- A rise in left atrial pressure is limited by the presence of the foramen ovale. If left atrial pressure should tend to increase, flow through the foramen ovale would be reduced, thus preventing significant elevation of left atrial pressure.
- The intrathoracic pressure is positive in the fetus because intraamniotic pressure is transmitted to the fluid-filled lung. Postnatally, intrapleural pressure becomes negative, thus increasing the pressure differences across capillaries and favoring fluid transudation.

Increased fluid accumulation in the lung of the fetus is manifested as pulmonary lymphangiectasia. This occurs only in those conditions in which pulmonary venous pressure can be raised to high levels, such as total pulmonary venous drainage with obstruction and aortic or mitral atresia with a small or closed foramen ovale.

Table 1.5 Cardiovascular disturbances associated with the development of fetal hydrops.

Obstructive lesions
Small or closed foramen ovale
Constricted ductus arteriosus
Atrioventricular valve insufficiency
High cardiac output states
Sacrococcygeal teratoma
Parasitic fetus
Twin-to-twin transfusion
Anemia
Decreased myocardial function
Arrhythmias

Factors contributing to hydrops in the fetus

The fetus is greatly affected by even small increases in venous pressure. This is due to several features that favor accumulation of fluid in fetal tissues, as compared with postnatally. Body water content is considerably greater in the fetus than in the adult. Furthermore, the proportion of extracellular fluid is much larger in the fetus. The lower the gestational age, the greater the relative amount of body water, as well as the proportion of extracellular fluid (Figure 1.13). The extracellular space in the fetus is capable of accommodating a much greater volume as compared with postnatally, with a lower tissue pressure, because tissue turgor is less.

The factors regulating movement of fluid between the circulation and the extravascular or extracellular space are expressed in the Starling law of the capillary:

$$Q_s = K_f[(P_c - P_i) - \sigma(\pi_c - \pi_i)]$$

where Q_s represents fluid movement across the capillary, K_f fluid filtration coefficient (mL/min per

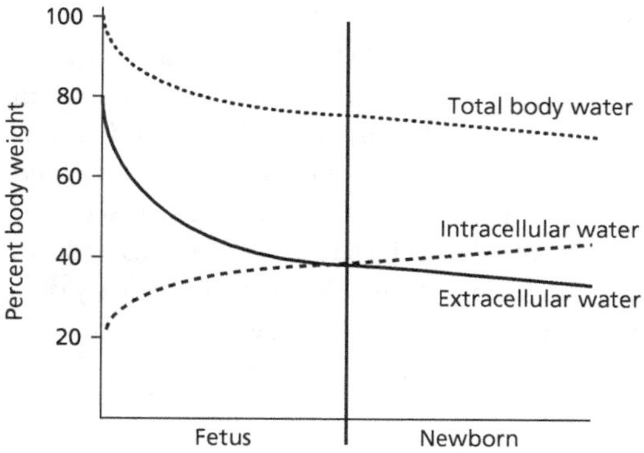

Figure 1.13 Changes in total body water, extracellular fluid and intracellular fluid during prenatal and postnatal development.

mmHg), P_c capillary hydrostatic pressure, P_i interstitial hydrostatic pressure, σ reflection coefficient, π_c capillary osmotic pressure, and π_i interstitial osmotic pressure.

In the adult, pressure at the arterial end of the capillary is about 45 mmHg and at the venous end about 15 mmHg. No measurements are available for the fetus, but based on arterial and venous pressures, they can be estimated to be about 30 mmHg at the arterial end and about 5 mmHg at the venous end of the capillary (Figure 1.14). Colloid osmotic pressure is largely related to plasma albumin concentration, which is considerably lower in the fetus than postnatally. The albumin concentration increases with gestational age so that the younger the fetus, the lower the colloid osmotic pressure. In Figure 1.14 the osmotic pressure in the fetus is depicted as being considerably lower in the fetal than the adult capillary.

Tissue turgor in the fetus is not known, but it is considerably lower than postnatally; it has been assumed to be 2 mmHg in Figure 1.14. In the adult capillary, there is a balance of hydrostatic and osmotic pressures so that most fluid transferred to the tissue space at the arterial end returns to the intravascular space at the venous end (Figure 1.14). Only a small volume is removed from the extracellular fluid by the lymphatic system. However, in the fetus, based on information regarding the volume of lymph flow (see below), a relatively large amount is removed by this means. It is therefore likely that there is a net movement of fluid out of the capillary into the extracellular space.

The filtration coefficient (see Chapter 1) is determined by the capillary membrane; in the fetus, the capillary is more permeable not only to fluid but also to protein. An elevation of venous pressure will increase the force driving fluid into the tissue space, which has a very large capacity in the fetus. In addition, the low colloid osmotic pressure may be further reduced by movement of albumin across the capillary membrane into the tissue space. Compared with the adult, where the difference in hydrostatic and colloid osmotic pressure is about 15 mmHg, the difference in the fetus is less. Therefore, elevation of venous pressure by only 2–3 mmHg, which does not appear to be very significant, may have a profound influence in increasing extracellular fluid volume.

An additional mechanism by which increased venous pressure may exaggerate the amount of extracellular fluid is by reducing lymphatic flow. In the adult sheep, left thoracic duct lymph flow is about 50 mL/kg per 24 hours; in the fetal lamb, it is

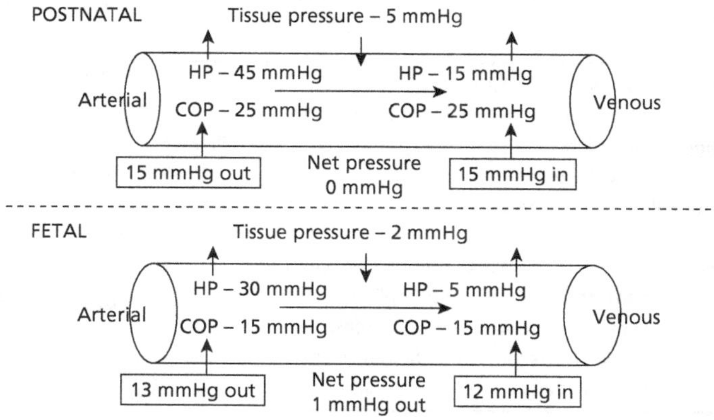

Figure 1.14 Factors affecting fluid transfer across capillary membranes during the postnatal and prenatal periods. COP, colloid osmotic pressure; HP, hydrostatic pressure.

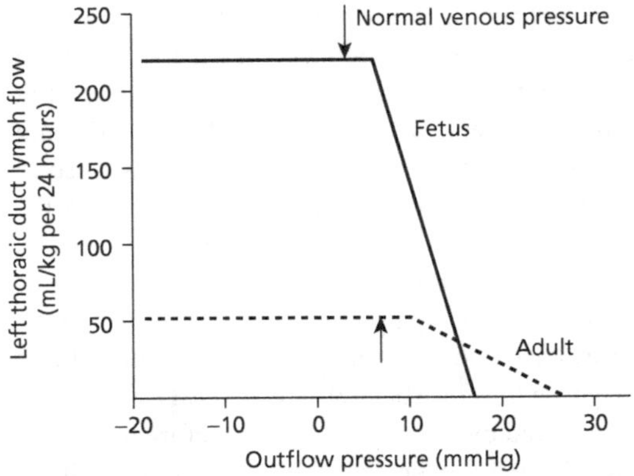

Figure 1.15 Effects of increasing venous pressure on left thoracic lymph flow in the fetal and adult sheep.

about 250 mL/kg per 24 hours. Elevation of venous pressure has a much greater effect in reducing lymph flow in the fetus than in the adult. This has been well demonstrated by Brace and is depicted in Figure 1.15. Not only does a similar increase in venous pressure have a more dramatic effect in reducing lymph flow in the fetus, but flow ceases at venous pressures of about 15 mmHg, whereas in the adult flow stops at pressures of 25–30 mmHg [34,35].

Thus any cardiovascular disturbance that increases fetal systemic venous pressure is likely to induce fetal edema. The factors that contribute to the development of hydrops as a manifestation of fetal cardiac failure are shown in Table 1.6.

Hormonal factors may also play a role in the increase in extracellular fluid volume. An increase in fetal venous pressure induces elevation of plasma arginine vasopressin (AVP) and atrial natriuretic peptide (ANP) concentrations. The reduction in arterial pressure that may occur if fetal cardiac output falls results in elevation of plasma AVP and angiotensin II concentrations. AVP decreases urinary output and, in the late-gestation fetus, reduces lung fluid production. ANP increases urinary output, but increases capillary permeability. Angiotensin II increases fetal fluid accumulation.

Table 1.6 Factors contributing to edema formation in the fetus.

Factor
High compliance of interstitial space: allows accommodation of large volume at low tissue pressure
High capillary filtration coefficient: allows large water flux at low vascular pressure
Low colloid osmotic pressure: reduces fluid movement from interstitium to capillary
High capillary permeability to protein: reduces fluid movement from interstitium to capillary
Sensitivity of lymphatic drainage to increased venous pressure: decreases removal of fluid from interstitium via lymphatic channels

Congenital cardiovascular malformations and the fetal circulation

It has long been recognized that congenital cardiovascular malformations may influence the development of the fetal circulation. In recent years ultrasound examination has provided the opportunity to assess the changes in circulatory development associated with advancing gestation. It has also become apparent that gestational changes in development and responses of the fetal circulation may affect the influence of various cardiovascular anomalies. The principal mechanisms by which congenital cardiovascular anomalies may affect fetal circulatory development are discussed in this section. Detailed considerations of these effects are presented in the chapters dedicated to individual lesions.

Cardiovascular malformations may:

- cause hydrops fetalis by increasing venous pressure (discussed above);
- change the volume or direction of blood flow;
- cause obstruction to blood flow;
- alter the oxygen saturation of blood delivered to various organs.

Changes in blood flow

Ventricular development

Interference with blood flow into or out of the left or right ventricle has for some time been thought to interfere with its development. Restriction of the foramen ovale or mitral orifice reduces blood flow into the left ventricle and results in hypoplasia as a result of the decreased volume in the chamber.

Experimental reduction of inflow of blood into the left ventricle of the fetal lamb for at least several days interferes with growth of the chamber [36].

Obstruction of outflow from a ventricle postnatally restricts ejection and induces enlargement as a result of the increased end-systolic volume. Atrial filling pressure increases and this helps to maintain stroke volume of the ventricle. Hypertrophy then ensues but ventricular volume is not significantly different from normal. In the fetus, the foramen ovale provides a large communication between the right and left atria. Aortic or pulmonary stenosis interferes with outflow of the left or right ventricle respectively and restricts the stroke volume of the affected chamber. Ventricular muscle mass increases in response to the increased systolic pressure. However, unlike postnatally, left or right atrial pressure does not increase significantly because of the presence of the foramen ovale. Venous return is diverted away from the ventricle with obstructed outflow and preferentially enters the ventricle with the greater diastolic compliance.

The total CVO can be maintained at normal levels, but ejection is increased from the normal ventricle and reduced from the obstructed chamber. We induced outflow obstruction of the left ventricle in fetal lambs by placing a constriction around the ascending aorta; this resulted in increased left ventricular muscle mass but a substantial reduction in the size of the left ventricle within just a few days [36]. These studies are discussed in Chapter 10. We induced pulmonary stenosis in fetal lambs at about 60 days' gestation by placing a band around the pulmonary trunk. The lambs were allowed to develop *in utero* and studied at about 120 days' gestation. Right ventricular muscle mass was greatly increased but, in the majority of fetuses, the size of the cavity of the ventricle, as well as the diameter of the tricuspid valve, were markedly reduced. The findings are reviewed in detail in Chapter 15.

Ascending aorta and aortic arch development

In fetal lambs, the left ventricle ejects about one-third of CVO, and about two-thirds of blood entering the ascending aorta is distributed to the brain and upper body. Thus only about 10% of CVO passes through the aortic isthmus. The relatively low blood flow through this segment is reflected by the fact that the diameter of the isthmus is only about half that of the ascending aorta.

In the human fetus, the left ventricle ejects about 45% of CVO. The volume passing through the aortic isthmus is not known, but it appears to be similar to that in the lamb and thus accounts for the fact that the diameter of the isthmus is also about 75% of that of the ascending aorta.

The diameter of the ascending aorta is affected by the magnitude of blood flow. Thus in the fetus with aortic atresia, no blood enters the aorta from the left ventricle, but flow occurs retrograde from the ductus arteriosus across the arch to the ascending aorta. The flow conducted by the ascending aorta is only that passing to the coronary circulation and the vessel is quite hypoplastic (see Chapter 11).

In the fetus with pulmonary atresia, no blood can be ejected by the right ventricle. All blood returning to the right side is directed through the foramen ovale and joins pulmonary venous return to the left atrium. Thus the total CVO is ejected into the ascending aorta. In the lamb, this would represent a flow about three times normal and in the human fetus a flow somewhat higher than twice normal. This high flow is associated with an aortic diameter considerably greater than normal (see Chapter 15).

Ductus arteriosus size and orientation

Normally, almost 60% of CVO traverses the ductus arteriosus from the pulmonary trunk to the descending aorta in the fetal lamb. In the late-gestation human fetus, flow is also exclusively from the pulmonary trunk to the descending aorta, although only about 30% of CVO passes through the ductus. Because a large volume is ejected by the right ventricle, the pulmonary trunk is large and, as a result of the direction of flow through the ductus, the inferior angle between the ductus and the descending aorta is oblique.

When RVO is markedly reduced, or completely obstructed, as with pulmonary atresia, flow into the pulmonary trunk is relatively low and is supplied by retrograde flow from the descending aorta across the ductus arteriosus. This results in poor development of the main pulmonary artery, and possibly the ductus arteriosus and the direction of flow in the ductus results in an acute inferior angle of the ductus with the descending aorta.

Conversely, severe reduction or curtailment of LVO, as in the presence of aortic atresia, results in hypoplasia of the ascending aorta (see above). If LVO is completely obstructed, the right ventricle ejects a much larger volume than normal, equivalent to the CVO. The blood flow through the ductus arteriosus is markedly increased, because the total cardiac output, excluding that distributed to the pulmonary circulation, passes through the ductus to provide both systemic and umbilical–placental flows. The ductus is large and connects with the descending aorta with a wide oblique inferior angle (see Chapter 6).

Effect of obstruction

The effect of obstruction of left or right ventricular output on blood flow into and out of the ventricle and on development of chamber size has been discussed above. Two other sites of obstruction that may affect fetal development are in the ductus arteriosus and in the aortic arch proximal to the ductus.

Ductus arteriosus obstruction and the pulmonary circulation

Pulmonary arterial and aortic pressures are similar in the fetus. Studies in fetal lambs have shown that constriction of the ductus arteriosus elevates pulmonary arterial pressure. This may result from constriction by mechanical means [37,38]. We have also shown that persistent compression of the ductus arteriosus in fetal lambs induces an increase in the medial smooth muscle layer of small pulmonary arteries, resulting in increased pulmonary vascular resistance [39]. The increased smooth muscle development may interfere with the normal fall in pulmonary vascular resistance after birth; studies in lambs have confirmed these observations [37,38].

Constriction of the ductus arteriosus *in utero* may result from administration of nonsteroidal antiinflammatory agents to the mother. One of the mechanisms that maintains patency of the ductus in the fetus is the relaxant effect of prostaglandin on ductus smooth muscle. Nonsteroidal antiinflammatory agents inhibit prostaglandin production and have been shown to constrict the ductus in both the sheep and human fetus (see Chapter 6). The resulting induction of an increase in the amount of pulmonary vascular smooth muscle could interfere with the postnatal fall in pulmonary vascular resistance and be responsible for the syndrome of persistent pulmonary hypertension of the newborn infant.

Constriction of the ductus reported in some fetuses with aortopulmonary transposition is discussed in Chapter 18.

Aortic arch obstruction and cerebral blood flow

In fetuses with aortic atresia, there is no blood ejected from the left ventricle into the ascending aorta. Blood flow to the head is derived from blood traversing the ductus arteriosus and then passing retrogradely across the aortic arch to the carotid arteries. Aortic atresia is frequently associated with coarctation of the aorta adjacent to the ductus arteriosus. As discussed in Chapter 12, it has been proposed that the coarctation is a result of the very high flow through the ductus; the junction between the aortic isthmus and the ductus arteriosus acts as a branch point and narrowing results at this site. Infants with aortic atresia have been reported to show a high incidence of neurodevelopmental problems as well as cerebral lesions on imaging and it has been suggested that reduced cerebral blood flow during fetal life may be responsible.

Effects of changes in blood oxygen content

Increased oxygen saturation of pulmonary arterial blood

Several congenital cardiovascular malformations alter the pattern of blood flow in the circulation in the fetus. These changes in the course of the circulation could potentially modify the oxygen saturation of blood delivered to various organs. In the normal fetus, well-oxygenated umbilical venous blood passing through the ductus venosus is preferentially directed through the foramen ovale to the left atrium and ventricle, which ejects it into the ascending aorta. However, in the fetus with aortopulmonary transposition, the pulmonary artery arises from the left ventricle. I previously speculated that the pulmonary circulation is exposed to blood with a higher oxygen content than normal and, because it is very reactive to small changes in oxygen, pulmonary vascular resistance and vascular development could be affected [40]. Jouannic *et al.* [41] reported that infants with transposition who had developed serious clinical deterioration soon after birth were identified to have had a small foramen ovale and/or a constricted ductus arteriosus during fetal life.

I have proposed that the observations of the abnormal foramen ovale and ductus could be related to the high oxygen saturation of blood entering the pulmonary circulation. The increased oxygen saturation will induce pulmonary vasodilatation, increase pulmonary blood flow, and result in increased pulmonary venous return to the left atrium. This will elevate left atrial pressure and tend to shift the flap of the foramen ovale to the right, thus reducing the size of the foramen. With the increase in LVO passing through the pulmonary circulation, a smaller proportion would be available to traverse the ductus arteriosus; this could account for the smaller ductus observed in some fetuses with transposition. Also, because the ductus is exposed to blood passing from the pulmonary trunk to the descending aorta, in the fetus with transposition it is subjected to a higher Po_2, which may further contribute to the constriction. These changes in the circulation in the fetus with aortopulmonary transposition are discussed in detail in Chapter 18.

Decreased oxygen saturation of ascending aortic blood

In the normal fetus, ascending aortic blood is derived from the left ventricle and has an oxygen saturation of about 65%. However, with aortopulmonary transposition, the aorta arises from the right ventricle and ascending aortic blood oxygen saturation will be considerably lower, probably about 45–50%. Whether this lower oxygen saturation will affect the cerebral circulation is open to speculation. Ultrasound studies have indicated that cerebral vascular resistance is decreased [42], suggesting that cerebral blood flow is increased to compensate for the lower oxygen saturation and thus maintain oxygen delivery. It is possible, though, that if the fetus is subjected to intrauterine stress, oxygen supply to the brain would be more readily compromised than in the normal fetus (see Chapter 18).

References

1 Bristow J, Rudolph AM, Itskovitz J. A preparation for studying liver blood flow, oxygen consumption, and metabolism in the fetal lamb in utero. J Dev Physiol 1981;3:255–266.

2 Lind J, Stern L, Wegelius C. Human Foetal and Neonatal Circulation. Springfield, IL: Charles C Thomas, 1964.

3 Edelstone DI, Rudolph AM, Heymann MA. Liver and ductus venosus blood flows in fetal lambs in utero. Circ Res 1978;42:426–433.

4 Bristow J, Rudolph AM, Itskovitz J, Barnes RJ. Hepatic oxygen and glucose metabolism in the fetal lamb: response to hypoxia. J Clin Invest 1983;71:1047–1061.

5 Edelstone DI, Rudolph AM. Preferential streaming of ductus venosus blood to the brain and heart in fetal lambs. Am J Physiol 1979;237:H724–H729.

6 Schmidt KG, Silverman NH, Rudolph AM. Assessment of flow events at the ductus venosus–inferior vena cava junction and at the foramen ovale in fetal sheep by use of multimodal ultrasound. Circulation 1996;93: 826–833.

7 Rudolph AM, Heymann MA, Teramo KAW, Barrett CT, Raiha NCR. Studies on the circulation of the previable human fetus. Pediatr Res 1971;5:452–465.

8 Reuss ML, Rudolph AM. Distribution and recirculation of umbilical and systemic venous blood flow in fetal lambs during hypoxia. J Dev Physiol 1980;2: 71–84.

9 Rudolph AM, Heymann MA. Circulatory changes with growth in the fetal lamb. Circ Res 1970;26:289–299.

10 Kenny J, Plappert T, Doubilet P *et al.* Changes in intracardiac blood flow velocities and right and left ventricular stroke volumes with gestational age in the normal human fetus: a prospective Doppler echocardiographic study. Circulation 1986;74:1208–1216.

11 De Smedt MCH, Visser GHA, Meijboom EJ. Fetal cardiac output estimated by Doppler echocardiography during mid- and late gestation. Am J Cardiol 1987;60: 338–342.

12 Sutton MS, Groves A, MacNeill A, Sharland G, Allan L. Assessment of changes in blood flow through the lungs and foramen ovale in the normal human fetus with gestational age: a prospective Doppler echocardiographic study. Br Heart J 1994;71:232–237.

13 Chaoui R, Heling KS, Taddei F, Bollmann R. Dopplerechokardiographische Analyse des Blutflusses über den fetalen Aorten und Pulmonalklappen in der zweiten Hälfte der Schwangerschaft. Geburtshilfe Frauenheilkd 1995;55:207–217.

14 Rasanen J, Wood DC, Weiner S, Ludomirski A, Huhta JC. Role of the pulmonary circulation in the distribution of the human fetal cardiac output during the second half of pregnancy. Circulation 1996;94:1068–1073.

15 Mielke G, Benda N. Cardiac output and central distribution of blood flow in the human fetus. Circulation 2001;103:1662–1668.

16 Rasanen J, Wood DC, Debbs RH, Cohen J, Weiner S, Huhta JC. Reactivity of the human fetal pulmonary circulation to maternal hyperoxygenation increases during the second half of pregnancy: a randomized study. Circulation 1998;97:257–262.
17 Kiserud T, Ebbing C, Kessler J, Rasmussen S. Fetal cardiac output, distribution to the placenta and impact of placental compromise. Ultrasound Obstet Gynecol 2006;28:126–136.
18 Dekaban AS, Sadowsky D. Changes in brain weights during the span of human life: relation of brain weights to body heights and body weights. Ann Neurol 1978; 4:345–356.
19 Behrman RE, Lees MH. Organ blood flows of the fetal, newborn and adult rhesus monkey: a comparative study. Biol Neonate 1971;18:330–334.
20 Acharya G, Wilsgaard T, Rosvold Berntsen GK, Maltau JM, Kiserud T. Reference ranges for umbilical vein blood flow in the second half of pregnancy based on longitudinal data. Prenat Diagn 2005;25:99–111.
21 Van Lierde M, Oberweis D, Thomas K. Ultrasonic measurement of aortic and umbilical blood flow in the human fetus. Obstet Gynecol 1984;63:801–805.
22 Haugen G, Kiserud T, Godfrey K, Crozier S, Hanson M. Portal and umbilical venous blood supply to the liver in the human fetus near term. Ultrasound Obstet Gynecol 2004;24:599–605.
23 Rudolph AM, Heymann MA. The circulation of the fetus in utero. Circ Res 1967;21:163–184.
24 Kessler J, Rasmussen S, Hanson M, Kiserud T. Longitudinal reference ranges for ductus venosus flow velocities and waveform indices. Ultrasound Obstet Gynecol 2006;28:890–898.
25 Rudolph AM, Heymann MA. Cardiac output in the fetal lamb: the effects of spontaneous and induced changes of heart rate on right and left ventricular output. Am J Obstet Gynecol 1976;124:183–192.
26 Gilbert RD. Control of fetal cardiac output during changes in blood volume. Am J Physiol 1980;238: H80–H86.
27 Hawkins J, Van Hare GF, Schmidt KG, Rudolph AM. Effects of increasing afterload on left ventricular output in fetal lambs. Circ Res 1989;65:127–134.
28 Friedman WF. The intrinsic physiologic properties of the developing heart. Prog Cardiovasc Dis 1972;15: 87–111.
29 Mahony L, Jones LR. Developmental changes in cardiac sarcoplasmic reticulum in sheep. J Biol Chem 1986;261: 15257–15265.
30 Itskovitz J, LaGamma EF, Rudolph AM. Baroreflex control of the circulation in chronically instrumented fetal lambs. Circ Res 1983;52:589–596.
31 Shinebourne EA, Vapaavuori EK, Williams RL, Heymann MA, Rudolph AM. Development of baroreflex activity in unanesthetized fetal and neonatal lambs. Circ Res 1972;31:710–718.
32 Itskovitz J, Rudolph AM. Denervation of arterial chemoreceptors and baroreceptors in fetal lambs in utero. Am J Physiol 1982;242:H916–H920.
33 Boekkooi PF, Baan J Jr, Teitel D, Rudolph AM. Chemoreceptor responsiveness in fetal sheep. Am J Physiol 1992;263:H162–H167.
34 Brace RA. Effects of outflow pressure on fetal lymph flow. Am J Obstet Gynecol 1989;160:494–497.
35 Brace RA, Valenzuela GJ. Effects of outflow pressure and vascular volume loading on thoracic duct lymph flow in adult sheep. Am J Physiol 1990;258:R240–R244.
36 Fishman NH, Hof RB, Rudolph AM. Models of congenital heart disease in fetal lambs. Circulation 1978;58: 354–364.
37 Wild LM, Nickerson PA, Morin FC III. Ligating the ductus arteriosus before birth remodels the pulmonary vasculature of the lamb. Pediatr Res 1989;25:251–257.
38 Abman SH, Shanley PF, Accurso FJ. Failure of postnatal adaptation of the pulmonary circulation after chronic intrauterine pulmonary hypertension in fetal lambs. J Clin Invest 1989;83:1849–1858.
39 Levin DL, Hyman AI, Heymann MA, Rudolph AM. Fetal hypertension and the development of increased pulmonary vascular smooth muscle: a possible mechanism for persistent pulmonary hypertension of the newborn infant. J Pediatr 1978;92:265–269.
40 Rudolph AM. Aortopulmonary transposition in the fetus: speculation on pathophysiology and therapy. Pediatr Res 2007;61:375–380.
41 Jouannic JM, Gavard L, Fermont L *et al.* Sensitivity and specificity of prenatal features of physiological shunts to predict neonatal clinical status in transposition of the great arteries. Circulation 2004;110:1743–1746.
42 Kaltman JR, Di H, Tian Z, Rychik J. Impact of congenital heart disease on cerebrovascular blood flow dynamics in the fetus. Ultrasound Obstet Gynecol 2005;25:32–96.

2

CHAPTER 2

Perinatal and postnatal changes in the circulation

After birth, the process of gas exchange is transferred from the placenta to the lungs. An adequate pulmonary blood flow must be established to provide for oxygen uptake and carbon dioxide removal when the umbilical–placental circulation is abolished. The separation of the systemic and pulmonary circulation, characteristic of the postnatal circulation, is achieved by closure of the ductus arteriosus and foramen ovale. During fetal life, the mother maintains fetal body temperature, but after birth the neonate must increase metabolism to maintain temperature. Measurements in fetal and neonatal lambs have demonstrated that fetal oxygen consumption is 6–8 mL/min per kg body weight. After birth it increases to 15–20 mL/min per kg, the value depending on environmental temperature. Cardiac output tends to be closely related to metabolism, reflected by oxygen consumption; in the lamb there is a considerable increase in cardiac output after birth (see below). In comparing postnatal cardiac output with fetal cardiac output, it should be appreciated that cardiac output in the fetus is usually expressed as combined ventricular output, whereas postnatal cardiac output represents the output of one ventricle. This must also be considered when expressing organ blood flow as a proportion of cardiac output.

Changes in cardiac output

Combined ventricular output in fetal lambs *in utero* is about 450 mL/min per kg body weight; about 300 mL/kg is ejected by the right ventricle and 150 mL/kg by the left ventricle. Cardiac output in awake, resting neonatal lambs is about 300–425 mL/min per kg. The values in newborns are determined to a large extent by environmental temperature; cardiac output is higher in lower temperatures. Postnatally, cardiac output represents the volume of blood flowing through the pulmonary and systemic circulation in series. Therefore the combined output of the right and left ventricles is 600–850 mL/min per kg. This represents a 30–80% increase over fetal values. Left ventricular output increases dramatically by threefold to fivefold. The mechanisms responsible for this marked increase in cardiac output after birth have not been fully defined.

The immediate events occurring at the time of birth include delivery of the fetus, ventilation, and separation of the umbilical–placental circulation. The process of ventilation includes physical expansion of the lung with air and removal of the fluid in the airways, as well as an increase in alveolar oxygen concentration. Because the events at birth occur almost simultaneously, it has been difficult to define the importance of individual processes in inducing perinatal circulatory changes. The separate roles of lung expansion, increased alveolar oxygen concentration, and elimination of the placental circulation have been examined in fetal lambs that were not delivered from the uterus [1,2]. We studied the lambs *in utero* after recovery from surgery to implant vascular catheters, a tube in the trachea, and an occluding balloon around the umbilical cord. Rhythmic expansion of the lungs with 3% oxygen and 5% carbon dioxide did not significantly change fetal blood gases (descending arterial Po_2 of ~21 mmHg and Pco_2 of ~40 mmHg). Subsequent ventilation with oxygen raised fetal arterial Po_2 to 40–60 mmHg. Then, while ventilating with oxygen the umbilical cord was occluded.

Congenital Diseases of the Heart, 3rd edition. By A. Rudolph
© 2009 Blackwell Publishing, ISBN: 9781405162456

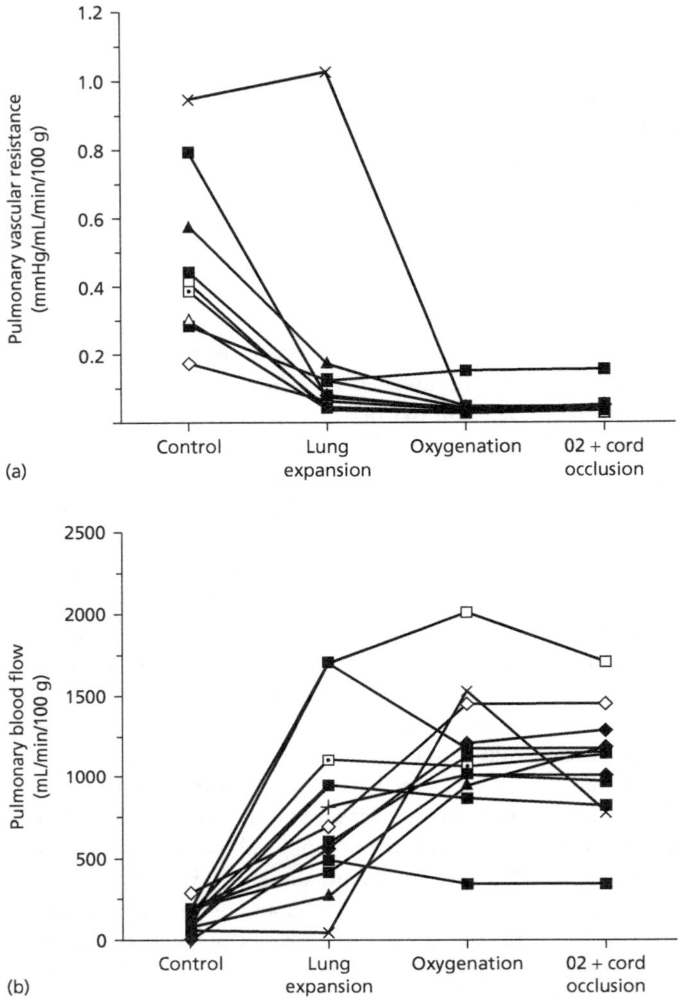

Figure 2.1 Changes in (a) pulmonary vascular resistance and (b) pulmonary blood flow resulting from physical expansion of the lung, ventilation with oxygen, and umbilical cord occlusion in fetal lambs *in utero*.

Lung expansion with no change in arterial blood gases resulted in a marked decrease in pulmonary vascular resistance and an increase in pulmonary blood flow (Figure 2.1). The changes in the course of blood flow and the amounts flowing through various chambers and great vessels are shown in Figure 2.2. The proportion of right ventricular output distributed to the lungs increased and the amount traversing the ductus arteriosus to the descending aorta fell. Flow through the foramen ovale into the left atrium decreased. Although pulmonary vascular resistance decreased, pulmonary arterial pressure did not fall; this suggests that the ductus arteriosus remained widely patent. Left ventricular output increased and was only slightly lower than right ventricular output.

During ventilation with oxygen, pulmonary vascular resistance decreased further and the rise in pulmonary blood flow was greater. Almost all the blood ejected by the right ventricle entered the pulmonary circulation and only a small amount passed through the ductus arteriosus. A small shunt from the aorta to the pulmonary artery through the ductus arteriosus could be detected. Left ventricular output now exceeded right ventricular output, as a result of the small left-to-right shunt through the ductus arteriosus. Flow across the foramen ovale was completely eliminated; this was probably

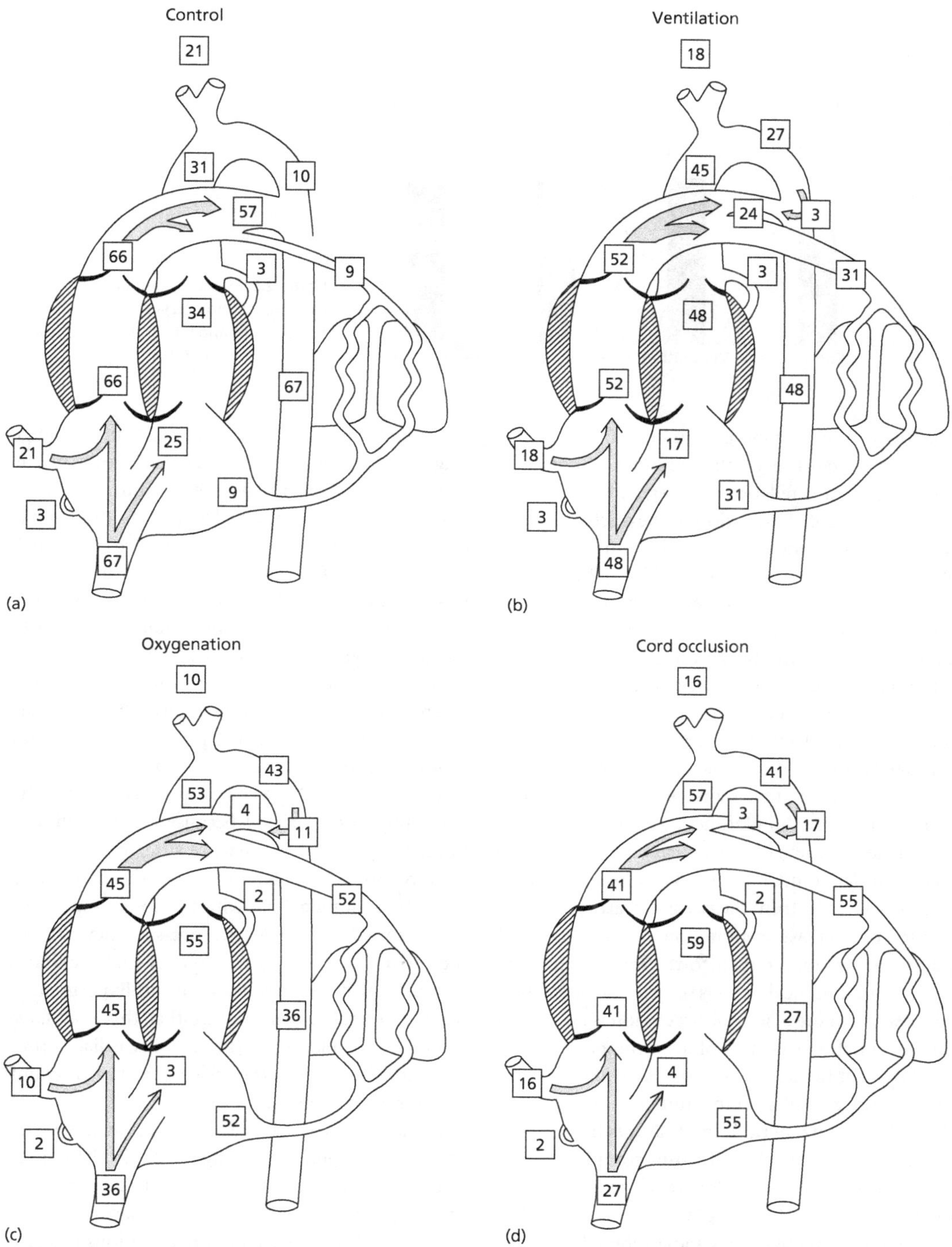

Figure 2.2 Effects of birth events on the proportions on combined ventricular output flowing through the cardiac chambers and great vessels in fetal lambs. (a) Control fetal circulation; (b) effect of ventilation (physical expansion of the lungs with no change of blood gases); (c) effect of ventilation with oxygen; (d) effect of umbilical cord occlusion.

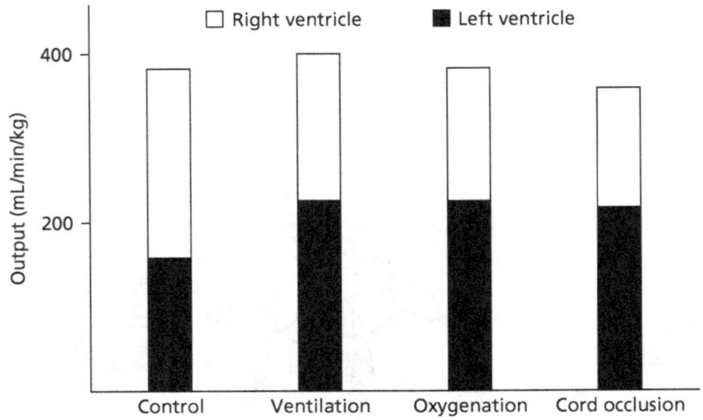

Figure 2.3 Effects of simulated birth events on combined ventricular output and on right and left ventricular output in fetal lambs *in utero*.

due to a 2–3 mmHg increase in left atrial pressure, resulting in closure of the foramen. Pulmonary arterial pressure fell progressively, probably as a result of gradual constriction of the ductus arteriosus. Subsequent occlusion of the umbilical cord eliminated umbilical–placental blood flow. This resulted in no further changes in pulmonary blood flow, but caused a rise in arterial pressure with a small increase in the flow from the aorta into the pulmonary artery through the ductus arteriosus.

Thus it is apparent that the circulatory adjustments associated with birth are largely the result of ventilation-induced decrease in pulmonary vascular resistance. The mechanisms by which physical expansion of the lung alone and ventilation with oxygen affect the pulmonary circulation are discussed in detail in Chapter 5. Closure of the foramen ovale results from the rise in left atrial pressure due to the increase in pulmonary blood flow and pulmonary venous return to the left atrium. The decrease in umbilical venous return associated with elimination of the placental circulation is not necessary for functional closure of the foramen ovale.

Closure of the ductus arteriosus proceeds slowly in the lamb, as well as in the human infant. During the early neonatal period, small shunts through the ductus may occur before it closes completely. The mechanisms involved in closure of the ductus arteriosus are discussed in Chapter 6.

However, in these studies, the combined ventricular output did not increase significantly. Left ventricular output increased from about 140 mL/min per kg to about 210 mL/min per kg; this was associated with a fall in right ventricular output, so that combined ventricular output did not change (Figure 2.3). At birth, the fetus is removed from the warm temperature in the uterus, into the cooler environment of room air. The possibility that the change in environmental temperature after birth could account for the increase in cardiac output was examined by delivering the lamb fetus into a water bath while allowing placental circulation to be maintained. Combined, as well as left and right, ventricular output did not change significantly when the bath temperature was 39 or 25°C, indicating that environmental temperature alone is not responsible for the increase in output [3].

The hypothesis has been proposed that fetal cardiac output is restricted because cardiac filling is limited by a high pericardial pressure, resulting from compression of the fetal chest by the uterus and maternal abdomen. Following the onset of spontaneous ventilation, a negative pressure develops in the pleural and pericardial spaces that facilitates venous return and increases output. Experimental studies in fetal lambs indicate that this may have some role in explaining an increase in cardiac output after birth, but it is not known whether it can account fully for the postnatal increase in output [4].

In the studies of the role of ventilation and environmental temperature change at birth, the fetuses were delivered by cesarean section 1–2 weeks prior to term gestation. In the sheep, fetal plasma triiodothyronine (T_3) and cortisol concentrations increase prior to delivery. The fetuses had therefore not been exposed to the increase in circulating concentrations of these hormones. Plasma T_3 concentration normally rises rapidly after birth and because

T_3 administration increases cardiac output in adults, it was hypothesized that the postnatal increase in cardiac output could be the result of the rise in T_3 concentration. Studies were conducted in three groups of lambs, all of which had surgery at about 130 days' gestation [5]. In the control group nothing further was done; in the second group thyroidectomy was performed at the time of surgery; and in the third group, the thyroid was removed at the time of delivery. In the control group, plasma T_3 concentration increased from 1 to 3–4 ng/mL within 30–60 min after birth. Left ventricular output increased from about 170 mL/min per kg in the fetus to about 340 mL/min per kg and oxygen consumption rose to 23 mL/min per kg within 60 min after birth. In the group that had thyroidectomy at 130 days' gestation, T_3 was not detectable in fetal plasma, or after birth; neither cardiac output nor oxygen consumption increased after delivery. In the lambs in which the thyroid was removed immediately before delivery, plasma T_3 concentration was about 1 mg/mL but did not increase after delivery. Cardiac output and oxygen consumption increased to the same levels as in the control group. These studies demonstrate that the normal postnatal increase in T_3 concentration is not responsible for the increase in cardiac output, but that prenatal thyroid action is necessary for cardiac output and oxygen consumption to increase after birth. Lack of T_3 could affect myocardial function through several mechanisms.

The myocardium of the lambs that underwent thyroidectomy about 2 weeks prior to birth had about half the normal number of β-adrenoceptors and showed a greatly reduced adenylate cyclase response to isoproterenol. Thyroid hormone is also known to increase Na^+/K^+-ATPase activity and to modify cardiac heavy-chain myosin. It is apparent that prenatal activity of thyroid hormone is necessary for the postnatal increase in cardiac output, but the exact mechanism of action is still not defined.

The possibility that cortisol may affect myocardial development and function also has to be considered. Fetal plasma cortisol concentration increases dramatically a few days before normal delivery of the lamb. Cortisol does affect myocardial growth as manifested by its effect on DNA and protein concentrations in fetal myocardium (see below).

Following the initial increase in cardiac output in the lamb, the cardiac output then falls in relation to body weight, paralleling the decrease in oxygen consumption relative to weight. Oxygen consumption falls from about 16–20 mL/min per kg immediately after birth to about 6–8 mL/min per kg by 8–10 weeks. Cardiac output falls from about 300–425 mL/min per kg to about 150–170 mL/min pr kg over the same period. This can be partly explained on the basis of the changes in surface area relative to body weight, because oxygen consumption is related to body surface area (see Chapter 3). The changes are likely to be less significant in the human infant because the changes in growth and body habitus are less striking in the postnatal period.

Another factor that may account for the relative decrease in cardiac output over the first few postnatal weeks is a change in sympathetic nerve activity. Myocardial contractility has been shown to fall over the first four to five postnatal weeks in the lamb and this is associated with a progressive increase in response to β-adrenoceptor stimulation [6]. This suggests that immediately after birth the myocardium is being subjected to high resting inotropic stimulation by catecholamines and that as the resting inotropic stimulation recedes myocardial contractility is reduced but the response to β-adrenoceptor stimulation increases.

The relatively high resting cardiac output in the early neonatal period reduces the reserve of the heart to respond to increased requirements. In fetal lambs, cardiac output per kilogram body weight increases by about 35% in response to volume loading, whereas in the 6–8-week-old lamb, cardiac output increases by about 65–70% above resting levels [7]. The actual cardiac output per kilogram achieved in the older lamb is no greater than in the neonate, but the resting output per kilogram is considerably lower. Thus there is greater reserve in the older animals.

Ductus venosus and hepatic blood flows

Following birth, elimination of umbilical venous return drastically reduces flow to the liver and through the ductus venosus. The mechanisms involved in closure of the ductus venosus have not yet been fully defined. A sphincter has been described at the origin of the ductus venosus from the umbilical vein, and it has been suggested that some degree of constriction of this sphincter is responsible for the high flow velocity in the vessel. There is little evidence for the role of a sphincter. It has been suggested that the ductus reacts passively to the intraluminal pressure, and that closure after birth is merely the result of the fall in blood flow associated with removal of umbilical venous return. However, contemporary research has shown that the ductus venosus is affected by prostaglandins. Administration of the prostaglandin synthesis inhibitor indomethacin to fetal lambs results in constriction of the ductus venosus; this can be reversed by infusion of PGE_1 [8,9]. It is thus possible that the patency of the ductus venosus in the fetus is maintained by circulating prostaglandins. The ductus venosus in the human is also regulated by PGE; infusion of PGE results in relaxation of the ductus in infants with total anomalous pulmonary venous drainage to the portal vein (see Chapter 13). In studies in both the lamb and the human infant, the ductus venosus has been shown to be patent for as long as 6–11 days after birth. In the early postnatal period, considerable amounts of portal venous flow traverse the ductus but by 3–4 days the amounts are negligible.

Associated with the elimination of umbilical venous return, hepatic blood flow falls rapidly, and then increases as gastrointestinal flow is established [10]. In the lamb, hepatic flow falls from the fetal level of 420 to about 100 mL/min per 100 g liver weight after delivery. Portal venous flow in the fetus is about 55 mL/min per 100 g liver weight. By 2 hours it increased to 140 mL/min per 100 g liver weight and by 10 hours to 300 mL/min per 100 g liver weight. Associated with the increase in portal venous flow, ductus venosus flow into the inferior vena cava increased to 150 mL/min per 100 g liver weight. Hepatic flow progressively increases after birth and by 7 days after birth reaches levels of about 250 mL/min per 100 g liver weight; by this time there is no flow through the ductus venosus.

Changes in organ blood flows

While *in utero*, the fetus is bathed in amniotic fluid at maternal body temperature. Fetal temperature is, in fact, slightly higher than maternal temperature, because heat is produced by the fetus and is transferred to the mother, perhaps through the amniotic fluid by conduction and convection but probably largely through the placental circulation. Because environmental temperature is high and no evaporation from the skin surface occurs, skin temperature is high and the arterioles, as well as the veins, are dilated. After birth, surface temperature decrease in environmental temperature and evaporation from the skin surface results in peripheral vasoconstriction of arteries and veins, with an increase in systemic vascular resistance.

The postnatal rise in systemic arterial Po_2 also has a marked effect on the vascular resistance in several organs. The coronary circulation is very sensitive to changes in Po_2. Before birth, the coronary vessels are perfused by blood with a Po_2 of about 25–28 mmHg, whereas after birth Po_2 of arterial blood rises to 80–90 mmHg. In lambs myocardial blood flow falls rapidly to 50% or less of the prenatal level. Fetal myocardial flow is about 200–250 mL/min per 100 g of muscle, and in the newborn lamb is about 100–125 mL/min per 100 g. However, despite the decrease in coronary blood flow, oxygen delivery to the myocardium is similar because, with the rise in arterial oxygen saturation from about 60–65% in the fetus to greater than 90% after birth, oxygen content increases [11].

Oxygen consumption per unit weight of myocardium is similar in the fetal and adult heart; it is somewhat higher in the neonatal period, probably due to high resting sympathetic activity. During fetal life the myocardium utilizes carbohydrate almost exclusively as an energy source [11]. The metabolic substrates are predominantly glucose and lactate and a small amount of pyruvate. In the adult, fatty acids constitute a major source of energy for the myocardium. It is not known when after birth the change in substrates used by the myocardium occurs. Nor is it known whether the fetal myocardium does not utilize fatty acid because fetal arterial concentrations of fatty acids are low, or because myocardial enzymes that assist in metabolism are not yet well developed in the fetus.

The cerebral circulation is also sensitive to changes in Po_2 of perfusing blood. In fetal lambs, hypoxemia increases cerebral blood flow and raising arterial Po_2 by ventilating the lamb with oxygen results in a marked decrease in cerebral blood flow. However, because oxygen content of the perfusing blood increases, oxygen delivery is maintained or even increased.

Changes in hemoglobin and tissue oxygen delivery

In the human, the higher hemoglobin level compared with maternal blood facilitates oxygen uptake by the fetus in the placenta. Most hemoglobin in the fetus is of fetal type (HbF). The oxygen dissociation curve of fetal red cells is shifted to the left compared with adult red cells (see Chapter 3). In the sheep, this difference in dissociation curves is related to the different affinities of HbF and adult hemoglobin (HbA) for oxygen. In the human, the dissociation curves for HbF and HbA are similar. However, there is a difference in the dissociation curves of intact red cells. This is related to the fact that HbF has much less affinity for organic phosphates such as 2,3-diphosphoglycerate (2,3-DPG) and ATP than does HbA. These phosphates, which are present in red blood cells, compete with oxygen for binding to hemoglobin. The difference in binding of fetal and adult hemoglobin is important in facilitating oxygen transfer from mother to fetus in the placenta.

In adult red cells, the preferential binding of 2,3-DPG to hemoglobin tends to release oxygen, which in the placenta readily binds to HbF. The affinity of reduced hemoglobin for 2,3-DPG is greater than that of oxyhemoglobin. At the tissue site, where oxygen diffuses from the capillary, hemoglobin is reduced and the binding of 2,3-DPG facilitates removal of oxygen from the blood to be available for the tissues. Because HbF does not have a high affinity for 2,3-DPG, this effect is less significant.

The human newborn infant has a high hemoglobin level (~16 g/dL), so that oxygen capacity is quite high, and the total amount of oxygen that can be transported to the tissues is large. However, because HbF levels are still high, the facilitation of oxygen delivery at the tissue site by 2,3-DPG is not as great as in adults. The lower extraction of oxygen would result in a relatively low arteriovenous oxygen difference across the systemic circulation, with a mixed venous oxygen saturation higher than in the adult. High levels of HbF in the newborn period may be disadvantageous in infants with heart disease who have a decrease in the amount of oxygen being transported to tissues as a result of reduced systemic blood flow or low arterial oxygen saturation (see Chapter 3).

Over the first 8–10 weeks after birth, hemoglobin concentration falls to 10–11 g/dL. This is accompanied by loss of HbF and almost 100% of hemoglobin is of the adult type. The decrease in hemoglobin concentration reduces oxygen delivery to the tissues, but HbA facilitates removal of oxygen so that extraction is increased (see Figure 3.5).

Myocardial growth before and after birth

Morphological studies of fetal and adult heart muscle show considerable differences in the myocytes, as well as in the extracellular tissue and capillaries. The adult myocardium shows little interstitial tissue between myocytes, and the myocytes are organized in a parallel arrangement. The diameter of the myocyte in the adult sheep is about 15–25 μm (Table 2.1). The nucleus is relatively small and polyploidy is quite frequently noted. In the fetal heart, however, there is more intercellular

Table 2.1 Myocyte size and numbers and the estimated total number of myocytes in the left ventricular free wall in the fetal lamb at 0.8 and 0.98 gestation and in the adult sheep.

	Fetus 0.8 gestation	*Fetus 0.98 gestation*	*Adult*
Myocyte diameter (μm)	5.1	5.5	15.5
Cross-sectional area (μm^2)	22	30	168
Length (μm)	25	25	50
Volume (μm^3)	550	750	8400
Left ventricular free wall			
Weight (g)	5.5	8.0	65
Total cell number	1×10^{10}	1.1×10^{10}	7.7×10^9

space between the myocytes and the cells are less well organized; the nuclei are large and polyploidy is unusual. The diameter of the myocyte in the fetal sheep heart is only 5–7 μm. The diameter of the myocyte increases by only a small amount during gestational development, so that the increase in muscle mass during prenatal growth is almost exclusively the result of increase in cell numbers, or *hyperplasia*. Following birth there is a rapid decrease in myocyte mitosis; a small increase in cell number occurs during the first few weeks after birth, but beyond this early neonatal period, essentially all myocardial growth is the result of increase in myocyte size, or *hypertrophy*. In addition to the differences in myocyte size, the arrangement of the sarcomeres changes during development. In the adult, the sarcomeres are well organized and parallel with each other. In the early-gestation fetus, the longitudinal orientation of the sarcomeres is more random, and with advancing gestation they align in a more parallel arrangement [12].

In addition to the morphological changes, the concentrations of DNA and protein in the myocardium reflect the changes in pattern of growth before and after birth. In the fetus the concentration of DNA is relatively high and the concentration of protein relatively low as compared with adult myocardium. This indicates a relatively large number of nuclei in fetal myocardium. The factors involved in the change in myocardial growth after birth have not been fully defined, but cortisol is at least one factor that has a significant role. Administration of cortisol into the coronary artery of fetal lambs resulted in a decrease in myocardial DNA concentration, and relative increase in protein concentration, simulating the changes occurring normally after birth [13].

Recently it has been proposed that the change in myocyte growth begins to occur to a limited extent from about 120 days' (0.8) gestation in the sheep. This is based on the observation that binucleate myocytes are seen in greater number [14]. Since polyploidy suggests that the myocytes have terminally differentiated, it appears that the increase in myocardial mass is at least partly due to increase in size of differentiated myocytes. This process is quite limited, so that increase of myocardial mass in the latter part of gestation is still largely due to hyperplasia of myocytes.

Since left ventricular output increases by about 25% after birth and systemic arterial pressure is similar to the prenatal level, the work of the left ventricle increases. However, the right ventricle ejects about 30% less volume after birth; also, as pulmonary vascular resistance falls, pulmonary arterial and right ventricular pressures decline, so that the work of the right ventricle drops rapidly. These changes in right and left ventricular work are reflected in changes in muscle development. The left ventricle increases rapidly in thickness and in weight. Right ventricular output and pressure fall after birth, so there is less stimulus for right ventricular myocardium to develop. It was thought that the right ventricle actually undergoes a decrease in muscle mass, so-called physiological atrophy. However, more recent studies in both the pig and the human have shown that right ventricular mass does not decrease but remains stationary for about a week after birth. However, the ratio of left to right ventricular weight increases rapidly due to left ventricular growth. After about a week, associated with growth, both left and right ventricular weights increase.

Postnatal circulatory changes in the premature infant

Little information is available regarding the circulation and its responses in the infant born prematurely. As mentioned above, the term lamb shows some increase in systemic arterial pressure as a result of the rise in systemic vascular resistance associated with removal of the low resistance umbilical–placental circulation. Also, the increase in pulmonary blood flow and venous return to the left atrium and ventricle raises left ventricular output after birth. Thus the level of arterial pressure cannot be assumed to reflect the magnitude of systemic blood flow. Arterial pressure is determined by both vascular resistance and blood flow.

It is well recognized that preterm infants have lower arterial blood pressures than infants born at term. The pressure is also related to the gestational age at the time of birth; the earlier the gestation, the lower the pressure. However, there are no established standards for actual pressures, but it has been commonly assumed that a mean blood pressure below 30 mmHg represents hypotension.

Subsequently, it was suggested that the level of mean arterial blood pressure that can be considered to be normal is equal to the gestational age in weeks [15]. This is somewhat arbitrary and has not been confirmed by any reliable observation. The concept was also commonly held that arterial mean pressures below the conceived norms were related to inadequate left ventricular output and reduced flow to various fetal organs. This was thought to contribute to mortality and also to the high incidence of cerebral insults in very premature infants.

In attempts to raise arterial pressure and left ventricular output, fluids with either electrolytes or volume expanders (e.g., albumin or plasma) were administered and catecholamines, particularly dopamine or dobutamine and less commonly epinephrine, were infused. In a review, Dempsey and Barrington [16] found no evidence that blood volume was reduced in preterm infants with blood pressures considered to be low, and stated that "the routine use of fluid boluses in hypotensive preterm babies in the first days of life is not supported by any empirical data, has no physiologic basis and is associated with worse outcomes."

Recognizing that arterial pressure is determined by both vascular resistance and blood flow, Evans [17] has attempted to examine systemic blood flow as well as arterial pressure in preterm infants. Several difficulties are encountered in measuring systemic flow in the early neonatal period in preterm infants. A major problem is that left ventricular output, as measured by ultrasound assessment of ascending aortic velocity, frequently does not represent systemic blood flow, as left-to-right shunt through the ductus arteriosus also contributes to left ventricular output. Although right ventricular output, which would measure systemic venous return, is more likely to represent systemic blood flow, it also may not be reliable, particularly if a large ductus left-to-right shunt is present. The enhanced venous return to the left atrium will raise left atrial pressure and if the foramen ovale is incompetent, or is stretched, an atrial left-to-right shunt may raise right ventricular output to levels above those of systemic venous return (see Chapter 4). In view of the great concern that circulatory compromise in the preterm infant may result in cerebral damage, Evans has measured superior vena cava (SVC) flow in these infants to reflect systemic blood flow to the brain and upper body. Kluckow *et al.* [18] have reviewed these observations. It is estimated that about 75% of SVC flow is derived from the brain. About one-third of all infants born at less than 30 weeks' gestation had SVC flows below the estimated normal levels recorded within 24 hours of birth, predominantly in the postnatal period of 5–12 hours. In their studies there was a poor relationship between systemic arterial hypotension and the magnitude of SVC flow. There was, however, an excellent relationship between the observation of reduced SVC flow and the development of periventricular/intraventricular hemorrhage. Evidence of the cerebral lesions were first noted during or after the increase of SVC flows to normal levels.

The factors responsible for the reduced SVC flow in these preterm infants have not been fully delineated. The lower the gestational age of the infant, the more likely is SVC flow to be low; other associations are lung disease requiring high positive-pressure ventilation, which may interfere with systemic venous return, and persistent patency of the ductus arteriosus. The possibility that the left ventricle of the preterm infant of less than 30 weeks is immature and not able to sustain an increase in output after birth has been suggested. We have shown in fetal lambs that the left ventricle is very sensitive to afterload and that at constant filling pressure, elevation of aortic pressure results in a dramatic fall in stroke volume [19]. It was suggested that preterm infants had decreased left ventricular contractility soon after birth and that this would limit their ability to increase output with increased filling pressure [20]. However, in studies in prematurely delivered lambs in which the ductus arteriosus was maintained patent by formalin injection of the wall, left ventricular output was dramatically increased because a large left-to-right shunt developed after the lungs were ventilated [21]. However, systemic blood flow was reduced and blood flow to many organs was compromised.

Based on the above discussion, it appears likely that the ductus arteriosus has a major role in the cardiovascular compromise in the early postnatal period in very premature infants. Ventilation results in a fall of pulmonary vascular resistance and if the ductus is patent, a left-to-right shunt develops. Possibly the pulmonary vascular resistance falls to very low levels in the very immature infant, facilitating the ductus shunt. To maintain systemic blood flow, the ventricular output has to increase dramatically to compensate for the shunt; this places a large volume load on the ventricle. If the ventricle is not capable of sustaining the increased output, systemic blood flow will be reduced, because blood is preferentially directed to the low resistance pulmonary circulation. Systemic arterial pressure may be maintained if systemic vascular resistance increases, but if systemic flow is severely compromised, pressure will fall.

Numerous therapies have been used to treat these infants. As mentioned above, fluid infusions, as either boluses or continuous administration, have been used almost routinely, although there is no evidence that they are effective and they possibly have adverse effects. Several catecholamines have been administered. Dopamine has been favored to increase arterial pressure and systemic blood flow. When infused at a rate of 5 μg/kg per min or more, it induces peripheral vasoconstriction; although it may raise arterial pressure, systemic flow may fall even though left ventricular output may be maintained but left-to-right shunt will increase. Dobutamine, which has an inotropic effect on the heart but does not induce significant peripheral vasoconstriction, may increase systemic flow a small amount, but does not raise arterial pressure. Epinephrine, which has been used less frequently, appears to induce a small increase in both systemic flow and pressure. In reviewing the results of the catecholamine infusions, Dempsey and Barrington [16] came to the same conclusion as they did for the effects of intravascular fluid infusions, namely that they did not appear to have any beneficial effect and could in fact be harmful. Corticosteroids, which have been known to produce a modest increase in arterial pressure, have also been recommended, although there is no convincing evidence that they are effective and potentially could have adverse effects.

Recently Paradisis *et al.* [22] instituted pilot studies to assess the effect of prophylactic administration of milrinone to prevent the fall in SVC blood flow they had recorded in the very preterm infants. Milrinone is a phosphodiesterase type III inhibitor with a positive inotropic effect on the myocardium; it is also a vasodilator. It had been shown to have some beneficial effect in improving cardiac output in patients with low output following surgery. Although initial observations of the effects of milrinone in preterm infants were encouraging, this has not been confirmed and it does not appear to have a beneficial effect.

Although less attention is being directed to blood pressure values in the very premature infant, one consideration of possible importance is the effect of low pressure on coronary blood flow. Myocardial perfusion of the left ventricle occurs predominantly in diastole, and flow is related to the pressure difference in the aorta and the intraventricular pressure during diastole. In the presence of a patent ductus arteriosus with a large left-to-right shunt, the left ventricle is handling a large volume load and pressure in the atrium and ventricle in diastole may be increased, With the large ductus shunt, aortic diastolic pressure may be reduced considerably and thus coronary blood flow may be compromised. This may be of particular importance because, with the increased workload on the left ventricle, oxygen requirements will be greater and, if coronary flow is reduced, ventricular function could be affected.

In considering the possible approaches to cardiovascular compromise in these very preterm infants, it would seem that if the shunt through the ductus arteriosus could be reduced, systemic blood flow could be enhanced. This could be accomplished by reducing the size of the ductus, increasing pulmonary vascular resistance, or reducing systemic vascular resistance. The problem with attempting to increase pulmonary vascular resistance is that in the preterm infant, pulmonary vessels appear to be less reactive than in term infants. Reducing systemic vascular resistance by use of vasodilators could be readily accomplished, but a major concern would be that coronary flow could be compromised. Current methods of pharmacological closure of the ductus with nonsteroidal antiinflammatory agents have the drawback that they are often not effective in very preterm infants and may not act rapidly enough, because the main fall in SVC flow has been observed at about 5–12 hours after birth.

Changes in childhood and adolescence

After the rapid adaptations of the circulation in the perinatal period, more gradual adjustments occur

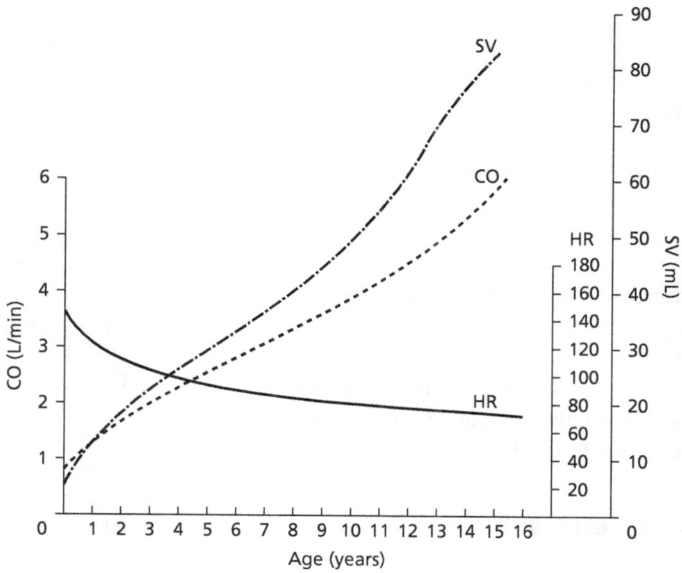

Figure 2.4 Changes in cardiac output (CO), heart rate (HR), and stroke volume (SV) during infancy, childhood and adolescence.

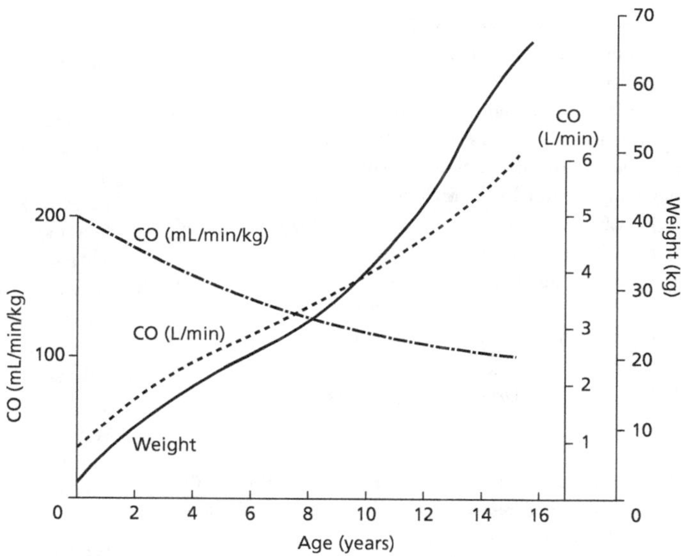

Figure 2.5 Relationships between changes after birth in body weight, actual cardiac output (CO) and cardiac output in mL/min per kg body weight.

in relation to changes in body size and configuration, and exertion. Based on reported measurements in humans, the changes in heart rate, cardiac output, and blood pressure during infancy, childhood and adolescence are shown in Figures 2.4 and 2.5. Resting heart rate decreases progressively and cardiac output increases and is fairly linearly related to body surface area over the whole age spectrum. The actual level of cardiac output at rest is about 3.5 L/min per m^2 of body surface. In view of the disproportion between body weight and body surface area, cardiac output is not directly related to body weight. During the first few years, cardiac output expressed as mL/min per kg body weight falls fairly rapidly. Immediately after birth, cardiac output is about 200 mL/min per kg; it first falls rapidly and then more slowly, reaching a level of about 100 mL/min per kg at rest in the adolescent age group. This decrease in cardiac output per kilogram of body weight while cardiac output per square meter of body surface area is constant can be explained on the basis of a change in body configuration. Associated with body growth there is an increase in stroke volume.

Figure 2.4 shows that stroke volume increases relatively more than cardiac output in relation to age. This is due to the fact that heart rate decreases with advancing age. Because cardiac output is linearly related to body surface area, but heart rate decreases with increasing age, stroke volume per square meter of body surface also increases with growth.

Systemic arterial pressure increases with growth, and systemic vascular resistance also increases when related to body surface area.

References

1 Teitel DF, Iwamoto HS, Rudolph AM. Effects of birth-related events on central blood flow patterns. Pediatr Res 1987;22:557–566.
2 Teitel DF, Iwamoto HS, Rudolph AM. Changes in the pulmonary circulation during birth-related events. Pediatr Res 1990;27:372–378,
3 van Bel F, Roman C, Iwamoto HS, Rudolph AM. Sympathoadrenal, metabolic, and regional blood flow responses to cold in fetal sheep. Pediatr Res 1993;34:47–50.
4 Grant DA, Kondo CS, Maloney JE, Walker AM, Tyberg JV. Changes in pericardial pressure during the perinatal period. Circulation 1992;86:1615–1621.
5 Breall JA, Rudolph AM, Heymann MA. Role of thyroid hormone in postnatal circulatory and metabolic adjustments. J Clin Invest 1984;73:1418–1424.
6 Teitel DF, Sidi D, Chin T, Brett C, Heymann MA, Rudolph AM. Developmental changes in myocardial contractile reserve in the lamb. Pediatr Res 1985;19:948–955.
7 Klopfenstein HS, Rudolph AM. Postnatal changes in the circulation and responses to volume loading in sheep. Circ Res 1978;42:839–845.
8 Adeagbo AS, Coceani F, Olley PM. The response of the lamb ductus venosus to prostaglandins and inhibitors of prostaglandin and thromboxane synthesis. Circ Res 1982;51:580–586.
9 Paulick RP, Meyers RL, Rudolph CD, Rudolph AM. Venous and hepatic vascular responses to indomethacin and prostaglandin E1 in the fetal lamb. Am J Obstet Gynecol 1990;163:1357–1363.
10 Townsend SF, Rudolph CD, Rudolph AM. Changes in ovine hepatic circulation and oxygen consumption at birth. Pediatr Res 1989;25:300–304.
11 Fisher DJ, Rudolph AM, Heymann MA. Myocardial oxygen and carbohydrate consumption in fetal lambs in utero and in adult sheep. Am J Physiol 1980;238:H399–H405.
12 Friedman WF. The intrinsic physiologic properties of the developing heart. Prog Cardiovasc Dis 1972;15:87–111.
13 Rudolph AM, Roman C, Gournay VA. Perinatal myocardial DNA and protein changes in the lamb: effect of cortisol in the fetus. Pediatr Res 1999;46:141–146.
14 Jonker SS, Zhang L, Louey S, Giraud GD, Thornburg KL, Faber JJ. Myocyte enlargement, differentiation, and proliferation kinetics in the fetal sheep heart. J Appl Physiol 2007;102:1130–1142.
15 Levene M, Chiswick M, Field D *et al.* Development of audit measures and guidelines for good practice in the management of neonatal respiratory distress syndrome. Arch Dis Child 1992;67:1221–1227.
16 Dempsey EM, Barrington KJ. Treating hypotension in the preterm infant: when and with what: a critical and systematic review. J Perinatol 2007;27:469–478.
17 Evans N. Assessment and support of the preterm circulation. Early Human Develop 2006;82:803–810.
18 Kluckow M, Evans N, Osborn DA. Low systemic blood flow and brain injury in the preterm infant. NeoReviews 2004;5:E98–E108.
19 Hawkins J, Van Hare GF, Schmidt KG, Rudolph AM. Effects of increasing afterload on left ventricular output in fetal lambs. Circ Res 1989;65:127–134.
20 Takahashi Y, Harada K, Kishkurno S, Arai, Ishida A, Takada G. Postnatal left ventricular contractility in very low birth weight infants. Pediatr Cardiol 1997;18:112–117.
21 Clyman RI, Mauray F, Heymann MA, Roman C. Cardiovascular effects of patent ductus arteriosus in preterm lambs with respiratory distress. J Pediatr 1987;111:579–587.
22 Paradisis M, Evans N, Kluckow M, Osborn D, McLachlan AJ. Pilot study of milrinone for low systemic blood flow in very preterm infants. J Pediatr 2006;148:306–313.

CHAPTER 3

Oxygen uptake and delivery

Oxygen in blood

Disturbances in oxygen uptake in the lungs, or in supply of adequate amounts of oxygen to the tissues, are common features of many congenital heart lesions. In this chapter, I review some of the factors influencing the amount of oxygen in the blood and the oxygen content in different locations in the circulation. The uptake of oxygen and its distribution to the tissues both prenatally and postnatally is described, and the effects of oxygen deprivation are considered. Also the potential advantages and disadvantages of oxygen administration are considered.

Oxygen capacity

Oxygen capacity refers to the maximal amount of oxygen that can be taken up by hemoglobin in blood. Traditionally, it has been measured by the manometric method of Van Slyke and Neill. A volume of blood is exposed to air and rotated gently for several minutes to allow the hemoglobin to combine with the maximal amount of oxygen. The amount of oxygen in the blood is then measured by the manometric method. The volume of oxygen dissolved in solution in blood is subtracted, thus providing a measure of the amount of oxygen combined with hemoglobin. Oxygen capacity is expressed as mL/100 mL (vol% or mL/dL) or sometimes as mL/L of blood. It should be appreciated that if any abnormal hemoglobins, such as sulfhemoglobin or methemoglobin, which do not have the same affinity for oxygen, are present, the oxygen capacity will not be representative of total hemoglobin content when measured by the manometric method [1]. Spectrophotometric methods for measuring oxygen capacity are reliable and simpler than the manometric method. They are based on the measurement of hemoglobin level. One method consists of diluting a small, accurately measured volume of blood with a solution of potassium cyanide, potassium ferrocyanide, and sodium bicarbonate (Drabkin solution), which converts all hemoglobin to cyanmethemoglobin. The concentration of hemoglobin is determined by spectrophotometry from standard curves at a wavelength of 540 nm. Estimates of the maximal amount of oxygen that can be attached to hemoglobin vary from about 1.34 to 1.39 mL/g hemoglobin [2].

It is now customary to multiply hemoglobin concentration in g/dL by 1.36 to determine oxygen capacity. Since all hemoglobin, including methemoglobin, is converted to cyanmethemoglobin, the oxygen capacity measured by this method may provide a falsely high reading if significant quantities of abnormal hemoglobins which do not have the usual high affinity for oxygen are present.

Oxygen content

Oxygen content is a term that indicates the amount of oxygen present in a blood sample. It is expressed as mL/dL (vol%) or as mL/L of blood, and refers to the total quantity, both combined with hemoglobin and dissolved in plasma. When oxygen is extracted from a blood sample and its quantity measured by the manometric method of Van Slyke and Neill, by the volumetric method of Roughton and Scholander or by gas chromatography, the volume of oxygen per unit volume of blood is obtained; this provides a true measure of oxygen content. Because these techniques are cumbersome and time-consuming, oxygen content is usually determined from the measurement of hemoglobin concentration and oxygen saturation

Congenital Diseases of the Heart, 3rd edition. By A. Rudolph

and addition of the amount of dissolved oxygen (see below).

Oxygen saturation

Oxygen saturation is a measure of the ratio of oxygen actually combined with hemoglobin to the total amount of oxygen that can be taken up by hemoglobin in a blood sample. It usually is expressed as a percentage. It is important to appreciate that the terms "oxygen saturation" and "oxygen capacity" concern only oxygen attached to hemoglobin and do not consider dissolved oxygen. The relationship between oxygen saturation, oxygen content and oxygen capacity is as follows:

$$O_2 \text{ saturation } (\%) = \frac{O_2 \text{ content} - \text{dissolved } O_2}{O_2 \text{ capacity}} \times 100$$

The importance of the quantity of dissolved oxygen in this equation will be discussed further in relation to hemoglobin levels and oxygen tension.

Oxygen saturation can be calculated by measuring oxygen content and capacity manometrically and using the above equation. This is very time-consuming and it has become customary to use a spectrophotometric method. This is based on the different spectral curves for oxyhemoglobin and reduced hemoglobin. At a wavelength in the red range of about 630–660 nm, the transmission of light by similar concentrations of oxyhemoglobin and reduced hemoglobin is quite different. However, at wavelengths in the green range (~510 nm) and in the infrared range (805 nm), transmission is similar for the two hemoglobins. Most methods currently used measure optical density of blood at about 650–660 nm to indicate the ratio of oxyhemoglobin to reduced hemoglobin, and optical density at 805 nm for total hemoglobin. From these readings, the amount of oxyhemoglobin as a percentage of total hemoglobin can be calculated, and this represents oxygen saturation.

There are several different methods by which this basic principle may be applied. When optical density is measured in a spectrophotometer by transmission of light of a specific wavelength through a cuvette containing the solution (absorbance spectroscopy), it is necessary to hemolyze blood so that red cells do not interfere with light transmission. This may be accomplished by rapid freezing and rethawing, but is accomplished more effectively with a saponin–NaOH solution or by a detergent solution. Triton X100 solution has been used quite extensively. If reflected light is used, however, the presence of intact red cells does not interfere with the measurements and thus whole blood can be used. The reflectance oximeter is simple to operate, and oxygen saturation can be measured on small blood samples (0.2 mL).

Oxygen saturation can also be derived quite accurately from measurement of oxygen tension (Po_2), pH and Pco_2 and hemoglobin or hematocrit levels; these measurements can all be made on less than 0.5 mL of blood. This method is based on the relationship between oxygen partial pressure and oxygen saturation of hemoglobin, designated the oxygen dissociation curve.

Oximetry

Oxygen saturation can be measured noninvasively by the use of oximeters. The same principles are used as for measuring saturation in blood samples. An oximeter probe consists of two diodes emitting light at wavelengths of 660 and 805 nm, with the amount of light transmitted or reflected being measured by photoelectric detectors on the opposite side of the probe. Most oximeters currently used measure transmittance and the probe is applied to a finger, toe, earlobe, or in small infants the palm of the hand. Reflectance oximeters have the emitting diodes and the photosensors next to one another and can therefore be applied to a flat surface, such as the scalp. To try to avoid the effects of absorbance by tissues other than blood, only the variation of absorption with the surge of arterial blood during each heart beat is measured, hence the description "pulse oximeter" is applied to this instrument. If an adequate pulse is not present, as in patients with poor perfusion due to shock, or obstruction to flow as in infants with aortic coarctation, the measurements may not be possible or may be unreliable.

Measurement of arterial oxygen saturation by oximetry is most reliable at higher levels of saturation; with decreasing oxygen saturation levels, the measurement is less reliable. Thus at oxygen saturation levels above about 90%, the saturation varies by about 2%. At levels of 70–90%, variation is

3–4%, whereas below 70%, variability may be 5% or even higher.

Arterial oxygen saturation in infants

Prior to the introduction of noninvasive oximetry, little information was available regarding arterial oxygen saturation in normal infants. It was generally accepted that beyond 2 days after birth, arterial oxygen saturation was above 95%, but that within the first 2 days saturations of 92–93% were acceptable. This was believed to be the result of inadequate expansion of the lungs, or small right-to-left shunts through the foramen ovale or ductus arteriosus. In a study of 50 normal newborn infants in whom right upper and lower extremity oxygen saturations were measured using pulse oximetry, Toth *et al.* [3] found that, at 2 min after birth, mean oxygen saturations in the right arm were 73% (range 44–95%) and in the right leg 67% (range 34–93%). Oxygen saturations were greater than 95% in the right arm within 12 min (range 2–55 min) and in the right leg within 14 min (range 3–55 min). Rabi *et al.* [4] found that oxygen saturations in the right arm were 87% (range 80–95%) at 5 min after vaginal delivery and 81% (range 75–83%) in infants delivered by cesarean section. A median oxygen saturation above 90% was reached in both groups by 8 min after birth.

Based on these and other observations, oxygen saturations in quietly resting infants breathing room air are above 92% within 10 min and above 97% by 24 hours after birth in both right arm and lower extremities.

Oxygen saturation differences between right arm and legs

It has long been recognized that oxygen saturation may be lower in the legs than in the arms in newborn infants as a result of shunting of poorly saturated pulmonary arterial blood through the ductus arteriosus into the descending aorta. This right-to-left shunt through the ductus occurs because pulmonary vascular resistance has not yet achieved postnatal levels, so the pulmonary arterial pressure is still somewhat elevated and the ductus arteriosus has not closed. Although the ductus right-to-left shunt results in lower saturation in the lower extremities compared with right and left arms, not infrequently the left arm oxygen saturation level is between that in the right arm and the leg. This is explained by the fact that the left subclavian artery arises from the descending aorta just above the junction of the ductus arteriosus. A small amount of the shunted blood may enter the subclavian artery, thus reducing left arm oxygen saturation somewhat compared with that in the right arm. Because the right subclavian artery arises from the brachiocephalic trunk (innominate artery), it receives blood only from the ascending aorta. In detecting differences it is therefore preferable to measure right arm and leg oxygen saturations. Noninvasive oximetry in the newborn infant has become standard procedure in many medical centers in the USA, but it is not standard practice to measure oxygen saturation in both the right arm and the legs. Routine measurement of oxygen saturation in both right arm and a leg should be encouraged because detection of a difference may be very helpful in assessment. Technically, it is preferred that both right arm and leg saturations be measured simultaneously. If a difference is detected, the oximeters and probes should be interchanged to confirm that the difference is real and not due to technical error. As mentioned above, oximetry is more reliable at higher oxygen saturations; at saturations above 80–85% a 2–3% difference is suspicious and a 5% difference is significant. At saturations below 80%, a 5% difference is suspicious and a 10% difference is significant.

Only recently has it been appreciated that, in normal babies, this difference is not apparent beyond about 10 min after birth. A difference detected beyond this time usually denotes the presence of pulmonary or cardiovascular abnormality. When a difference is detected, most commonly the right arm saturation is higher, but occasionally the lower limb saturation is higher than that in the right arm. A lower saturation in the leg results from shunting of less well oxygenated pulmonary arterial blood across the ductus arteriosus to the descending aorta. This may result from maintenance of a high pulmonary vascular resistance and pulmonary arterial pressure after birth with persistent patency of the ductus arteriosus. A higher oxygen saturation in the legs can only occur if oxygen saturation in the pulmonary artery is higher than that in the

Table 3.1 Oxygen saturation differences between the right arm and the lower extremities.

Oxygen saturation higher in right arm than in legs (result of shunting of poorly oxygenated pulmonary arterial blood through the ductus arteriosus to the descending aorta)
Elevated pulmonary vascular resistance
Lung disease with hypoxic pulmonary vasoconstriction
Persistent pulmonary hypertension of the newborn
Aortic arch obstruction
Aortic arch interruption
Coarctation of the aorta
Decreased left ventricular output
Aortic stenosis
Left ventricular dysfunction
Oxygen saturation higher in legs than in right arm (result of shunting of highly oxygenated pulmonary arterial blood through the ductus arteriosus to the descending aorta)
Aortopulmonary transposition
Taussig–Bing anomaly
Total anomalous pulmonary venous connection to superior vena cava
Truncus arteriosus with interrupted aortic arch

ascending aorta and is diagnostic of congenital cardiovascular malformation. The causes of arterial saturation differences between the right arm and lower extremity are shown in Table 3.1.

Alveolar hypoxia resulting from poor expansion, atelectasis, consolidation or airway obstruction may induce pulmonary vasoconstriction and pulmonary arterial hypertension with shunting of pulmonary arterial blood through the ductus arteriosus and thus reduce oxygen saturation in the descending aorta. Persistent pulmonary hypertension of the newborn is also associated with elevated pulmonary vascular resistance as a result of prenatal influences (see Chapter 5). The magnitude of the difference in oxygen saturation depends on several factors, including the degree of elevation of pulmonary vascular resistance, the size of the ductus arteriosus, and the oxygen saturation of blood in the ascending aorta and pulmonary artery. Thus, even if there is a large shunt of pulmonary arterial blood into the descending aorta, there may be a relatively small difference in saturation if ascending aortic blood saturation is reduced. This may occur with lung disease because pulmonary venous oxygen saturation is low, or with both lung disease and persistent pulmonary hypertension of the newborn as a result of right-to-left shunting through the foramen ovale. The saturation difference may be exaggerated in infants with lung disease by administering oxygen, because pulmonary venous and thus ascending aortic oxygen saturation may be increased.

Blood flow to the ascending aorta in infants with interruption of the aortic arch is provided by ejection from the left ventricle, but descending aortic flow is provided exclusively from the pulmonary artery through the ductus arteriosus. In infants with coarctation of the aorta, although saturation differences between the right arm and the legs may occur, they are usually small, because the postnatal development of aortic obstruction is associated with constriction of the ductus arteriosus and thus the ductus diameter is relatively small when the clinical features become manifest (see Chapter 12). Infants with severe aortic stenosis, as well as some with poor left ventricular function, have a reduction of flow into the ascending aorta, with adequate flow into the ascending aortic branches, but reduced flow across the aortic isthmus. Blood to the lower body is provided through the ductus arteriosus into the descending aorta and thus a saturation difference often occurs. Because the oxygen saturation difference depends on the saturation of pulmonary arterial and ascending aortic blood, under some circumstances, even though the shunt across the ductus is quite large, only a small difference may be detected because pulmonary arterial oxygen saturation is increased. This frequently occurs in infants with aortic arch interruption because an associated ventricular septal defect allows a large left-to-right shunt, increasing pulmonary arterial saturation. It may also occur in infants with aortic stenosis or aortic coarctation as a result of elevation of left atrial pressure, stretching of the foramen ovale, and left-to-right shunt at the atrial level (see Chapter 12). An unusual circumstance in which there may be a large difference between oxygen saturations in the ascending and descending aorta, but with no detectable difference between right arm and leg, is when the right subclavian artery originates from the descending aorta, so that it does not reflect ascending aortic saturation.

A higher oxygen saturation in the legs than in the right arm indicates that pulmonary arterial saturation is higher than that in the ascending aorta. This is most commonly encountered with aortopulmonary transposition (see Chapter 18). Shunting from the pulmonary artery to the descending aorta through the ductus arteriosus is most prominent in the early postnatal hours and is unlikely to be detected after a few days. After birth, while pulmonary vascular resistance is still somewhat elevated, pulmonary arterial pressure is also maintained. If the ductus is still patent, bidirectional shunting can be observed. During systole, the kinetic force associated with systole directs blood through the ductus to the descending aorta, but during diastole, because pulmonary vascular resistance has fallen to levels below systemic vascular resistance, blood shunts from the descending aorta into the pulmonary circulation. Continuing decrease in pulmonary vascular resistance results in a further fall in pulmonary arterial pressure; if the ductus remains open, blood is shunted only from the aorta into the pulmonary artery.

Pulmonary arterial may be higher than ascending aortic oxygen saturation in Taussig–Bing anomaly (double outlet right ventricle with the pulmonary artery related to the ventricular septal defect, so that blood ejected by the left ventricle passes through the ventricular septal defect preferentially into the pulmonary artery). If saturation in the leg is higher than that in the right arm, the presence of a lower blood pressure in the leg than the right arm is helpful in distinguishing Taussig–Bing anomaly from aortopulmonary transposition, because aortic coarctation is often associated with Taussig–Bing anomaly but not with transposition. A higher oxygen saturation in the legs than in the right arm has been observed rarely in two other congenital cardiovascular malformations. In the infant with total anomalous drainage of all the pulmonary veins via the superior vena cava (SVC), the well-oxygenated blood will pass into the right ventricle and pulmonary artery. Poorly oxygenated inferior vena cava (IVC) blood may shunt through the foramen ovale into the left atrium and ventricle, leading to a lower saturation in the ascending aorta and thus the right arm. In the infant with truncus arteriosus and interrupted aortic arch, well-oxygenated blood from the left ventricle may be directed preferentially to the pulmonary arteries and through the ductus arteriosus, resulting in a higher saturation in the leg than the right arm.

If there is a small difference in oxygen saturation between the right arm and leg, the difference may be exaggerated by administration of oxygen. Also, if oxygen saturation differences are small, measurement of oxygen tensions during oxygen administration may show large differences (see Chapter 3).

Relationship between oxygen partial pressure (tension) and oxygen saturation of hemoglobin: the oxygen dissociation curve

Figure 3.1 shows the relationship between the Po_2 to which a hemoglobin solution or blood is exposed, and the degree of saturation of hemoglobin. They are related in the form of an S-shaped curve, which has a fairly flat portion in the upper ranges of oxygen saturation, above about 85%. This permits hemoglobin to be almost fully saturated in the lungs even when there is a somewhat reduced Po_2 due to inadequate ventilation. The curve is quite steep in the mid-portion; this is advantageous for release of oxygen at the tissue site, as small reductions in Po_2 result in considerable release of oxygen from hemoglobin.

It was believed for some time that there was a marked difference in the curves for adult and fetal

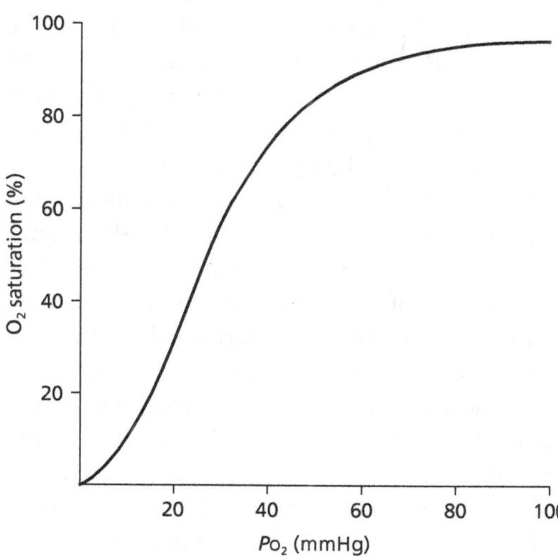

Figure 3.1 Oxygen dissociation curve for normal adult human blood.

hemoglobin, with the fetal hemoglobin curve being steeper and to the left. This would result in a much greater oxygen saturation at the same Po_2, and thus aid in uptake of oxygen by fetal blood from maternal blood at the placental site. However, it has been shown in recent years that the oxygen dissociation curves for human fetal and adult hemoglobin are almost identical when the hemoglobin is in solution. However, in other species, such as the sheep and goat, there is a marked difference between the dissociation curves of adult and fetal hemoglobin.

Recently, it has also been shown that the amount of organic phosphate in the red cells has a profound effect on the oxygen dissociation curve of hemoglobin. These organic phosphates decrease the affinity of hemoglobin for oxygen by competing with oxygen for binding to hemoglobin. 2,3-Diphosphoglycerate (2,3-DPG) is the more important phosphate, being present in adult erythrocytes in a concentration of about 5 μmol/mL, whereas adenosine triphosphate (ATP), which exerts a similar effect, is found in a concentration of 1 μmol/mL. An increase in 2,3-DPG in blood shifts the oxygen dissociation curve to the right, thus facilitating delivery of oxygen at the tissue site (see Figure 3.2). The binding of 2,3-DPG is increased when hemoglobin is in a reduced state. In the tissues, hemoglobin becomes reduced by removal of oxygen; this results in increased binding of 2,3-DPG and thus facilitates release of oxygen.

Fetal hemoglobin has considerably less affinity for 2,3-DPG than does adult hemoglobin. In human blood, the affinity of fetal hemoglobin for 2,3-DPG is only about 40% that of adult hemoglobin. This makes fetal hemoglobin behave as if 2,3-DPG levels are low; therefore, the oxygen dissociation curve is shifted to the left. Although fetal red cells do contain 2,3-DPG, the poor binding of 2,3-DPG by fetal hemoglobin is an important factor in facilitating transport of oxygen across the placenta from mother to fetus. On the maternal side of the placenta, the reduction of hemoglobin effectively shifts the curve to the right, increasing oxygen release. On the fetal side, 2,3-DPG does not interfere with the affinity of fetal hemoglobin for oxygen and thus the uptake of oxygen by fetal erythrocytes.

The oxygen dissociation curve is shifted to the left when H^+ ion concentration is decreased (or if pH is increased, i.e., alkalemia) and to the right

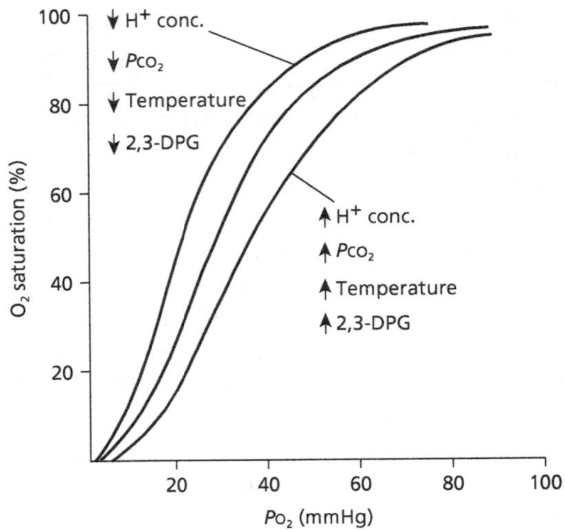

Figure 3.2 Effects of changes in H^+ ion concentration, Pco_2, temperature, and 2,3-diphosphoglycerate (2,3-DPG) concentration on oxygen dissociation curve of blood.

with increased H^+ ion concentration (or decreased pH, i.e., acidemia). It is also shifted to the left when temperature is decreased and when Pco_2 is reduced and vice versa (Figure 3.2). Whether the effect of the change in Pco_2 is independent of the change in pH which results from the increase or decrease in Pco_2 has not been resolved. Changes in Pco_2 do facilitate uptake or release of oxygen; this is known as the Bohr effect. Thus, in the lungs, CO_2 diffuses from blood into the alveoli resulting in a fall in Pco_2 and an increase in pH; this shifts the dissociation curve to the left and tends to facilitate oxygen uptake. In the tissues, CO_2 enters the blood in the capillaries and increases Pco_2 and decreases pH, thus moving the curve to the right and facilitating oxygen release.

To express the position of the oxygen dissociation curve, the parameter "P_{50}" has been used. This indicates the Po_2 at which hemoglobin is 50% saturated with oxygen. The higher the P_{50} value, the greater the shift to the right and the less the affinity of hemoglobin for oxygen.

Although it has long been known that the oxygen dissociation curve is shifted by changes in pH and Pco_2, the magnitude of the change with specific alterations has not been appreciated. In 2004, in studies of adult blood, Hamilton *et al.* [5] found that there was a linear relationship between changes in pH and the shift of the curve. When pH increased from 7.40 to 7.47, the maximum decrease of P_{50} (leftward shift) was 6.4 mmHg (range 0.6–6.4), whereas a decrease in pH from 7.40 to 7.24 was associated with a maximum increase of P_{50} (rightward shift) of 7.5 mmHg (range 2.9–7.5).

Although these changes in P_{50} were substantial, the effect on oxygen saturation varied greatly, depending on the level of saturation. Thus in arterial blood with high oxygen saturation levels, a shift of P_{50} had only minor effects on oxygen saturation, because the dissociation curves are fairly flat in this range. However, at venous oxygen saturation levels, shifts of P_{50} had dramatic effects on saturations. Thus with a right shift of 7.5 mmHg at a pH of 7.24, oxygen saturation was 13% lower at the same Po_2. In this report, the relationship between pH and change in P_{50} was observed to be linear in the pH range 7.2–7.5. If linearity extends below this pH range, I have estimated that at pH 7.0 there would be a shift of P_{50} of about 20 mmHg to the right (Figure 3.3). These relationships between the actual level of oxygen saturation and the effects of changes in P_{50} are potentially of great importance in patients with cyanotic congenital cardiovascular malformations, because frequently arterial oxygen saturations are similar to or lower than venous levels encountered in adults; in this range of oxygen saturation an increase in P_{50} of 20 mmHg could potentially reduce oxygen saturation at a blood Po_2 of 25 mmHg from about 50% to about 25%. If arterial oxygen saturation is considerably reduced, an

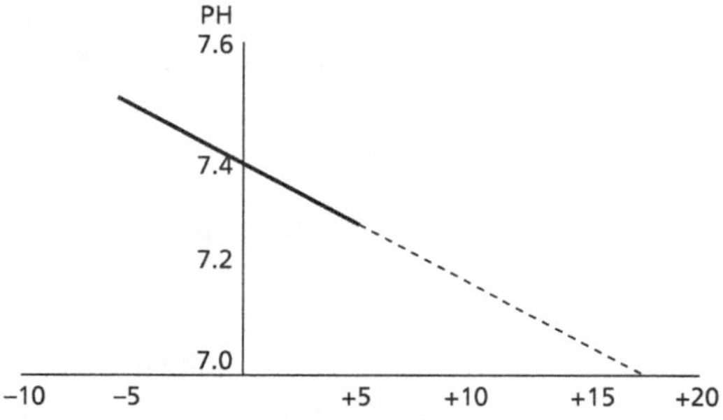

Figure 3.3 Relationship between change in P_{50} with change in pH. The bold line shows the relationship described in Ref. 5. The broken line extension shows the change with further reduction in pH, assuming the relationship is linear in this pH range.

increase in P_{50} associated with acidemia could dramatically reduce oxygen saturation at any given Po_2 and thus markedly reduce oxygen content of blood delivered to the tissues.

It has also frequently been stated that an increase in P_{50} associated with acidemia in an infant may be beneficial, because it would facilitate release of oxygen at the tissue site and provide higher oxygen delivery. This would be correct if arterial blood is at higher levels of oxygen saturation, because a high P_{50} would not affect oxygen saturation significantly. At the venous level, acidemia would significantly reduce the oxygen saturation if pH is reduced and thus oxygen extraction by tissues would be higher. If, however, arterial blood has an oxygen saturation that is greatly reduced, and the dissociation curve is shifted to the right, there would be no advantage in oxygen extraction and in fact extraction could be reduced because the curve would tend to be flatter. The potential impact of the development of acidemia on oxygen delivery in infants with cyanosis has not been fully appreciated. Whether the effect of acidemia on P_{50} is the same for fetal as for adult hemoglobin has not been determined. This knowledge would be important because if the behavior is similar, perhaps acidemia should be treated aggressively in severely hypoxemic infants.

Relation between oxygen attached to hemoglobin and dissolved oxygen

The amount of oxygen dissolved in blood is related to the partition coefficient, the partial pressure of oxygen, and temperature. The solubility of oxygen is 0.00003 mL/mL blood per mmHg at 37°C. A convenient way to remember the amount of dissolved oxygen is that at a Po_2 of 100 mmHg at 37°C, there is 0.3 mL/dL. The amount dissolved is linearly related to Po_2 (Figure 3.4). At the usual systemic arterial Po_2 of about 100 mmHg, most of the oxygen in blood is attached to hemoglobin, which is almost 100% saturated, and only 0.3 mL/dL is present in dissolved form. The amount dissolved is related to Po_2 in a linear manner, so that at lower Po_2 levels, a quite insignificant amount of oxygen is dissolved in plasma; in fetal arterial blood, where Po_2 is only 20–25 mmHg, there is a negligible amount of dissolved oxygen. In terms of oxygen

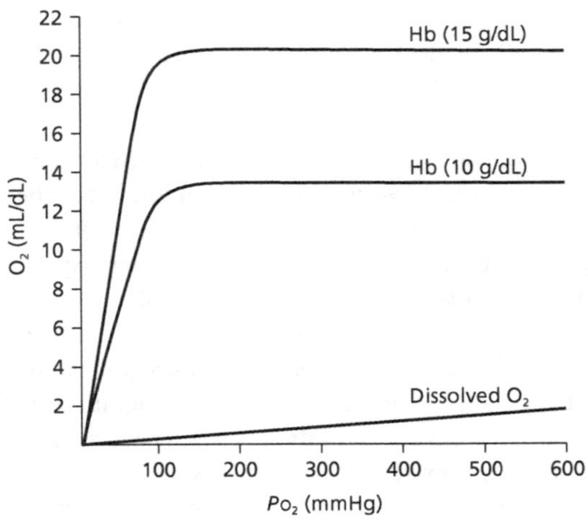

Figure 3.4 Oxygen dissociation curves are expressed as oxygen content rather than oxygen saturation in relation to Po_2, thus demonstrating the important influence of the level of hemoglobin in determining the amount of oxygen that can be taken up at any Po_2. Also, the small amount of oxygen physically dissolved is noted.

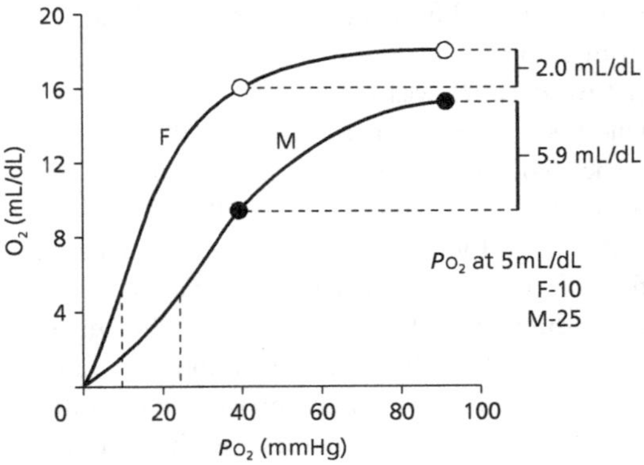

Figure 3.5 Effect of shifting the oxygen dissociation curve to the left or right on the amount of oxygen delivered at the tissue site. Although at high Po_2 the amount of oxygen attached to hemoglobin is similar for both curves, at a venous Po_2 of about 40 mmHg, the amount of oxygen that would be extracted in the case of curve F (fetal; shift to the left) is considerably less than for curve M (maternal).

transport and supply, the quantity of hemoglobin is thus the most important factor. At low hemoglobin concentrations, a greater proportion of the total oxygen in blood is present in dissolved form, and at higher levels a much smaller proportion is dissolved.

When Po_2 is increased by raising the oxygen fraction of inspired air (FIO_2), the amount of dissolved oxygen is increased. Because hemoglobin is almost fully saturated at a Po_2 of 100 mmHg, insignificant quantities of additional oxygen are taken up by hemoglobin at levels above this. Thus, the proportion of dissolved oxygen is much greater. At a Po_2 of 600 mmHg, dissolved oxygen in the blood comprises 1.8 mL/dL.

In considering the availability of oxygen to the tissues, it is important to take into account not only oxygen saturation of blood but also the hemoglobin concentration (oxygen capacity), because this is crucial in determining the total amount of oxygen that can be carried by each volume of blood. The oxygen dissociation curve then may be drawn as shown in Figure 3.4, using oxygen content rather than oxygen saturation on the ordinate.

These important facts concerning oxygen supply and delivery are depicted in Figures 3.4 and 3.5. Figure 3.4 shows the effects of oxygen capacity (hemoglobin level) on oxygen content and the importance of dissolved oxygen as a proportion of total oxygen at different levels of Po_2. When hemoglobin is 15 g/dL at a Po_2 of 100 mmHg and full oxygen saturation, oxygen bound to hemoglobin comprises 20.4 mL/dL and dissolved oxygen about 0.3 mL/dL of plasma or about 1.5% of total oxygen. If, however, hemoglobin is reduced to 10 g/dL at a Po_2 of 100 mmHg, oxygen bound to hemoglobin comprises 13.6 mL/dL and dissolved oxygen 0.3 mL/dL or about 2.5%.

If the oxygen concentration of inspired air is increased so that Po_2 is 600 mmHg, the amount of oxygen combined with hemoglobin does not change significantly. However, dissolved oxygen increases to 1.8 mL/dL, representing about 9% of total oxygen when hemoglobin is 15 g/dL, but as much as about 14% of total oxygen content when hemoglobin is 10 g/dL.

In Figure 3.5 the effects of the shape of the oxygen dissociation curve on oxygen delivery at the tissues are shown. In the case of curve M, which approximates a normal curve for adult (maternal) blood, decreasing the Po_2 from 100 mmHg (the level usually present in arterial blood) to 40 mmHg (the level in venous blood) results in a release of oxygen amounting to about 5 mL/dL. If, however, the curve is shifted to the left, depicted by curve F (fetal blood), a decrease in Po_2 from 100 to

40 mmHg results in a release of oxygen amounting to only about 2 mL/dL.

This relationship may have very important implications in the newborn period. If an infant at birth has a large percentage of fetal hemoglobin, the oxygen dissociation curve is shifted to the left, so that oxygen delivery to the tissues is decreased. In newborn infants with severe hypoxemia associated with cyanotic congenital heart disease, if hypothermia develops, shifting the curve to the left may result in a reduction in oxygen release at the tissue site. Metabolic acidemia, which often develops in these infants, would have the opposite effect of shifting the curve to the right and would tend to facilitate oxygen release at the tissue level.

Contrast medium used for angiography (organic iodide solutions) has been shown to produce a shift in the oxygen dissociation curve to the left. *In vivo*, the effect is maximal within about 1 min after injection into the vascular system, but may last up to about 15 min. This is not due to a direct effect of the contrast medium on hemoglobin, because contrast agents shift the curve to the right when added to a hemoglobin solution. The shift to the left *in vivo* could possibly interfere with oxygen delivery to the tissues in cyanotic patients or in patients with markedly reduced cardiac output after angiography.

Levels of oxygen in cardiac chambers and great vessels

Changes in oxygen levels in cardiac chambers were used early in the experience with cardiac catheterization to detect the level of shunts in patients with congenital heart disease. Differences in oxygen content were used in the evaluation but now it is customary to compare oxygen saturations. It is more reliable to compare oxygen saturation rather than oxygen content in assessing shunts, because it is not influenced by differences in oxygen capacity.

With a shunt of the same magnitude there is a smaller increase or decrease in oxygen content, the lower the oxygen capacity. Thus, at low oxygen capacities, a small change in oxygen content may not be considered a significant shunt, whereas at high oxygen capacity, a fairly large change in oxygen content may be considered indicative of a shunt, but it may in fact not be significant. However, the change in oxygen saturation due to a shunt is not dependent on the level of oxygen capacity. This is easily demonstrated in the following examples.

- If a volume of arterial blood with oxygen saturation 100% is shunted so as to be added to an equal volume of venous blood with an oxygen saturation of 60%, it would raise the saturation to 80%. This rise of 20% in oxygen saturation would not be influenced by the oxygen capacity.
- However, when oxygen content differences are measured, if oxygen capacity were 15 mL/dL, the oxygen content of arterial blood would be 15 mL/dL and of venous blood $(60 \times 15)/100$ or 9 mL/dL. The oxygen content of mixed blood would be $(80 \times 15)/100$ or 12 mL/dL; thus, an increase in oxygen content of 3 mL/dL would occur.
- If oxygen capacity were 25 mL/dL, the oxygen content of arterial blood would be 25 mL/dL, of venous blood $(60 \times 25)/100$ or 15 mL/dL, and of the final mixture $(80 \times 25)/100$ or 20 mL/dL, and the difference in oxygen content would be 5 mL/dL.

In considering oxygen saturation differences between chambers, it is important to appreciate that the amount of change that occurs is not only related to the volumes of blood mixing but also to the initial oxygen saturation levels of the blood. Consider, for example, the case of a quantity of pulmonary venous blood with an oxygen saturation of 100% being shunted so as to mix with an equal quantity of venous blood. If the oxygen saturation of venous blood is 40%, the oxygen saturation of the mixture would be 70%, whereas if the oxygen saturation of venous blood is 80%, the final saturation would be 90%. For the same magnitude of shunt there is a 30% increase in oxygen saturation in the first instance and only a 10% increase in the second. This principle is very important for detecting left-to-right shunts from oxygen saturation differences in those patients who possibly have two or more sites of shunting. If there is an increase in oxygen saturation at one level and a small increase at a second level, it may be difficult to determine the presence or absence of a second shunt. Again, an example demonstrates the problem.

> If three volumes of pulmonary venous blood of 100% oxygen saturation are shunted to the right atrium and mix with one volume of venous blood of 72% saturation, the final oxygen saturation will be $(3 \times 100) + (1 \times 72)/4 = 93\%$. If, now, a ventricular left-to-right shunt also occurs with one volume of left ventricular blood of 100% oxygen saturation mixing with one volume of right atrial blood of 93% oxygen saturation, the final saturation would be 96.5%. This further increase of 3.5% oxygen saturation is in the questionable range for indicating a shunt.

The above-mentioned considerations must therefore be taken into account in evaluating differences in oxygen saturation between chambers or in detecting shunts.

In evaluating oxygen saturation differences between chambers, it is important to compare samples obtained as close in time as possible. Therefore, it is rather pointless to compare samples taken an hour or two apart, especially if medications have been given between samplings or if the patient's status has changed. Similarly, comparing oxygen saturations of samples obtained while an infant is crying may be quite unreliable. Variability in oxygen saturation may be due to changes in blood flow, oxygen consumption, ventilation and other factors in the patient; it may also be related to inaccuracy of the method of measurement.

In comparing oxygen saturations between chambers, it is usual to take all factors into account in developing guidelines for what constitutes significant differences. In view of the many factors that may influence this, it is desirable to obtain more than one sample from each site. Clearly, a difference in oxygen saturation would be more significant if it were found in two or more sets of comparisons rather than only in one. In general, in considering left-to-right shunts, a similar small difference in oxygen saturation is more significant in the higher ranges of saturation, in view of the greater accuracy of the oximeter in this range and since oxygen saturation is usually less variable in the higher range.

Vena cava oxygen saturation

The oxygen saturation in the IVC is variable, largely due to the difficulty in obtaining a good mixed venous sample. The oxygen saturation of renal veins is relatively high whereas that of hepatic veins is quite low. There is a short segment of IVC between the right atrium and the hepatic veins, so that there is not adequate distance for mixing to occur. Even if repeated samples are withdrawn in the IVC below the hepatic veins, variable oxygen saturations may be obtained at the same level if the catheter is rotated, because selective sampling from different streams may occur. It has also been noted that the oxygen saturations may be different in inspiration and expiration.

SVC oxygen saturation is also variable, but usually is not subject to the wide variations noted in the IVC. Right atrial blood refluxes a short distance into the superior and inferior vena cava during atrial systole. For this reason, it is useful to obtain a sample in the high SVC just below the junction of the left innominate vein and a low SVC sample just above the right atrial–SVC junction.

SVC or IVC oxygen saturations are usually in the range 65–75%, but saturations in the 75–80% range are common in infants and in anxious older children. In children, oxygen saturations below 65% are usually related to a low cardiac output, severe anemia, or systemic arterial hypoxemia. If the SVC oxygen saturation is greater than 80%, it is advisable to explore further to obtain measurements in the jugular vein and left innominate vein in order to exclude the possibility of a shunt from anomalous pulmonary venous drainage or arteriovenous fistulae.

IVC samples are not particularly useful. However, if right atrial oxygen saturation is higher than in the SVC, a high IVC oxygen saturation could explain the rise in oxygen saturation at the atrial level. In this circumstance, it may be necessary to use other techniques to determine whether there is a left-to-right shunt at the atrial level.

Hepatic venous oxygen saturation may be helpful in diagnosing total pulmonary venous return to the portal veins. If there is no ductus venosus flow, all the portal venous blood, including pulmonary venous return, must pass through the liver and return via hepatic veins. In infants with this anomaly, hepatic venous oxygen saturation is the highest that can be obtained. In infants in whom the diagnosis is entertained, the catheter should be manipulated into a hepatic vein early in the procedure, as it is most valuable in excluding or confirming the diagnosis immediately.

Right atrial oxygen saturation

Oxygen saturation is often variable in different parts of the chamber due to inadequate mixing of IVC, SVC, and coronary sinus streams. The most consistent values are obtained by sampling in the midlateral position, which is the midportion of the atrium along the right cardiac border. A significant increase in oxygen saturation in the right atrium, as compared with the SVC, indicates a left-to-right shunt. An increase of at least 8–10% can be considered to be significant in one set of samples. If two sets are compared, an increase of 6–7% is significant. However, increases of as much as 10% have been encountered at the right atrial level in the absence of a left-to-right shunt detectable by other means. This is particularly likely to be noted in patients in whom SVC saturation is low.

An increase in right atrial oxygen saturation is most often due to a shunt across an atrial septal defect, but it may be associated with other lesions. These include anomalous pulmonary venous drainage to the right atrium or coronary sinus, left ventricular to right atrial communication, sinus of Valsalva fistula to the right atrium, and coronary arteriovenous fistula draining to the right atrium. An increase in right atrial oxygen saturation is commonly found in patients with left-to-right shunts at the ventricular level, with no cause for atrial shunting, due to regurgitation of blood across the tricuspid valve. This is particularly likely to be noted in infants with large ventricular septal defects with cardiomegaly and cardiac failure.

Complete admixture of pulmonary and systemic venous returns may occur in the right atrium, in which case oxygen saturations in the right atrium and in both ventricles and the aorta and pulmonary artery are all almost identical. This occurs when there is total anomalous pulmonary venous connection to the systemic venous system, although differences in pulmonary and systemic arterial oxygen saturations may occur due to selective SVC and IVC streaming (see Chapter 13). It is also noted in mitral atresia with or without a hypoplastic left ventricle. If right atrial oxygen saturation is at systemic levels, it is important to enter the left atrium. In mitral atresia, left atrial oxygen saturation is higher; also, left atrial pressure is higher than right atrial pressure. In total anomalous pulmonary venous drainage, left and right atrial saturations are similar, and right atrial pressure is higher than left atrial pressure. In cases of common atria, there may be almost equal oxygen saturations in the right and left atria, but usually left atrial saturation is slightly higher, and also systemic arterial saturation is slightly higher than pulmonary arterial oxygen saturation.

Right ventricular oxygen saturation

Oxygen saturation in the right ventricle often is slightly lower (3–4%) than that in the midlateral right atrium in normal individuals. This is probably due to addition of coronary sinus blood, which has a low oxygen saturation (30–40%) and tends to stream directly across the tricuspid valve. An increase in oxygen saturation of about 6–8% on a single set of samples and of 4–5% on two or more sets of samples is considered significant. Right ventricular samples should be collected from the body of the right ventricle and from the outflow region (infundibulum).

An increase in right ventricular oxygen saturation is most commonly due to a left-to-right shunt through a ventricular septal defect; however, it could be associated with other lesions, such as sinus of Valsalva fistula or rupture into the right ventricle or a coronary arteriovenous fistula entering the right ventricle. Not uncommonly, a large increase in right ventricular oxygen saturation occurs in patients with atrial left-to-right shunts due to streaming into the right ventricle. This is especially likely to occur in defects low in the atrial septum, in which case only a small increase in oxygen saturation may be noted in the midlateral right atrium; the major increase is noted in the body of the right ventricle. Also, in patients with ventricular septal defects high in the septum, and particularly in subpulmonary (supracristal) defects, there may be only a small increase in oxygen saturation in the body of the right ventricle but a large increase in the outflow region. An increase in oxygen saturation in the right ventricle, especially in the outflow region, may also be noted in the absence of any ventricular shunt when there is a large left-to-right shunt into the pulmonary artery and regurgitation into the right ventricle across the pulmonary valve. This is most likely to occur when there is pulmonary hypertension with a large dilated pulmonary artery.

Pulmonary arterial oxygen saturation

Normally, most venous blood is quite well mixed by the time the ventricle is reached; an increase of 3% or more in oxygen saturation in pulmonary arterial compared with right ventricular blood is significant. An increase in oxygen saturation in the pulmonary artery is most commonly associated with a patent ductus arteriosus. Other causes include left-to-right shunts from other lesions, such as aortopulmonary fenestration, coronary arteriovenous fistula draining into the pulmonary artery, or anomalous origin of the left coronary artery from the pulmonary artery (due to collateral flow from the right coronary arterial system). Not uncommonly, an apparent increase in oxygen saturation in the pulmonary artery is associated with a ventricular septal defect, especially if it is in the subpulmonary region. During systole, the shunt is directed through the infundibulum and pulmonary valve directly into the pulmonary artery. If a right ventricular sample is obtained just below the pulmonary valve, it will be quite obvious that there is a large oxygen saturation increase at this level, but if a sample is obtained in the ventricular body, it may appear that the shunt is at the pulmonary arterial level. A similar problem frequently occurs in patients with double-outlet right ventricle with subpulmonary ventricular septal defect, in whom left ventricular blood is preferentially ejected into the pulmonary artery, where the oxygen saturation is considerably higher than in the right ventricular body.

Oxygen saturations in the main and branch pulmonary arteries are usually similar in patients with no shunt or with atrial or ventricular shunts. They may, however, differ by 2–3% or even as much as 5–6% in patients with patent ductus arteriosus. In the main pulmonary artery, depending on the direction from which the catheter enters the vessel, variable measurements may be obtained. If the pulmonary artery is catheterized retrogradely from the aorta through the ductus arteriosus, the catheter tip is directed toward the pulmonary valve, and the sample obtained may give a falsely low oxygen saturation due to preferential sampling of the right ventricular stream. In older patients, particularly when the ductus arteriosus is not very large, there is often preferential streaming of shunted blood into the left pulmonary artery, so that a higher oxygen saturation is measured in the left compared with the main, or right, pulmonary artery. When the catheter is passed into the main pulmonary artery from the right ventricle, its tip may be directed to the entrance of the ductus to measure an unusually high oxygen saturation.

Pulmonary venous and left atrial oxygen saturation and Po_2

The oxygen dissociation curve is relatively flat in the upper ranges of oxygen saturation, so that changes in Po_2 of considerable degree may not be appreciated from oxygen saturation measurements. Therefore, it is advisable to routinely measure Po_2 as well as oxygen saturation in samples obtained from the left side of the heart and the systemic arterial circulation.

It is not always possible to sample all the pulmonary veins, and it is important to recognize that there may be marked variation in Po_2 in different veins, depending on ventilation–perfusion relationships. In a pulmonary vein draining an atelectatic lobe, Po_2 may be reduced to near venous levels. Although these major differences are to be expected in some individuals in whom there is obvious evidence of major lung disease, smaller differences are frequently noted in patients with cardiac failure, with marked cardiomegaly and with less obvious pulmonary problems. In infants with large hearts and with large pulmonary arteries there may be areas of atelectasis or hyperinflation due to bronchial compression, which also produce large differences in pulmonary venous Po_2 and oxygen saturation.

Pulmonary venous oxygen saturation is normally 97–100% and the Po_2 90–105 mmHg in individuals at sea level, but at altitude they are lower due to the lower partial pressure of oxygen in inspired air. The Po_2 may be reduced by various pulmonary diseases, but also by disturbance in ventilation–perfusion relationships. If there is alveolar hypoventilation, as frequently occurs in patients who have been sedated, pulmonary venous Po_2 will be reduced, often to levels of 80–85 mmHg and sometimes lower and oxygen saturation may be 88–94%. In children with very large pulmonary blood flows, as in large atrial septal defects, pulmonary venous oxygen saturation is commonly reduced to 92–94% and Po_2 to 85–90 mmHg. This is probably related to the high velocity of flow across the pulmonary capillary bed which, with normal alveolar ventilation, does not permit normal oxygen uptake.

Simultaneous measurement of Pco_2 and H^+ concentration in pulmonary venous blood is often also helpful: when there is pulmonary disease or alveolar hypoventilation, Pco_2 and H^+ concentration may be increased.

Pulmonary venous Po_2 may be reduced by an anatomic intrapulmonary shunt, such as with pulmonary arteriovenous fistulae or some types of destructive lung disease. Physiological shunting, in which there are no abnormal arteriovenous connections but perfusion occurs through unventilated or poorly ventilated areas, can also reduce Po_2. It is often possible to differentiate the mechanism for the reduced Po_2 by administering 100% oxygen for a period of 15 min. If the lowered Po_2 is due to hypoventilation, it will rise to normal levels of 500–600 mmHg. However, it is important that either a tight-fitting mask or a hood with a high flow of oxygen be used for a period of 15 min in order that all alveoli that are being ventilated have the opportunity to equilibrate with the high oxygen. Using this method it is not possible to differentiate between true anatomic shunts and perfusion of portions of the lung that are completely unventilated, as in both these conditions Po_2 will increase but will not reach normal levels.

In newborn infants who have been sedated, pulmonary venous Po_2 is often only 80–85 mmHg and oxygen saturation 90–94%; this may be due to hypoventilation or inadequate expansion of some areas of the lung. With 100% oxygen breathing, the systemic arterial Po_2 may not increase to more than 400–500 mmHg in apparently normal infants. In older infants with cardiac failure, pulmonary venous Po_2 is often reduced to 80–90 mmHg, with an oxygen saturation of 88–92%, and Pco_2 is frequently increased to 42–48 mmHg; pH may be reduced to 7.25–7.35.

Pulmonary venous Po_2 is often increased in severely cyanotic infants with severe hypoxemia while breathing room air. The systemic arterial hypoxemia, often accompanied by an increase in H^+ ion concentration, stimulates the respiratory center, resulting in hyperventilation. If pulmonary perfusion is normal, but particularly if it is decreased, alveolar ventilation is increased relative to perfusion and pulmonary venous Po_2 may be increased to 110–115 mmHg. Pco_2 is reduced, sometimes to as low as 15–20 mmHg. Associated with the lowered Pco_2 there is respiratory alkalosis of pulmonary venous blood, and pH may be increased to 7.45 or more. There is a marked contrast between the low Pco_2 and normal or increased pH in the pulmonary venous blood and the normal or slightly increased Pco_2 and often reduced pH in systemic arterial blood.

In normal individuals, left atrial oxygen saturation and Po_2 are similar to those in the pulmonary vein. A lower oxygen saturation in the left atrium is usually due to right-to-left shunting through an atrial septal defect or patent foramen ovale, but it may be caused by anomalous drainage of the superior or inferior vena cava into the left atrium. In evaluating a small decrease in oxygen saturation at the left atrial level, it should be appreciated that it may not be due to atrial right-to-left shunting but to differences in pulmonary venous oxygen saturations. If the pulmonary vein or veins sampled have normal oxygen saturations but other pulmonary veins have a lower oxygen saturation, the left atrial oxygen saturation could be reduced.

In certain congenital heart lesions there is complete admixture of pulmonary and systemic venous returns at the left atrial level. This occurs in tricuspid atresia or in pulmonary atresia, when all the systemic venous blood crosses the atrial septum. Under these circumstances, the oxygen saturations are equal in the left atrium, the left ventricle, and the pulmonary and systemic arteries.

Left ventricular oxygen saturation

Normally, oxygen saturation in the left ventricle is similar to that in the pulmonary veins and the left atrium. A decrease in oxygen saturation in the left ventricle relative to the left atrium occurs as a result of right-to-left shunting through a ventricular septal defect. A blood sample obtained at the left ventricular apex may not show a decrease in oxygen saturation, but it is detected in the outflow region or in the aorta. This is due to the fact that blood shunted from the right ventricle through the ventricular septal defect streams toward the aorta during systole. With right-to-left shunting across the atrial septum, left ventricular oxygen saturation is often lower than that in the left atrium, due to the lack of adequate mixing in the atrium. If a sample is obtained near a pulmonary vein entering the left atrium, this will show a higher oxygen saturation than the left ventricular sample.

Systemic arterial oxygen saturation and Po_2

Normally, systemic arterial oxygen saturation and Po_2 are similar to those in the pulmonary veins. However, oxygen saturation may be 2–3% and Po_2 2–5 mmHg lower, due to the fact that there is addition of a small amount of coronary venous blood in the left ventricle through drainage of thebesian veins. The discussion above concerning the effects of ventilation–perfusion relationships on pulmonary venous blood also pertains to systemic arterial blood. A decreased systemic arterial Po_2 or oxygen saturation may be due to pulmonary factors or to right-to-left shunting at the atrial or ventricular level. Arterial oxygen saturation is commonly lower than that in the left ventricle when there is systolic streaming of right ventricular blood through a ventricular septal defect into the aorta. This occurs in lesions such as ventricular septal defect with severe pulmonic stenosis or markedly increased pulmonary vascular resistance. It is also noted when the aorta arises from the right ventricle, as in double-outlet right ventricle, aortopulmonary transposition with ventricular septal defect, or truncus arteriosus communis.

With aortopulmonary transposition and ventricular septal defect, the aortic oxygen saturation is reduced but higher than that in the right ventricle. An aortic oxygen saturation higher than that in the right ventricle and lower than that in the left ventricle could be associated with a transposed aorta and a high ventricular septal defect.

Differences between oxygen saturation or Po_2 levels in the ascending aorta and its branches and the descending aorta and its branches are noted frequently when there is right-to-left shunting through a patent ductus arteriosus from the pulmonary artery. When the aorta and pulmonary artery arise normally from the ventricles, ductal right-to-left shunting results in a lower oxygen saturation in the descending aorta (see above).

Bidirectional shunting may occur through the patent ductus arteriosus when pulmonary vascular resistance is somewhat lower than systemic vascular resistance, particularly in newborn infants. The right-to-left shunting occurs during systole, when right ventricular ejection tends to direct blood through the ductus; also, the high velocity of flow in the descending aorta may tend to create a Bernoulli effect, favoring passage of blood from the pulmonary trunk to the aorta. During diastole, left-to-right shunting will predominate. This bidirectional shunting occurs when the ductus arteriosus is widely patent and pulmonary arterial pressure is elevated. When the ductus is small, and pulmonary arterial pressure low, shunting is exclusively left to right.

With aortopulmonary transposition, oxygen saturation in the pulmonary artery may be higher than that in the ascending aorta, and ductus right-to-left shunting causes oxygen saturation in the descending aorta to be higher than that in the ascending aorta. Po_2 levels in the ascending and descending aorta or their branches should be measured if ductus right-to-left shunting is suspected, as this is more reliable in showing differences if arterial oxygen saturations are relatively high. This is related to the shape of the oxygen dissociation curve, which is fairly flat at higher Po_2; therefore, with only a small difference in saturation, Po_2 differences would be much greater.

Oxygen supply and requirements

Oxygen requirements are determined by metabolic activity. Basic cellular functions such as ionic transport and electrical activity consume minimal amounts of oxygen, and cardiac contraction and normal respiration require relatively small amounts of oxygen. In homeothermic animals, a large proportion of oxygen consumption is directed toward heat production to maintain body temperature. Physical activity is also an important factor in increasing metabolic activity and oxygen consumption. Thus heavy exertion may increase oxygen consumption as much as fivefold.

In the fetus, body temperature is maintained in the moist environment of the amniotic fluid by the mother. There is therefore no oxygen consumption necessary for metabolism for heat production. In addition, although fetal breathing movements and limb motion occur, they are intermittent and contribute minimally to oxygen utilization. Fetal oxygen consumption is therefore low compared with postnatally: fetal lambs consume 7–8 mL/kg per min compared with about 20 mL/kg per min in the resting postnatal lamb [6].

Oxygen delivery

Oxygen is supplied to the fetus from the mother across the placenta. As mentioned above, the high percentage of fetal hemoglobin, with its low P_{50}, facilitates uptake of oxygen. For example, in the sheep, at a Po_2 of about 35 mmHg, umbilical venous blood oxygen saturation is 85–90%, whereas oxygen saturation of maternal uterine venous blood is only about 40%. An important mechanism employed by the fetus to increase oxygen delivery is to raise hemoglobin concentration, which occurs as a response to chronic hypoxemia.

Oxygen delivery is determined by umbilical blood flow ($\dot{Q}uv$) and oxygen content of umbilical venous blood ($Cuvo_2$):

$$\text{Fetal } O_2 \text{ delivery (mL/kg/min)} = \dot{Q}\text{uv (dL/kg/min)} \times Cuvo_2 \text{ (mL/dL)}$$

In the sheep, with an umbilical venous flow of about 200 mL/kg per min and an umbilical venous oxygen content of about 10 mL/dL, oxygen delivery is about 20 mL/kg per min. However, the oxygen content of blood delivered to the tissues is lower, because umbilical venous blood mixes with systemic venous blood before being distributed to fetal aorta. Also, because of shunting in the heart and great vessels, the oxygen content of blood passing to upper and lower body organs is different (see Chapter 1).

Postnatally, sympathoadrenal stimulation produces a marked increase in brown fat metabolism and in oxygen consumption. This is an important mechanism for maintaining body temperature in response to lowered environmental temperature. Brown fat stimulation results from sympathoadrenal stimulation and is due to β-adrenoceptors. However, there is a limitation in the ability of the fetus to increase its oxygen supply. In the fetal lamb, only a modest increase in oxygen consumption of 15% results from maximal β-adrenoceptor stimulation [7]. It has also been suggested that a high circulating level of adenosine in the fetus limits the lipolysis and thus the rise in oxygen consumption with catecholamine stimulation [8].

Even though β-adrenoceptor stimulation produces only a 15% increase in oxygen consumption in the fetal lamb, arterial hypoxemia with lactic acidemia and a fall of pH results. β-Adrenoceptor stimulation by infusion of isoproterenol increases umbilical blood flow by 15%, but total oxygen delivery to the fetus does not change because umbilical venous oxygen content falls. There appears to be a diffusion limitation for oxygen, so that when umbilical blood flow increases, the decreased transit time in the placenta results in a fall in oxygen uptake.

Postnatally, oxygen uptake occurs in the lungs. The amount of oxygen taken up is dependent on pulmonary blood flow ($\dot{Q}p$) and pulmonary venous oxygen content ($Cpvo_2$):

$$O_2 \text{ uptake} = \dot{Q}\text{p (L/min)} \times Cpvo_2 \text{ (mL/L)}$$

Thus, in a 3.5-kg infant with a body surface area of 0.2 m^2, pulmonary blood flow is about 600 mL and $Cpvo_2$ is about 200 mL/L (assuming hemoglobin concentration is 15.5 mL/dL and pulmonary venous oxygen saturation 100%). Oxygen uptake is therefore 0.6×200 or 120 mL; this is equivalent to about 35 mL/kg body weight.

Normally, all pulmonary venous blood passes to the left atrium and ventricle and is ejected into the aorta and systemic circulation. Thus all oxygen taken up in the lungs is distributed to the systemic circulation. The term *systemic oxygen transport* (SOT) has been used to designate the amount of oxygen delivered to the body. It is the product of systemic blood flow ($\dot{Q}s$) and oxygen content of systemic arterial blood ($Csao_2$):

$$\text{SOT (mL/min)} = \dot{Q}\text{s (L/min)} \times Csao_2 \text{ (mL/L)}$$

With some congenital heart lesions, SOT may differ from the total amount of oxygen in pulmonary venous blood. Thus, when a left-to-right shunt is present, a proportion of pulmonary venous blood recirculates through the lungs, and SOT will thus be lower than the amount of oxygen in pulmonary venous blood. Similarly, in the presence of a right-to-left shunt, SOT will be higher than the amount of oxygen in pulmonary venous blood, because venous blood shunted into the arterial system contains some oxygen.

SOT may be reduced by (i) a decrease in systemic blood flow, or (ii) a reduction in arterial oxygen content due to decreased arterial oxygen saturation or reduction of hemoglobin concentration (as with anemia). Aortic atresia (see Chapter 11) provides an example of the situation in which total pulmonary uptake of oxygen is normal, but SOT may be reduced. In the presence of aortic atresia, systemic blood flow is dependent entirely on flow through the ductus arteriosus. Constriction of the ductus would decrease systemic flow, and even if arterial oxygen content is within the normal range, oxygen delivery would be reduced.

Pulmonary blood flow may be reduced in lesions in which there is obstruction on the right side of the heart. In infants with pulmonary atresia, for example, pulmonary blood flow is derived from the aorta via the ductus arteriosus. Constriction of the ductus arteriosus results in a decrease in pulmonary blood flow and oxygen uptake. Systemic blood flow is maintained by right-to-left shunting through either an atrial or ventricular septal communication. Because systemic venous blood contains oxygen, albeit in lower concentrations than arterial blood, SOT would be higher than pulmonary uptake and is expressed as:

$$\text{SOT} = (\dot{Q}\text{p} \times C\text{pvo}_2) + (\dot{Q}_{\text{R-L}} \times C\text{mvo}_2)$$

where $\dot{Q}$p represents pulmonary blood flow, $C\text{pvo}_2$ pulmonary venous oxygen content, $\dot{Q}_{\text{R-L}}$ right-to-left shunt, and $C\text{mvo}_2$ mixed venous oxygen content.

It is a common misconception that the degree of hypoxemia in patients with pulmonary atresia is determined by the magnitude of the right-to-left shunt. If oxygen consumption by the tissues is constant and pulmonary blood flow does not change, an increase in right-to-left shunt will result in an immediate fall in arterial oxygen saturation. However, because the total amount of oxygen delivered to the body will increase, a smaller proportion will be consumed by tissues and the venous blood returning to the heart will have a higher oxygen saturation. After a short period the systemic arterial oxygen saturation will stabilize at the original level. Rather, the balance between pulmonary blood flow, which determines oxygen uptake in the lungs, and tissue oxygen consumption influences the systemic arterial oxygen saturation. If consumption of oxygen exceeds that taken up in the lungs and delivered to the body, oxygen saturation of venous blood will be reduced and thus systemic arterial saturation will fall.

In recent years, it has become common practice to measure arterial oxygen tension ($P\text{ao}_2$), rather than oxygen saturation and oxygen content. This is not a good indication of oxygen delivery in infants, especially preterm infants, because the P_{50} varies with the amount of fetal hemoglobin present. Thus at the same $P\text{o}_2$, if P_{50} is low because a high percentage of fetal hemoglobin is still present, oxygen saturation of blood would be higher, and oxygen delivery greater. At the same $P\text{o}_2$ in a 3-month-old infant, in whom P_{50} is higher because fetal hemoglobin concentrations are lower, oxygen delivery would be lower, assuming that systemic blood flows are similar.

Oxygen consumption

As mentioned above, in the absence of physical activity and need for thermal regulation, oxygen consumption in the fetus is relatively low (7–8 mL/kg per min). Because all oxygen exchange occurs across the placenta, fetal oxygen consumption ($\dot{V}\text{o}_2$) is readily measured:

$$\dot{V}\text{o}_2 = \dot{Q}\text{uv} \times (C\text{uvo}_2 - C\text{uao}_2)$$

where $\dot{Q}$uv represents umbilical blood flow, and $C\text{uvo}_2$ and $C\text{uao}_2$ are umbilical venous and umbilical arterial oxygen contents.

In the sheep fetus, the liver consumes about 25% of the total oxygen consumption of 7–8 mL/kg per min [9]; consumption by other organs is shown in Table 1.2 (see Chapter 1). It has also been estimated that about 33% of oxygen consumption is directed toward metabolism related to fetal growth [10]. In the fetus, almost no fatty acids are used as an energy source, and metabolism involves predominantly carbohydrates, as glucose and lactate, and amino acids.

Postnatally, as mentioned above, oxygen consumption increases markedly in association with increased metabolism associated with maintaining body temperature. In the lamb born from the intrauterine environment into air with a room temperature of 20–22°C, oxygen consumption is raised to 20–25 mL/kg per min in the resting state [11]. Physical activity causes a further increase in oxygen consumption.

Factors affecting postnatal oxygen consumption

Body temperature is regulated by balancing heat production and heat loss. Heat production is largely provided by two mechanisms: shivering, and increasing metabolism, particularly of fat. Shivering occurs in the newborn in some species, but most heat production is from brown fat metabolism, which is associated with increase in oxygen consumption. Inability of the animal to increase oxygen consumption adequately to provide enough energy for heat production will result in a fall in body temperature.

With infants, the environmental conditions under which oxygen consumption is increased have been termed the *neutral thermal environment*; neutral temperature is about 33°C. A reduction in temperature below this level, or rise of environmental temperature above this level, will be associated with an increase in oxygen consumption. Factors that influence heat loss from the body surface, such as humidity, conduction, convection, and radiation, will also modify oxygen consumption.

Because heat loss is proportional to body surface area, oxygen consumption is related to body surface area (about 120–150 mL/min per m^2). The smaller the animal, the larger the surface area relative to body weight. It is well known that oxygen consumption per kilogram body weight is considerably higher in animals such as mice and guinea pigs compared with dogs and especially horses and cattle. For this reason, oxygen consumption per kilogram body weight is considerably higher in newborn infants compared with adults. In a 70-kg adult with a surface area of 1.7 m^2, oxygen consumption at 150 mL/min per m^2 amounts to 255 mL/min or 3.6 mL/kg per min. In a 3-kg infant with a surface area of 0.22 m^2, oxygen consumption would be 33 mL/min or 11.0 mL/kg per min. In a premature infant, oxygen consumption in relation to body weight is even larger.

Adult animals have the capacity to increase metabolism and oxygen consumption markedly in response to cold stress, and thus are able to maintain body temperature unless temperatures are extremely low. However, newborns, although they increase oxygen consumption, are less capable of producing the same magnitude of response and are therefore likely to demonstrate a fall in core body temperature [10]. This has been termed a *hypometabolic response* but, as discussed below, it probably represents a lower reserve in ability to raise oxygen consumption.

Oxygen extraction

Oxygen extraction represents the proportion of oxygen delivered that is consumed. In the lamb fetus, with an oxygen delivery of about 22 mL/kg per min and oxygen consumption of 7–8 mL/kg per min, the oxygen extraction ratio is about 0.3 or 30% [12].

The extraction ratio varies considerably in different organs, being dependent both on total oxygen delivery and on metabolism. Thus the fetal liver receives a large volume of well-oxygenated blood from the umbilical vein, and despite its relatively high rate of metabolism, displays a low extraction ratio for oxygen. However, the fetal heart, even though supplied by a high myocardial flow, normally shows an oxygen extraction ratio of 65–70% [13].

In the fetus, arterial blood supplied to organs other than the liver has a relatively low Po_2. Ascending aortic blood has a Po_2 of 25–28 mmHg and descending aortic blood has a Po_2 of about 22 mmHg and an oxygen saturation of about 50%. Venous blood from the peripheral circulation in the lower extremities has a Po_2 of about 15 mmHg with an oxygen saturation of about 30%. In the sheep fetus, with a hemoglobin concentration of about 8 g/dL, oxygen capacity is about 10.5 mL/dL. The amount of oxygen taken up in the extremities is therefore:

$$[(50 \times 10.5)/100] - [(30 \times 10.5)/100] \\ = 2.1 \text{ mL/dL blood flow}$$

Even at the low Po_2 in fetal arterial blood, with an arteriovenous Po_2 difference of only 7 mmHg, a reasonable amount of oxygen can be extracted because the P_{50} is low, as most of the hemoglobin is of the fetal type. Although the fetus has an arteriovenous Po_2 difference of only 7 mmHg, it is capable of increasing oxygen extraction significantly under hypoxemic conditions. Studies in fetal lambs have shown that oxygen extraction can be increased to 65–70% under conditions of stress. If fetal arterial Po_2 is reduced to about 15 mmHg, with an oxygen saturation of about 30%, venous oxygen saturation may fall to 10% with a Po_2 of 8–10 mmHg.

Postnatally, systemic arterial Po_2 increases to more than 90 mmHg. Oxygen saturation of hemoglobin, and the actual amount of oxygen attached to hemoglobin, increases. In the adult, oxygen extraction is also about 0.3 or 30%, with oxygen delivery of 450–500 mL/min per m^2 and oxygen consumption of about 150 mL/min per m^2. Arterial oxygen saturation is 95–98% with a Po_2 of 100 mmHg and mixed venous oxygen saturation is about 65% at a Po_2 of 35–40 mmHg. In the adult sheep with a hemoglobin concentration of about 8 g/dL and oxygen capacity of 0.5 mL/dL, oxygen uptake would be:

$$[(100 \times 10.5)/100] - [(65 \times 10.5)/100] = 3.7 \text{ mL/dL blood flow}$$

In the adult, oxygen extraction can also be increased to about 70% under conditions of stress, and this is associated with a decrease in venous Po_2. A fall in venous Po_2 has been used as a fairly sensitive indicator of inadequacy of oxygen supply to the tissues. The presence of fetal hemoglobin during the postnatal period is somewhat disadvantageous in terms of tissue oxygen uptake. Because the P_{50} of fetal hemoglobin is low, it is fully saturated with oxygen at a relatively low Po_2. Thus at a Po_2 of 35 mmHg, fetal lamb blood has an oxygen saturation of about 90%. When Po_2 is raised above this level, little additional oxygen is attached to hemoglobin.

Thus in the newborn lamb, if all hemoglobin is of the fetal type, hemoglobin concentration is 8 g/dL (oxygen capacity 10.5 mL/dL), arterial blood Po_2 is 100 mmHg, and venous blood Po_2 35 mmHg, the amount of oxygen extracted would be:

$$[(100 \times 10.5)/100] - [(90 \times 10.5)/100] = 1.05 \text{ mL/dL blood flow}$$

To provide adequate oxygen for tissue needs, the blood flow could be raised. Possibly, venous Po_2 could be reduced to increase oxygen extraction. It appears, however, that an attempt is made to maintain venous Po_2 at about 35 mmHg, and when it falls below that level, there is the likelihood for lactate production with the development of metabolic acidemia.

In newborn animals, if fetal blood is exchanged with blood with hemoglobin with a high P_{50}, the oxygen uptake per unit of blood flow is increased and cardiac output falls [14]. This indicates that if hemoglobin is mainly of the fetal type in the neonate, oxygen extraction is low and cardiac output is maintained at relatively high levels, in order to provide adequate oxygen to the tissues (see Figure 3.5).

Effect of reducing oxygen supply

It has become common practice to use the term *hypoxia* to indicate inadequate oxygenation. However, it should be used to specify inadequate oxygen to permit aerobic metabolism in tissues. *Hypoxemia* is the term that indicates a reduction in arterial oxygen saturation. The term *asphyxia* describes the condition in which oxygen uptake as well as CO_2 removal is affected. Inadequate oxygen supply to tissues may result from mechanisms that differ in the fetus and postnatally.

Oxygen supply to the fetus may be reduced acutely by several mechanisms.

1 Decreased oxygen delivery to the placenta: maternal hypoxemia decreases oxygen delivery to the placenta because oxygen content of umbilical arterial blood is reduced. The umbilical venous Po_2 falls but Pco_2 does not change. A reduction in uterine blood flow will also reduce oxygen delivery to the placenta. This results in a fall in both umbilical venous Po_2 and a rise in Pco_2.

2 Interference in diffusion of oxygen across the placental membranes or an inadequate placental exchange surface will reduce fetal oxygen delivery. Umbilical venous blood will show a fall in Po_2 and a rise in Pco_2.

3 Decrease in umbilical blood flow: when umbilical venous blood flow is reduced, umbilical venous Po_2 and oxygen saturation may increase slightly because uterine flow at the placental site is higher than umbilical blood flow. This perfusion–perfusion relationship is similar to the ventilation–perfusion relationship in the lung postnatally.

Responses to acute hypoxemia

The responses to acute hypoxemia have been studied in some detail in late-gestation fetal lambs.

Table 3.2 Fetal responses to hypoxemia induced by maternal hypoxemia.

Heart rate	Decreased
Cardiac output	Decreased
Systemic arterial pressure	Increased
Umbilical–placental blood flow	Unchanged
Vascular resistances	
Cerebral	Decreased
Coronary	Decreased
Adrenal	Decreased
Pulmonary	Increased
Peripheral	Increased
Gastrointestinal	Increased
Splenic	Increased
Renal	Increased
Hepatic	Increased
Umbilical–placental	Increased

Characteristically, there is rapid onset of bradycardia, a fall in combined ventricular output, and slower development of arterial hypertension. There is "centralization" of the circulation, with reduction in blood flow to the nonvital organs, such as the peripheral circulation (skin, muscle, bone), lung and kidneys, gastrointestinal tract, liver, and spleen. Blood flow in vital organs such as the brain, heart, and adrenal gland is increased. These responses to hypoxemia are summarized in Table 3.2 [15].

The mechanisms responsible for the responses to hypoxemia are complex and the effects are the result of interacting influences. The main mechanisms involved include chemoreflex responses, hormonal effects, direct local vascular responses, and baroreflex responses.

Chemoreceptor stimulation

Hypoxemia affects the carotid bodies predominantly. This results in bradycardia, mediated by reflex simulation of the vagus nerve. The magnitude of the bradycardia response is related to the fall in carotid arterial oxygen level. Chemoreceptor activity also stimulates the sympathoadrenal system. Reflex sympathetic nervous system stimulation is probably partly responsible for many of the vascular responses, such as vasoconstriction in the peripheral circulation, gastrointestinal tract and some other organs, and also for coronary vasodilatation. Carotid chemoreceptor stimulation is also responsible for catecholamine release from the adrenal glands, probably through sympathetic nerve pathways.

The decrease in combined ventricular output is mainly the result of the bradycardia, but the increase in afterload on the heart, associated with pulmonary and peripheral vasoconstriction, may contribute to the fall in cardiac output.

Hormonal effects

Concentrations of several vasoactive hormones in plasma are increased during fetal hypoxemia. Catecholamine concentrations increase dramatically. The major stimulus to adrenal medullary secretion is chemoreceptor activity. However, hypoxemia produces direct stimulation of catecholamine secretion by the adrenal gland when arterial Po_2 falls markedly to below 15–16 mmHg. In the fetus, norepinephrine concentrations increase from 200–400 pg/mL to as high as 4000–6000 pg/mL, whereas epinephrine concentrations increase only by a relatively small amount, from about 50 pg/mL to 500–800 pg/mL.

In addition to the rise in catecholamine concentrations, plasma arginine vasopressin (AVP) concentrations rise during hypoxemia. This response could be due to chemoreflex stimulation. Both catecholamines and AVP contribute to the vasoconstrictor responses; catecholamines may also be involved in coronary vasodilatation. Plasma angiotensin concentrations increase only slightly during fetal hypoxemia, in contrast with the large increase associated with small reductions in blood volume.

Direct local vascular responses

Changes in oxygen concentration in blood perfusing various organs may directly alter vasoreactivity. In many instances, release of some vasoactive substances, or inhibition of the release of others, has been shown to be involved in the responses. There is also some evidence to support the concept that oxygen levels may directly affect vascular smooth muscle cells. The vascular response is determined by the summation of the effects of the various factors influencing the vessels.

In the cerebral and coronary circulations, hypoxemia causes vasodilatation. The magnitude of the response is related to the level of oxygen content rather than the Po_2. In the brain, if CO_2

content also increases, as during fetal asphyxia associated with decreased uterine blood flow, cerebral blood flow is further enhanced. The increase in flow with hypoxemia is, at least in part, related to nitric oxide mechanisms [16].

In the myocardium, although blood flow under normoxic conditions is very high, coronary blood flow increases markedly during hypoxia by as much as threefold to fourfold. The direct local vasodilatation could also partly involve nitric oxide release, but adenosine appears to be the more important mediator for the vasodilatation. In addition to the local effects of hypoxemia, the increase in circulating catecholamine concentrations contributes to coronary vasodilatation by stimulating β-adrenoceptors.

A decrease in the oxygen concentration of blood perfusing the lung in the fetus causes marked vasoconstriction. Nitric oxide is a very effective pulmonary vasodilator. Nitric oxide is, at least in part, responsible for the maintenance of pulmonary blood flow during normoxemia, because administration of the inhibitor *N*-ω-nitro-L-arginine results in vasoconstriction. It is thus possible that inhibition of nitric oxide release during hypoxia could contribute to the vasoconstriction. Recently it has been suggested that hypoxia may exert its effect by directly affecting oxygen-sensitive potassium channels. Blocking these potassium channels results in vasoconstriction, and hypoxia inhibits K^+ currents on pulmonary smooth muscle cells. The pulmonary vascular system and its responses are discussed in more detail in Chapter 5.

Baroreflex response

Baroreflexes arising from the aortic sinuses and carotid artery are well developed in the sheep fetus by 0.6 gestation. The increase in arterial blood pressure resulting from peripheral vasoconstriction during hypoxemia could contribute to the bradycardia. However, the chemoreflex is responsible for the immediate bradycardia associated with hypoxemia, because the rise in arterial pressure is delayed for at least 30–60 s.

Influence of mode of reduction in oxygen delivery

To assess the possible role of the method of reducing oxygen delivery on fetal responses, the effects of decreasing oxygen delivery by 50% were studied in fetal lambs [17]. As mentioned above, with maternal hypoxemia, as with acute reduction of uterine blood flow, the oxygen content of umbilical venous blood falls whereas umbilical blood flow does not change significantly. Therefore, reducing umbilical venous oxygen content by 50% will reduce fetal oxygen delivery by 50%. A 50% decrease in umbilical blood flow will also cause a 50% reduction in oxygen delivery, because umbilical venous oxygen content does not change significantly when umbilical blood flow falls.

The fall in oxygen delivery associated with maternal hypoxemia or reduced uterine blood flow results in marked cerebral and coronary vasodilatation, and peripheral vasoconstriction. However, a similar decrease in oxygen delivery resulting from reduced umbilical blood flow results in only modest cerebral and coronary vasodilatation, and only mild peripheral vasoconstriction. These differences in response can be explained by patterns of blood flow in the fetal circulation (see Chapter 1). Umbilical venous blood passes through the ductus venosus, and ductus venosus blood is preferentially directed through the foramen ovale into the left atrium and ventricle. With reduced umbilical blood flow, umbilical venous blood oxygen content does not fall, and thus the blood entering the left ventricle and ejected into the ascending aorta manifests only a modest fall in oxygen saturation. However, when umbilical venous oxygen content is decreased, as with reduced uterine blood flow or maternal hypoxemia, the fall in ascending aortic oxygen saturation is marked, and thus coronary and cerebral vasodilatation are prominent. The lower oxygen content to which the aortic and carotid chemoreceptors are exposed also results in greater stimulation, and this can account for the more prominent peripheral vasoconstriction.

Fetal oxygen consumption during oxygen deprivation

Oxygen delivery can be reduced considerably without significantly affecting oxygen consumption. This is due to the ability of the fetus to increase oxygen extraction from about 30% to about 70%. Thus umbilical blood flow can be reduced acutely by almost 50% with no fall in oxygen consumption. Further decreases result in a rapidly progressive fall in $\dot{V}O_2$, and lactic acidemia develops. Similarly, uterine blood flow or maternal arterial oxygen content can be reduced considerably before fetal $\dot{V}O_2$ falls.

There may be a lesser ability for $\dot{V}O_2$ to be maintained as readily with reduced uterine flow or maternal hypoxemia, because at the considerably lower levels of arterial oxygen content, extraction may be somewhat limited in some organs by the level to which venous oxygen content may fall.

Postnatal response to reduced oxygen supply

As described above, hypoxemia in the fetus causes bradycardia; it also results in a cessation or depression of fetal breathing movements. In the adult, hypoxemia causes a marked increase in respirations and tachycardia. The increased respiratory effort is the result of carotid chemoreceptor stimulation. However, chemoreflex stimulation in anesthetized ventilated animals results in bradycardia. It has now been proposed, based on experimental studies, that the tachycardia resulting from hypoxemia is due to a reflex arising from the lungs or chest in association with the increased respiratory effort; this overrides the bradycardia resulting from chemoreceptor stimulation.

In 1-week-old lambs, hypoxemia also causes increased respiration. Although the tachycardia is not as marked as in the adult, heart rate does increase modestly, and in contrast with the fetal response to hypoxemia, a small increase in cardiac output occurs. In addition, the animals become anxious and restless; this is the alarm reaction resulting from chemoreflex stimulation. With increasing age of the lamb, there is a progressive increase in the tachycardia and cardiac output response to the same degree of hypoxemia; the adult-type response is manifested by 8–10 weeks of age.

The responses of vasculature in various organs are similar to those in the fetus; vasodilatation occurs in the myocardium and brain, whereas vasoconstriction occurs in the peripheral circulation, gastrointestinal tract, kidneys, and spleen, as well as in the lung.

Oxygen consumption during hypoxemia

In the adult, oxygen consumption is maintained during hypoxemia of mild or moderate degree, but falls with a more severe fall in arterial oxygen saturation. Newborn infants and animals decrease their oxygen consumption with even relatively mild hypoxemia. With more severe hypoxemia, $\dot{V}O_2$ falls markedly, and core body temperature may fall. It has been suggested that hypoxemia reduces metabolism in neonates by an as yet undefined mechanism; this has been termed *hypoxic hypometabolism*. The different responses of the newborn and adult can probably be explained by the difference in the ratio of body surface area to body weight. In the adult, with a small body surface area relative to weight, the oxygen consumption required for metabolism to maintain body temperature is low, and the animal is able to preserve $\dot{V}O_2$ by maintaining oxygen delivery by means of increased heart rate and cardiac output. In the newborn, with relatively large body surface area and limited ability to increase cardiac output, the large amount of oxygen required for maintenance of body temperature cannot be provided, and thus $\dot{V}O_2$ falls. With severe hypoxemia, $\dot{V}O_2$ and metabolism are so reduced that body temperature falls. This phenomenon would be even more prominent in the preterm infant, in whom the ratio of body surface area to weight is even larger.

The combined influence of a cool environment and hypoxemia is of particular importance in the neonate. When the infant is not in an optimal environment, oxygen consumption will be increased to maintain body temperature. If hypoxemia occurs under these conditions, there is little or no reserve, and $\dot{V}O_2$ falls and core body temperature will also fall. Furthermore, in view of the competition for available oxygen for basal metabolic needs and metabolism for thermogenesis, lactic acidemia is likely to develop.

Prenatal and postnatal chemoreflex responses

During the discussion of hypoxia, the important role of chemoreflexes has been stressed, in both the fetus and the newborn. It has been clearly demonstrated in fetal lambs that the carotid chemoreceptor reflex is responsible for the bradycardia and is a major contributor to the sympathoadrenal response to hypoxemia [18].

The sensitivity of the chemoreceptors is related to the level of oxygenation, but whether PO_2, oxygen saturation, or oxygen content is the determining factor has not been resolved. In the fetal lamb, for the same drop in oxygen saturation, the degree of bradycardia is less marked when resting carotid arterial oxygen saturation is relatively high (about 60%) than when resting oxygen saturation is lower (35–40%). Furthermore, when the resting carotid arterial oxygen saturation is raised to above 80%, by ventilating the fetus *in utero* with air or oxygen, the cardiovascular response to chemoreceptor stimulation by chemical means (cyanide) is completely ablated.

Fetal carotid arterial Po_2 is normally about 25 mmHg, with an oxygen saturation of about 65%. After birth, Po_2 increases to 90–95 mmHg and oxygen saturation to above 95%. At these oxygen levels, the chemoreceptors are relatively insensitive, and a response occurs only with severe hypoxemia. The receptors reset over the first few days after birth, so that by 7–10 days they are responsive to modest decreases in oxygen saturation from normal postnatal levels.

This relative insensitivity of the peripheral chemoreceptors in the early postnatal period probably explains the fact that infants with cyanotic congenital heart disease with quite marked hypoxemia appear comfortable, do not have significantly increased respiratory effort, and do not have bradycardia. Studies in newborn lambs in which the carotid and aortic chemoreflexes have been ablated by sectioning the afferent nerves show that during hypoxemia they do not show an alarm reaction, do not develop increased respiration, and show no increase in heart rate or cardiac output. They develop progressive metabolic acidemia. This response is reminiscent of some descriptions of sudden infant death syndrome (SIDS). The possibility that SIDS may result from lack of postnatal resetting of the chemoreceptor is a concept for consideration.

Of great interest is whether the chemoreceptors reset after birth if there is persistent hypoxemia due to congenital heart disease or if the infant is born at high altitude. Also, if resetting does occur, the time course at which this occurs after birth is of great interest.

It is known that chemoreflex sensitivity is somewhat depressed in children with cyanotic heart disease, in whom cyanosis has persisted after birth, but the degree of depression has not been well defined. Since chemoreflex activity is depressed in cyanotic patients, one might wonder if they are more susceptible to SIDS than normally oxygenated infants.

Metabolic effects of oxygen deprivation

As mentioned above, oxygen deprivation may result from inadequate ventilation, reduced pulmonary venous oxygen content, reduced pulmonary blood flow, or decreased SOT resulting from inadequate systemic blood flow or from a reduction in arterial oxygen content due to anemia or hypoxemia (see Chapter 3). Any of these mechanisms will reduce oxygen supply to the tissues, and when this is severe enough, hypoxia results. When this occurs, the effects are similar no matter what the cause. Figure 3.6 shows the sequence of events.

Energy supply during inadequate oxygen supply is maintained by anaerobic metabolism. The substrate predominantly used for anaerobic glycolysis is glucose, and thus hypoglycemia is very likely to occur in infants with cyanotic congenital heart disease. Preterm infants, who frequently have

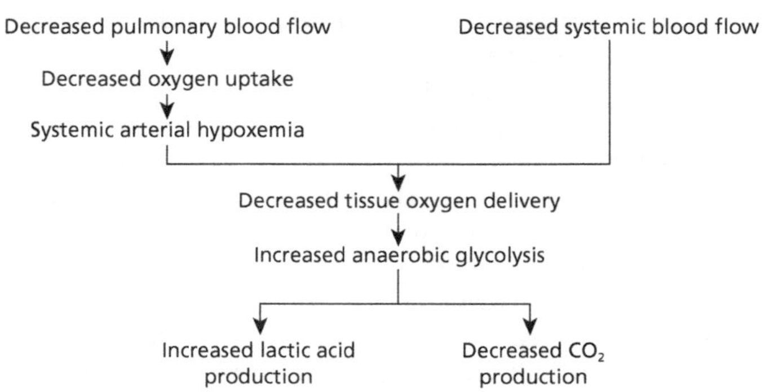

Figure 3.6 Sequence of events associated with inadequate oxygen supply to tissues resulting in metabolic acidemia and decreased CO_2 production.

postnatal hypoglycemia, would have a problem in maintaining energy supply during hypoxia.

Infants with congenital heart disease who develop hypoxia do not usually have elevated arterial Pco_2 levels. This could be related to the fact that CO_2 readily diffuses across the alveolar–capillary membrane, and even though pulmonary blood flow may be markedly decreased in some lesions, adequate pulmonary stimulation is achieved. An additional important factor is that CO_2 production in the tissues is reduced. Lactate is normally metabolized by oxygen to CO_2 and water. However, with hypoxia, lactate metabolism is depressed and thus CO_2 is not generated. The presence of a normal or decreased arterial Pco_2 may be useful in differentiating between heart disease and lung disease in a cyanotic infant.

Effects of oxygen administration

It is universal practice to administer oxygen by inhalation to infants with cardiorespiratory distress. Also, administration of oxygen is often used to attempt to distinguish between the various causes of cyanosis. This is the oxygen test, and it has been taught that if the test is positive, it suggests a pulmonary cause for the cyanosis.

During air breathing, with normal ventilation and normal lungs, the Po_2 of pulmonary venous blood is 98–100 mmHg. Administration of 100% oxygen will result in a large increase in Po_2. After breathing oxygen for 10–15 min, almost all nitrogen in the airways is eliminated and the alveoli contain oxygen, water vapor, and carbon dioxide. Thus, at sea level, with a barometric pressure of 760 mmHg, the maximal partial pressure for oxygen is 760 – [47 (water vapor pressure) + ~40 (CO_2 pressure)] or about 670 mmHg. Because some alveoli may be collapsed but perfused and because there is a small alveolar–pulmonary venous diffusion gradient for oxygen, pulmonary venous Po_2 usually reaches 500–600 mmHg. In neonates, probably because the lungs may not yet be fully expanded, pulmonary venous Po_2 often does not exceed 400–450 mmHg during 100% oxygen, with spontaneous ventilation.

If ventilation is depressed or there is partial collapse of a lung segment, the pulmonary venous Po_2 is reduced during air breathing. Administration of 100% oxygen significantly increases alveolar and pulmonary venous Po_2. If a segment of lung is completely atelectatic but is perfused, the pulmonary venous blood will have a similar Po_2 to blood entering this segment, because no gas exchange is occurring.

Generally, it is not practical to measure oxygen in pulmonary venous blood, so measurements are made on systemic arterial blood or oxygen saturation is recorded on the skin surface. Po_2 and oxygen saturation may be slightly lower in systemic arterial blood than in the pulmonary veins because a small amount of blood with low oxygen levels may enter the left ventricle from thebesian veins. Marked differences result from right-to-left shunts at the atrial or ventricular level. Right-to-left shunting through the ductus arteriosus produces lower levels of oxygenation in the descending aorta and its branches compared with the ascending aorta and its branches (see Chapter 3). It is now customary to compare Po_2 or oxygen saturation levels in the right arm and a lower extremity to detect a ductus arteriosus right-to-left shunt. The measurement is preferably made in the right arm, because the left subclavian artery arises close to the junction of the ductus arteriosus with the descending aorta. Blood shunted right to left through the ductus arteriosus may pass into this vessel, thus reducing the measured difference between the upper and lower extremity.

Potential benefits and adverse effects of oxygen administration

In patients with alveolar hypoventilation due to respiratory depression or lung disease, oxygen administration will increase pulmonary venous and arterial oxygen levels.

Reduced pulmonary blood flow

In infants with congenital heart lesions associated with reduced pulmonary blood flow, or in whom pulmonary blood flow is decreased by persistent pulmonary hypertension syndrome, the response to oxygen is dependent on the magnitude of pulmonary flow. The lower the pulmonary blood flow, the less the benefit. Oxygen uptake depends on pulmonary flow and oxygen content of pulmonary venous blood. When breathing air, with normal ventilation, there will be a high ventilation–perfusion ratio, or relative hyperventilation, and pulmonary venous Po_2 may be slightly above the normal 95–98 mmHg, with an oxygen saturation of 100%. If pulmonary venous Po_2 is raised to about 500 mmHg by administering 100% oxygen, no additional oxygen can be taken up by hemoglobin, so oxygen content will be raised by 1.2 mL/dL of blood. This represents the increase in the dissolved oxygen with an increase of Po_2 from 100 to 500 mmHg, and dissolved oxygen of 0.3 mL/dL per 100 mmHg.

If hemoglobin concentration is 15 g/dL, the amount of oxygen taken up in the lungs by hemoglobin would be about 20 mL/dL of blood flow. Thus 100% oxygen administration would augment oxygen uptake by only 6%. In striking contrast is the large increase in oxygen uptake that can be achieved by increasing hemoglobin concentration. For each 1 g/dL increase in hemoglobin concentration, oxygen uptake would be raised by 1.35 mL/dL of pulmonary blood flow. It is thus apparent that if an infant with cyanotic heart disease with decreased pulmonary flow does not respond adequately to oxygen administration, and if pulmonary blood flow cannot be increased, blood transfusion to raise hemoglobin concentration could be beneficial.

Although oxygen administration results in only a small increase in oxygen uptake, especially when pulmonary flow is greatly reduced, this additional amount could be adequate to avoid rapidly progressive hypoxia. Thus in a newborn infant with an oxygen consumption of 25 mL/min, if pulmonary blood flow is reduced by 50% to about 400 mL/min, 100% oxygen administration could add oxygen amounting to 1.2 mL/dL or 8.8 mL/min. This represents about one-third of the oxygen requirement of the infant.

The concern is frequently raised that administration of 100% oxygen to a severely cyanosed infant with pulmonary blood flow derived through the ductus arteriosus could be dangerous because it could constrict the ductus and result in deterioration. However, there is almost no risk that this could occur, because the ductus is subjected to the Po_2 of blood passing through it from the aorta. Ductus constriction would not occur until Po_2 is increased above 30–35 mmHg, but significant constriction would occur at higher levels. At this level of Po_2, a newborn infant with mainly fetal hemoglobin would be adequately oxygenated. Also, if ductus constriction did tend to occur, pulmonary flow would fall, Po_2 would decrease, and the ductus would open again.

Reduced systemic blood flow

When systemic blood flow is reduced because of shock, or low cardiac output due to myocardial failure, oxygen administration will increase oxygen delivery to the tissues, because dissolved oxygen levels will be raised.

In several congenital heart lesions, such as interruption of the aortic arch (Chapter 12) or aortic atresia (Chapter 11), the systemic blood flow to the lower body, or to the whole body, is dependent on flow from the pulmonary artery to the aorta via the ductus arteriosus. Pulmonary blood flow is normal or increased. Administration of 100% oxygen will increase the total oxygen uptake in the lungs considerably because potentially, if pulmonary venous Po_2 is raised by 400 mmHg, additional oxygen of 1.2 mL/dL of pulmonary blood flow would be taken up. If pulmonary flow is three times the normal (2000–2500 mL/min), additional oxygen of 20–25 × 1.2 or 24–30 mL/min would be taken up in the lungs. Also, systemic arterial oxygen saturation would be close to 100% and Po_2 could be raised well above 100 mmHg.

In aortic atresia, in which there is complete admixture of pulmonary and systemic venous return, oxygen saturation and Po_2 of arterial blood would be in the higher ranges because of the high ratio of pulmonary to systemic blood flow (see Chapter 4). Administration of 100% oxygen frequently raises oxygen saturation to 100% and arterial Po_2 will often exceed 100 mmHg. With very low systemic blood flows, Po_2 levels of 250–300 mmHg may be achieved. However, if oxygen saturation is already almost 100%, oxygen administration could increase arterial oxygen content by increasing dissolved oxygen but only by 0.3 mL/dL per 100 mmHg rise in Po_2.

Systemic oxygen transport depends on systemic blood flow and arterial blood oxygen content. Thus if systemic blood flow is markedly reduced, relatively little increase in oxygen delivery to the tissues could be achieved by oxygen administration.

Oxygen administration could be deleterious when systemic blood flow is derived from flow from the pulmonary artery via the ductus arteriosus. The increase in Po_2 of blood passing through the ductus could be considerable and cause constriction, resulting in a decrease in systemic arterial pressure and systemic blood flow (see Chapters 11 and 12). Even though Po_2 of arterial blood may be 200–300 mmHg, systemic blood flow may be so low that tissue hypoxia occurs, with lactic acid accumulation and metabolic acidemia.

References

1 Van Slyke DP, Neill JM. The determination of gases in blood and other solutions by vacuum extraction and manometric measurement. J Biol Chem 1924;61:523.

2 Clauvel M, Schwartz K. Blood oxygen capacity. Technical difficulties of its determination by the Van Slyke method and comparison with hemoglobin content. Clin Chem 1968;14:253–261.

3 Toth B, Becker A, Seelbach-Göbel B. Oxygen saturation in healthy newborn infants immediately after birth measured by pulse oximetry. Am J Obstet Gynecol 2002;266:105–107.

4 Rabi Y, Yee W, Chen SY, Singhal N. Oxygen saturation trends immediately after birth. J Pediatr 2006;148:590–594.

5 Hamilton C, Steinlecher B, Gruber E, Simon P, Wollenek G. The oxygen dissociation curve: quantifying the shift. Perfusion 2004;19:141–144.

6 Sidi D, Kuipers JRG, Teitel D, Heymann MA, Rudolph AM. Developmental changes in oxygenation and circulatory responses to hypoxemia in lambs. Am J Physiol 1983;245:H674–H682.

7 Gournay VA, Roman C, Rudolph AM. Effect of beta-adrenergic stimulation on oxygen metabolism in the fetal lamb. Pediatr Res 1999:45:432–436.

8 Ball KT, Gunn TR, Power GG, Asakura H, Gluckman PD. A potential role for adenosine in the inhibition of non-shivering thermogenesis in the fetal sheep. Pediatr Res 1995;37:303–309.

9 Bristow J, Rudolph AM, Itskovitz J, Barnes RJ. Hepatic oxygen and glucose metabolism in the fetal lamb: response to hypoxia. J Clin Invest 1983;71:1047–1061.

10 Sidi D, Kuipers JR, Heymann MA, Rudolph AM. Effects of ambient temperature on oxygen consumption and the circulation in newborn lambs at rest and during hypoxemia. Pediatr Res 1983;17:254–258.

11 Toubas PL, Hof RP, Heymann MA, Rudolph AM. Effects of hypothermia and rewarming on the neonatal circulation. Arch Franc Pediat (Suppl) 1978;34:84–92.

12 Itskovitz J, LaGamma EF, Rudolph AM. The effects of reducing umbilical blood flow on fetal oxygenation. Am J Obstet Gynecol 1983;145:813–818,

13 Fisher DJ, Rudolph AM, Heymann MA. Myocardial oxygen and carbohydrate consumption in fetal lambs in utero and in adult sheep. Am J Physiol 1980;238: H399–H405.

14 Teisseire BP, Ropars C, Vallez MO, Herigault RA, Nicolau C. Physiological effects of high-P50 erythrocyte transfusion on piglets. J Appl Physiol 1985;58:1810–1817.

15 Cohn HE, Sacks EJ, Heymann MA, Rudolph AM. Cardiovascular responses to hypoxemia and acidemia in fetal lambs. Am J Obstet Gynecol 1974;120:817–824.

16 van Bel F, Sola A, Roman C, Rudolph AM. Role of nitric oxide in the regulation of the cerebral circulation in the lamb fetus during normoxemia and hypoxemia. Biol Neonate 1995;68:200–210.

17 Jensen A, Roman C, Rudolph AM. Effects of reducing uterine blood flow on fetal blood flow distribution and oxygen delivery. J Dev Physiol 1991;15:309–323.

18 Bartelds B, van Bel F, Teitel DF, Rudolph AM. Carotid, not aortic, chemoreceptors mediate the fetal cardiovascular response to acute hypoxemia in lambs. Pediatr Res 1993;34:51–55.

CHAPTER 4
Functional assessment

Congenital cardiac defects influence the circulation in several ways. They may impose an excessive volume load on one or both ventricles, as with left-to-right shunt lesions, valvar regurgitation, or when one ventricle is absent or hypoplastic. They may place a pressure load on a ventricle by causing obstruction to its outflow, as with semilunar valve stenosis or aortic coarctation. If lesions are severe, cardiac output may be compromised. Lesions that cause cyanosis may seriously interfere with oxygen supply to the body; the influences of hypoxemia and hypoxia are discussed in Chapter 3. To assess the severity of congenital heart lesions, in addition to careful evaluation of clinical symptoms and signs, a number of functional aspects of the heart and circulation may be examined. In this chapter, some of these are reviewed: measurement of intravascular pressures, assessment of cardiac output and shunts, calculation of vascular resistances, evaluation of valve orifice and pressure gradients, and assessment of cardiac chamber size and performance.

Intravascular pressures

Pressures in the heart and great vessels are still usually measured routinely with a fluid-filled catheter and an external transducer. The operator should always check the pressure tracings or the oscilloscope during the procedure to ensure that the recorded tracing is not damped. There are many factors that might interfere with the recording of a pressure tracing, even when the system has been tested previously. Most commonly, a small or large air bubble in the catheter, stopcock, connecting tube or transducer itself may cause damping. This can be overcome by flushing saline in both directions to remove bubbles. A small clot in the tip of the catheter may also interfere with frequency response. Another common cause of interference is a small leak in the system, which allows blood to enter the catheter, particularly when the tip is in a high-pressure area. The presence of blood in the catheter is particularly likely to produce marked damping of the pressure tracing when the catheter lumen is narrow and the length great. Repeated forceful flushing of the catheter with small amounts of heparinized saline is most helpful in preventing damping of pressure recordings.

It is customary to refer all intravascular pressures to atmospheric pressure, and the midpoint of the anteroposterior chest diameter is used as the zero reference level. Routinely, all pressures are measured at end expiration, as this seems to be least affected by changes in respiratory pattern. However, if an infant is grunting or an older child is having expiratory difficulty, the end-expiratory pressure may be raised considerably and not be reliable.

Vena cava and right atrial pressures

Pressure in the superior vena cava (SVC) is similar to that in the right atrium except when there is an obstruction at the SVC–right atrial junction. Inferior vena cava (IVC) pressure within the thoracic cavity is also similar to right atrial pressure. In all these sites, pressure decreases during inspiration and increases with expiration. When the catheter is in the IVC below the diaphragm, there is modification of respiratory changes; pressure alterations are less prominent and there is also usually a slight increase during inspiration and a decrease during expiration.

The contour typical of right atrial pressure is shown in Figure 4.1. The *a* wave is due to atrial systole, the *c* wave is associated with onset of ventricular

Congenital Diseases of the Heart, 3rd edition. By A. Rudolph
© 2009 Blackwell Publishing, ISBN: 9781405162456

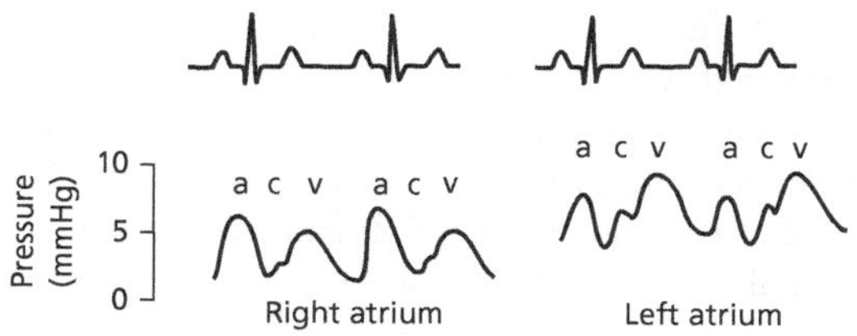

Figure 4.1 Normal pressure contours and levels in the right and left atria.

systole, and the *v* wave is associated with atrial and ventricular filling. The *a* wave is the dominant wave, and in the right atrium is almost always taller than the *v* wave. When the heart rate is rapid, the *c* wave is often not identifiable.

In older children, mean right atrial pressure is about 2–6 mmHg, with an *a* wave of 5–10 mmHg and a *v* wave of 4–8 mmHg. In infants, the mean pressure is usually 0–4 mmHg, with correspondingly lower *a* and *v* waves. In premature infants, right atrial pressure tends to be even lower. The *a* wave is increased with right ventricular hypertrophy, tricuspid stenosis or atresia, and in any condition that decreases compliance of the right ventricle such as constrictive pericarditis. It is also frequently increased in arrhythmias. The classic example is the "cannon" *a* wave found in complete atrioventricular dissociation, when the atrium contracts against a closed tricuspid valve and *a* wave pressures of 15–25 mmHg may be developed. However, it can also be found in other arrhythmias.

The right atrial *c* wave may be increased and occur late in the cycle in patients with tricuspid insufficiency and blends with the *v* wave to form a large *cv* wave. In mild insufficiency there may be only a limited increase in the size of the *c* and *v* waves. The waves also may not be very prominent if the regurgitated volume is accommodated in a large and compliant atrium and venous system. The *v* wave is also increased when right ventricular compliance is decreased, and also in cardiac failure, as part of the general increase in right atrial pressures. In patients with large atrial septal defects, the *a* and *v* waves are often of similar height, and there may be a deep *x* and *y* descent.

Diastolic pressure differences between the right atrium and right ventricle should be measured, particularly in early diastole during the rapid inflow phase and in late diastole at the time of the *a* wave, in order to assess the presence of tricuspid stenosis. This is done ideally with two catheters, measuring both pressures simultaneously. Since this is often not feasible, a rapid pressure tracing can be recorded at high amplification as the catheter is withdrawn from the right ventricle into the right atrium. Comparison of the pressures during the same phase of the respiratory cycle can detect abnormal pressure gradients.

Right ventricular pressure

Right ventricular systolic pressure is usually about 15–25 mmHg in normal children and adults, and the end-diastolic pressure is equal to or slightly lower than the atrial *a* wave. If the heart rate is rapid or the PR interval short, the end-diastolic pressure is equal to the *a* wave, but when the PR interval is long, the *a* wave begins to descend before ventricular systole commences.

In the infant, right ventricular systolic pressure is normally higher than in older children and adults. At birth, the pressure is similar to that in the systemic arteries but it falls rapidly, paralleling the postnatal fall in pulmonary arterial systolic pressure.

Right ventricular systolic pressure is increased when there is a large ventricular septal defect, pulmonary stenosis, or increased pulmonary vascular resistance. End-diastolic pressure is increased in heart failure, severe pulmonary outflow obstruction, and with decreased compliance as in constrictive pericarditis and tamponade. When the ventricular septum is intact and there is moderate to severe right ventricular outflow obstruction, the pressure contour is modified, showing a slower rise and fall and thus appearing more triangular in shape than usual. The more severe the stenosis, the more triangular the contour.

On careful withdrawal of the catheter from the pulmonary artery to the tricuspid valve, it is usually possible to determine the site of obstruction in the right ventricle (Figure 4.2).

Pulmonary arterial pressure

Pulmonary arterial systolic pressure is normally similar to right ventricular systolic pressure; pulmonary arterial diastolic pressure in the older child is about 8–12 mmHg and mean pressure about 10–16 mmHg. Few reliable measurements of

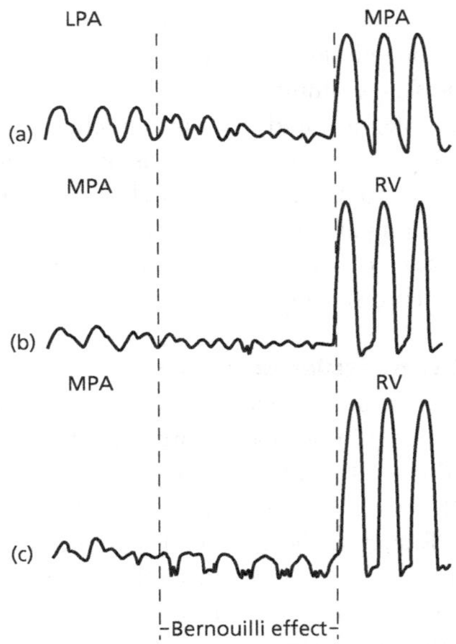

Figure 4.2 (a) Pressure recorded during withdrawal of a catheter from the left pulmonary artery (LPA) into the main pulmonary artery (MPA) across a stenotic area. (b, c) Pressures recorded during withdrawal from the main pulmonary artery into the right ventricle (RV) across a stenotic valve. In (a) and (b) the systolic pressure falls just beyond the stenosis, but in (c) there is actually a negative systolic pressure. All represent examples of the Bernoulli effect. Note also the low diastolic pressure in the main pulmonary artery, characteristic of peripheral pulmonary stenosis.

normal pulmonary arterial pressure have been obtained in infants immediately after birth and at various ages after birth. However, on the basis of observations in animals and a limited number of measurements in human babies, it appears that at birth, prior to ventilation, the pulmonary arterial pressure is about (65–80)/(35–50) mmHg, with a mean pressure of 40–70 mmHg. The pressure falls postnatally, at first rapidly and then more gradually (see Chapter 5). Pulmonary arterial systolic pressure is increased if there is a large communication between the two ventricles or the aorta and pulmonary artery; in the latter case, diastolic pressure is also equal to aortic pressure if the communication is very large. If pulmonary vascular resistance is low, the pulmonary arterial diastolic pressure may be considerably lower than aortic diastolic pressure in patients with large ventricular septal defect, even though systolic pressures are similar.

Systolic, diastolic, and mean pressures are increased when pulmonary vascular resistance is elevated by vascular or pulmonary disease and when pulmonary venous pressure is elevated. The level of pulmonary arterial diastolic pressure may be quite valuable as a guide to the level of pulmonary vascular resistance in patients with large communications between the two ventricles or when both great vessels arise from the same ventricle. If pulmonary arterial diastolic pressure is two-thirds of systolic pressure or more, it is likely that pulmonary vascular resistance is high; if it is one-third to half of systolic pressure, pulmonary vascular resistance is likely to be only slightly or moderately increased (see Chapter 5).

In assessing whether the pulmonary circulation responds to vasodilators, the response of diastolic pressure is helpful. With a large ventricular septal defect, even though pulmonary vascular resistance may fall, the right ventricular and pulmonary arterial systolic pressure will remain equal to aortic systolic pressure. However, if pulmonary vascular resistance is reduced, pulmonary arterial diastolic pressure will fall; if the pulmonary circulation does not respond to vasodilators, pulmonary arterial diastolic pressure will not change significantly. This analysis of pulmonary vascular resistance based on diastolic pressure is, of course, of no value in the presence of pulmonary valvar insufficiency.

In newborn infants, there is frequently a pressure drop between the main pulmonary artery and the left and right branches, probably related to the normal difference in size of the vessels. The main pulmonary artery in the fetus leads directly into the large ductus arteriosus, and the two pulmonary arteries arise as branches from this large trunk. After birth, when the ductus closes, this pattern persists and gradually assumes the adult configuration after 3–6 months. The pressure difference is normally quite small, only up to about 10–15 mmHg systolic and 5–8 mmHg mean pressure. However, if there is increased pulmonary blood flow due to left-to-right shunts, larger pressure differences can occur (see Chapter 5).

Pulmonary valvar or peripheral pulmonary artery stenosis may produce a change in pressure contour related to the Bernoulli phenomenon. This is manifested by a decrease in, or actual negative, systolic pressure just beyond the stenosis as the catheter is withdrawn from the periphery through the stenotic area (Figure 4.2). It is related to the high velocity of blood flowing through the orifice past the catheter lumen. In patients with main pulmonary artery stenosis, the pressure tracing in the proximal segment between the valve and the stenosis usually shows a very low diastolic pressure even in the absence of valvar insufficiency (Figure 4.2).

Pulmonary artery wedge, pulmonary venous, and left atrial pressures

Pulmonary arterial wedge pressure is obtained either by passing an end-hole catheter distally into a pulmonary artery to occlude the branch or by inflating a balloon proximal to the tip of an end-hole catheter (Swan–Ganz catheter). This provides a pressure that is similar to that in the pulmonary veins and left atrium. The pulmonary wedge pressure usually shows damping of the *a* and *v* waves and usually has a mean level 2–3 mmHg higher than pulmonary venous pressure. It is more likely to be representative of pulmonary venous pressure when the latter is increased; when it is low, no phasic pressure may be noted in the wedge position.

Pulmonary venous and left atrial pressures are similar in contour and level. Whereas the right atrium usually shows a dominant *a* wave, the left atrium shows a dominant *v* wave (see Figure 4.1). This dominance of the *v* wave is not related to the connection with the left ventricle and systemic circulation but is transmitted from the pulmonary arteries and is related to pulmonary blood flow. In patients in whom a pulmonary vein drains into the right atrium, *v* wave dominance is noted in the vein, up to a region near its entry into the right atrium, where it assumes the characteristic of the right atrial pressure contour, with the *a* wave becoming prominent. Also, in patients with total anomalous pulmonary venous drainage, if a catheter can be inserted into the pulmonary veins, a dominant *v* wave is observed. If pulmonary blood flow is high, the *v* wave may be transmitted to the junction of the common pulmonary venous trunk with the systemic veins. Also, in these individuals, if the right atrium shows a dominant *a* wave, similar dominance is seen in the left atrium, which receives all its blood from the right atrium.

In patients with large left-to-right shunts, the *v* wave is usually increased in amplitude relative to the *a* wave. Frequently, there is also a pressure difference between the pulmonary vein and the left atrium in infants and small children with large left-to-right shunts, probably related to the high flow and possibly associated with the presence of the catheter in a vein of relatively small diameter. When pulmonary blood flow is low, as in patients with pulmonary atresia, the pulmonary venous and left atrial pressure contours do not show the prominent *v* wave.

The mean left atrial pressure in older children is normally about 5–10 mmHg, with the *a* wave about 6–12 mmHg and *v* wave about 8–15 mmHg. In infants, the mean pressure is usually only 3–6 mmHg, with correspondingly lower *a* and *v* waves.

Pressure differences between left and right atrium

In many patients, particularly in those with cyanotic congenital heart disease, and in most infants, it is possible to pass the venous catheter across an atrial opening into the left atrium. In these instances, it is customary to measure the pressure differences between the left and right atrium. In view of the fact that there are often marked respiratory variations in pressure, comparisons are best made in pressures recorded simultaneously with a catheter in each chamber. Since this is usually not practical, especially in infants, tracings of the two pressures at the same phase of respiration and heart rate can be compared by superimposition.

Frequently it has been assumed that if left and right atrial mean pressures are equal, there is a large communication between the atria; this assumption may be erroneous. Because atrial pressures are determined by compliance of the atrial wall and venous return, and by ventricular compliance, it is quite possible to have equal mean pressures with only a small septal opening. Phasic pressures between the atria may be quite different under these circumstances.

A pressure difference between the right and left atrium may be noted with tricuspid atresia and total anomalous pulmonary venous drainage; in these lesions the total systemic output passes from the right to the left atrium across the septum. The mean pressure may be only 1–2 mmHg higher in the right atrium but it may reach differences of 5 mmHg or greater if the atrial opening is small. If the opening is small, there usually is a tall *a* wave, greater than 15 mmHg, in the right atrium. With mitral or aortic atresia, total pulmonary venous return passes across the atrial septum from the left to the right atrium. Left atrial pressure is higher than the right, and if the atrial opening is small, a prominent *a* wave as well as *v* wave may be seen. Although equal mean pressures in the two atria are not helpful in excluding the possibility that the atrial opening is small, a large pressure difference is positive evidence of the fact that the opening is not large. A large left-to-right atrial pressure difference in infants with patent ductus arteriosus, coarctation of the aorta or aortic stenosis, in whom there is often a large atrial left-to-right shunt, indicates that the atrial septal opening is small and that it may represent a dilated foramen ovale.

Pulmonary venous wedge pressure

In some patients, it may not be possible to manipulate a catheter into a pulmonary artery. This may occur in patients who have undergone the original Fontan procedure (atria to pulmonary artery connection) and the catheter cannot be manipulated past the anastomosis. It may be possible to enter one pulmonary artery but not the other, because unilateral pulmonary stenosis is present. It may be important to know the level of pulmonary arterial pressure to assist in making decisions about therapy. A technique that has been helpful is measurement of pulmonary venous wedge pressure. If an end-hole catheter or balloon catheter with an end-hole can be manipulated into a pulmonary vein, wedging it in the vein in the periphery of the lung can provide a reliable estimate of mean pulmonary arterial pressure [1]. The technique is most unreliable when pulmonary arterial mean pressure is elevated above 40 mmHg; pulmonary venous wedge pressure is considerably lower, presumably because the small pulmonary vessels are markedly narrowed and this interferes with adequate transmission of pulmonary arterial pressure.

Left atrial to left ventricular pressure differences

Pressure differences between the left atrium and ventricle during diastole are best demonstrated by simultaneous recording with two catheters. If the left atrium cannot be entered, pulmonary arterial wedge pressure may be recorded, although it is not as reliable. A pressure difference is noted in mitral stenosis, both in the rapid inflow phase and during atrial systole. A gradient may also be noted when there is a large diastolic flow across the mitral valve, as in large left-to-right shunts and in mitral regurgitation. This is most prominent in the rapid inflow phase in early diastole.

Left ventricular and systemic arterial pressure

Left ventricular and aortic systolic pressures are normally equal. In the mature newborn infant, the systolic pressure is usually 65–80 mmHg and arterial diastolic pressure is 45–60 mmHg, with a mean arterial pressure of 60–65 mmHg. The pressures are normally considerably lower in premature infants, depending on gestational age. In an infant of 30 weeks' gestation, the pressure is in the range 40–50 mmHg systolic, 25–35 mmHg diastolic, and 30–35 mmHg mean. It increases fairly linearly with gestational age to the levels given for mature infants. After birth there is also a gradual increase in arterial pressures. By 1 year after birth, the systolic pressure averages 90–110 mmHg and diastolic pressure 65–75 mmHg, with a mean pressure of 70–80 mmHg.

Left ventricular systolic pressure is increased when there is outflow obstruction. Left ventricular end-diastolic pressure is increased in left ventricular failure, decreased left ventricular compliance, left ventricular outflow obstruction, mitral insufficiency, and any condition in which there is a marked increase in pulmonary venous return to the left ventricle due to left-to-right shunting.

The pressure contour in the ascending aorta is normally quite different from that in the descending aorta and the major peripheral arteries. Systolic pressure is usually lower and diastolic pressure higher. As the catheter is withdrawn peripherally, there is usually an increase in systolic pressure and a decrease in diastolic pressure, although mean pressures are similar. This difference is related to several hemodynamic factors, such as pressure pulse transmission, flow velocity, and pressure waves reflected from the peripheral vascular resistance. The importance of this phenomenon is that if left ventricular and systemic arterial systolic pressures are being examined to assess the presence of obstruction in the outflow tract, mild degrees of aortic stenosis may not be recognized if central aortic pressure is not measured. The systolic pressure in a femoral or brachial artery may be as much as 20–30 mmHg higher than that in the ascending aorta. Thus, if a needle or cannula is inserted into the peripheral artery to compare arterial with left ventricular pressure to assess the presence of aortic stenosis, an incorrect interpretation of its presence, or severity, may be made.

The aortic pressure contour is altered by any condition in which there is increased diastolic runoff, such as in aortopulmonary shunts, arteriovenous fistulae, low peripheral vascular resistance, and aortic insufficiency. The pressure rises very sharply, falls rapidly and has a low dicrotic notch, and diastolic pressure is reduced. In aortic stenosis, when severe, the upstroke is delayed and there may be an anacrotic notch; the pulse pressure is often also narrowed.

In several conditions in which the velocity of left ventricular ejection may be increased, a rapid rise in aortic pressure may be seen, with normal diastolic pressures. This accounts for the palpation of a peripheral pulse that has a sharp upstroke and may be mistaken for a wide pulse pressure. It is noted in ventricular septal defect and mitral insufficiency.

A pressure difference between the ascending and descending aorta is noted in aortic coarctation. The nature of the pressure difference varies with the severity and the collateral circulation. In mild coarctation there may be only a small difference of 15–20 mmHg in systolic pressure, with no diastolic pressure difference. In severe stenoses with little or no collateral circulation, a large systolic and diastolic pressure difference occurs, and the systolic pressure in the descending aorta may be lower than the diastolic pressure in the ascending aorta. This is usually observed during infancy. However, if collateral arteries are well developed, even in severe obstruction, the diastolic pressure in the descending aorta may be only slightly lower than that in the ascending aorta, and there may be a systolic pressure difference of as little as 20–30 mmHg. The descending aortic pressure does show a very slow upstroke. However, in view of these pressure findings, it is important to realize that the severity of a coarctation cannot be assessed from pressure differences alone, except when a large difference is present.

Systolic pressure differences between the ventricles and the aorta and the pulmonary artery

Normally, systolic pressures in the left ventricle and aorta are considerably higher than those in the right ventricle and pulmonary artery. In the presence of a large ventricular or aortopulmonary communication, these pressures are equal. A comparison of left- and right-sided ejection pressures is therefore valuable in assessing the size of the communication. In a patient with a ventricular septal defect, right ventricular and pulmonary arterial systolic pressures may be increased to the level in the left ventricle by increased pulmonary flow or increased pulmonary vascular resistance. Differences in left and right ventricular systolic pressures, even intermittently, suggest that the communication is not very large. When left and right ventricular systolic pressures are equal, separation may be induced by administering a pulmonary vasodilator, which may result in a fall in pulmonary arterial and right ventricular systolic pressure below left ventricular systolic pressure. Induction of ventricular ectopic beats by manipulating the catheter against the wall of the ventricle may also demonstrate differences in systolic pressures. However, if right and left ventricular systolic pressures remain identical with all maneuvers, it is indicative of the fact that the ventricular septal defect is very large (at least the diameter of the aortic orifice).

Cardiac output and intravascular shunts

Cardiac output was first measured in humans by application of the Fick technique, involving measurement of oxygen consumption and the arteriovenous oxygen difference across the lungs. This technique has been used extensively in the assessment of congenital heart disease; for this reason, it is presented in some detail.

Fick technique

Measurement of oxygen consumption

Oxygen consumption must be measured if blood flows are to be calculated by the Fick method using oxygen content of blood samples. Oxygen consumption is now usually measured by the open circuit method (see Chapter 4). In the past it was measured by collecting expired air, and in some centers this method is still preferrred in older children and adults. The technique involves collecting a timed sample of expired air by having the patient breathe through a respiratory valve attached to a mouthpiece while the nostrils are clamped. The expired air may be collected in either a Douglas bag or a Tissot spirometer. Similar collections can be made in newborn infants using a nasal valve. These closed-system methods for measuring oxygen consumption cannot readily be used in infants and children and have been largely replaced by open or flow-through systems, which are easily constructed or are commercially available. The method of making the calculations for the closed systems is briefly presented because it explains the principles on which the measurement is based.

Some of the standard terms for designating gas volumes and proportions are shown in the box below; the proportions of individual gases in a mixture are usually given as a fraction of the total volume. Usually, V_I, or inspired air volume, is not measured but V_E alone is collected and measured.

V_I	Total volume of inspired air
$\dot{V}_I$	Volume of air inspired per minute
V_E	Total volume of expired air
$\dot{V}_E$	Volume of air expired per minute
$\dot{V}O_2$	Volume of oxygen consumed per minute
$\dot{V}CO_2$	Volume of carbon dioxide produced per minute
F_I	Fraction of gas in inspired air
F_IO_2, F_ICO_2, F_IN_2	Fractions of oxygen, carbon dioxide, and nitrogen in inspired air
F_E	Fraction of gas in expired air
F_EO_2, F_ECO_2, F_EN_2	Fractions of oxygen, carbon dioxide, and nitrogen in expired air

Calculation of oxygen consumption from expired air
The amount of oxygen consumed can be derived from the folowing equation:

$$\dot{V}O_2 = \dot{V}_I F_IO_2 - \dot{V}_E F_EO_2 \quad (4.1)$$

However, while oxygen is consumed, carbon dioxide is eliminated into expired air, and the volumes of oxygen consumed and carbon dioxide eliminated may be different, so that $\dot{V}_I$ is not necessarily equal to $\dot{V}_E$.

Apart from very minute quantities of other gases, inspired and expired air consist largely of oxygen, carbon dioxide, and nitrogen. Thus,

$$V_I F_IN_2 + V_I F_IO_2 + V_I F_ICO_2 = V_E F_EN_2 + V_E F_EO_2 + V_E F_ECO_2 \quad (4.2)$$

Since nitrogen does not exchange across the lungs during respiration,

$$\dot{V}_I F_IN_2 = \dot{V}_E F_EN_2$$

or

$$\dot{V}_I = \dot{V}_E F_EN_2 / F_IN_2 \quad (4.3)$$

In order to substitute for $\dot{V}_I$ in equation (4.1), the following can be applied if the fraction of carbon dioxide in expired air is measured:

$$\dot{V}_E = \dot{V}_E F_EN_2 + \dot{V}_E F_EO_2 + \dot{V}_E F_ECO_2$$

Thus,

$$\dot{V}_E F_EN_2 = \dot{V}_E(1 - F_EO_2 - F_ECO_2) \quad (4.4)$$

Room air contains 20.93% or a fraction of 0.2093 of oxygen, and 0.03% or a fraction of 0.0003 of carbon dioxide. The fraction of nitrogen in inspired air is thus 1 – 0.2093 – 0.0003 or 0.7904.

Substituting in equation (4.3)

$$\dot{V}_I = \frac{\dot{V}_E(1 - F_EO_2 - F_ECO_2)}{0.7904}$$

and substituting in equation (4.1)

$$\dot{V}O_2 = \left[\frac{\dot{V}_E(1 - F_EO_2 - F_ECO_2)}{0.7904}\right] F_IO_2 - \dot{V}_E F_EO_2$$

In room air $F_IO_2 = 0.2093$

$$\dot{V}O_2 = \dot{V}_E\left[\left(1 - F_EO_2 - F_ECO_2 \times \frac{0.2093}{0.7904}\right) - F_EO_2\right]$$

$$\dot{V}O_2 = \dot{V}_E[0.265(1 - F_EO_2 - F_ECO_2) - F_EO_2] \quad (4.5)$$

If F_ECO_2 is not measured and equation (4.1) is used and it is assumed that $\dot{V}_I = \dot{V}_E$, a reasonably accurate measurement of $\dot{V}O_2$ will be obtained but there will be a small error. The magnitude of the error will depend on the difference between $\dot{V}CO_2$ and $\dot{V}O_2$. This is related to body metabolism and the respiratory exchange ratio (RER):

$$RER = \dot{V}CO_2/\dot{V}O_2$$

If there is predominantly carbohydrate metabolism, the RER is close to 1 and $\dot{V}CO_2 = \dot{V}O_2$ and the error using equation (4.1) is minimal. However, if there is largely fat metabolism, as in starvation, RER is reduced to near 0.7 and the error would then be larger but still not more than about 6–7% of actual oxygen consumption.

If F_{ECO_2} is measured, $\dot{V}CO_2$ can be calculated easily if the patient is breathing room air, because

$$\dot{V}CO_2 = \dot{V}_E F_{ECO_2} - \dot{V}_I F_{ICO_2}$$

Since F_{ICO_2} in room air is 0.0003, it is negligible and therefore

$$\dot{V}CO_2 = \dot{V}_E F_{ECO_2} \quad (4.6)$$

It is customary to express the volumes of oxygen consumed and carbon dioxide produced in terms of volumes of dry gas at standard temperature and pressure dry (STPD). When expired air leaves the nose or mouth it is at body temperature and pressure and fully saturated with water vapor (BTPS). When it is collected in a bag or spirometer, the temperature falls to room temperature, the volume measured is at ambient temperature and pressure, and it is still saturated with water vapor (ATPS).

The volume of expired gas as measured must therefore be converted from ATPS to STPD. The principles embodied in Boyle's law and Charles law are used in this conversion:

$$\frac{P_1V_1}{T_1} = \frac{P_2V_2}{T_2} \quad (4.7)$$

where V_1 and V_2 represent volumes of gas, P_1 and P_2 gas pressures, and T_1 and T_2 temperatures. Standard pressure is 760 mmHg and standard temperature is 273 K. The collected sample gas pressure is the same as barometric pressure (P_B) but, because it is saturated with water vapor, this water vapor pressure must be deducted. Water vapor pressures at various temperatures can be obtained from published tables. The room temperature or spirometer temperature should be measured also. This is usually measured in degrees Celsius and 273 is added to convert it to degrees Kelvin.

Using equation (4.7), if the volume V_1 is to be determined at STPD, $P = 760$ mmHg and $T = 273$ K. Thus,

$$= \frac{V_2 \times (P_B - P_{H_2O})}{T_2}$$

or

$$V_1 = V_2 \times \frac{273}{T_2} \times \frac{P_B - P_{H_2O}}{760} \quad (4.8)$$

Tables have also been published that provide a factor with which to multiply the measured volume, V_2, to convert it to STPD. It is usually very close to 0.9 and, in general, if $\dot{V}_E$, measured at ATPS, is multiplied by 0.9, it will provide a reasonably close measure of the STPD volume.

The most common problem in measurement of oxygen consumption by these methods is that there may be loss of some of the expired air, usually because the nostrils are not completely closed or because children do not hold their lips tightly enough around the mouthpiece. Another source of leak is if the inspiratory side of the valve allows expired air to escape. A second major problem is rebreathing. If the expiratory side of the valve leaks and allows expired air to be inhaled during inspiration, the F_{IO_2} and F_{ICO_2} will be different from the figures for room air that are used in the calculations. A similar problem will arise if the dead space of the valve is too large for the subject in whom it is being used.

Open-circuit method

Using the open-circuit method, oxygen consumption can readily be measured in young children and infants of any age or size. A hood is placed over the child's head and a stream of air is pulled over the head using a pump that will maintain a constant rate of airflow, at least four to five times the expected tidal volume, so that expired air does not collect in the hood. In this method, the child's expired air is mixed with several volumes of room air.

When the open-circuit method is used for measurement of oxygen consumption in infants, the expired oxygen fraction (F_{EO_2}) is continuously measured by sampling using a very sensitive oximeter. This is important, because the oxygen difference between air and expired air will be small. The inspired oxygen fraction ($F\text{IO}_2$) is room air. The oxygen difference is thus easily determined by subtraction. The volume of air being removed by the pump is measured in the expiratory side. Although there is a small difference in $V\text{I}$ and $V\text{E}$, depending on RER, this can be disregarded in the open-circuit method, because of the huge volume of room air that dilutes the expired air volume. However, it is necessary to correct the total expired volume from ATPS to STPD using the method outlined above.

An example demonstrates how $\dot{V}\text{O}_2$ is calculated.

> Assume the following: measured expired volume withdrawn by the pump is 10 L/min; temperature is 27°C and barometric pressure 755 mmHg; measured oxygen in the air withdrawn by the pump is 20.43% or 0.2043; and water vapor pressure derived from the appropriate table is 5.5 mmHg. The calculation using equation (4.8) would be
>
> Volume of gas withdrawn (converted to STPD)
>
> $$= 10 \times \frac{273}{300} \times \frac{755 - 5.5}{760} = 8.97 \text{ L/min}$$
>
> Assuming the room air oxygen fraction as 0.2093, oxygen fraction difference is 0.2093 − 0.2043 = 0.005. Correction factor for the RER of 0.9 is 1.02:
>
> $$\dot{V}\text{O}_2 = 8.97 \times 0.005 \times 1.02$$
> $$= 0.0457 \text{ L/min or } 45.7 \text{ mL/min}$$

If it is technically impossible to measure oxygen consumption because of lack of cooperation, oxygen consumption can be assumed on the basis of measurement of oxygen consumption. In normal infants and children at various ages, it has been established that oxygen consumption is related to body surface area (see below). However, it should be appreciated that $\dot{V}\text{O}_2$ may vary greatly under different circumstances and may also be altered by cardiac failure and possibly by marked hypoxemia; therefore, it is always desirable to make actual measurements.

Calculation of cardiac output and shunts using the Fick method

The Fick principle is easily understood if one considers a situation in which a known amount of some indicator (I) is added to a volume of fluid (V). If the concentrations of the indicator in the fluid before (C_{I_1}) and after (C_{I_2}) this addition are known, the volume of fluid can be calculated:

$$\text{Since } VC_{I_2} - VC_{I_1} = I, \text{ then } V = \frac{I}{C_{I_2} - C_{I_1}}$$

In a similar mann.er, if there is a constant flow of a liquid, the volume flow per unit time can be calculated from the following equation:

$$\dot{Q} = \frac{I}{C_{I_2} - C_{I_1}} \tag{4.9}$$

where $\dot{Q}$ represents the flow rate, I any substance added or removed, and C_{I_1} and C_{I_2} the concentra tions before and after the site of exchange.

Although any indicator substance may be used, the method has been applied most frequently using the normal physiological uptake of oxygen as the indicator. In the individual with normal circulation, oxygen is taken up by blood in the lungs and the flow is represented by the following equation:

$$\dot{Q} = \frac{\dot{V}\text{O}_2}{\text{CaO}_2 - \text{C}\bar{v}\text{O}_2} \tag{4.10}$$

where $\dot{V}\text{O}_2$ represents oxygen consumption per unit time, CaO_2 arterial oxygen content, and CvO_2 mixed venous oxygen content. Since normally right and left ventricular outputs are equal, $\dot{Q}$ represents cardiac output (CO). The units usually applied are as follows:

$$\text{CO (L/min)} = \frac{\dot{V}\text{O}_2 \text{ (mL/min)}}{\text{CaO}_2 \text{ (mL/L)} - \text{CvO}_2 \text{ (mL/L)}} \tag{4.11}$$

Cardiac output changes with age and weight

As shown in Figures 2.4 and 2.5 (see Chapter 2), cardiac output increases with advancing age and increasing weight. It is thus inconvenient to compare cardiac output in individuals of various ages without knowledge of the values for output at different ages and body size. The most important factor in the Fick equation that changes with growth is oxygen consumption, which is linearly related to body surface area. It has thus become customary to express cardiac output in relation to body surface area. *Cardiac index* is the term used for cardiac output per square meter of body surface area. Flow measurements for pulmonary and systemic circulations and for ventricular stroke volumes are also expressed in relation to body surface area. Body surface area is estimated from graphs based on various formulae that take into consideration the individual's height and weight. The reliability of these estimates in infants and particularly premature infants is somewhat questionable. Normal cardiac index is considered to be 2.5–3.5 L/min per m^2 of body surface area.

In calculating cardiac output by the Fick method, it is desirable that oxygen consumption be measured. However, particularly in infants, this is not done routinely and assumed oxygen consumption based on reported values related to body surface area is used. Many laboratories use the data derived by LaFarge and Miettinen [2] in 1970 or others [3,4] to assume oxygen consumption from estimated body surface area. Although oxygen consumption relates fairly well to body surface area, there are differences related to age and sex. Although in adults, oxygen consumption is about 10–20% higher in males than in females, this difference is not apparent in infants and children. In adults and adolescents, oxygen consumption is assumed to be 120–180 mL/min per m^2 body surface area. In children aged about 2–8 years, it is assumed to be 150–200 mL/min per m^2, whereas in infants under 3 months old it is lower, about 120–130 mL/min per m^2.

Considering these variabilities, it is not surprising that correlations between measured and assumed oxygen consumptions are poor. The calculation of cardiac output or blood flows by the Fick method based on assumed oxygen consumption is therefore likely to yield unreliable estimates.

In measuring cardiac output by the Fick method, several other potential errors that may arise require consideration. It is assumed that the volume of oxygen being taken up in the body is in equilibrium with the volume of oxygen being taken up from air in the lungs. Therefore, there must be a steady state of oxygen exchange during the whole period over which the measurement is being made. Since, at rest, it is customary to collect a timed expired air sample for about 3 min, there should be a steady state for a short period before and during the whole collection period. During this period and for some time before, there should be a steady state between the respiratory quotient in the tissues and the RER, because otherwise the relationship RER = $\dot{V}\text{CO}_2/\dot{V}\text{O}_2$ may be altered and thus make $\dot{V}\text{O}_2$ erroneous.

An additional problem is that it is not practical to obtain a continuous measurement of oxygen content of the arterial and mixed venous samples over the whole period, so it is assumed that they are constant. Any change in oxygen content could be a source of error. In the past, samples were usually withdrawn slowly over about a 1-min period in the middle of the expired air collection to try to obtain a sample representative of the whole period. In recent years, however, because very small volumes of blood are required for measurement of oxygen, the blood sample is representative of only a short period of the time over which oxygen consumption is measured.

The arterial blood sample is collected from any systemic artery and the venous sample from the pulmonary artery, as this represents the best mixed venous sample obtainable in the normal individual. Samples from the venae cava or right atrium may not be well mixed and may differ, and thus introduce errors in flow calculation.

Vascular shunts

When shunting of blood occurs in the heart and great vessels, the Fick method has been used to calculate pulmonary and systemic blood flows and the magnitude of the shunts. The equations used are as follows:

$$\dot{Q}\text{p} = \frac{\dot{V}\text{O}_2}{C\text{pvo}_2 - C\text{pao}_2} \qquad (4.12)$$

$$\dot{Q}\text{s} = \frac{\dot{V}\text{O}_2}{C\text{sao}_2 - C\text{mvo}_2} \qquad (4.13)$$

where $\dot{Q}$p represents pulmonary flow, $C\text{pvo}_2$ and $C\text{pao}_2$ oxygen content of pulmonary venous and pulmonary arterial blood respectively, $\dot{Q}$s systemic flow, and $C\text{sao}_2$ and $C\text{mvo}_2$ oxygen content of systemic arterial and mixed venous blood respectively.

In making these calculations, it is assumed that $\dot{V}\text{O}_2$ as measured by uptake in the lungs is equal to the amount of oxygen being used in the body tissues and that there is a steady state during the collection and measurement of blood oxygen content.

When blood is shunted from the left side of the heart to the right, it is added to the systemic blood flow returning from the veins and recirculates through the lungs, increasing pulmonary blood flow by the amount shunted. Thus,

$$\dot{Q}p = \dot{Q}s + \dot{Q}_{L\text{-}R}$$

or

$$\text{Left-to-right shunt } \dot{Q}_{L\text{-}R} = \dot{Q}p - \dot{Q}s \quad (4.14)$$

Similarly, blood shunted from the right side of the heart is added to that returning from the lungs to enter the systemic circulation and therefore

$$\dot{Q}s = \dot{Q}p + \dot{Q}_{R\text{-}L}$$

or

$$\text{Right-to-left shunt } \dot{Q}_{R\text{-}L} = \dot{Q}s - \dot{Q}p \quad (4.15)$$

In some complicated cases of congenital heart disease, blood may be shunted left to right at one level and right to left at another level or even in a bidirectional manner through the same defect. In order to attempt to assess the magnitude of shunt in each direction, the concept of *effective pulmonary blood flow* has been introduced. Effective pulmonary blood flow ($\dot{Q}ep$) is the quantity of mixed venous blood that eventually reaches the lungs to be oxygenated. It can be calculated from the following equation:

$$\dot{Q}ep = \frac{\dot{V}O_2}{CpvO_2 - CmvO_2} \quad (4.16)$$

To calculate left-to-right and right-to-left shunts, the following approach is considered.

If the proportion of mixed venous blood that passes through the lungs is represented by effective pulmonary flow, the rest of the blood flowing through the lung is that which is already oxygenated and is recirculating through the lungs; therefore, physiologically it represents a left-to-right shunt. Total pulmonary flow is a combination of effective pulmonary flow and left-to-right shunt. Thus,

$$\dot{Q}_{L\text{-}R} = \dot{Q}p - \dot{Q}ep \quad (4.17)$$

The total volume of mixed venous blood returning to the right side of the heart usually represents systemic blood flow. There is an exception to this in the presence of a peripheral arteriovenous shunt (see below). The effective pulmonary blood flow is the portion that eventually gets to the lungs to be oxygenated; the remainder enters the systemic arterial circulation without being oxygenated and represents the right-to-left shunt:

$$\dot{Q}_{R\text{-}L} = \dot{Q}s - \dot{Q}ep \quad (4.18)$$

It should be appreciated that these shunt calculations provide estimates of physiological shunting, i.e., the amount of systemic venous blood that reaches the systemic arterial circulation without being oxygenated and the amount of pulmonary venous blood that recirculates through the lungs. The actual anatomic shunts, or actual volumes of blood shunted, may be somewhat larger. For example, if systemic venous blood passes through an atrial septal defect into the left atrium and there is a left-to-right shunt at the ventricular level, some of the systemic venous blood that passed in a right-to-left direction will now pass in a left-to-right direction. This will reach the lungs and therefore will not be calculated as shunt in physiological terms.

Calculation of the ratio of pulmonary to systemic blood flow

In many congenital heart lesions it is convenient to consider the relationship between pulmonary and systemic blood flows. Except for some unusual situations of severe cardiac failure or hypoxia, systemic blood flow does not vary greatly at rest, and the ratio gives an indication of the magnitude of increase or decrease in pulmonary blood flow. The ratio can easily be estimated from measurements of oxygen saturation of pulmonary venous ($SpvO_2$) and arterial ($SpaO_2$) blood and systemic arterial (SaO_2) and mixed venous ($SmvO_2$) blood. If there is no evidence for right-to-left shunting, pulmonary venous and systemic arterial oxygen saturations will be similar.

From equations (4.12) and (4.13)

$$\frac{\dot{Q}p}{\dot{Q}s} = \frac{\dot{V}O_2}{CpvO_2 - CpaO_2} \times \frac{CsaO_2 - CmvO_2}{\dot{V}O_2}$$

Oxygen content is equal to (oxgen capacity × oxygen saturation) + dissolved oxygen. If the patient is breathing room air, dissolved oxygen is small and similar above and below the equation and therefore can be disregarded. Then,

$$\frac{\dot{Q}p}{\dot{Q}s} = \frac{(Sao_2 \times O_2\ capacity) - (Smvo_2 \times O_2\ capacity)}{(Spvo_2 \times O_2\ capacity) - (Spao_2 \times O_2\ capacity)}$$

or

$$\frac{\dot{Q}p}{\dot{Q}s} = \frac{Sao_2 - Smvo_2}{Spvo_2 - Spao_2} \quad (4.19)$$

and if there is no right-to-left shunt

$$\frac{\dot{Q}p}{\dot{Q}s} = \frac{Sao_2 - Smvo_2}{Sao_2 - Spao_2} \quad (4.20)$$

A $\dot{Q}p/\dot{Q}s$ ratio of 1:1 would indicate no shunting in either direction or a bidirectional shunt of equal magnitude. A ratio of 2:1 implies that there is a left-to-right shunt equal to systemic blood flow; a ratio of 4:1 indicates the left-to-right shunt is three times systemic blood flow. A $\dot{Q}p/\dot{Q}s$ ratio less than 1:1 indicates that there is a right-to-left shunt. Thus a ratio of 0.8:1 signifies that pulmonary blood flow is 20% less than systemic blood flow.

Left-to-right shunt through a peripheral arteriovenous malformation

A peripheral arteriovenous malformation allows well-oxygenated arterial blood to enter the venous system and to return to the lungs without passing through the tissues supplied by the systemic arteries; this represents a left-to-right shunt. Considerable confusion has been created by the suggestion that, in patients with arteriovenous malformations, the volume of blood ejected by the left ventricle and returning to the right atrium represents systemic blood flow. This concept is inappropriate.

Systemic blood flow is the volume of blood that passes through the tissues where oxygen and carbon dioxide exchange occurs. Therefore, with arteriovenous malformations, systemic blood flow is the left ventricular output minus the volume of arterial blood shunted into the venous system. This is similar to the hemodynamics in the presence of a patent ductus arteriosus. The blood shunted from the aorta to pulmonary artery is the left-to-right shunt; thus the systemic blood flow is the left ventricular output minus the volume of the left-to-right shunt. It is interesting to note that it is not possible to calculate systemic blood flow reliably by the Fick method in patients with arteriovenous malformations because it is impossible to obtain a representative mixed venous sample. Blood returning to the right atrium will include blood shunted through the arteriovenous malformation. Systemic blood flow can be estimated by using SVC blood if the arteriovenous shunt is in the lower body, or IVC blood if the arteriovenous shunt is in the head or upper body, as the best estimate of mixed venous blood.

Importance of the ratio of pulmonary to systemic blood flow in admixture lesions

The hemodynamics of many congenital heart lesions are characterized by complete or almost complete admixture of the pulmonary and systemic venous returns. Conditions include those listed in Table 4.1. In these conditions, the blood being distributed to the lungs and to the systemic circulation will have the same oxygen saturation. A similar situation prevails in patients in whom pulmonary blood flow is derived entirely from aortic blood. This occurs in individuals with pulmonary atresia when pulmonary blood flow is derived through a patent ductus arteriosus or an aortopulmonary shunt such as a Blalock–Taussig, Potts or Waterston anastomosis. Also, when the pulmonary arteries are absent, pulmonary blood flow is derived from major aortopulmonary collateral or bronchial arteries. In these circumstances, the

Table 4.1 Congenital heart lesions characterized by complete or almost complete admixture of the pulmonary and systemic venous returns.

Admixture at the systemic venous or right atrial level
Total anomalous pulmonary venous drainage
Mitral atresia
Aortic atresia with intact ventricular septum
Admixture at the left atrial level
Tricuspid atresia
Pulmonary atresia with intact ventricular septum
Admixture at the ventricular or great vessel level
Single ventricle
Pulmonary or aortic atresia with ventricular septal defect
Truncus arteriosus communis

oxygen saturation of both systemic and pulmonary arterial blood is largely determined by the $\dot{Q}p/\dot{Q}s$ ratio. Unless there is significant pulmonary disease, the pulmonary venous blood is usually fully or almost fully saturated with oxygen; the other variable factor, then, is systemic mixed venous oxygen saturation. A series of curves can be drawn relating systemic arterial oxygen saturation to the $\dot{Q}p/\dot{Q}s$ ratio at any systemic venous oxygen saturation, assuming that pulmonary venous blood is fully saturated.

If pulmonary venous oxygen saturation is 100% and mixed venous oxygen saturation is 50%

$\dot{Q}p/\dot{Q}s$ ratio	Final saturation
0.5:1	66.6%
1:1	75%
2:1	83.3%
3:1	87.5%
4:1	90%

If pulmonary venous oxygen saturation is 100% and mixed venous oxygen saturation is 70%

$\dot{Q}p/\dot{Q}s$ ratio	Final saturation
0.5:1	80%
1:1	85%
2:1	90%
3:1	92.5%
4:1	94%

These relationships are shown graphically in Figure 4.3. It is quite clear that at lower $\dot{Q}p/\dot{Q}s$ ratios, a small increase in the ratio results in a large increase in arterial oxygen saturation, but at higher ratios a much smaller increase in oxygen saturation occurs with a similar increase in the ratio. This concept is extremely important in therapeutic palliative operations to increase or decrease pulmonary blood flow. If pulmonary blood flow is reduced and systemic arterial oxygen saturation is very low, a shunt that results in a small increase in pulmonary flow and $\dot{Q}p/\dot{Q}s$ ratio will produce a large increase in oxygen saturation. Larger increases in flow produce only relatively small further rises in saturation. However, these large increases in pulmonary blood flow will significantly increase volume load on the heart. Similarly, in a patient with very high pulmonary blood flow, high $\dot{Q}p/\dot{Q}s$ ratio, and

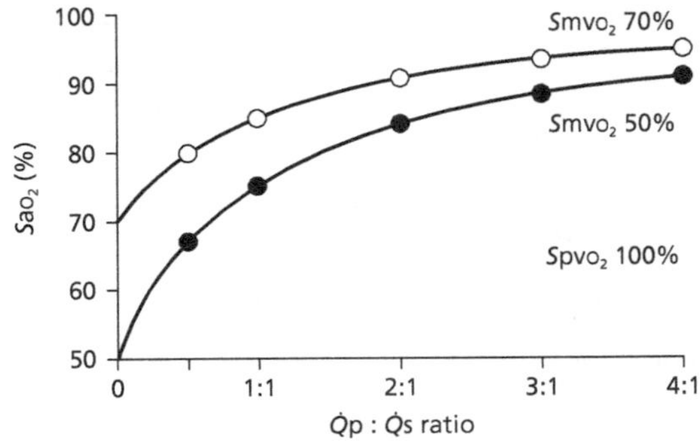

Figure 4.3 Effect of the pulmonary–systemic ratio ($\dot{Q}p$:$\dot{Q}s$) on systemic arterial oxygen saturation (Sa_{O_2}) when there is complete admixture of both systemic and pulmonary venous returns. It is assumed that pulmonary venous oxygen saturation (Spv_{O_2}) is 100%; two curves are drawn, assuming mixed venous oxygen saturation (Smv_{O_2}) at 50% and 70%, respectively.

cardiac failure due to volume loading, pulmonary blood flow can be markedly reduced by a pulmonary artery banding procedure without greatly decreasing arterial oxygen saturation.

Problems and errors in calculating flows and shunts by the Fick method

Some of the general problems in applying the Fick method to calculation of flows have been discussed above, but certain difficulties arise in specific congenital cardiovascular malformations.

Systemic blood flow

A mixed venous blood sample is best obtained from the pulmonary artery in the absence of a left-to-right shunt. When a left-to-right shunt is present, blood obtained in the cardiac chamber proximal to the shunt is used as a mixed venous sample. Thus, with a left-to-right shunt into the pulmonary artery, right ventricular blood is used and this usually reliably represents mixed venous blood. With shunting into the right ventricle, right atrial blood is used; this is not reliable because venous streams from the SVC and IVC are not well mixed and oxygen measurements in different locations of the atrium may vary considerably. Not uncommonly, some degree of tricuspid regurgitation is present and some of the well-oxygenated blood shunted into the right ventricle may be ejected into the atrium. With a left-to-right shunt into the right atrium, it is not possible to obtain a reliable mixed venous sample. SVC and IVC blood samples may have very different oxygen saturations. It has been suggested that mixed venous oxygen saturation be calculated from levels in each cava. Because it has been estimated that venous return through the IVC represents about two-thirds and through the SVC about one-third of total venous return to the heart in adults, mixed venous oxygen saturation is calculated with this assumption. Thus mixed venous oxygen saturation is calculated using two-thirds IVC oxygen saturation and one-third SVC oxygen saturation. This proportioning of SVC and IVC return is different in infants because of differences in body configuration. It has been suggested that in infants an equal upper and lower body venous return be assumed. I know of no recommendations for children at ages between infant and adult. An additional problem in measurement of IVC oxygen saturation is that it may vary greatly depending on the site where the sample is obtained because of streaming. The hepatic veins enter the IVC just below the connection to the right atrium. Renal venous blood has a relatively high oxygen saturation, whereas hepatic venous blood has a relatively low oxygen saturation. Sampling above or below hepatic venous entry can result in large differences in measurement. When one or more pulmonary veins drain into the SVC or IVC, venous blood has to be collected before their entry.

Oxygen saturations in the ascending and descending aorta may be different when there is a right-to-left shunt through the ductus arteriosus. It is therefore not possible to calculate systemic blood flow, because the proportions of flow to the ascending and descending aorta are not known. If it is assumed that the proportions of descending and ascending aortic flows are similar to those of IVC and SVC returns, similar assumptions, as mentioned above, may be used. However, if there is a large difference in oxygen saturations, SVC and IVC oxygen saturations may be different, and since the relative $\dot{V}O_2$ of the upper and lower body is not known, major errors may be involved in attempts to make these calculations.

Pulmonary blood flow

Pulmonary venous oxygen saturation may be similar in all the veins, but if there are differences that are great, it is quite impossible to obtain a true mixed pulmonary venous sample. Even if all pulmonary veins could be sampled, since oxygen consumption in each lobe cannot be measured, it is not possible to measure total pulmonary blood flow accurately. If there is no atrial right-to-left shunting, a left atrial sample is more representative of mixed pulmonary venous blood. In some patients it is not possible to collect pulmonary venous blood. If there is atrial right-to-left shunting, it is commonly assumed that the oxygen saturation in pulmonary venous blood is 96–98% while the patient is breathing room air, but it is quite evident that errors may be involved in this assumption.

Pulmonary arterial oxygen saturation may be different in the left and right pulmonary artery in patients with patent ductus arteriosus, and without knowing the $\dot{V}O_2$ in each lung, it is not possible to calculate pulmonary blood flow accurately. It is also not possible to calculate blood flow to either lung when one lung receives its blood from a pulmonary artery arising from the right ventricle and the other receives its blood supply from bronchial vessels or a pulmonary artery arising from the aorta.

A major and often unrecognized potential error in calculation of pulmonary blood flow may occur when there are large bronchial arterioles anastomosing with distal pulmonary arterioles. When the pulmonary artery arises from the right ventricle, samples obtained in the major pulmonary arteries would have oxygen saturations lower than those in the aorta and bronchial arteries. If there is a large bronchial flow, the true oxygen saturation of precapillary blood would be considerably higher than that measured in the pulmonary arteries. The pulmonary flow calculated from the measured pulmonary arterial oxygen saturation would be considerably lower than the true pulmonary flow. In patients with aortopulmonary transposition with a large bronchial flow, errors in the opposite direction would occur. Oxygen saturation in the pulmonary artery would be higher than that in the aorta and bronchial arteries. With a large bronchial flow, the true pulmonary arterial oxygen saturation of blood perfusing the lungs would be lower and the flow calculated from the oxygen saturation measured in the pulmonary artery would be higher than the actual flow.

Magnitude of arteriovenous difference

The accuracy of calculation of flow by the Fick method is determined, among other factors, by the accuracy with which $\dot{V}o_2$ and arteriovenous oxygen difference can be measured. When the arteriovenous oxygen difference is large, the errors inherent in measuring oxygen content or saturation do not result in major errors in calculation of flow. However, when arteriovenous difference is small, small errors in measurement may result in large errors of flow measurement. The following example demonstrates the problem.

If $\dot{V}o_2$ is 150 mL/min, $Cpvo_2$ 200 mL/L, and $Cpao_2$ 150 mL/L:

$$\dot{Q}p = \frac{150}{200 - 150} = 3 \text{ L/min}$$

If $Cpao_2$ was 5% lower, i.e., 142.5 mL/L:

$$\dot{Q}p = \frac{150}{200 - 142.5} = 2.6 \text{ L/min,}$$

a difference of 7.5%

However, if $\dot{V}o_2$ is 150 mL/min, $Cpvo_2$ 200 mL/L, and $Cpao_2$ 180 mL/L:

$$\dot{Q}p = \frac{150}{200 - 180} = 7.5 \text{ L/min}$$

If $Cpao_2$ was 5% lower, i.e., 171 mL/L:

$$\dot{Q}p = \frac{150}{200 - 171} = 5.2 \text{ L/min,}$$

a difference of 30%

These potential errors would be of particular importance in calculation of pulmonary flow where very large left-to-right shunts are present, and also in aortopulmonary transposition, when pulmonary arterial oxygen saturation is quite high. Similar errors arise in calculating systemic blood flow in patients with severe hypoxemia, in whom systemic arteriovenous differences may be quite small.

Calculation of flow during oxygen administration

Special mention is made of this problem because errors have been, and still are, frequently made in calculation of flows while a patient is breathing oxygen. In fact, there are numerous publications in the scientific literature in which the results are questionable because of incorrect flow calculations.

It has become common practice to derive oxygen content by measuring oxygen saturation and multiplying it by oxygen capacity (see Chapter 3). When a patient is breathing room air and a systemic arterial or pulmonary venous Po_2 is about 100 mmHg, oxygen saturation is almost 100% and dissolved oxygen is only about 0.3 mL/dL or 3 mL/L. If there is a moderately large left-to-right shunt, with a relatively high oxygen saturation of 85% in the pulmonary artery, and if $\dot{V}o_2$ is 150 mL/min and oxygen capacity 200 mL/L, then, if oxygen contents are derived from oxygen saturation:

$$Cpvo_2 = (100/100) \times 200 + 3.0 \text{ (dissolved)} = 203 \text{ mL/L}$$

$$Cpao_2 = (85/100) \times 200 + 2.5 \text{ (dissolved)} = 172.5 \text{ mL/L}$$

$$\dot{Q}p = 150/(203 - 172.5) = 4.9 \text{ L/min}$$

If dissolved oxygen is not taken into account, $Cpvo_2$ is 200 mL/L, $Cpao_2$ 170 mL/L, and $\dot{Q}p$ 5.0 L/min. Thus, little error is produced during breathing of room air.

If the patient is breathing 100% oxygen and pulmonary arterial oxygen saturation is 92%, true oxygen content derived from oxygen saturation can be estimated only if Po_2 is also known. If Po_2 in pulmonary venous blood is 550 mmHg and in pulmonary arterial blood 100 mmHg:

$$Cpvo_2 = (100/100) \times 200 + [5.5 \times 3.0 \text{ (dissolved)}] = 216.5 \text{ mL/L}$$

$$Cpao_2 = (92/100) \times 200 + [1 \times 3.0 \text{ (dissolved)}] = 187.0 \text{ mL/L}$$

$$\dot{Q}p = 150/(216.5 - 187) = 5.1 \text{ L/min}$$

However, if dissolved oxygen is not considered, $Cpvo_2$ is 200 mL/L, $Cpao_2$ 184 mL/L, and $\dot{Q}p$ 150/(200 – 184) or 9.4 L/min. This represents an overestimate of pulmonary blood flow of almost 100%.

Thus in calculation of blood flows by the Fick method during administration of oxygen, it is most reliable to measure oxygen content in the blood samples, but if oxygen saturations are measured, it is imperative that Po_2 also be measured to correct for dissolved oxygen. It should also be realized that not only calculation of flows but also of shunts and pulmonary–systemic flow ratios are in error if these facts are not considered.

Calculation of pulmonary blood flow in special circumstances

Not infrequently, in certain congenital heart lesions it is impossible to pass a catheter into the pulmonary artery, or the flow through the lungs is derived from bronchial vessels. In many of these lesions there is complete admixture of pulmonary and systemic venous returns and the blood perfusing the lungs has the same oxygen saturation as systemic arterial blood. In these conditions, therefore, it is possible to calculate pulmonary blood flow even though a catheter cannot be passed into a pulmonary artery.

$$\dot{Q}p = \frac{\dot{V}o_2}{Cpvo_2 - Cpao_2}$$

However, since $Cpao_2 = Csao_2$

$$\dot{Q}p = \frac{\dot{V}o_2}{Cpvo_2 - Csao_2}$$

$$\dot{Q}s = \frac{\dot{V}o_2}{Csao_2 - Cmvo_2}$$

Indicator dilution techniques

A variety of indicators may be used for quantitative measurement of cardiac output as well as for qualitative assessment of flow patterns. Indicator techniques that have been used include dyes that change optical density of blood, thermodilution, radioisotopes, and radiographic contrast media. These techniques are being used much less frequently in recent years. I do not propose to discuss these techniques in detail, but merely to present the principles involved in their use.

Dye dilution curves

Various dyes, when injected into the circulation, increase the optical density of the blood in specific wavelengths. Blue dyes, such as Evans blue (T-1824) and indigo-carmine, increase optical density in the 620–650 nm range, and indocyanine green increases optical density in the infrared range (± 810 nm). The dye is injected into one part of the circulation and sampled at another site by continuous withdrawal through a cuvette, which senses changes in optical density at the appropriate wavelength. In view of the fact that optical density of blood changes markedly when hemoglobin is oxygenated or reduced, the baseline optical density before dye is injected tends to vary considerably in the 620–650 nm range, particularly in cyanotic patients. In the infrared range, optical densities of reduced hemoglobin and oxyhemoglobin are similar and therefore baseline variation is negligible; indocyanine green dye is thus preferred.

In the absence of a left-to-right or right-to-left shunt, cardiac output can be measured by injecting an indicator into a central vein, the right atrium, a ventricle, or a pulmonary artery and sampling in a peripheral artery. In order to measure cardiac output, it is necessary to calibrate the sensing device for a known concentration of the indicator in blood.

Thermodilution

Blood flows may be determined quantitatively by using cold solutions as the indicator and measuring the change in temperature by means of a rapidly responsive thermistor on a catheter. The advantage of the method is that the indicator may be room-temperature saline and the sensor can be a very tiny thermistor at the tip or on one side of a catheter. The thermistor can be inserted retrogradely through a peripheral artery into the central aorta and injections of saline of known temperature made into the right atrium or pulmonary artery. Little temperature loss occurs across the lungs, accounting for the success of the method. However, if the thermistor is in a peripheral artery, considerable temperature equilibration occurs with surrounding tissues, producing erroneous results.

It is possible to measure flow by the thermodilution method using a single catheter with a thermistor near the tip and a lumen a variable distance proximal to the tip. The thermistor is positioned in the pulmonary artery and the lumen in the SVC or IVC. Room-temperature saline is injected and the curve obtained from the thermistor in the pulmonary artery is used for calculating cardiac

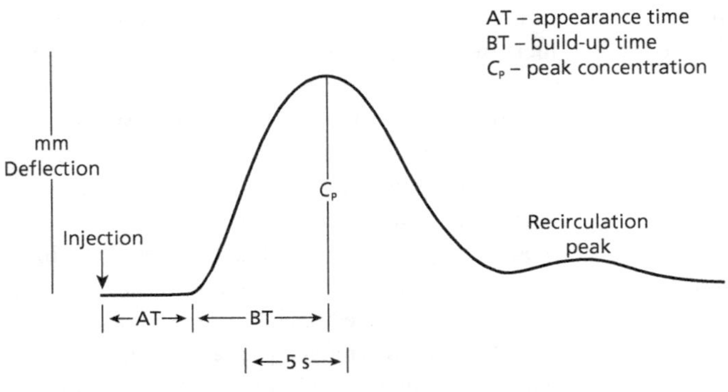

Figure 4.4 Normal dye dilution curve showing appearance time, build-up time, peak concentration, and recirculation.

output. Although this technique is reliable in adults with no shunts, it is often difficult to use in infants and young children because of the problem in placing the injection lumen at an appropriate site when the thermistor is positioned in the pulmonary artery.

Other indicators

Other indicators, particularly radioisotopes, have been used, with external monitoring either by means of crystals for detection of gamma emission over an isolated area or by a scintillation gamma camera to monitor over the whole chest. These techniques are not described in detail here, but the principles are similar to those of dye dilution and thermodilution.

Calculation of cardiac output

The concentration curve of the indicator has the shape shown in Figure 4.4. Based on the Stewart Hamilton principle, cardiac output (CO) can be calculated by dividing the amount of indicator (I) injected by the mean concentration of the indicator ($\bar{C}$) over the period that the concentration curve is inscribed before recirculation occurs:

$$\text{CO} = \frac{I\ (\text{mg})}{\bar{C}\ (\text{mg/mL}) \times t\ (\text{s})}$$

This will give CO in mL/s; in order to measure it in L/min, the equation would be:

$$\text{CO (L/min)} = \frac{I\ (\text{mg}) \times 60}{\bar{C}\ (\text{mg/L}) \times t\ (\text{s})}$$

Because the recirculation peak appears before the indicator concentration falls to near zero, in order to calculate CO it is assumed that the concentration falls exponentially. Difficulty arises in many patients with congenital heart disease with a large left-to-right shunt. Recirculation is so rapid that it is not possible to define the downslope to describe the single circulation curve without interference from recirculation.

In order to overcome this, a method has been designed to calculate flows from the first portion of the curve. This is known as the *forward triangle method* and it makes the assumption that there is a reasonably consistent relationship between the portion of the curve from the onset to the peak and the remaining portion. By dropping a vertical line from the peak concentration (C_p) to baseline, a triangle is formed that has the upward deflection as one side, the vertical line as a second, and the distance between the appearance of the indicator and the peak concentration, known as build-up time (BT), as the third (Figure 4.5). The area of this triangle is $^1/_2 C_p \times$ BT.

It has been shown that, in normal circulations, the area occupied by this triangle is about 0.37 of

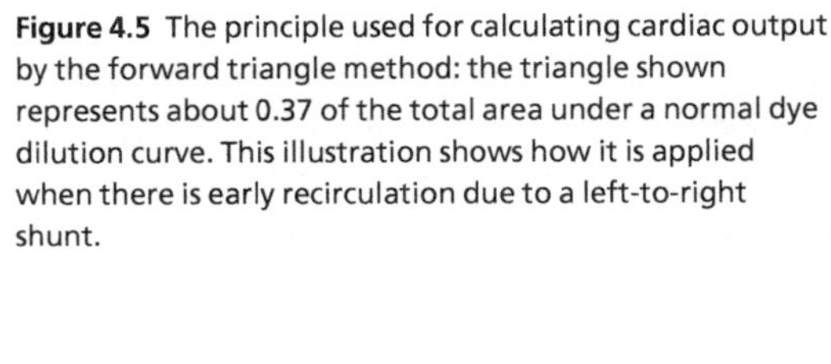

Figure 4.5 The principle used for calculating cardiac output by the forward triangle method: the triangle shown represents about 0.37 of the total area under a normal dye dilution curve. This illustration shows how it is applied when there is early recirculation due to a left-to-right shunt.

the total area of the curve as computed by conventional methods. If this is used as a correction factor, the cardiac output then can be calculated from the following equation:

$$CO = \frac{I \times 60}{\frac{1}{2}C_p \times BT} \times 0.37$$

The figure 0.37 has been derived when injections are made into the central circulation and it is modified if injections are made into peripheral veins. This is the correction necessary for adults, but the factor may be somewhat different in infants and children, and also in the presence of various cardiovascular abnormalities.

There are several potential errors in calculation of cardiac output by the indicator dilution method that make it accurate only to within 15–20% of actual flow. I will not discuss these problems in detail here, but some of the factors that may present difficulties include the following.

- Flow must be constant throughout the withdrawal period.
- Withdrawal must be absolutely constant.
- There must be adequate mixing of indicator with the flowing blood.
- The amount of indicator injected must be measured accurately.
- If the downslope of the curve is very delayed (as occurs in valvar insufficiency), the output calculation may be much more inaccurate.
- If circulation is very slow, the curve inscribed is spread out and because recirculation from some parts of the circulation appears early, it is difficult to delineate the curve for a single circulation and the measurements of output are quite inaccurate.

Indicator curves may also be used qualitatively to demonstrate patterns of blood flow. Thus, the rapid recirculation curve noted with left-to-right shunt results in a curve that may show a sudden change in the downslope just beyond the peak; the earlier this occurs, the larger the left-to-right shunt (Figure 4.6). An early appearance of indicator is indicative of a right-to-left shunt.

It is also possible to detect the level of right-to-left shunting by sampling from a peripheral artery and selectively injecting indicator into different chambers. Thus, if there is an atrial right-to-left shunt, normal curves will be seen with injections into the pulmonary artery or right ventricle, but an early appearance will be noted with injections into the right atria or vena cava. The proportion of right-to-left shunt can be expressed as that percentage of total systemic venous return that is shunted. This can be calculated from an indicator-dilution curve applying the forward triangle method (Figure 4.7).

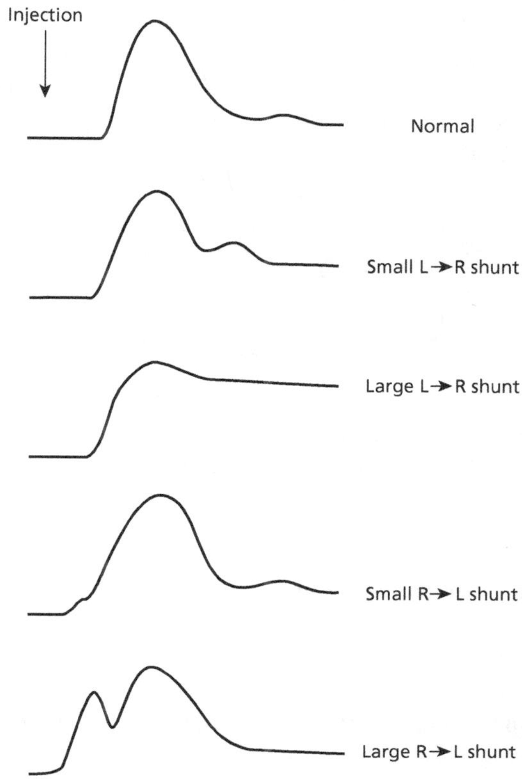

Figure 4.6 Changes in the contour of dye dilution curves produced by left-to-right and right-to-left shunts.

The initial part of the curve represents that proportion of the indicator-labeled blood that is shunted and the second curve is produced by the blood and indicator that pass normally through the circulation. Using the forward triangle method, the shunt flow could be derived from the initial triangle and normal flow from the second triangle. The normal appearance time, needed to calculate BT_2, is derived by extending the upslope of the second curve to the baseline (see Figure 4.7). The sum of the two represents total systemic blood flow.

The right-to-left shunt as a percentage of systemic venous return can then be calculated from the following equation:

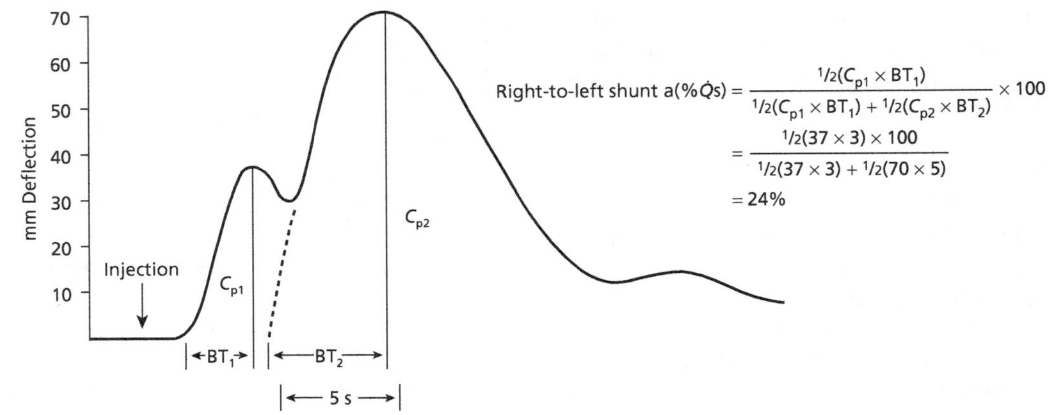

Figure 4.7 The forward triangle method can be used to calculate the right-to-left shunt as a percentage of total systemic venous return by comparing the area of the triangle of the initial curve with that of the major curve.

Right-to-left shunt (%$\dot{Q}$s)

$$= \frac{1/2(C_{p1} \times BT_1)}{1/2(C_{p1} \times BT_1) + 1/2(C_{p2} \times BT_2)} \times 100$$

In applying this type of analysis, it is important to ensure that there is adequate mixing of indicator before the site of the right-to-left shunt.

Vascular resistance

General considerations

The concept of vascular resistance has been used extensively in circulatory physiology to provide an estimate of the response of the vascular bed to various pharmacological and physiological influences. It is based on the Poiseuille equation relating flow, pressures, and the cross-sectional area of the tube through which the fluid flows:

$$Q = \frac{\Delta P \pi r^4}{8 \eta l}$$

where Q is flow, ΔP the pressure difference across the tube, r the radius of the tube, η the viscosity of the fluid, and l the length of the tube. This principle has been applied to assess the cross-sectional area of vascular beds by making certain assumptions. If, in the Poiseuille equation, it is assumed that η, the viscosity of the fluid, and l, the length of the major resistance vessels, are constant, then, since π is a constant,

$$Q \propto \Delta P r^4 \text{ or } \frac{Q}{\Delta P} \propto r^4$$

In the latter relationship, the greater the radius r, the greater the flow, and the term *conductance* has been applied to the ratio $Q/\Delta P$. The larger this value, the larger the cross-sectional area. However, if the reciprocal relationship is considered, then $\Delta P/Q \propto 1/r^4$ and the smaller the radius, the less the flow at any given pressure differential. The ratio $\Delta P/Q$ has been used to express the degree of *resistance* (R) to blood flow; the larger the value, the smaller the cross-sectional area. The equation $R = \Delta P/Q$ has been used extensively; if ΔP is expressed in mmHg and flow in L/min, then resistance is derived as mmHg/L per min and is termed a resistance unit.

The figures derived from this calculation take many major assumptions into account, only some of which are mentioned below.

- In applying the Poiseuille equation, flow is laminar and continuous. In the vascular system, flow is pulsatile, and although it is probably laminar in the small vessels in which resistance is measured, this is not definitely known. In order to apply the varying pulsatile pressure to analysis, a mean pressure is used on either side of the vascular bed in calculating ΔP.
- The Poiseuille relationship was established for saline or other Newtonian fluids. Since blood is a non-Newtonian fluid, there may be marked

differences in patterns of flow in small vessels of different geometry.

• It is generally assumed that viscosity is reasonably constant. Blood viscosity is largely influenced by hematocrit, and the relationship is curvilinear. Over the usual range of hematocrit of 35–45%, little change in viscosity occurs, but with increases beyond 50%, viscosity increases dramatically with small changes in hematocrit. This is important, because in infants with high hematocrits after birth and in older children with cyanotic congenital heart disease, the viscosity factor must be taken into account in considering vascular resistance. A high vascular resistance figure may be calculated and may not reflect the size of the vascular bed but the high hematocrit.

• In the original description, Poiseuille used rigid glass tubes to develop his equation. However, since the vascular system is not rigid, changes in vessel diameter may occur as transmural pressures are changed. Furthermore, the problem is compounded by the fact that with pulsatile pressures there may be alternating changes in vessel diameter and this will be influenced by the compliance of the vessel wall. The influence of transmural pressures is of great importance in interpreting vascular resistance. It has become customary to use the concept of vascular resistance to delineate the state of constriction of the vascular bed, as a constricted bed will have narrow vessels and thus a high resistance. However, it must be realized that resistance is an expression of cross-sectional area and not vessel tone or constriction.

If transmural pressure changes, the calculated figure for vascular resistance may reflect a change in cross-sectional area of the vessels rather than any change in the degree of active constriction or dilatation. An example of this is shown below.

> If mean arterial pressure is 40 mmHg, venous pressure 5 mmHg, and flow 5 L/min, the calculated vascular resistance is (40 – 5)/5 or 7 units. If venous pressure is raised to 15 mmHg, the vessels will be distended by the greater transmural pressure, and for the same flow of 5 L/min, an arterial pressure of only 45 mmHg may be required. The calculated resistance would be (45 – 15)/5 or 6 units.

This is related purely to physical changes in pressure–flow relationships and does not necessarily indicate that there has been vasodilatation on an active basis. Thus, in comparing vascular resistance between different individuals, between one condition and another, and in the same individual at different times, it is necessary to consider the actual levels of arterial and venous pressures, as well as the magnitude of flow.

Calculated resistances in the pulmonary and systemic circulations are often used to compare the state of tone in the vascular bed from one individual to another and in the same individual at different times. However, a problem arises in comparing resistances in individuals of different weights and ages. During the first 6–8 weeks after birth, the pulmonary vasculature is changing from fetal to postnatal morphology; this is associated with a normal fall in pulmonary vascular resistance. Beyond this period, pulmonary arterial pressures change only modestly. Systemic arterial pressure increases slowly with advancing age beyond infancy. The factor in the Poiseuille equation that changes most significantly with weight and age is the flow.

Resistance has therefore been calculated in relation to body surface area, because this provides a figure that is reasonably constant for all ages, except the neonatal period. This is discussed in more detail in the following sections on systemic and pulmonary vascular resistance.

Systemic vascular resistance

Systemic vascular resistance (R_s) is calculated from the following equation:

$$R_s = \frac{Psa\text{ (mean)} - Pra\text{ (mean)}}{\dot{Q}s}$$

where *P*sa is mean systemic arterial pressure (mmHg), *P*ra mean right atrial pressure (mmHg), and $\dot{Q}$s systemic blood flow (L/min).

Normal R_s is about 20 units/m^2 in children, but it varies markedly between about 15 and 30 units/m^2. In newborn infants, arterial pressure is relatively lower and systemic blood flow is similar to that in older children in relation to body surface area. Systemic vascular resistance is lower, in the range 10–15 units/m^2; this gradually rises, reaching a level averaging about 20 units/m^2 at 12–18 months after birth. Thereafter, only a gradual small rise occurs.

The systemic vascular resistance varies greatly in response to sympathetic activity, degree of sedation, and administration of drugs or radiographic contrast medium and is therefore not a particularly useful measurement.

It is not possible to calculate systemic vascular resistance in the presence of aortic coarctation with different ascending and descending aortic pressures, because differential flow to the upper and lower body cannot be calculated. It is also not possible to calculate systemic vascular resistance when there is a right-to-left shunt through the ductus arteriosus, because the respective flows to the upper and lower body are not known.

Pulmonary vascular resistance

The calculated pulmonary vascular resistance is used frequently as a guide to the degree of constriction or obstruction of the pulmonary vascular bed. Often, great reliance is placed on this figure in deciding whether a patient with congenital heart disease should or should not have surgery. This is most unfortunate, as there are many potential errors concerned in making the calculation; this should be recognized in applying the measurement in making decisions. Pulmonary vascular resistance (R_p) is calculated from the following equation:

$$R_p = \frac{Ppa\ (\text{mean}) - Ppv \text{ or } Pla\ (\text{mean})}{\dot{Q}p}$$

where Ppa is mean pulmonary arterial pressure (mmHg), Ppv or Pla mean pulmonary venous or left atrial pressure (mmHg), and $\dot{Q}p$ pulmonary blood flow (L/min).

In older children and adults, normal R_p is 1–3 units/m^2. In the first week after birth, it is considerably higher and normally may be 8–10 units/m^2. It then falls rapidly and by about 6–8 weeks after birth it has reached adult levels. It has been suggested that comparison of pulmonary vascular resistance from one individual to another on the basis of body surface area is inappropriate, as it gives a false impression of the true state of the pulmonary vascular bed. However, we have found it convenient to use the figure of pulmonary vascular resistance per square meter of body surface area in comparisons between different individuals and in following the condition of the pulmonary circulation in the same individual with advancing age.

In making these comparisons, it is important to note the actual level of left atrial pressure. If it is higher than normal, it can be assumed that the pulmonary vessels are being distended to some degree by the increased transmural pressure, and thus the calculated pulmonary vascular resistance would in fact be higher if left atrial pressures were reduced to normal levels. This concept may be important in patients with large ventricular or aortopulmonary left-to-right shunts, in whom left atrial pressure is often elevated. The pulmonary vascular resistance obtained after the defect has been closed and left atrial pressure decreased may be higher than the previous figure, even though the pulmonary vessels have not undergone any change in anatomy.

Another possible example in which actual figures of pulmonary vascular resistance could be misinterpreted is in an infant with a large ventricular left-to-right shunt. The measurement is first made when the infant is in severe heart failure and left atrial pressure is high. After the baby is treated, left atrial pressure may fall; the calculated pulmonary vascular resistance could then increase, giving the false impression that there has been an increase in pulmonary vasoconstriction or vessel pathology even though no actual change had occurred.

In analyzing the effects of pharmacological agents on the pulmonary circulation, it is important to consider changes in pulmonary arterial and left atrial pressure and in pulmonary blood flow. It is possible that the drug may alter pressure or flow and cause a change in calculated vascular resistance, without having a direct local effect on the pulmonary blood vessels. An example of the way in which effects on the pulmonary vessels may be confused is shown by the action of methoxamine (Vasoxyl), an α-adrenoceptor agonist. Methoxamine has been shown to cause mild vasoconstriction when applied directly to the pulmonary vessels; however, it does produce marked systemic vasoconstriction, a rise in systemic arterial pressure, and a rise in left ventricular end-diastolic and left atrial pressure. As a result of the rise in left atrial pressure, pulmonary vessels will be distended and the *calculated* pulmonary vascular resistance may not change or may actually fall slightly suggesting, erroneously, that methoxamine is a pulmonary vasodilator.

Responsiveness of the pulmonary circulation

When pulmonary vascular resistance is elevated, the decrease in cross-sectional area of the pulmonary vascular bed may be due to constriction of the medial muscular component of the small pulmonary vessels, to actual organic changes of hyalinization and fibrosis of the medial and intimal layers, or to intimal proliferation with thrombosis and intraluminal obstruction. It is important to know what the nature of the vascular obstruction is, because the decision regarding the operability of a patient with congenital heart disease may be determined by the pulmonary vascular reactivity. If it can be shown that pulmonary vascular resistance is due to organic changes, it is less likely that surgical correction of the defect will result in a major fall in vascular resistance. However, if the increase is due to vasoconstriction related to medial hypertrophy of smooth muscle, the prospects for improvement in the vessels are good.

There are no good methods for accurately assessing pulmonary vascular responsiveness, but a reasonable evaluation may be made by administering pulmonary vasodilator agents. Inhalation of 100% oxygen has been found to produce a fall in pulmonary vascular resistance in some patients. I believe that the effect of oxygen in reducing pulmonary vascular resistance is significant only when pulmonary venous Po_2 is reduced. When pulmonary venous Po_2 is normal, oxygen produces only mild to modest vasodilatation. In many patients with large pulmonary blood flows, particularly in infants, mild pulmonary edema and mild hypoxia is common; it is in these patients particularly that oxygen may reduce pulmonary vascular resistance.

A common error when evaluating the effects of oxygen on pulmonary vascular resistance is the use of oxygen saturation to calculate pulmonary flow before and after oxygen administration. As mentioned above, if dissolved oxygen is not considered, the calculated oxygen content for pulmonary venous blood would be underestimated, thus giving a very low pulmonary arteriovenous difference, with an erroneously high pulmonary blood flow and an apparent marked reduction in pulmonary vascular resistance (see above).

One of the first pharmacological agents used for assessing pulmonary vascular reactivity was tolazoline hydrochloride (Priscoline), which is a reasonably effective pulmonary vasodilator. It is injected slowly, in doses of 1 mg/kg, through a catheter positioned in the main pulmonary artery. Tolazoline also produces peripheral vasodilatation, with flushing and warmth, and its effect on the pulmonary vessels is fairly short-lived, usually lasting only 15–30 min or sometimes less. Other vasodilators that have been used include prostacyclin, adenosine and magnesium sulfate, and nitric oxide (discussed in Chapter 5).

Assessment of response of pulmonary circulation to vasodilators

When there is a large communication between the left and right ventricles or the aorta and the pulmonary artery, the pulmonary and systemic arterial systolic pressures are equal. As mentioned above, if pulmonary vascular resistance is decreased, pulmonary arterial systolic pressure remains at systemic levels but diastolic pressure may fall. The more important factor to assess is whether pulmonary blood flow increases. In patients with ventricular septal defect, it is possible to measure all the variables necessary to calculate pulmonary vascular resistance before and after administering the vasodilator. In those patients who have lesions that result in complete admixture of pulmonary and systemic circulations, it is possible to obtain an indication of the effects of dilator agents on pulmonary vascular resistance merely by measuring peripheral arterial oxygen saturation. If pulmonary vascular resistance falls more than systemic vascular resistance, the ratio of pulmonary flow to systemic flow will increase, resulting in a rise in oxygen saturation. A marked change is indicative of a very responsive pulmonary circulation. A change in pulmonary vascular resistance of only 1–2 units/m^2 cannot be regarded as significant, in view of the many variables involved in its calculation.

Pulmonary vascular resistance cannot be calculated in conditions in which there is branch stenosis of a pulmonary artery or in which there is a shunt preferentially directed to one artery (as in patent ductus arteriosus). It is also not possible to calculate pulmonary vascular resistance when there is a large bronchial collateral flow or major aortopulmonary collateral arteries; a falsely high value will be obtained, because flow across the pulmonary vascular bed is larger than that calculated by the Fick method.

Calculation of valve area

It was common practice to calculate the valve area from measurements of left ventricular and aortic pressure tracings and blood flow, because it was thought to be a more reliable indicator of the severity of aortic stenosis than pressure gradient alone. Currently, however, most of the recommendations for surgery are based on the magnitude of the systolic pressure gradient and valve area is not commonly estimated. I present the method of calculating valve area because it provides useful information in understanding the dynamics of flow across a stenotic valve.

In a stenotic area, the severity of the obstruction and the magnitude of the flow determine the pressure required to produce flow across it. In an attempt to relate the measured pressures across valve orifices, Gorlin and Gorlin [5] derived a formula to calculate the area of the orifice. This is based on observations in hearts perfused at autopsy. The basic formula used is as follows:

$$A = \frac{Q}{K\sqrt{\Delta P}}$$

where A is orifice area, Q flow, K a constant, and ΔP the mean pressure gradient across the orifice. For the aortic and pulmonary valves, flow occurs only in systole, so the mean flow during systole is calculated. This is performed as follows. The time of the cardiac cycle during which the semilunar valve is open is measured on the aortic or pulmonary arterial pressure curve. This is the systolic ejection time. This is multiplied by the heart rate to give the systolic ejection period, or the time (in s/min) that the valve orifice is open and during which flow occurs. The cardiac output (in mL/min) is divided by this number to give an estimate of the mean systolic flow or the flow rate during systole (in mL/s).

The mean systolic pressure gradient is calculated from the pressures in the left ventricle and aorta, or right ventricle to pulmonary artery. This is best done on tracings obtained simultaneously with two catheters, but if this is not possible, tracings obtained at different times can be superimposed. The mean pressure difference can be measured in two ways (Figure 4.8).

1 Mean systolic pressure can be estimated by drawing a horizontal line across the pressure tracing so that the area above the line equals the two small areas outside the curve below the line. This is shown in the first left ventricular and aortic pressure pulse in Figure 4.8.

2 It can also be done by measuring the height of the pressure curve at numerous equidistant points during systole and dividing by the number of observations made. This is shown as the second pressure pulse in Figure 4.8.

The factor K for the aortic and pulmonary valves is 44.5. A sample calculation is shown in Figure 4.8. For the mitral valve, mean diastolic flow is calculated by measuring the time the valve is open, i.e., when left atrial pressure exceeds left ventricular pressure. The mean diastolic pressure difference is calculated. The K factor for the mitral valve is 31.5.

Valve areas vary with age and weight, and in order to compare one individual with another, it is convenient to express valve area in relation to body surface area. For the aortic and pulmonary valves, an area of about 2.5 cm^2/m^2 is considered normal.

Because the calculation of mean systolic pressure difference requires considerable time, attempts have been made to simplify the method. Bache described a formula for calculating aortic valve area that used peak left ventricular–aortic pressure differences (peak systolic pressure difference or PSPD). The formula is similar to the Gorlin formula:

$$A = \frac{Q}{37.8\sqrt{\text{PSPD} + 10}}$$

Quantitative ultrasound techniques

Ultrasound procedures provide a great deal of information about cardiovascular function. Cardiac chamber size, ventricular wall thickness, and rate and effectiveness of ventricular contraction can all be measured. Numerous indices have been developed to assess ventricular performance during systole and relaxation. Isovolumic relaxation time affords an evaluation of diastolic function. These techniques are discussed in detail in texts on echocardiography. The application of

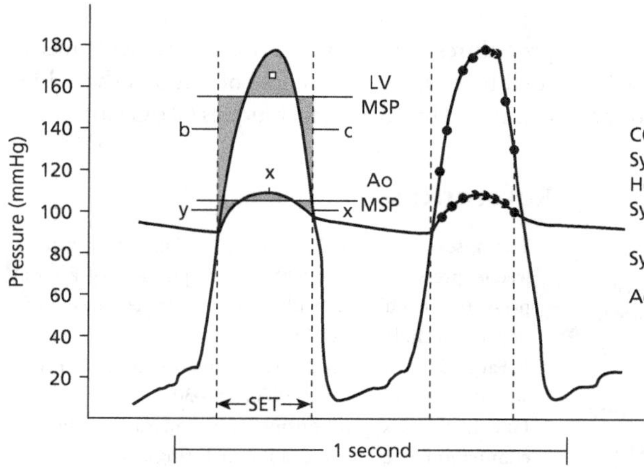

CO (measured) = 3000 mL/min

Systolic ejection time (SET) = 0.25 s

Heart rate = 120/min

Systolic ejection period (SEP) = 120 × 0.25 = 30 s/min

Systolic flow = 3000/30 = 100 mL/s

Aortic valve area

$$= \frac{Q\ (\text{systolic})}{44.5\sqrt{\text{LV MSP} - \text{Ao MSP}}} = \frac{100}{44.5\sqrt{156 - 107}} = \frac{100}{44.5\sqrt{49}} = 0.3\ \text{cm}^2$$

Figure 4.8 Gorlin and Gorlin method for calculating aortic valve area. The simultaneous left ventricular and aortic pressure tracings show a large systolic pressure difference. Mean systolic pressure (MSP) of the left ventricle (LV) and aorta (Ao) can be calculated by one of two methods. The duration of systole (systolic ejection) is indicated by the interval between the onset of the aortic systolic pressure rise and the dicrotic notch in the aortic tracing. The first method used for calculating mean systolic pressure is shown in the first set of pressures. A line is drawn on the left ventricular pressure so that area *a* equals area *b* and area *c*. This can be done by transcribing the pressure tracings onto graph paper with 1-mm squares. The aortic mean systolic pressure is measured by drawing a line so that area *x* equals area *y* and area *z*. The second method used is to measure the pressure at numerous equidistant points along the pressure tracing over the period of systole and to divide the sum of the heights by the number of points taken; this is done for the left ventricle and the aorta separately. The cardiac output (CO) is measured by one of the techniques described and heart rate is recorded during the pressure measurements. The duration of systole in each minute is calculated by multiplying systolic ejection time (SET) by the heart rate to give the systolic ejection period (SEP). Cardiac output is divided by SEP to provide the mean flow across the valve during systole. To calculate valve area, the mean systolic flow is divided by a constant (for the aortic valve *K* is 44.5) multiplied by the square root of the mean systolic pressure difference between the left ventricle and the aorta.

Doppler ultrasound has been of great value in providing assessment of blood flow, so that cardiac output can be measured. It has also permitted the estimation of pressure drops across obstructions, so that the severity of stenosis can be assessed by noninvasive techniques.

Measurement of blood flow

Blood flow is calculated from the product of mean velocity and cross-sectional area. The mean velocity can be determined by integrating the velocity at a specific site, usually the ascending aorta above the sinuses of Valsalva. The average velocity can be measured over the whole cardiac cycle for a specific time period to provide mean velocity. The technique frequently used is to obtain the integral of the velocity of each beat. This, multiplied by cross-sectional area, provides a measure of stroke volume; cardiac output is obtained by multiplying this by heart rate. Values for cardiac output obtained by this technique compare favorably with estimates from other techniques. It is important to recognize some of the problems with the technique.

Vessel diameter is determined from either M-mode or two-dimensional echocardiograms. The assumption is made that the vessel is circular in order to calculate cross-sectional area. If the vessel is not circular at the site of insonation, considerable error could be introduced. It is also important that the angle of incidence of the ultrasound signal and the direction of flow be as low as possible. If the angle is greater than 20–30°, considerable error could be introduced. Flow has been measured by this method in both the aorta and the pulmonary artery. It has also been measured through the mitral valve, using the velocity signal during diastolic flow. A major problem with measurement of flow is that the diameter of the atrioventricular valve changes considerably with phases of the cardiac cycle, so that this may introduce considerable error into the calculation, depending on the diameter used.

Estimation of pressure gradient

The Bernoulli equation has been modified to estimate pressure drop across an orifice (ΔP), using the peak velocity measured in the jet just distal to the stenosis (V_{max}):

$$\Delta P = 4(V_{max})^2$$

Because the Bernoulli equation applies to obstructions in which well-formed jets are developed, gradients measured across stenoses longer than about 5–8 mm are probably not reliable. Estimates of systolic pressure gradients across the pulmonary and aortic valves by Doppler technique correlate quite well with those measured by cardiac catheterization. However, there is frequently a considerable overestimate. This is related to the fact that the gradient measured by ultrasound is at the peak velocity, which temporally occurs prior to the peak of the pressure gradient. The ultrasound technique is of great value in assessing severity of stenosis and in following progress of the lesion. However, because current recommendations for valvotomy or other procedures are based on pressure gradients measured by catheter, the degree of stenosis should be confirmed by invasive techniques (see Chapter 10).

References

1 Thompson J, Moore P, Teitel DF. Pulmonary venous wedge pressures accurately predict pulmonary arterial pressures in children with single ventricle physiology. Pediatr Cardiol 2003;24:531–537.

2 LaFarge CG, Miettinen OS. The estimation of oxygen consumption. Cardiovasc Res 1970;4:23–30.

3 Lindahl SG. Oxygen consumption and carbon dioxide elimination in infants and children during anaesthesia and surgery. Br J Anaesth 1989;62:70–76.

4 Lundell BP, Casas ML, Wallgren CG. Oxygen consumption in infants and children during heart catheterization. Pediatr Cardiol 1996;17:207–213.

5 Gorlin R, Gorlin SG. Hydraulic formula for calculation of the area of the stenotic mitral valve, other cardiac valves, and central circulatory shunts. Am Heart J 1951;4:1–29.

5

CHAPTER 5

Prenatal and postnatal pulmonary circulation

It is well established that pulmonary vascular resistance is very high during fetal life and that this accounts for the relatively low blood flow through the lungs. Because gas exchange is accomplished in the placenta, there is little requirement for pulmonary flow for metabolic purposes and the major proportion of the output of the right ventricle is diverted through the ductus arteriosus (see Chapter 1). This diversion of blood away from the lungs serves the important role of reducing the pulmonary venous return to the left atrium and ventricle, thus diminishing the volume load on the left ventricle. Should the poorly oxygenated blood ejected by the right ventricle be directed through the lungs, this same blood would again be ejected by the left ventricle (without having increased its oxygenation in the lung). Thus the low pulmonary flow reduces the total workload on the fetal heart. Although the fetal lung does not have a role in gas exchange, it may have important functions in other aspects of metabolism, including hormonal regulation.

Postnatal survival of the fetus, after the placental circulation has been eliminated, is dependent not only on the achievement of adequate alveolar ventilation but also on the establishment of a pulmonary blood flow large enough for gas exchange. Dramatic functional and structural changes occur in the pulmonary blood vessels after birth, and it has been shown clearly that these pulmonary vascular changes are crucial in determining the hemodynamic adjustments and consequent clinical manifestations in infants with congenital heart disease. It has also become evident that the presence of congenital heart lesions may modify the normal maturational changes in the pulmonary circulation. In this chapter, the fetal pulmonary circulation and its developmental changes after birth are discussed. The possible changes in the pulmonary circulation that may be produced in the fetus by the presence of congenital heart lesions are considered and the effects of various congenital heart lesions on the normal postnatal maturation of the pulmonary vessels are presented.

Fetal pulmonary circulation

Morphological features

The lung arises from the embryonic foregut; in the human this occurs during the first week of development. The lung bud divides into the two lung sacs, which further divide to form the bronchopulmonary segments. By 16 weeks' gestation, the bronchial tree is essentially fully developed, and further growth is accomplished by growth of new acini, or respiratory units.

As the lung buds develop, they are ensheathed by a mesenchymal layer. The first pulmonary vessels are traditionally thought to form from vasculogenesis, resulting in the formation of tubes which created an isolated plexus. This plexus, it is believed, develops connections with the main pulmonary artery and its hilar branches form from the left sixth branchial arch; the right sixth arch remains as the proximal portion of the right pulmonary artery. The connections from these vessels with the pulmonary vascular plexus develop early; in the human, there is continuity from at least 38 days' gestation [1]. The development of the capillary plexus within the mesenchyme by vasculogenesis has been closely associated with the formation of bronchoalveolar units and it has generally been assumed that the vascular development follows the

Congenital Diseases of the Heart, 3rd edition. By A. Rudolph
 ISBN: 9781405162456

growth of alveolar units. As stated by Hall *et al.* [1] from a study of human embryos, "The airways would seem to act as a template for pulmonary artery development."

Recently, however, Parera *et al.* [2], based on studies of mouse embryos, have proposed that at the earliest sign of lung development, the lung vascular network is already connected to the embryonic circulation. They also suggest that extension of the vasculature into the developing lung results from growth of new capillaries from preexisting vessels, namely by angiogenesis. Further to these newer concepts about pulmonary vascular development, there is now increasing evidence that, at least postnatally, angiogenesis promotes alveolar development and may be responsible for maintenance of alveolar integrity. Administration of agents that inhibit angiogenesis or inhibition of vascular endothelial growth factor (VEGF) receptors in infant rats interferes with vascular development and also with alveolarization [3]. Also in newborn rats in which lung injury was produced by hyperoxia, VEGF gene therapy stimulated angiogenesis and limited the severity of alveolar disruption associated with hyperoxia [4]. The concept that vascular growth influences pulmonary airway development has raised interesting speculation regarding the interference with lung development in preterm infants with bronchopulmonary dysplasia and disturbed growth resulting from oxygen toxicity.

Pulmonary vascular smooth muscle cells have a diverse origin, being derived from three different sites: bronchial smooth muscle, perivascular mesenchyme, and endothelial cells [1]. This could explain the findings of Frid *et al.* [5] that fetal and adult bovine pulmonary arteries show the presence of several phenotypically distinct smooth muscle populations.

The development of pulmonary venous connection to the left atrium has been examined in human fetuses. There had been some question whether the pulmonary veins developed from the embryonic systemic sinus venosus, but Webb *et al.* [6], from examination of human embryos, excluded this possibility. They noted that the pulmonary vein canalizes as a single vessel within the mediastinum; this connects to the pulmonary vascular plexus and then to the left atrium as four separate veins.

The main pulmonary trunk is relatively large in the fetus, reflecting the fact that the larger proportion of combined ventricular output (CVO) is ejected into it from the right ventricle. The main trunk continues directly into the ductus arteriosus, and the left and right pulmonary arteries arise as branches of the pulmonary trunk–ductus arteriosus conduit. The left and right pulmonary arteries are quite large at their origin, but rapidly decrease in size as they enter the lung. The branching pattern of the vessels is similar to that in the adult by mid-gestation and further growth during fetal and postnatal life is characterized by development of additional terminal respiratory units with associated blood vessels. The pulmonary trunk and the major pulmonary arteries are thick-walled, similar to the aorta, and the walls are composed of numerous layers of elastic fibers, mainly circumferentially arranged, with only few smooth muscle cells and few collagen fibers.

The elastic composition of the arterial wall extends to the preacinar vessels, but in the smaller preacinar and larger acinar arteries (30–200 μm diameter), the medial layer is composed largely of smooth muscle cells. In vessels of 30–50 μm diameter, the thickness of the muscle layer is about 15% of the external vessel diameter. In the smaller acinar arteries, the muscular layer is only partial and more distal intraacinar arteries have no muscular component. There has been some confusion regarding possible changes in the thickness of the muscular medial layer of the small pulmonary arteries during fetal development. It had been proposed that the thickness of the medial muscular layer increased progressively over the last 3 months of gestation in the human fetus. Studies in fetal lambs which related the thickness of the muscle layer to the external diameter of the arterioles indicate that there are no significant changes from about 60 days' gestation to term (about 140 days) [7]. More recent studies in the human confirm that the thickness of the pulmonary arterioles does not change significantly over the latter period of gestation [8]. The muscular development of the pulmonary arterioles in the fetus is of considerable importance, as it determines the reactivity of the circulation to many of the physiological and abnormal influences to which it may be subjected.

Growth of the fetal lung is characterized by development of new vessels and respiratory units. The composition of the arteries with regard to the smooth muscle component continues to reflect their size and their relationship to the airways. It has been shown in the lamb lung that not only does the total number of muscular arteriolar vessels increase with lung growth, but vessel numbers increase per unit volume of lung tissue. These changes result in a dramatic increase in cross-sectional area of the pulmonary vascular bed [7].

Examination of lungs of stillborn animal and human fetuses has shown that the muscular arteries have a small lumen and a thick intimal layer, in which the endothelial cells are rounded and tend to overlap. Also, the smooth muscle cells in the media are rounded. However, it is likely that these vessels may not have these characteristics *in vivo*, and that these features are the result of constriction of the muscle layer with a drop of intraluminal pressure from the high fetal levels to atmospheric pressure. In preparations in fetal lambs in which the arterial tree was fixed while being perfused at fetal pressures, although the intima was somewhat thickened, the endothelial cells were flattened and the lumen was not slit-like, as had been described in the stillborn fetuses.

Functional aspects

Gestational changes in flow

Normally, blood flow through the fetal lung is quite low. Most of our knowledge of fetal pulmonary circulation is derived from lambs; we have measured pulmonary blood flow in lambs in the normal *in utero* environment. In lambs of 0.4–0.7 gestation (60–110 days), the lungs receive only about 4% of CVO, or about 18–20 mL/min per kg fetal body weight. During later gestation there is a modest actual and relative increase in pulmonary blood flow most prominent from about 120 days' gestation [9]. Near term (140–150 days), the lungs receive about 8–10% of CVO, or about 35–45 mL/min per kg fetal body weight. Figure 5.1 depicts the changes in pulmonary blood flow, pulmonary arterial pressure, and pulmonary vascular resistance during the last trimester of gestation in the fetal lamb. It is evident that pulmonary arterial pressure rises gradually, paralleling the similar increase in aortic pressure. Total pulmonary vascular resistance falls gradually; this is probably related to the increase in

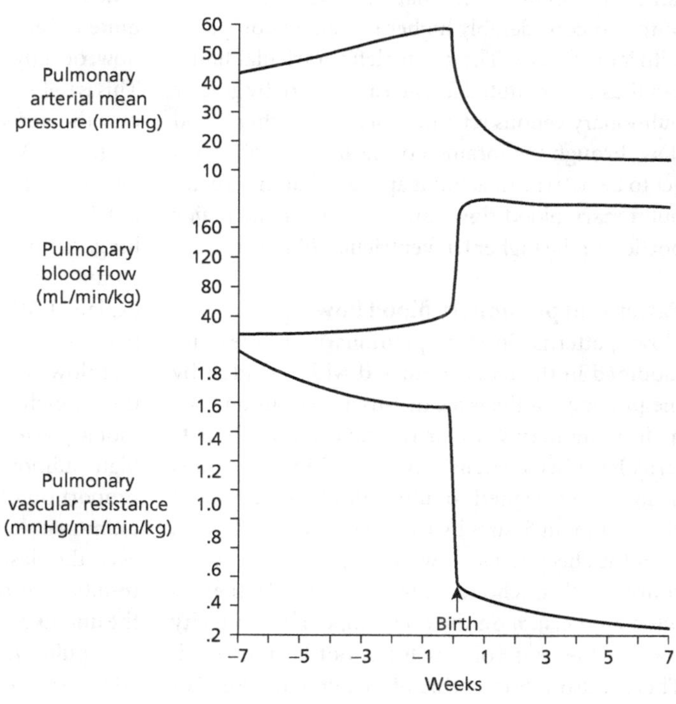

Figure 5.1 Changes in pulmonary arterial pressure, pulmonary blood flow, and calculated pulmonary vascular resistance during the 7 weeks preceding birth, at birth, and 7 weeks postnatally. The prenatal data were derived from lambs and the postnatal data from other species.

vessel numbers, although it could also be explained by relaxation of the muscle wall. However, if changes in pulmonary vascular resistance are related to changes in lung weight, there is an increase in resistance in late gestation, suggesting that pulmonary vascular tone has increased progressively to term.

Pulmonary blood flow has been measured in human fetuses using Doppler ultrasound blood velocity waveforms in the left and right pulmonary arteries. However, there has been considerable variation in the magnitude of pulmonary blood flow in human fetuses in published reports. At about 20 weeks' gestation, it was estimated that pulmonary blood flow was about 13% of CVO, but by 30 weeks it was about 20% of CVO [10]. Although the flows could not be accurately related to fetal weight, in the latter quarter of gestation pulmonary flows were estimated to be at least double those measured in fetal lambs. Values of about 100 mL/min per kg estimated fetal weight were recorded in human fetuses compared with about 45 mL/min per kg in lambs. It was also reported by Sutton *et al.* [11] that pulmonary blood flow was about 22% of CVO in the human fetus. However, Mielke and Benda [12] found that pulmonary flow was only 11% of CVO, a level much closer to that in the fetal lamb. As discussed in Chapter 1, left ventricular output is considerably higher in human compared with lamb fetuses. The greater left ventricular filling can thus be accounted for, at least in part, by greater pulmonary venous return. Whether a higher blood flow through the foramen ovale also contributes is yet to be determined, but it appears that the greater pulmonary blood flow can account for the major portion of the higher left ventricular filling.

Patterns of pulmonary blood flow

Flow patterns in the pulmonary arteries are modified in the fetus compared with the adult by the presence of the large ductus arteriosus and the high pulmonary vascular resistance. Velocity patterns have been extensively studied in fetal lambs using electromagnetic or ultrasonic flowmeters and also in human fetuses by Doppler ultrasound.

In the sheep fetus, flow in the pulmonary trunk continues throughout the whole of systole: there is often an incisura on the downslope of the velocity tracing, the cause of which has not been defined. There is also a short period of backflow at the end of systole (Figure 5.2). Flow through the ductus arteriosus is also continuous throughout systole. The flow contour in the branch pulmonary arteries is quite different. There is a short period of forward flow, occupying only about the first third of systole. This is followed by backflow, which extends throughout the remainder of systole and into diastole (Figure 5.2). It is not known what accounts for this pattern of flow in the branch pulmonary arteries, but I believe the high peripheral resistance in the lung, the ductus arteriosus, and the relatively low compliance of the large pulmonary arteries can explain it. With the onset of systole, blood is ejected from the right ventricle into the pulmonary trunk and flows through the ductus arteriosus and into the branch pulmonary arteries. The large pulmonary arteries are distended, but because of the high pulmonary vascular resistance, only a small proportion of the blood passes into the peripheral pulmonary circulation. As systole continues, however, the elasticity of the major pulmonary arteries results in recoil and this pushes blood back toward the ductus arteriosus and descending aorta.

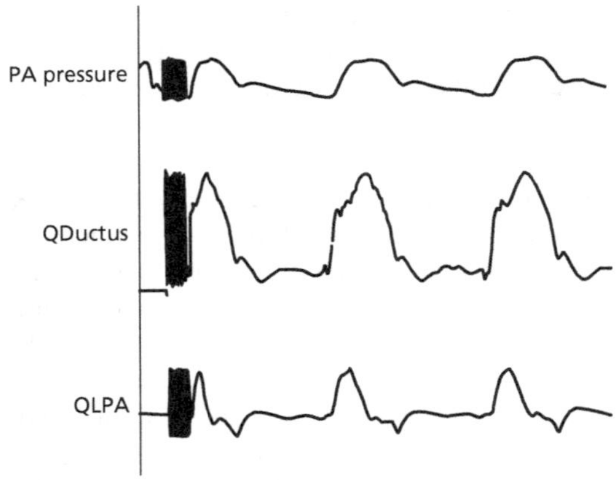

Figure 5.2 Pulmonary arterial pressure (PA pressure) and blood flow patterns in the ductus arteriosus (QDuctus) and the left pulmonary artery (QLPA) were recorded in a fetal lamb *in utero* at 125 days' gestation. Flow recordings were obtained with ultrasonic flowmeters. Note that flow through the ductus arteriosus from the pulmonary artery to the descending aorta occurs continuously throughout systole. The flow contour in the left pulmonary artery is quite different. There is a period of forward flow for a short period, occupying only about the first half of systole. This is followed by backflow, which extends throughout the remainder of systole and into diastole.

If pulmonary vascular resistance is reduced by administration of a vasodilator such as acetylcholine, the duration and magnitude of the forward flow area are increased and those of the backflow are decreased. Ventilation of the lungs with air results in a flow contour similar to that seen postnatally. However, pulmonary vasoconstriction, as with fetal hypoxemia, decreases the duration and magnitude of forward flow and enhances the backflow.

In the human fetus, velocity patterns in branch pulmonary arteries are similar to those recorded in lambs, but in conformance with the relatively lower pulmonary vascular resistance, the initial forward flow is more prolonged and larger, and there is either minor or no backflow.

Regulation of pulmonary vascular tone

Studies in the adult have consistently shown that responses of the pulmonary circulation to a variety of stimuli are considerably less than those of the systemic circulation. In the fetus numerous factors have been shown to produce dramatic pulmonary vasomotor responses. Cassin *et al.* [13] demonstrated some role of the autonomic nervous system in influencing fetal pulmonary vessels during hypoxia. However, there is little evidence for the role of the autonomic nervous system in normal vasoregulation, because sympathetic blockade with phentolamine (α-adrenoceptor blocker), propranolol (β-adrenoceptor blocker), or parasympathetic blockade with atropine causes no change in pulmonary vascular resistance at any gestational age.

Responses to changes in Po_2

The fetal pulmonary vasculature is extremely sensitive to many physiological and pharmacological influences. One factor that has been studied intensively is the response of the circulation to changes in oxygen environment. In many of the earlier studies, the main interest was in assessing the role of physical expansion of the lung as compared with the effects of oxygen in producing the pulmonary vascular changes at the time of birth (see below). However, many subsequent studies have shown that in the *in utero* fetus, in which the lungs have not been ventilated, changes in oxygen levels have a profound effect on the pulmonary circulation. Thus increasing the Po_2 of fetal blood by placing the ewe in a hyperbaric oxygen chamber results in a marked increase in pulmonary blood flow in the fetus *in utero* [14]. We have also examined the response of the pulmonary circulation in chronic fetal lamb preparations, in which an electromagnetic flowmeter transducer was implanted around the main or left pulmonary artery to measure total or left lung pulmonary blood flow [15]. Po_2 of the pulmonary arterial blood was varied from the resting level of about 18 mmHg while the ewe was breathing air to 25–28 mmHg by 100% oxygen inhalation and down to 10–12 mmHg by administering nitrogen and air mixtures to the ewe. Pco_2 and pH were not changed during the studies. Since there is no alveolar ventilation in the fetus, the levels of pulmonary arterial blood gases and pH represent those to which the pulmonary vessels are exposed. We found that even over this relatively small range of Po_2 variation, pulmonary blood flow and pulmonary vascular resistance changed dramatically. The relationship of pulmonary vascular resistance to pulmonary arterial Po_2 was curvilinear (Figure 5.3) and it appears that the response in the later-gestation lamb is much greater than in the younger lamb. This is of considerable interest, because the thickness of the media does not change significantly over the latter half of gestation. This suggests that either the mechanisms by which oxygen affects vasodilatation are not fully developed, or that the pulmonary vascular smooth muscle does not have the same contractile capacity in the younger fetus.

Responses of pulmonary blood flow and pulmonary vascular resistance to hypoxemia have not been reported in the human fetus. However, there

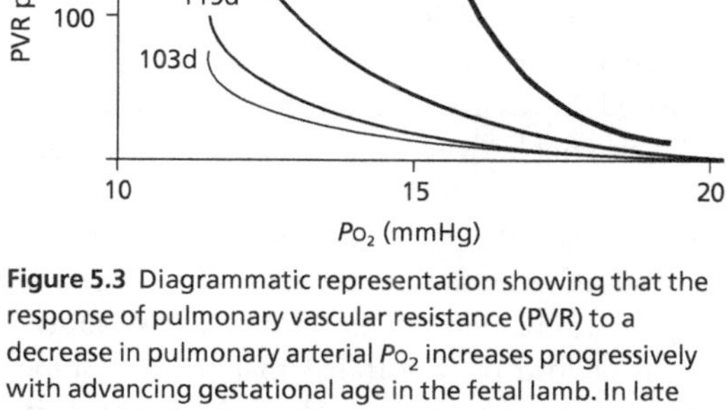

Figure 5.3 Diagrammatic representation showing that the response of pulmonary vascular resistance (PVR) to a decrease in pulmonary arterial Po_2 increases progressively with advancing gestational age in the fetal lamb. In late gestation the fetal pulmonary circulation is very sensitive to small changes in Po_2.

is some evidence indicating that fetal pulmonary vascular resistance may be responsive to small increases in Po_2 resulting from administration of 60% oxygen to the mother. No change in pulmonary blood flow was reported in fetuses less than 25 weeks' gestation, but a small increase in flow occurred in fetuses above 30 weeks' gestation [10]. This suggests that the pulmonary vasculature in the human, as in the lamb, is poorly responsive early in gestation and becomes more reactive in later gestation.

The greater responsiveness of the pulmonary vasculature to hypoxia with advancing gestation could be related to several factors. It is possible that the number of smooth muscle cells in the media increases with advancing gestation, or that the smooth muscle cells are individually more responsive to hypoxia. Isolated pulmonary arterial smooth muscle cells contract when exposed to hypoxia [16]. Thus, at least in part, the gestational change in response could be due to an inherent change in the smooth muscle cell. The possibility that there could be changes in sensitivity or function in oxygen-sensitive K^+ channels or Ca^{2+}/K^+ channels in the cell membrane should be entertained (see below). Possibly, there is also an increase in the capability for release of vasoconstrictor substances, such as endothelin. A further possibility is that production of vasodilator agents such as prostacyclin or endothelial-derived relaxing factor (nitric oxide) is more markedly inhibited by hypoxia in older than younger fetuses.

The role of pH changes in influencing the response to hypoxemia in the fetus has not been established. It has been clearly shown in the newborn that there is an interrelationship between hypoxemia and acidemia in potentiating pulmonary vasoconstriction [17]. In the fetus, acidemia alone does not significantly modify pulmonary vascular resistance, but it is quite likely that acidemia does increase the fetal vasoconstrictor response to decreased Po_2, as in the newborn (see below).

It is also not known how much of the pulmonary vascular response during hypoxia is due to local direct effects of the perfusing blood or how much is the result of reflex autonomic effects from chemoreceptor stimulation. Studies from Dawes' laboratory in Oxford demonstrated that there is some degree of autonomic control of the pulmonary circulation in the fetal lamb [13] and that some of the vasoconstriction in response to severe asphyxia is mediated through the autonomic nerves. Sympathetic stimulation produced mild vasoconstriction, and vagus nerve stimulation mild vasodilatation in late-gestation lambs. However, studies in fetal lambs suggested that the major vasoconstrictor effect was from local change in Po_2, because sympathetic or parasympathetic blockers did not significantly alter the hypoxic response.

The fact that fetal pulmonary vessels react to small Po_2 changes raises the interesting question as to whether persistent changes in Po_2 of blood perfusing the lung may alter normal pulmonary circulatory development. This is a very important consideration if certain congenital heart lesions are present during fetal life. In a number of lesions, such as aortopulmonary transposition, the normal pattern of distribution of umbilical venous and of inferior and superior vena cava blood to the ascending aorta and pulmonary artery may be disturbed, and the pulmonary circulation could be exposed to a higher than normal Po_2. The question for speculation is whether this may result in a decrease in pulmonary vascular resistance and increase in pulmonary blood flow. This is discussed in Chapter 18. It is also interesting to speculate whether this may alter the development of the pulmonary arterioles. It is possible that a higher Po_2 in the blood perfusing the lungs would relax pulmonary vessels and that there would be less stimulus for the growth of the medial smooth muscle layer. A media with fewer smooth muscle cells could make the pulmonary vessels less reactive to various stimuli both before and immediately after birth.

Regulation of pulmonary vascular responses

A summary of smooth muscle contraction and relaxation is helpful in understanding the mechanisms influencing pulmonary vasomotion. A brief review has been presented by Webb [18].

Contraction results from the interaction of myosin light chain (MLC) with actin, with energy being provided from adenosine triphosphate (ATP) through the action of myosin ATPase. The interaction between MLC and actin is facilitated by phosphorylation of MLC by MLC kinase. This process is initiated by an increase in the cytosolic concentration of Ca^{2+} which combines with the protein calmodulin. The Ca^{2+}–calmodulin complex stimulates MLC kinase activity, thus phosphorylating MLC. The intracellular Ca^{2+} concentration may be increased by release of Ca^{2+} from sarcoplasmic reticulum, or by passage from the extracellular space through Ca^{2+} channels. Vasoconstrictors such as norepinephrine, angiotensin II, and endothelin 1 act on membrane receptors and, through a mechanism involving guanine nucleotide regulatory proteins (G proteins), stimulate phopholipase C activity. Phospholipase C induces the production of two second messengers, diacylglycerol (DAG) and inositol 1,4,5-trisphosphate (IP_3). DAG activates phosphokinase C that affects Ca^{2+} channels and IP_3 binds to receptors on sarcoplasmic reticulum and stimulates release of Ca^{2+} that is then available to combine with calmodulin. The contraction induced by the phosphorylation of MLC by MLC kinase is not sustained because myosin phosphatase reduces the phosphorylation of MLC and thus relaxation would occur. However, contraction is sustained by the action of Rho kinase, which inhibits myosin phosphatase.

Vascular smooth muscle relaxation is accomplished largely by reduction of cytosolic Ca^{2+} concentrations, so that there is less Ca^{2+}–calmodulin complex to induce MLC kinase activity. It may also result from increased MLC phosphorylase activity, because this will dephosphorylate MLC and reduce its binding with actin. Cytosolic Ca^{2+} may be reduced by movement of Ca^{2+} into the sarcoplasmic reticulum or by passage across the cell membrane into the extracellular space. Several mechanisms may be involved in these transfers: Ca^{2+}/Mg^{2+}-ATPase is important in both the sarcoplasmic reticulum and the cell membrane; Na^{+}/Ca^{2+} exchangers in the cell membrane are also important in decreasing cytosolic Ca^{2+}.

Vasoconstrictor or vasodilator agents exert their effects through several mechanisms. Many achieve their effects through binding with receptors in the smooth muscle cell membrane that are coupled through G proteins to adenylate cyclase, an enzyme that, when stimulated, induces production of cyclic adenosine monophosphate (cAMP). This exerts its effects through various protein kinases. Thus stimulation of the prostacyclin (PGI_2) receptor activates protein kinases that activate K^{+} channels and increases Ca^{2+} uptake into sarcoplasmic reticulum, thus inducing relaxation. Agents that bind to β-adrenergic receptors increase cAMP, which activates protein kinase A (PKA) that decreases the affinity of MLC kinase to the Ca^{2+}–calmodulin complex and thus induces relaxation.

Vasodilator agents may exert their effect through a cyclic guanosine monophosphate (cGMP) mechanism. Thus nitric oxide (NO), produced in endothelial cells adjacent to smooth muscle cells, diffuses directly into the muscle cells and stimulates the enzyme guanylyl cyclase to produce cGMP. As with cAMP this activates protein kinases that exert various actions, such as reduction of cytosolic Ca^{2+} concentration both by movement across the cell membrane or transfer to the sarcoplasmic reticulum, thus resulting in vasodilation. The cGMP is hydrolyzed to 5′-GMP by cyclic nucleotide phosphodiesterase. Several phosphodiesterases have been identified, but in vascular smooth muscle phosphodiesterase V is important; by degrading cGMP, it limits the relaxation of smooth muscle. Phosphodiesterase inhibitors limit or prevent the degradation of cGMP and thus either maintain or possibly enhance the vasodilator action.

Recently, vasodilation has been achieved through a mechanism not involving a reduction of cytosolic Ca^{2+} concentration. The G protein RhoA induces Rho kinase activity that inhibits the activity of MLC phosphatase. As mentioned above, MLC phophatase, by interfering with the phosphorylation of MLC, limits the contraction stimulated by the action of MLC kinase. Inhibition of Rho kinase by the pharmacological agent fasudil results in vascular relaxation in animal studies [19].

Many of the factors responsible for vasomotor regulation of the pulmonary circulation also have effects on development and morphology of the pulmonary blood vessels. This is discussed below.

Vasoactive agents affecting the pulmonary circulation

As mentioned above, the autonomic nervous system does not appear to exert any significant effect on the pulmonary circulation in the normal fetus [13]. However, fetal pulmonary vessels are constricted by norepinephrine and high doses of epinephrine, and are dilated by isoproterenol or other β-adrenoceptor agonists. Parasympathetic blockade with atropine causes vasodilation. The endothelium has a major role in regulating pulmonary vascular resistance. Numerous vasodilator and vasoconstrictor agents are derived from endothelial cells, including NO, PGI_2, prostaglandin (PG)E, leukotrienes, endothelin, and bradykinin (see below). Many biological agents have been implicated in pulmonary vascular responses to hypoxia, pulmonary arterial distension, and increased pulmonary blood flow, but as yet no single mechanism has been proven to be the sole factor responsible for a specific response.

Vasodilators

A number of agents have been shown to dramatically reduce pulmonary vascular resistance in the fetus. Acetylcholine injected in very small amounts into the fetal pulmonary artery produces an immediate increase in pulmonary blood flow. However, repeated injections of similar amounts of the drug every few minutes results in tachyphylaxis, a progressive diminution in the response. Similarly, continuous infusion of acetylcholine produces a dramatic immediate response of flow, but after a variable period of 10–30 min, the flow drops to control levels. Responsiveness is restored an hour or more after the administration of acetylcholine has been stopped. Tolazoline, bradykinin, adenosine, and histamine all produce responses similar to those of acetylcholine.

These agents all exert their action through endothelial cells, and endothelium is required for their vasodilator effect. They act on the endothelial cells to produce endothelial-derived relaxing factor (EDRF), which then stimulates an increase in cGMP concentration in smooth muscle cells; this has a relaxing effect. It has been shown that EDRF is identical to NO, which is derived from L-arginine in the endothelial cell facilitated by the action of the enzyme nitric oxide synthase (NOS). Administration of *N*-ω-nitro-L-arginine blocks the production of NO and inhibits the effects of the endothelium-dependent vasodilator agents. NO diffuses into the smooth muscle cell and stimulates cGMP directly rather than via membrane receptors. The mechanism responsible for the loss of vasodilator effect with continued or repeated administration of the endothelium-dependent agents has not been determined. It is possible that the ability of the cell to produce NO is limited, or that stimulation of cGMP production in smooth muscle cells by NO wanes.

Some vasodilators produce relaxation of pulmonary vascular smooth muscle by a direct effect on K^+ channels; the drug lemakalim opens these channels and causes vasodilatation. Other agents, such as sodium nitroprusside, atrial natriuretic peptide (ANP), and 8-bromo-GMP increase cGMP concentrations in smooth muscle cells directly. These agents result in prolonged vasodilatation, with no loss of response with continuing administration. Both ANP and brain natriuretic peptide (BNP) are pulmonary vasodilators, although ANP appears to be more effective. C-type natriuretic peptide also induces some vasodilation, but it is not as effective as ANP and BNP.

PGE_2 and PGD_2 are both vasodilators of the pulmonary circulation in the fetus. Postnatally PGE_2 produces mild vasodilation, but PGD_2 is a mild pulmonary vasoconstrictor [20]. PGI_2 is a somewhat more potent vasodilator than the other two prostaglandins, and it continues to exert a dilator action after birth. Furthermore, prolonged infusion of PGE_2 and PGI_2 is not associated with diminution of the vasodilator response.

Adrenomedullin, a 52-amino-acid peptide, has been found to have prominent vasodilator effects in many organs and, in some species, on the pulmonary circulation. This peptide is secreted by the adrenal gland but also by many other tissues, including vascular endothelium. In fetal lambs it produces a marked increase in pulmonary blood flow, to levels achieved normally after birth. Its effect does appear to be endothelium-dependent, because the vasodilatation is largely abolished by NO blockade. However, it differs from acetylcholine in that it has a more prolonged vasodilator effect and, with repeated doses, the effect is enhanced rather than diminished; the increase in pulmonary blood flow is maintained for 1–3 hours. The differences in these responses are yet to be explained.

Calcium channel blockers interfere with L-type voltage-gated calcium channels in muscle cells. Calcium channels in the cell membrane permit entry of extracellular Ca^{2+} into the cytoplasm and this, as discussed above, induces smooth muscle contraction. The dihydropyridine class of calcium channel blockers, which includes amlodipine, nifedipine and nimodipine, is more effective in interfering with transfer of extracellular Ca^{2+} across the membrane and in producing relaxation of vascular smooth muscle. Calcium channel blockers are beneficial in only few patients with pulmonary hypertension and potentially have serious side effects.

Phosphodiesterase inhibitors have been shown to have a relaxant action on pulmonary vascular smooth muscle. The phosphodiesterase that is most important in limiting cGMP activity in vascular smooth muscle is phophodiesterase V. Inhibitors of phosphodiesterase V, such as dipyridamole and sildenafil, are effective pulmonary vasodilators. In fetal lambs infusion of sildenafil decreased pulmonary vascular resistance [21].

The identification of the RhoA/Rho kinase effect in maintaining smooth muscle contraction by interfering with the action of myosin phosphatase (see above) has prompted investigation of the effect of Rho kinase inhibitors in promoting vasodilation in the pulmonary circulation. It has been shown that one such agent, fasudil, is quite effective in producing this response [22].

Vasoconstrictors

Pulmonary vascular resistance in the fetus is maintained at very high levels. Whether this is due to lack or absence of mechanisms that induce vasodilatation, or to continuous release of vasoconstrictor substances, has not been established. Apart from the demonstration that hypoxemia causes fetal pulmonary vasoconstriction, infusion of most vasoconstrictor agents, such as α-adrenergic agonists, produces a mild increase in pulmonary vascular resistance in fetal lambs.

The role of vasoconstrictors in normal regulation of pulmonary vascular tone has been demonstrated by administration of putative or specific blockers. Leukotrienes are derived from arachidonic acid through the lipoxygenase pathway. It has been postulated that leukotriene (LT)C_4 and LTD_4, which do cause pulmonary vasoconstriction, may be at least partly responsible for maintaining the high fetal pulmonary vascular resistance, because inhibition of leukotriene production or blockade of receptors results in a dramatic increase in pulmonary blood flow in fetal sheep.

A similar role has also been proposed for endothelin. In mammals, endothelin appears in three isoforms, ET-1, ET-2 and ET-3, the effects of which are mediated through the membrane receptors ET_A and ET_B. When stimulated, the membrane receptors couple with several G proteins and activate phospholipase, as well as protein kinases. ET_A receptors are located predominantly on vascular smooth muscle cells in humans and their stimulation induces contraction. ET_B receptors have been identified mainly on vascular endothelial cells; stimulation induces release of NO and prostanoids, which exert a relaxant effect on adjacent vascular smooth muscle cells. However, in animals these responses to stimulation of ET_A and ET_B receptors may vary with species and particular vascular beds. Several studies have documented the prominent effects of endothelin on the pulmonary circulation in the fetus. The role of endothelin in regulating pulmonary vascular tone in the fetus is controversial. In fetal lambs, injection of ET-1 into the pulmonary circulation resulted in a substantial fall in pulmonary vascular resistance, suggesting that ET_B receptors dominate in the response [23]. This is supported by the fact that an ET_B receptor agonist also markedly reduced pulmonary vascular resistance. However, the specific ET_A receptor blocker BQ 123 caused only a modest fall in pulmonary vascular resistance. This suggests that endothelin does not have an important role in maintaining the high pulmonary vascular resistance in the normal fetus.

However, there is evidence suggesting that endothelin may have an important role in the pulmonary vascular responses in pathological states. In fetal lambs, constriction of the ductus arteriosus results in pulmonary arterial hypertension and increased thickness of the media of resistance vessels. Chronic infusion of the selective ET_A receptor blocker BQ 123 limited the degree of pulmonary hypertension and also reduced muscularization of the pulmonary arterioles [24]. Also, BQ 123 reduced pulmonary vascular resistance in prematurely delivered lambs with pulmonary arterial hypertension related to hyaline membrane disease [25].

Endothelin receptor blockers have been available for clinical use for several years. Bosentan, a nonselective blocker that affects both ET_A and ET_B receptors, has been used as a pulmonary vasodilator in patients with pulmonary hypertension with moderate effectiveness. Because bosentan blocks ET_B as well as ET_A receptors, and therefore presumably inhibits the potential vasodilator effect of NO and prostanoid release, it was hoped that a selective ET_A blocker would be more effective as it would eliminate only the constrictor effect of endothelin. A selective ET_A blocker, sitaxsentan (Thelin), has been studied in Europe, but does not appear to be more effective than bosentan; it is currently undergoing trials in the USA.

There has been considerable interest in the role of free radicals, particularly superoxide (O_2^-), now generally termed reactive oxygen species (ROS), as a vasoconstrictor of pulmonary vessels. In 2001, Waypa *et al.* [26], from studies of perfused rat lungs, proposed that hypoxia increased the production of ROS by mitochondria and that this was responsible for the vasoconstriction resulting from hypoxia. This was supported by the fact that superoxide dismutase, which limits the production of ROS, inhibits hypoxic pulmonary vasoconstriction. The mechanism by which ROS induce vasoconstriction is still to be resolved, but one possibility that has been proposed is that ROS react with NO to produce peroxynitrite, a powerful vasoconstrictor. ROS have been implicated in causing pulmonary vasoconstriction in ventilated preterm lambs [27] and also in lambs ventilated with high oxygen gas mixtures.

Mechanical factors affecting pulmonary vessels

Increasing pulmonary arterial pressure constricts the ductus arteriosus and results in a rapid increase in pulmonary blood flow, with a progressive increase in flow over 30–60 min. Following this decrease in vascular tone, there is a gradual fall of flow to baseline values over 2–3 hours, while pulmonary pressure remains elevated, indicating that pulmonary vascular resistance has increased above its resting level [28]. Vasodilatation associated with the increase in pulmonary arterial pressure could be the result of physical distension of the pulmonary vasculature alone. However, it appears that the response is more complex, because the increase in pulmonary blood flow associated with partial ductus arteriosus constriction can be almost completely abolished by prior administration of an NO inhibitor. Thus pulmonary arterial pressure increase may result initially in a release of NO by the endothelium; the subsequent fall in flow may result from exhaustion of this mechanism, or from later release of a constrictor such as endothelin.

We have shown that chronic elevation of pulmonary arterial pressure results in an increase in the thickness of the wall of fifth-generation pulmonary arteries, similar to that observed in newborn infants with persistent pulmonary arterial hypertension [29]. In one fetus this resulted from constriction of the ductus arteriosus and the model of chronic constriction of the ductus is now widely used to study chronic pulmonary arterial hypertension in lamb fetuses, as well as simulation of persistent pulmonary arterial hypertension of the newborn (PPHN).

Changes in pulmonary circulation after birth

Postnatal increase in pulmonary blood flow

Breathing at birth is associated with a marked fall in pulmonary vascular resistance and an increase in pulmonary blood flow from about 35 to 160–200 mL/min per kg in the fetal lamb. This occurs within a few minutes after adequate ventilation has been established (see Figure 5.1). Pulmonary arterial pressure does not fall as rapidly and probably remains elevated while the ductus arteriosus is still widely patent. Calculated pulmonary vascular resistance falls within minutes from the prenatal level of about 1.6 to about 0.3 mmHg/mL per min per kg, a reduction of about 80%. After the ductus arteriosus begins to close, pulmonary arterial pressure also falls. In the human, the ductus arteriosus is functionally closed within 10–15 hours after birth, but in other species it may close earlier. Once the ductus has closed, pulmonary arterial pressure can vary independently of systemic arterial pressure.

Mechanisms for postnatal changes in pulmonary blood flow

Pulmonary blood flow increases markedly after birth, and the mechanisms responsible for the dramatic decrease in pulmonary vascular resistance have been studied extensively. Studies by Ardran *et al.* [30] demonstrated conclusively that expansion of the lungs with air resulted in a dramatic immediate increase in pulmonary blood flow. However, it was not apparent whether this was the result of simple physical expansion of the lungs with gas, or due to the increase in oxygen concentration to which the vessels were subjected. The separate effects of physical expansion and of oxygen have been demonstrated by an interesting series of studies by several investigators. In studies in fetal lambs exteriorized from the uterus, but with the umbilical–placental circulation maintained, the lungs were expanded by insufflation of the trachea with a mixture of 3% oxygen and 7% carbon dioxide in nitrogen [31]. This did not change the pH, Po_2, or Pco_2 of the fetal blood significantly, but there was a considerable reduction in pulmonary vascular resistance. When the lungs were then expanded with air, a much greater fall in pulmonary vascular resistance ensued. When fluid that had a Po_2, pH, and Pco_2 similar to fetal blood was instilled into the fetal trachea to expand the lungs, pulmonary vascular resistance did not change significantly, but if the Po_2 of this fluid was increased, the pulmonary vascular resistance fell [32]. All these studies indicate that Po_2 elevation, as well as physical expansion of the lungs with a gas but not by fluid, dilate the pulmonary vessels. These separate effects of physical expansion of the lungs with gas and of direct exposure to oxygen are of considerable interest, but the contribution of each and the exact mechanism by which each of these reduces pulmonary vascular resistance was not defined.

The vascular effects of alveolar distension could be related to the development of a gas–fluid interface on the alveolar walls. The surface forces would tend to collapse the alveoli, and this could exert a negative pressure on the alveolar septa and the small vessels running between alveoli, producing some degree of distension. This explanation would also be consistent with the lack of any vascular effect when the alveoli are distended with fluid, since no interface would develop.

Although some of the hypoxic vasoconstriction of the fetal pulmonary circulation appears to be mediated through chemoreflex mechanisms, reflexes and the autonomic nervous system do not appear to be involved in the decreased pulmonary vascular resistance response to oxygen. Complete pharmacological blockade of α- and β-adrenoceptors and of parasympathetic activity does not significantly alter the oxygen response.

To determine the relative importance of physical expansion by gas versus oxygenation in reducing pulmonary vascular resistance, we set up chronic preparations of late-gestation lambs *in utero*, in which an intratracheal tube was inserted into the fetus and pulmonary blood flow was measured by the radioactive microsphere technique [33]. Rhythmic ventilation of the fetal lungs with 3% oxygen and 7% carbon dioxide did not change fetal blood gases, but resulted in a dramatic increase in pulmonary blood flow. Subsequent ventilation with oxygen caused a further variable increase in pulmonary blood flow in some but not all lambs (see Figure 2.1, p. 26). All these studies have conclusively shown that physical expansion of the lungs and an increase in oxygen concentration in the alveoli can reduce pulmonary vascular resistance independently of each other. Numerous investigations have been conducted to attempt to elucidate the mechanisms by which each functions.

Expansion of the adult lung has been shown to result in liberation of prostaglandins. In the fetal lamb, expansion of the lung with gas results in an increase in PGI_2 concentration in pulmonary venous blood [34]. PGI_2 is a potent pulmonary vasodilator. Furthermore, blockade of prostaglandin production by administration of prostaglandin synthesis inhibitors, such as indomethacin, prior to ventilating the lungs markedly limits the fall in pulmonary vascular resistance. In some studies the fall in pulmonary vascular resistance was not abolished completely, so that the fall in vascular resistance could be related to the alveolar surface tension effect described above, or to some other factor.

However, Velvis *et al.* [35] found that prostaglandin synthesis inhibition completely abolished the fall in pulmonary vascular resistance associated with rhythmic ventilation of the lungs without altering Po_2 and Pco_2, but had no effect on the vasodilation resulting from ventilation with oxygenation. Thus whether there is a fall in pulmonary vascular resistance associated with lung expansion due to physical factors alone has yet to be resolved.

The pulmonary vasodilator effect of oxygenation of the lung is probably the result of NO liberation from the pulmonary vascular endothelium, because prior administration of the NO inhibitor *N*-ω-nitro-L-arginine markedly decreased the fall in pulmonary vascular resistance associated with oxygenation [36]. It has been proposed by Ivy *et al.* [37] that the NO effect of oxygenation could be at least partly related to stimulation of ET_B receptors, because blockade of these receptors with the selective ET_B receptor blocker BQ-388 attenuated the fall in pulmonary vascular resistance associated with oxygen ventilation. However, in their study, BQ-388 limited the fall in pulmonary vascular resistance during ventilation with both low and high oxygen gases, so the effect appears to be related to lung expansion and not specifically associated with oxygenation.

Another mechanism that has been considered a regulator of pulmonary vascular tone is the presence of oxygen-sensitive K^+ channels in the membrane of pulmonary vascular smooth muscle cells [38]. A decrease in oxygen levels inhibits these oxygen-sensitive, voltage-gated K^+ channels in pulmonary arterial smooth muscle cells. Inhibition of voltage-gated K^+ channels depolarizes membrane potential, and activates Ca^{2+} influx via voltage-gated calcium channels, inducing contraction [39]. Blockade of K^+ channels with glibenclamide causes constriction of pulmonary vascular smooth muscle, but opening K^+ channels with lemakalim results in reduced tone, as may be associated with an increase in oxygenation. The relationships between NO and membrane K^+ channels are yet to be determined.

Many other vasoactive agents have been considered to affect the postnatal increase in pulmonary blood flow. Exposure of pregnant ewes to hyperbaric oxygen greatly increases fetal blood Po_2 and markedly increases fetal pulmonary blood flow [14]. Bradykinin concentrations in left atrial blood increased to levels greater than those in the pulmonary artery, indicating that bradykinin was released in the lungs. Bradykinin produces marked vasodilatation of the fetal pulmonary circulation and possibly could have a role in the changes after birth. The possible role of other pulmonary vasodilators, such as acetylcholine, adenosine, natriuretic peptides, and calcitonin gene-related peptide, is still to be determined.

One of the perplexing questions that requires an answer is how an increase in alveolar oxygen level that would raise pulmonary venous Po_2 could dilate the precapillary pulmonary arterioles. It has been proposed that there are chemosensitive cells in the walls of the pulmonary veins that, through a local axon reflex, influence the precapillary vessels when Po_2 and Pco_2 changes occur; however, there is little convincing evidence for the existence of this mechanism. There is now good documentation that the precapillary vessels are influenced by diffusion of gas into them from surrounding alveoli through which they are coursing. Hydrogen inhaled into the lung can be detected almost instantaneously by means of a platinum-electrode catheter in a pulmonary artery as large as 2 mm diameter, indicating transport of gas from alveoli into large precapillary vessels. This has also been confirmed for oxygen in studies of rapidly frozen lung in which the living exposed lung has been instantaneously frozen with liquid propane. In these preparations, the blood in pulmonary arterioles can be seen to be partly oxygenated [40]. Thus, it is perfectly reasonable to assume that when the fetal lung is ventilated with air, the high level of Po_2 in the alveolar gas can produce pulmonary arteriolar dilatation.

Pulmonary vascular resistance and pulmonary arterial pressure continue to fall after the initial rapid decline, and these later changes appear to be related to regression of the medial muscle layer. The muscle layer thins very rapidly and the vessels resemble adult pulmonary vessels within a few weeks. Associated with the muscle changes, pulmonary vascular resistance falls rapidly during the first 10–14 days and reaches adult levels of about 0.08 mmHg/mL per min per kg about 6–8 weeks after birth (see Figure 5.1). A fall in pulmonary arterial pressure parallels this change. There is considerable variation in different species in the time course of these postnatal changes. In the puppy and lamb, the fall in pulmonary vascular resistance is quite rapid, the major drop occurring in 5–7 days; in the human infant it is slower, taking about 6–8 weeks, whereas in the calf it is delayed for 10–12 weeks. In addition to the early postnatal fall in pulmonary vascular resistance related to the change in the medial smooth muscle over the first 2 months, the growth of new vascular and alveolar units increases the cross-sectional area of the pulmonary vascular bed and this contributes to a continuing fall in vascular resistance (see below).

The fact that pulmonary vascular resistance does not immediately fall to adult levels is not due to a lack of complete vasodilator response, but most likely to a simple physical effect of the smooth muscle. The thicker wall of the pulmonary arterioles probably makes them less compliant, so that they are not as readily distended by increasing pulmonary blood flow as are adult vessels, and thus create a higher pulmonary vascular resistance. Pulmonary blood flow can be increased about threefold in the adult without causing any significant rise in pulmonary arterial pressure; this signifies that the vessels are very distensible and can accommodate an increased flow. In the newborn period, however, the vessels are not as distensible and therefore cannot accommodate an increased flow without elevation in pulmonary arterial pressure. In addition, there are relatively fewer vessels relative to alveoli in the infant lung, as mentioned below.

Postnatal morphological changes in pulmonary vessels

As mentioned above in the description of fetal pulmonary vessels, the preacinar arteries are muscularized, and the intraacinar arteries, which are associated with bronchioli, are partially muscular or nonmuscular. The arteries beyond this level are not muscularized. Also the lumen is small, the medial layer relatively thick, and the intimal layer also quite thick. Rapidly following expansion of the lungs, the pulmonary arteriolar lumen enlarges, the endothelium becomes flattened, and the medial diameter is decreased. This reduction in wall thickness appears to be due largely to a decrease in overlap of adjacent smooth muscle cells [41]. Within days to a few weeks, the arterioles develop the features characteristic of the adult lung, namely a thin wall with a very low ratio of lumen to wall diameter. Interestingly, there is also gradual distal extension of smooth muscle in the media of the intraacinar and alveolar duct arteries that occurs over months and years. It is not known whether these smooth muscle cells develop from pericytes or differentiate from fibroblasts. Postnatally, growth of the lungs is associated with an increase in the number of both pulmonary vessels and alveoli during infancy and childhood. As mentioned above, current evidence indicates that new vessel growth, stimulated by VEGF activity, precedes alveolar development. Initially, the increase in numbers of arteries exceeds that of the alveoli, so that the ratio of alveoli to arteries falls from about 20:1 in the neonatal lung to about 10:1 by 4–5 years of age. Subsequently, little further preferential growth of arteries occurs. Associated with this there is a gradual decrease in pulmonary vascular resistance for the first 4–5 years after birth. Since pulmonary vascular resistance is an indication of cross-sectional area, an increase in the number of vessels will increase the total area and decrease the calculated resistance.

It is interesting to speculate on the mechanisms responsible for the decrease in thickness of the wall of the vessels relative to lumen diameter. It was generally assumed that there was a decrease in the amount of smooth muscle in the pulmonary arterioles after birth. It was questioned whether there is loss of cells by apoptosis, or whether there is merely cessation of growth of new cells. The reduction in growth could be due to removal of a growth-stimulating factor such as endothelin, which is a very effective mitogen [42], or to increased production of heparin by endothelial cells, or other growth-inhibiting factors. However, the current concept is that there is no loss of smooth muscle cells but that the cells change configuration and that there is less overlap of cells (see above). Also, the intimal layer is thinner because endothelial cells become flattened.

The main pulmonary trunk and the left and right pulmonary arteries also undergo considerable change after birth. In the fetus, the pulmonary trunk continues into the ductus arteriosus, and the left and right pulmonary arteries arise as branches of the large channel. The diameter of the branches is much less than that of the trunk (Figure 5.4a). After birth, when the ductus arteriosus closes, the pulmonary trunk is still very large and presents as a dome, with the left and right branches arising posteriorly (Figure 5.4b). Although the branch vessels increase in size, there is, for several weeks after birth, a marked discrepancy between the large main pulmonary trunk and the branches. In some normal infants, a small pressure difference of up to 8–15 mmHg has been detected between the main pulmonary trunk and the left and right branches. However, if pulmonary blood flow is increased, as for example by a left-to-right shunt, the pressure difference may be twice that figure. This explains the frequent presence of a systolic or occasionally systolic and diastolic murmur over the upper left sternal border with radiation to the left and sometimes the right lung in newborn infants. We have termed this a *murmur of physiological peripheral pulmonary stenosis* [43]. With further growth, the left and right pulmonary arteries enlarge and

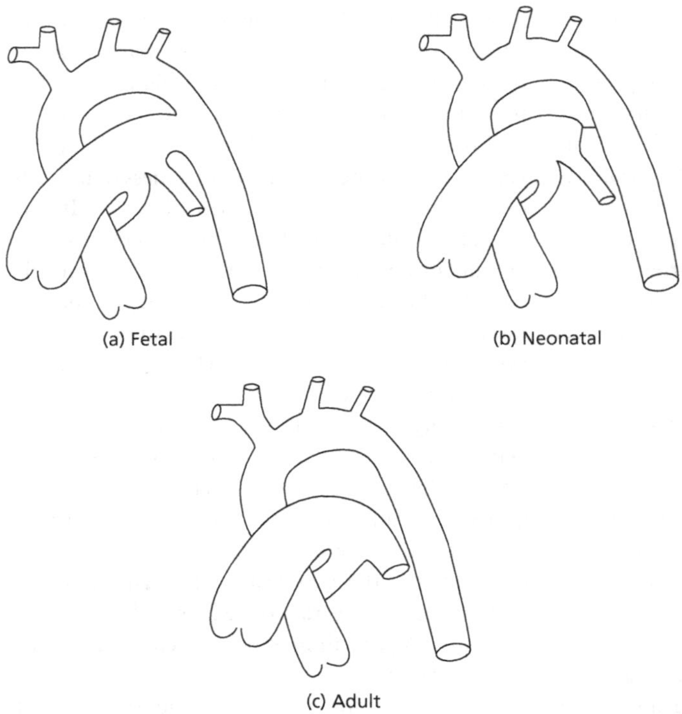

Figure 5.4 Changes in the configuration of the pulmonary trunk and its primary branching from fetal to adult life. In the fetus (a), the main pulmonary trunk is large and continues into the ductus arteriosus, which provides a large communication with the aorta. The branch pulmonary arteries are small in comparison with the trunk. In the newborn period (b), the ductus arteriosus has closed and the branch pulmonary arteries are disproportionately small compared with the pulmonary trunk. A pressure gradient may be noticed between the main and branch pulmonary arteries. In the adult (c), the branch pulmonary arteries have enlarged in response to the increased flow.

assume the adult configuration (Figure 5.4c); the pressure difference also gradually disappears, as does the murmur.

Associated with the reduction in pulmonary arterial pressure, the wall of the main pulmonary trunk becomes thinner, loses much of the smooth muscle cell component, and over the course of several months the elastic lamellae are largely replaced by collagen fibers.

Effects of acute and chronic hypoxia on pulmonary circulation

Acute hypoxia

During early infancy, the pulmonary circulation retains the marked constrictor response to hypoxia characteristic of the fetus. The effects of hypoxia in increasing pulmonary vascular resistance are markedly influenced by the blood H^+ concentration. The relationship between pulmonary vascular resistance and Po_2 and pH, as observed in studies of newborn calves, is shown in Figure 5.5. Although acidemia and hypoxia independently produce an increase in pulmonary vascular resistance, the pulmonary vasoconstriction is greatly increased when both oxygen lack and acidemia are present. Lung disease may interfere with alveolar oxygen uptake, with resultant hypoxia. Carbon dioxide concentrations in pulmonary venous blood may also be increased, resulting in a fall in pH. This will increase pulmonary vascular resistance, but it has been established that the effect is predominantly due to the increase in H^+ concentration that it causes rather than to the direct effects of Pco_2 change.

This relationship is of importance in infants with lung disease, because pulmonary vascular resistance may be increased to levels above systemic vascular resistance. If the ductus arteriosus is still patent, right-to-left ductus shunting occurs. This results in a lower Po_2 and oxygen saturation in blood in the descending aorta and its branches compared with the ascending aorta and its distribution. Right-to-left shunt may also occur through the foramen ovale, which is usually patent during infancy. Shunting at this site will aggravate the reduction in oxygen saturation and Po_2 in both ascending and descending aortic blood. Pulmonary blood flow is markedly reduced, thus further interfering with oxygen uptake in the lungs.

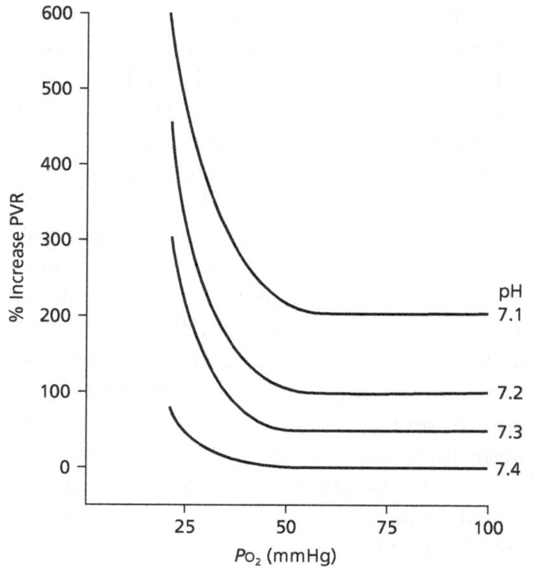

Figure 5.5 Effects of changes in Po_2, in pH alone, and in both combined on pulmonary vascular resistance (PVR) as derived from studies in newborn calves. Note that at a high Po_2 of 100 mmHg, decreasing pH increases pulmonary vascular resistance. When Po_2 is decreased, at a normal pH of 7.4 only a small increase in pulmonary vascular resistance occurs below a Po_2 of 50 mmHg. However, when Po_2 is decreased at low pH, there is a marked accentuation of the pulmonary vasoconstrictor effect.

The magnitude of the rise in pulmonary arterial pressure and pulmonary vascular resistance in response to acute hypoxia rapidly decreases after birth in the normal infant or animal. Whereas pulmonary arterial pressure may rise to systemic arterial levels during the first day, within a few days the mean pressure may increase only to levels of 20–25 mmHg from resting values of 15 mmHg. The rapidity with which the response to hypoxia decreases after birth varies greatly in different species; it falls rapidly in the lamb, so that within 3–4 days mean pulmonary arterial pressure may increase only a few mmHg with hypoxia. The change in the calf occurs much more slowly over several weeks. Although reliable measurements are not available in the normal human infant, the response appears to diminish rapidly over 1–2 weeks after birth. There also seems to be considerable variation in individuals in the same species.

It has often been suggested that systemic arterial hypoxemia is associated with an increase in pulmonary vascular resistance. As mentioned above in the section on fetal responses to hypoxia, there is only a relatively minor reflex effect of arterial chemoreceptor stimulation on pulmonary vascular resistance. The predominant effect of hypoxia is associated with changes in Po_2 in the pulmonary vessels. For this reason, in congenital heart lesions with systemic arterial hypoxemia but normal ventilation and normal pulmonary venous Po_2, such as aortopulmonary transposition or in pulmonary atresia with a patent foramen ovale or ventricular septal defect, the low systemic arterial Po_2 does not significantly increase pulmonary vascular resistance.

Mechanisms of response to hypoxia

Many vasoactive agents have been implicated in the pulmonary vasoconstrictor response to hypoxia. The possibilities considered are that vasoconstrictor substances are released, that production of vasodilators is inhibited, or that alteration of Po_2 directly affects smooth muscle cells.

Although endothelial cells release many vasoactive agents, hypoxia induces contraction of isolated pulmonary vascular smooth muscle cells [16]. This direct effect could be related to the influence of hypoxia on oxygen-sensitive K^+ channels, resulting in an increase in intracellular Ca^{2+}. Endothelin produced by endothelial cells could cause vasoconstriction by stimulation of ET_A receptors on smooth muscle cells. Bosentan, a nonselective endothelin blocker, limited the vasoconstrictor response to hypoxia in pigs [44], although other studies have not confirmed the role of endothelin in hypoxia. The role of NO is also somewhat controversial. NOS activity and NO production were inhibited by hypoxia in pulmonary vessels in rats. However, in a study of Tibetan sheep, inhibition of NOS resulted in greater pulmonary vasoconstriction at high altitude compared with low altitude. This suggests that with prolonged hypoxia, augmentation of endothelial NOS may have a regulatory role in the hypoxic response [45]. This upregulation of NOS in endothelial cells of the pulmonary vasculature during chronic hypoxia has been noted to be dependent on the increase in hypoxia-inducible factor (HIF)-1 [46]. Based on these studies, it is possible that NO activity is reduced in acute hypoxia, but that with more prolonged activity, NOS activity increases to limit severe pulmonary vascular changes. Whether reduced production or activity of other vasodilators such as PGI_2 is involved in the acute hypoxia response is yet to be resolved.

Many vasodilators limit the pulmonary vasoconstrictor response to hypoxia, but this could be related to a general vasodilator action and does not necessarily indicate that reduced production has a role in the hypoxic response. The earliest demonstration of this effect was the reduction of right ventricular hypertensive response to hypoxia by acetylcholine in puppies [47]. Attenuation of the pulmonary vasoconstrictor response has also been observed with other vasodilators, such as tolazoline, NO, sildenafil, and fasudil.

The normal pulmonary vascular changes after birth are partly related to the increase in Po_2. The effects of hypoxia on the pulmonary circulation are markedly influenced by the time after birth that the hypoxia is induced. Conditions that interfere with normal oxygenation after birth may delay the normal decrease in pulmonary vascular resistance and delay the maturation of the pulmonary vessels. It is now well recognized that when an infant is born, and continues to live, at high altitude, the lowered fraction of oxygen in the inspired air will influence pulmonary vascular changes. There is a close relationship between the altitude and the effect on the pulmonary vessels if large populations are examined; however, there is considerable individual variation in the level of pulmonary vascular resistance in different people living at the same altitude. The increased pulmonary vascular resistance persists through childhood and adult life if the individual remains at high altitude. In adult populations living at sea level, the mean pulmonary arterial pressure is about 12 mmHg. In individuals living at an altitude of 1800 m (6000 feet) it averages 16 mmHg; at 3400 m (11 000 feet) it is about 24 mmHg, and at 4300 m (14 000 feet) it is about 40 mmHg.

If the hypoxia is present immediately or very soon after birth, the pulmonary vessels retain the same features seen in fetal vessels. The wall is thick, the endothelial cells are not flattened, and the smooth muscle cells overlap. Furthermore, the smooth muscle cells do not undergo normal postnatal maturation but retain the features characteristic of fetal cells. There is also rapid extension of muscularization to more peripheral vessels that normally do not show smooth muscle cells in the wall. Collagen and elastin formation also increases.

If exposure to hypoxia occurs beyond the immediate neonatal period, the pulmonary circulation undergoes rapid morphological changes in response to hypoxia; these changes are discussed in two excellent reviews [48,49]. The changes involve not only the cellular components of the vessel wall (endothelial cells, smooth muscle cells, and fibroblasts) but also the proteins in the matrix (collagen and elastin). Smooth muscle cells in the media undergo both hypertrophy and hyperplasia and there is rapid peripheral extension of muscularization to intraacinar and alveolar duct arteries, as normally occurs slowly over the childhood years. In addition to the muscular changes, fibroblasts in the adventitia proliferate and there is a dramatic increase in the synthesis of collagen as well as elastin. Even relatively short periods of hypoxia postnatally for 3–5 days are associated with a reduction in the total number of pulmonary arterioles, as evidenced by an increase in the ratio of the numbers of alveoli to arteries.

At least in infancy, when the individual is brought down to sea level, there is a rapid reduction in pulmonary vascular resistance within 1–2 weeks, although it may not return to the same values as in infants born at sea level. Furthermore, there is a greater rise in pulmonary arterial pressure with acute hypoxia, or with increased pulmonary blood flow as during exercise, in young animals or infants exposed to hypoxia for a period of only a few days. These findings suggest that chronic hypoxia after birth may result in permanent effects on the pulmonary circulation. The increased smooth muscle in the medial layer regresses fairly rapidly in the higher oxygen environment, but the pulmonary vasculature is somewhat less compliant than normal because of the increased amount of elastin and collagen in the vessel wall. This causes an increase in pulmonary vascular resistance, which is further accentuated by the decrease in vessel numbers, which reduces the total cross-sectional area of the pulmonary circulation. If the individual is exposed to hypoxia for a considerable period after birth, the collagen changes and the reduction in vessel numbers are likely to be more severe. Under these circumstances, return to sea level will probably result in less dramatic reduction in pulmonary vascular resistance. The increased pulmonary vascular resistance and response to acute hypoxia are due to the persistence and proliferation of the medial muscle. With advancing age, progressive intimal damage, fibrous change, and luminal obstruction develop in a manner similar to that seen in some congenital heart lesions (see Chapter 5). Associated with these changes, the pulmonary vasculature becomes less responsive to both superimposed increased or decreased oxygenation.

Even relatively mild degrees of chronic hypoxia are sufficient to alter the normal pattern of pulmonary vascular maturation. This is somewhat contradictory to the studies of the effects of acute reduction in Po_2 in inspired air in newborn animals. In these experiments, it was found that it was necessary to reduce Po_2 of pulmonary venous blood to levels below about 50 mmHg before pulmonary vasoconstriction was stimulated. This apparent discrepancy may be explained on the basis of the magnitude of the response and its length of duration. If pulmonary vascular resistance is being examined acutely, fairly large changes are necessary before any definite conclusion can be drawn, so that marked reductions in pulmonary venous Po_2 are necessary. In chronic exposure at high altitude there may not be enough of an increase in pulmonary vascular resistance to give convincing documentation by physiological measurements, but mild pulmonary vasoconstriction may prevent normal maturation of the arteries.

However, it is also possible that morphological changes in pulmonary vessels may not be entirely related to the pulmonary vasoconstriction associated with acute hypoxia. It was generally assumed that the increase in smooth muscle in the media was due to pulmonary vasoconstriction. There is some evidence to support this view, because in a study by Rabinovitch *et al.* [50] in rats one pulmonary artery was constricted to prevent the increased pulmonary arterial pressure associated with chronic hypoxia. In this lung, there was no increase in pulmonary arterial smooth muscle, which did occur in the lung with pulmonary hypertension; however, there were other changes in the pulmonary vessels of the lung with the constricted pulmonary artery. It is now thought that although mechanical distension alone may induce some increase in smooth muscle growth, it is more likely that endothelial cells release growth factors on exposure to lower oxygen environments. These growth factors stimulate smooth muscle cell hyperplasia and hypertrophy, and may also stimulate fibroblastic activity.

As mentioned above, endothelial cells exposed to hypoxia produce endothelin, which is a potent mitogen; endothelin blockade has been shown to limit the vascular responses to hypoxia. It is also possible that endothelial damage by hypoxia may permit transport of growth-promoting factors such as insulin-like growth factor 1 from circulating blood into the subendothelial layers. A further possible effect of hypoxia is to inhibit the production of growth-inhibitory factors, such as heparin, by endothelial cells.

Two mechanisms that could be responsible for the pulmonary vascular changes have been proposed. Studies by Rabinovitch [51] have suggested that an enzyme with elastolytic activity, a vascular elastase, is responsible for many of the morphological changes associated with pulmonary arterial hypertension. This could arise from smooth muscle cells, and its production could be stimulated by some plasma factor that passes through the damaged intima. It induces hyperplasia and hypertrophy of the smooth muscle cells and also increases fibroblast activity. Administration of an antagonist to vascular elastase prior to hypoxia has been shown to reduce the severity of the vascular morphological changes. Attention has also been directed to the possible role of angiotensin. Although one study suggested that pulmonary vascular changes resulting from angiotensin infusion resulted from the increase in pulmonary arterial pressure, other studies have suggested that angiotensin II may directly affect smooth muscle cell growth, as well as stimulate fibroblastic activity. Blockade of angiotensin II receptors with losartan has also been effective in limiting the morphological changes resulting from hypoxia.

The effect of lowered alveolar Po_2 on the pulmonary vessels may occur in conditions other than altitude. It is common in infants with idiopathic respiratory distress syndrome and lung diseases of various types. Normal pulmonary vasodilatation may be prevented after birth if the lesion is present early; alternatively, if the lung disease develops in the first 2–3 months after birth, marked pulmonary vasoconstriction may occur. The pulmonary

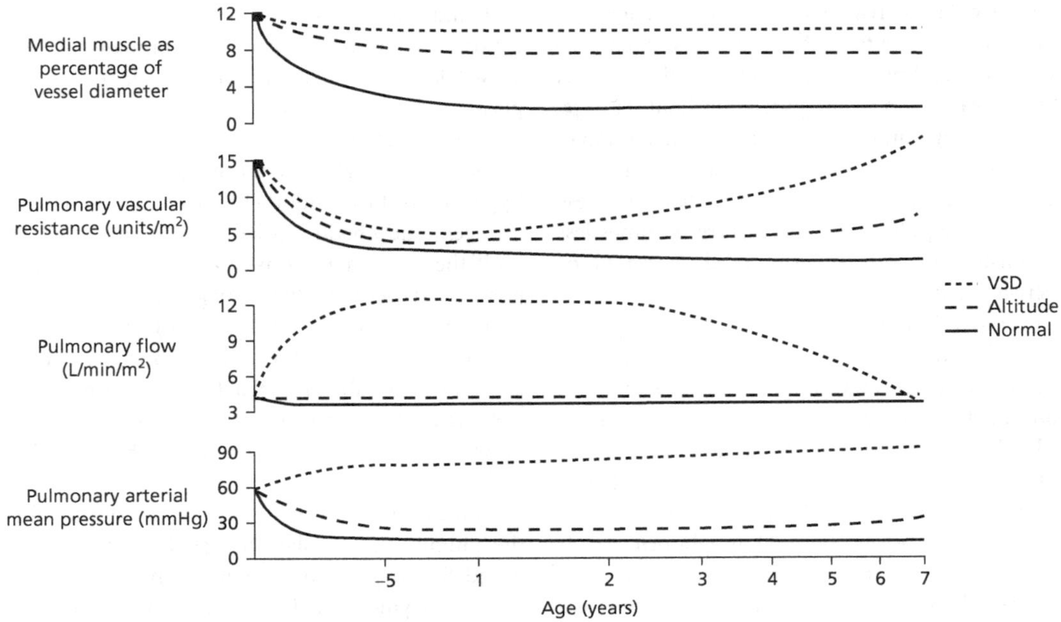

Figure 5.6 Comparison of the postnatal changes in infants with a large ventricular septal defect (VSD) and in infants born at high altitude, with the normal. The presence of a large VSD results in persistence of a high pulmonary arterial pressure. Pulmonary vascular resistance falls more slowly after birth and does not reach normal levels. Associated with the fall in pulmonary vascular resistance, pulmonary blood flow increases markedly due to left-to-right shunting. The medial muscle layer of the small pulmonary arteries does not undergo its normal regression. After a variable period, pulmonary vascular resistance begins to increase due to secondary intimal changes, and this is associated with a fall in pulmonary blood flow. In the infant born and contining to live at high altitude there is also a delay in the maturation of the small pulmonary vessel muscle layer, due to the effects of hypoxia in maintaining constriction. Pulmonary arterial pressure does not fall as rapidly as normal and remains somewhat elevated, the actual level of pressure being dependent on the altitude. In adult life, some intimal change may develop, with an increase in pulmonary vascular resistance and pulmonary arterial pressure.

vessels are much more responsive to the effects of Po_2 reduction in infants than in older children and adults, due to the greater amount of medial smooth muscle. If there is continuous hypoxia after birth, there is persistence of the medial muscle layer, of increased pulmonary vascular resistance, and of pulmonary hypertension (Figure 5.6). Thus the patient who has had persistent lung disease from birth will respond more dramatically to hypoxia with pulmonary vasoconstriction than will a normal individual.

Effects of congenital heart disease on the pulmonary circulation

Changes after birth: pressure–flow relationships

In many infants with congenital heart lesions there is a large communication between the aorta and the pulmonary artery or between the left and right ventricle. If the communication is large enough, after birth pulmonary arterial and right ventricular systolic pressure will continue to be maintained at systemic levels due to equalization across the large defect. With communications at the aortopulmonary level, diastolic pressures in the aorta and pulmonary artery may also be similar. In these infants there is retardation of the normal maturation of the pulmonary arterioles. The smooth muscle layer in the arterioles thins to some degree, but not to the extent noted normally, and the time period of the changes is prolonged. The persistence of the muscle interferes with the normal decrease in pulmonary vascular resistance. After the initial decrease resulting from postnatal expansion of the lung with air, pulmonary vascular resistance falls slowly over the first 3–4 months. It also does not reach the very low levels seen normally (see Figure 5.6). The pulmonary vascular resistance is maintained at levels of about two to four times the normal level, but it falls enough to permit a large pulmonary blood flow. Pulmonary blood flow increases as resistance falls, but pulmonary arterial systolic pressure remains high at systemic levels, as its level is determined by the size of the communication between the two sides of the heart and not by the pulmonary vascular resistance alone.

If the communication is smaller, pulmonary arterial pressure will fall after birth; the magnitude of the fall will be determined by the size of the communication as well as the change in pulmonary vascular resistance. If the defect is small, pulmonary arterial pressure will fall to normal or near-normal levels, and pulmonary vascular resistance will drop normally. With moderate-sized defects, pulmonary arterial pressure will be somewhat elevated and the fall in pulmonary vascular resistance will be delayed, although it may achieve normal levels at rest.

The mechanism responsible for the persistence of a thick smooth muscle layer and higher pulmonary vascular resistance is not known. Teleologically, it is quite clear that there must be precapillary vasoconstriction, as otherwise the high pulmonary arterial pressure would be transmitted to the capillaries and hemorrhage and massive transudation of fluid would occur. The persistence of the smooth muscle in the media of small pulmonary arteries was previously attributed to the high pressure which, it was thought, mechanically stimulated smooth muscle growth. This is in contrast to normal, in which pulmonary arterial pressure falls and the medial layer becomes thinner.

Experimental studies in newborn lambs in which a large aortopulmonary communication had been introduced surgically *in utero* suggest that, in association with increased blood flow and pressure postnatally, endothelial function is altered. Endothelium-dependent pulmonary vasodilation was impaired in lambs with shunts and the vasoconstrictor response to inhibition of NO was enhanced [52].

It is very likely that some of the mechanisms responsible for the changes during chronic hypoxia are also involved in congenital heart disease. It has been proposed that endothelin may be responsible for the pulmonary vascular changes associated with congenital cardiovascular malformations. Because it is a potent mitogen, it is possible that it is liberated from the endothelium and induces both smooth muscle and fibroblast stimulation. However, the role of endothelin is controversial. In lambs in which an aortopulmonary shunt had been placed *in utero*, endothelin abnormalities were noted before any morphological changes occurred [53]. ET-1 production in the lungs has been noted to be increased in children with lesions associated with increased pulmonary arterial pressure but not in those with increase pulmonary blood flow alone [54]. However, Adatia and Haworth found no abnormalities of endothelin prodiction in patients with congenital cardiac lesions with either increased flow or pulmonary vascular resistance [55]. It is possible that endothelin has a role early in the initiation of pulmonary vascular structural changes, or that it has a local effect and circulating levels do not reflect the local effects.

Endothelial damage may result from shear stress (see Chapter 5) and plasma growth factors may therefore pass more readily into the media. Also, it is possible that vascular elastase activity is stimulated (see Chapter 5) and this results in the medial changes.

In patients with atrial septal defect, pulmonary arterial pressure falls normally after birth, pulmonary vascular resistance falls normally, and the vessels undergo normal maturation with regard to the medial muscle layer. This suggests that large pulmonary blood flows may not alter the normal regression of the media of the pulmonary vessels. However, the development of a high pulmonary blood flow in atrial septal defect is dependent on the postnatal fall in pulmonary vascular resistance (see Chapter 8), so that the increased pulmonary blood flow follows the decrease in vascular smooth muscle.

If pulmonary blood flow is increased in the postnatal period, pulmonary vascular smooth muscle regression is delayed. This has been noted in both clinical and experimental situations. If one pulmonary artery is ligated in an adult animal, the pulmonary arterial pressure does not rise, due to distension of the vessels and decrease in pulmonary vascular resistance in the remaining lung. Thus, even though pulmonary blood flow is doubled through this lung, pressure is not increased. If, however, one pulmonary artery is ligated in a newborn animal, blood flow to the remaining lung will increase and pulmonary arterial pressure will rise [56]. This is related to the fact that the vessels with thick muscle walls are less compliant and the pulmonary vascular resistance cannot fall as readily as in the adult. Associated with the persistent pulmonary hypertension is a delay in normal vascular muscle regression. A similar phenomenon may be noted in infants born with an absence of one pulmonary artery or with the condition of so-called hemitruncus, in which one pulmonary artery arises normally from the right ventricle but the other arises from the aorta. Here, too, total systemic venous return is presented to one lung, and the high flow immediately after birth prevents normal pulmonary vessel maturation.

Another instance in which a large flow is presented to the lungs is where a left-to-right shunt occurs from a very high pressure to a low-pressure chamber (obligatory shunt; see Chapter 9). The high flow occurs independently of the changes in pulmonary vascular resistance, and since the pulmonary arterioles do not distend readily to accommodate the increased flow, pulmonary arterial pressure is maintained at a higher than normal level and the smooth muscle in the media is retained.

The three known factors associated with delayed maturation of the pulmonary arterioles, namely large systemic pulmonary communications, altitude, and increased pulmonary blood flow, all have one feature in common: increased pulmonary arterial pressure. If more than one of these disturbances occur in the same individual, the effects on the pulmonary vessels are additive. The combined effect of hypoxia produced by altitude and increased flow produced by ligation of one pulmonary artery soon after birth has been demonstrated in calves. When one pulmonary artery was ligated and the calves kept at sea level, only mild-to-moderate pulmonary arterial hypertension was noted. When animals were maintained at an altitude of about 1800 m with both pulmonary arteries intact, a mild degree of pulmonary hypertension also occurred. If, however, animals with one pulmonary artery ligated were exposed to altitude, severe pulmonary hypertension with a progressive increase in pulmonary vascular resistance developed [57]. A similar phenomenon has been noted in infants with large ventricular septal defects [58]. The ventricular septal defect interferes with normal regression of smooth muscle, but the additive effect of hypoxia, if the infant is born at high altitude, further impedes the postnatal changes in the pulmonary vascular smooth muscle, and pulmonary vascular resistance is maintained at high levels. This retards the development of large pulmonary blood flows, and thus cardiac failure is less frequent and of lesser severity in infants with systemic–pulmonary communications born at high altitude.

In early infancy, increased pulmonary vascular resistance with large systemic–pulmonary communications is associated with predominantly a thick medial muscle layer, but the more peripheral arterioles soon become muscularized. No obvious morphological changes in the endothelium are apparent although, as mentioned above, experimental studies suggest there may be early disturbance of endothelial function. If the large defect persists, further changes occur in the arterioles. The intimal layer begins to thicken initially by cellular proliferation, but subsequently fibrosis develops. The intimal changes are not always uniform and may be eccentric in the lumen. These secondary intimal changes result in a progressive decrease in lumen size and an increase in pulmonary vascular resistance. The intimal changes are unusual under the age of 1 year, but undoubtedly have been noted earlier, although they are not usually extensive in infants. Their rate of progression beyond the first year is quite variable, but by the age of 2–3 years there are usually prominent intimal changes.

The smooth muscle layer in the media also undergoes further change. The medial layer increases, with a progressive decrease in the lumen diameter to wall thickness ratio. It is likely that the increase in muscle mass is due to both hyperplasia and hypertrophy of smooth muscle cells, as occurs with hypoxia. The muscularization of the intra-acinar and alveolar arterioles also proceeds more rapidly than in the normal child. In addition there is a progressive increase in collagen formation in the media, and particularly the adventitia, of the arterioles. Heath and Edwards have classified the magnitude of the morphological changes as follows: grade I, early muscular changes; grade II, intimal proliferation; grade III, fibrous proliferative phase; and grade IV, more severe obstruction [59].

Pulmonary vascular resistance increases as a result of both the changes in the vessel wall, which greatly reduces the compliance of the vessel, and the encroachment of the lumen by the thickened intima. This reduces pulmonary blood flow and left-to-right shunt and the symptoms of cardiac failure may improve. The temporal changes in pulmonary arterial pressure, pulmonary blood flow, pulmonary vascular smooth muscle, and pulmonary vascular resistance are shown in Figure 5.6.

In patients with atrial septal defects, the pulmonary circulation responds quite differently. As I have mentioned, the pulmonary vascular smooth muscle and pulmonary vascular resistance follow normal developmental patterns after birth, and pulmonary arterial pressure falls rapidly to normal levels. Even with high pulmonary blood flow, these pulmonary vessels are relatively normal. Only in later life, usually beyond adolescence and often not before 20–40 years of age, do secondary changes occur in the pulmonary arterioles. These changes are almost exclusively localized to the intima; there is little medial muscle hypertrophy. The intimal changes are quite similar to those observed with large aortopulmonary communications, but they occur late in life.

The mechanism for the intimal changes and why they develop at different ages in patients with atrial septal defects compared to those with aortopulmonary communications is not known. It has been shown by Fry that a threefold increase in endothelial shearing force through segments of perfused artery demonstrates damage to the endothelial cells; he suggests that these changes result from the increased shear on the endothelial lining created by the higher velocity of flow [60]. These findings could provide an explanation for the intimal changes in the pulmonary circulation. In atrial septal defect, the pulmonary arterioles are thin-walled and widely dilated; over the course of many years, the increased velocity due to the large pulmonary blood flow may gradually result in progressive intimal damage and proliferation. Significant degrees of pulmonary vascular obstruction develop only after the changes are quite extensive. In patients with large systemic–pulmonary communications with pulmonary hypertension, the pulmonary arterioles are thick-walled due to medial muscle retention, and their lumina are narrower. For the same increase in pulmonary blood flow as occurs in atrial septal defect there is now a much greater increase in velocity, because the vessels are narrower. This will create greater wall shear with more severe intimal damage and more rapid onset of obliterative pulmonary vascular disease.

This mechanism could also explain the high incidence of pulmonary vascular disease in adults who are born and continue to live at high altitude. The persistence of the medial muscle coat makes the vessels less compliant and narrower, so that over the course of years the intima becomes damaged by even normal blood flows.

The role of blood hematocrit in the development of pulmonary vascular obstructive disease has not been considered seriously. There are two possible mechanisms by which increased hematocrit could contribute toward this. A high hematocrit increases blood viscosity; this effectively increases vascular resistance, as a greater pressure difference across the vascular bed is required to produce the same flow as at lower viscosity. Thus, there is an elevation in pulmonary arterial pressure that promotes retention of the medial muscle layer. The second mechanism relates to the possible effect of increasing shear on the endothelium. Usually, a layer of plasma lies on the endothelial cells when blood flow through a tube or vessel is laminar. However, when hematocrit is high, there could be increased shear on the intimal lining, with damage. A high hematocrit could contribute to the development of early pulmonary vascular obstruction in infants with severe cyanotic cardiac lesions, such as aortopulmonary transposition.

In all these situations in which pulmonary arterial pressure remains elevated after birth, the normal regressive changes in the main pulmonary trunk do not occur. The wall remains thick and the elastic fibers persist after birth. The histology of the pulmonary trunk provides a history of the development of pulmonary hypertension. If pulmonary hypertension has been present since birth, the pulmonary trunk shows persistence of the elastic tissue, as seen in patients with large communications between the ventricles or great arteries. If, however, pulmonary hypertension develops late in life, as in patients with atrial septal defect with pulmonary vascular disease, the main pulmonary trunk is thin and is composed largely of collagen. In view of the different structure, it is most unusual for aneurysmal dilatation of the main pulmonary artery to occur in patients with large ventricular or great vessel defects, but it may occur in adults with atrial septal defect and pulmonary vascular disease.

The possibility that genetic factors may be involved in determining the rapidity with which pulmonary vascular changes occur with congenital cardiac malformations has not been considered seriously. Interest in possible genetic factors has been renewed with the observation that mutations in the gene for bone morphogenetic protein receptor type II (BMPR2) may be associated with the development of primary pulmonary arterial hypertension in adults [61]. BMPR2 is a serine/threonine receptor kinase. Bone morphogenetic proteins are members of the transforming growth factor (TGF)-β superfamily of ligands; they serve several functions in cells, such as cell growth and differentiation, and are involved in osteogenesis. In the pulmonary vasculature BMPR2 inhibits the proliferation of vascular smooth muscle and disturbance in its activity is associated with pulmonary hypertension. A large number of mutations of the gene have now been detected and are found in about 25% of patients with sporadic primary pulmonary hypertension [62]. In a study of children and adults with congenital cardiac malformations and elevated pulmonary vascular resistance, BMPR2 mutations were detected in only 6% [63]. Several of the patients with BMPR2 mutations had atrioventricular communications, raising the question whether there is a genetic relationship between the cardiac lesions and pulmonary vascular abnormalities.

Pulmonary vascular responses in congenital heart disease

Normally there is a minor response of the pulmonary circulation to vasomotor agents and to oxygen administration in the adult. During early infancy, while there is still a considerable amount of smooth muscle in the media, hypoxia causes considerable elevation of pulmonary arterial pressure, and vasodilators produce some fall in pressure. As mentioned above, individuals born and continuing to live at altitude have persistence of smooth muscle and also show greater vascular reactivity. Children with congenital cardiac lesions associated with pulmonary vascular changes may also show considerable response to pulmonary vasodilators and to oxygen.

The responses to vasodilators appear to correlate with the amount of smooth muscle in the media. In an early study, in which tolazoline (Priscoline) was used as the vasodilator, infants and children had three types of response [64]. Those with normal or slightly increased pulmonary arterial pressure showed negligible response. Some with pulmonary arterial hypertension showed a marked increase in pulmonary blood flow, a fall in pulmonary arterial pressure, especially diastolic, and a decrease in pulmonary vascular resistance. This group of patients usually had moderate elevations of resting pulmonary vascular resistance and large or moderate left-to-right shunts. Infants or children with pulmonary arterial hypertension and very high pulmonary vascular resistance with little or no left-to-right shunt, or with some right-to-left shunt, showed little or no change in pulmonary vascular resistance.

The reactivity of the pulmonary circulation was considered to reflect the amount of smooth muscle in the media. In those children with no elevation of pulmonary arterial pressure, there was no significant increase in smooth muscle, hence the lack of response. Lack of a significant response in the presence of marked pulmonary hypertension suggested that the smooth muscle in the media had been largely replaced by fibrous tissue, and also that a considerable proportion of the increased pulmonary vascular resistance could be related to intimal thickening. Smooth muscle may undergo regression when closure of a large ventricular septal defect reduces pulmonary arterial pressure and flow. The magnitude of the response of pulmonary vascular resistance to vasodilators has been used to predict the likelihood that pulmonary vascular resistance will fall following closure of a communication between the ventricles or great arteries.

Although tolazoline was used for many years as a pulmonary vasodilator, other drugs have replaced it because of its side effects of tachycardia, nausea, and vomiting. It was generally administered in a single bolus, since its effects were variable when given as a continuous infusion. PGI_2 is an effective pulmonary vasodilator and it can be administered by continuous infusion. A combination of adenosine triphosphate and magnesium chloride (ATP-$MgCl_2$) has also been found to be comparable to tolazoline as a pulmonary vasodilator. It can be administered by continuous infusion and is not associated with significant side effects. These drugs have a significant vasodilator effect on the systemic circulation, and systemic arterial pressure should be monitored during their administration. A fall in systemic arterial pressure could result in a decrease in pulmonary arterial pressure without an effect on pulmonary vascular resistance.

Inhalation of NO has been used to assess whether pulmonary vascular resistance is responsive to vasodilators. This gas has a strong pulmonary vasodilator effect; because it has minimal effect on the systemic circulation at the concentration administered, it is now the preferred agent for examining pulmonary vascular responsiveness. Recently, the phosphodiesterase V inhibitor sildenafil has been shown to be a pulmonary vasodilator and is as effective as NO in assessing responsiveness of the pulmonary circulation.

The effect of oxygen on pulmonary vascular resistance has also been used to assess reactivity and infer the amount of muscularization of the vessels. In studies in newborn calves, administration of 100% oxygen had no effect on pulmonary vascular resistance when systemic arterial Po_2 was 90 mmHg or higher during air breathing. In many infants and children with increased pulmonary vascular resistance associated with large ventricular or aortopulmonary communications, administration of 100% oxygen lowers pulmonary vascular resistance, with an increase in pulmonary blood flow and left-to-right shunt. The most dramatic effects of oxygen are noted in those individuals with decreased systemic arterial oxygen saturation or Po_2. Oxygen saturation may be in the high 80s or low 90s, yet oxygen inhalation may have a dramatic effect. If the pulmonary veins can be catheterized, oxygen saturation may be evenly reduced, but often one or two of the veins show a considerable reduction to levels of about 80%. The reduced pulmonary venous saturation may result from a disturbance in ventilation–perfusion relationships; pulmonary blood flow is high, but alveolar ventilation is either normal, or may be reduced if some pulmonary edema or congestion is present. Diffusion may also be impaired by pulmonary edema. Additional factors that may affect alveolar ventilation are local areas of atelectasis resulting from airway compression by large pulmonary arteries, and pulmonary infection. Infants with Down syndrome and congenital cardiac lesions are particularly prone to pulmonary involvement, resulting in decreased pulmonary venous oxygenation and high pulmonary vascular resistance; inhalation of 100% oxygen often lowers resistance markedly.

Although the most dramatic responses to oxygen in patients with congenital heart lesions usually occur in those with impaired oxygenation, occasionally a modest reduction in pulmonary vascular resistance results in patients with normal arterial and pulmonary venous oxygen contents. It is difficult to explain this based on the fact that oxygen does not have a significant effect on pulmonary vascular resistance in normal well-oxygenated animals. The response to oxygen could be related to an effect on endothelial cells, because, as mentioned above, recent studies suggest endothelial dysfunction in newborn lambs with simulated aortopulmonary communications. Possibly oxygen decreases endothelin production or increases NO liberation in these circumstances. Perhaps oxygen could have a direct effect on smooth muscle cells by influencing oxygen-sensitive K^+ channels (see above).

Effects of pulmonary venous and left atrial hypertension

Pulmonary arterial hypertension is frequently associated with conditions that produce an increase in pulmonary venous pressure. Some degree of the increased pulmonary arterial pressure is merely passive, i.e., there is pressure elevation to compensate for the increased venous pressure and to maintain perfusion pressure across the vascular bed. However, frequently there is an elevation in pulmonary arterial pressure out of proportion to the increased pulmonary venous pressure, and pulmonary vascular resistance is increased. The mechanisms responsible for the increased pulmonary vascular resistance are not known. It is common to find that pulmonary vascular resistance is markedly increased in infants with increased pulmonary venous pressure due to lesions such as cor triatriatum and total anomalous pulmonary venous drainage with obstruction of the pulmonary veins. In infants with left heart failure due to severe aortic stenosis or aortic coarctation, pulmonary hypertension is also often encountered. It has been suggested that there may be some local axon reflex that causes pulmonary arteriolar constriction when pulmonary vascular pressure is increased, but there is no evidence for its existence. The more likely explanation is that the elevated pulmonary venous pressure is transmitted through the capillaries to the arterioles and the increased intraluminal pressure distends the vessel, stretching the smooth muscle and thus stimulating its contraction and persistence.

Another mechanism that has been proposed as being important in adults with mitral stenosis is bronchiolar compression. Elevation of left atrial and pulmonary venous pressure is associated with edema in peribronchial tissue and because the small bronchioles in this region are not supported by cartilage, they are readily compressed. I think that this mechanism could be important in the infant with increased pulmonary venous pressure due to any cause. The bronchiolar compression would interfere with ventilation to the lung segment, resulting in decreased Po_2 and possibly increased Pco_2, with resultant pulmonary vasoconstriction. If the bronchiolar compression was extensive enough, marked increase in pulmonary vascular resistance could occur.

Effects of prematurity

Premature infants with intracardiac or aortopulmonary communications behave somewhat differently from mature infants. They appear to develop large left-to-right shunts with cardiac failure earlier after birth, often within the first 2–3 weeks, as compared with onset after 3–6 weeks in the mature infant. This has been confirmed in premature infants with patent ductus arteriosus. The more premature the infant, the sooner after birth it develops large left-to-right shunts and cardiac failure. In infants weighing less than 1000 g, cardiac failure often develops within the first week after birth.

The most plausible explanation for this difference in behavior of premature infants is that although the morphology of the vessels is similar to that in more mature infants, pulmonary vascular responses are less well developed. The response of the pulmonary circulation to hypoxia, as well as to vasodilators, is less prominent in preterm fetal lambs (see above). It is thus also possible that, in the presence of a communication between the ventricles or great vessels, the pulmonary arteries in the preterm infant do not have the same capacity to react by maintaining constriction as those in the mature infant. Therefore pulmonary vascular resistance falls more rapidly.

Another interesting difference in behavior of the preterm infant is the response to left-to-right shunts. In the mature infant that develops a left-to-right shunt with a ventricular septal defect or an aortopulmonary communication, no significant symptoms occur until the shunt is quite large, usually with a pulmonary to systemic flow ratio of more than 2:1. However, premature infants who have had respiratory distress syndrome tolerate poorly even small left-to-right shunts, including those at the atrial level. It is not unusual for an infant with respiratory distress requiring assisted ventilation to be intolerant of withdrawal from the ventilator. Under this circumstance, it is important to determine if there is a cardiac lesion with a left-to-right shunt, because improvement in respiratory status is frequently readily accomplished by elimination of the shunt. Although there is often a reluctance to recommend surgery for a cardiac lesion in which the pulmonary to systemic blood flow ratio is only 1.5–2:1, in these infants it may result in rapid improvement in respiration.

The mechanisms by which small left-to-right shunts may have such significant effects in these infants have not been defined. A possible explanation is that blood flow to some areas of the lungs may be restricted because of poor aeration or atelectasis. Blood flow through perfused areas would therefore be greater than normal even in the absence of left-to-right shunting. If pulmonary blood flow is increased by the presence of a shunt, the flow through these areas would be even further enhanced. Poor reactivity of the precapillary vessels in the preterm infant could thus permit the arterial pressure to be transmitted to the capillaries and veins and result in pulmonary edema.

Effects of pulmonary vasculature on shunts (dependent and obligatory shunts)

In many communications between the systemic and pulmonary circulations, the relationship between the systemic and pulmonary vascular resistances is important in determining the size and direction of the shunt. After birth, when the placental circulation is removed, if there is a large communication between the aorta and pulmonary artery or between the ventricles, the pressures are essentially equal, and flow to the pulmonary and systemic circulations will be determined by their relative vascular resistances. Thus, as pulmonary vascular resistance falls after birth, there is increasing pulmonary blood flow with a left-to-right shunt. If pulmonary vascular resistance increases, as might occur if intimal proliferative changes occur, the left-to-right shunt will decrease, and if the changes become severe, right-to-left shunt develops. I have used the term *dependent shunting* to describe this.

In patients with atrial septal defect, the changes in afterload of the left and right ventricles are important in determining the amount of blood ejected by each ventricle and thus the amount and direction of shunt. Therefore, the shunt in atrial septal defect is also of the dependent type. In those lesions in which there is a communication between a very high pressure and a low-pressure chamber or great vessel, the relationship between systemic and pulmonary vascular resistances is not important in determining the magnitude of the shunt. In many endocardial cushion defects there is a mitral valve cleft and an atrial septal defect. Blood is essentially ejected from the left ventricle into the right atrium during ventricular systole. The pulmonary vascular resistance does not determine the size of the shunt. This is also noted in peripheral arteriovenous fistulae, and I have applied the term *obligatory shunting* to this type of shunt.

In patients with obligatory shunts, the left-to-right shunt is relatively independent of pulmonary vascular resistance. If the shunt is present soon after birth, a large left-to-right shunt will occur even while pulmonary vascular resistance is still high. This increased pulmonary blood flow will tend to delay normal pulmonary vascular maturation, so that there will be retention of smooth muscle. The risks of developing right-sided heart failure are great, since the right ventricle is presented with a large volume at high pressure. Also, there is a very significant risk that these individuals will develop early and severe pulmonary vascular disease.

Pharmacological treatment of increased pulmonary vascular resistance in congenital cardiac disease

It was generally believed that in patients with congenital cardiovascular malformations with high pulmonary vascular resistance, unless the lesion was amenable to surgery, the pulmonary vascular changes would progress. Compared with primary pulmonary hypertension, in which the severity of pulmonary vascular obstruction tends to progress fairly rapidly, the deterioration with congenital cardiac lesions is relatively slow. Little attention has therefore been directed to attempting to institute medical therapy. However, in recent years, newer pharmacological agents have proved quite effective in treating patients with primary pulmonary hypertension. These include calcium channel blockers, the nonselective endothelial receptor blocker bosentan and the specific ET_A blocker sitaxsentan, PGI_2 (epoprostenol) and its analogs treprostinil and beraprost, and phosphodiesterase V inhibitors such as sildenafil. Although they do not cure the disease, they may slow or even inhibit progression and greatly improve physical performance and longevity. Little has been published about the experience of these agents in patients with high pulmonary vascular resistance associated with congenital cardiac lesions.

Calcium channel blockers have been used quite effectively in patients with primary pulmonary hypertension. They have been noted to delay the rate of progression of the disease and to improve physical performance. They appear to be most effective in those patients who show an acute fall in pulmonary vascular resistance with administration of vasodilator agents. There are few reports of their use in patients with congenital cardiac lesions with high pulmonary vascular resistance. In one study of 10 children aged 3–12 years, seven of whom had Down syndrome, administration of nifedipine for 1–4 years resulted in a fall in pulmonary vascular resistance and some functional improvement [65]. Enthusiasm for the use of calcium channel blockers in primary pulmonary hypertension is waning, because other drugs appear to be more effective. There does not at present seem to be much justification for their use for pulmonary hypertension in congenital cardiac lesions.

The nonselective endothelin blocker bosentan was administered for a 16-week period to 37 patients with congenital cardiac lesions and severe elevation of pulmonary vascular resistance; 17 patients served as controls [66]. Bosentan reduced pulmonary arterial pressure and pulmonary vascular resistance and improved exercise capacity, but had no adverse effect on arterial oxygen saturation. Other studies have also shown improvement, but it remains to be seen how much improvement occurs and for how long it is sustained. Although it would seem likely that selective ET_A blockade would be desirable, there is as yet no evidence that the selective ET_A blocker sitaxsentan is more effective than bosentan.

PGI_2 has a short half-life, so to achieve an effect it is administered by continuous intravenous infusion. Rosenzweig *et al.* [67] studied the effects of chronic PGI_2 infusion in 20 patients (mean age 15 years) with various congenital cardiac malformations and pulmonary vascular obstruction, none of whom had shown a change in hemodynamics with acute infusion. There was considerable improvement, with a fall in pulmonary arterial mean pressure of about 20% and a decrease in pulmonary vascular resistance of almost 50%. Exercise capacity also increased substantially.

To overcome the inconvenience and problems of administration by chronic intravenous infusion, analogs of prostaglandin have been prepared. Treprostinil can be administered by subcutaneous injection, and appears to be as effective as PGI_2 when given by intravenous infusion. Because treprostinil has a longer half-life, accidental disruption of infusion for several hours does not have the adverse effect of interruption of prostaglandin infusion. When administered every 3 hours by subcutaneous injection, it has the same effect as intravenous infusion. The serious disadvantage is that many subcutaneous injections have to be given every day; the injections are painful and in many patients produce intense pain and erythema. It is especially difficult to recommend it for younger children. The experience with beraprost, the analog that can be administered orally, is quite limited. It has been used in Japan and to some extent in Europe. Preliminary studies suggest it is not as effective as the other two agents and this has resulted in a delay of trials in the USA, where it is not yet available.

The phosphodiesterase V inhibitor sildenafil has been used effectively as a pulmonary vasodilator in patients with primary pulmonary hypertension. It has also been administered orally in infants with persistent pulmonary hypertension of the newborn, with great effectiveness [68]. The prospect that it will be effective in patients with high pulmonary vascular resistance associated with congenital cardiac lesions is promising and several studies are now in progress. A recent review presents current concepts regarding management of pulmonary hypertension [69].

References

1 Hall SM, Hislop AA, Pierce CM, Haworth SG. Prenatal origins of human intrapulmonary arteries. Am J Respir Cell Mol Biol 2000;23:194–203.

2 Parera MC, van Dooren M, van Kempen M *et al.* Distal angiogenesis: a new concept for lung vascular morphogenesis. Am J Physiol 2005;288:L148–L149.

3 Jakkula M, Le Cras TD, Gebb S *et al.* Inhibition of angiogenesis decreases alveolarization in the developing rat lung. Am J Physiol 2000;279:L600–L607.

4 Thebaud B, Ladha F, Michelakis ED *et al.* Vascular endothelial growth factor gene therapy increases survival, promotes lung angiogenesis, and prevents alveolar damage in hyperoxia-induced lung injury: evidence that angiogenesis participates in alveolarization. Circulation 2005;112:2477–2486.

5 Frid MG, Moiseeva EP, Stenmark KR. Multiple phenotypically distinct smooth muscle cell populations exist in the adult and developing bovine pulmonary arterial media in vivo. Circ Res 1994;75:669–681.

6 Webb S, Kanani M, Anderson RH, Richardson MK, Brown NA. Development of the human pulmonary vein and its incorporation in the morphological left atrium. Cardiol Young 2001;11:632–642.

7 Levin DL, Rudolph AM, Heymann MA, Phibbs RH. Morphological development of the pulmonary vascular bed in fetal lambs. Circulation 1976;53:144–151.

8 Wagenvoort CA, Neufeld HN, Edwards JE. The structure of the pulmonary arterial tree in fetal and early postnatal life. Lab Invest 1961;10:751–762.

9 Rudolph AM, Heymann MA. Circulatory changes with growth in the fetal lamb. Circ Res 1970;26:289–299.

10 Rasanen J, Wood DC, Debbs RH, Cohen J, Weiner S, Huhta JC. Reactivity of the human fetal pulmonary circulation to maternal hyperoxygenation increases during the second half of pregnancy: a randomized study. Circulation 1998;97:257–262.

11 Sutton MS, Groves A, MacNeill A, Sharland G, Allan L. Assessment of changes in blood flow through the lungs and foramen ovale in the normal human fetus with gestational age: a prospective Doppler echocardiographic study. Br Heart J 1994;71:232–237.

12 Mielke G, Benda N. Cardiac output and central distribution of blood flow in the human fetus. Circulation 2001;103:1662–1668.

13 Cassin S, Dawes GS, Ross BB. Pulmonary blood flow and vascular resistance in immature foetal lambs. 1964;171: 80–89.

14 Heymann MA, Rudolph AM, Nies AS, Melmon KL. Bradykinin production association with oxygenation of the fetal lamb. Circ Res 1969;25:521–534.

15 Lewis AB, Heymann MA, Rudolph AM. Gestational changes in pulmonary vascular responses in fetal lambs in utero. Circ Res 1976;39:536–541.

16 Zhang F, Carson RC, Zhang H, Gibson G, Thomas HM. Pulmonary artery smooth muscle cell $[Ca^{2+}]_i$ and contraction: responses to diphenyleneiodonium and hypoxia. Am J Physiol 1997;273:L603–L611.

17 Rudolph AM, Yuan S. (1966) Response of the pulmonary vasculature to hypoxia and H^+ ion concentration changes. J Clin Invest 45, 399–411.

18 Webb RC. Smooth muscle contraction and relaxation. Adv Physiol Edu 2003;27:201–206.

19 Chitaley K, Weber DS, Webb RC. RhoA/Rho-kinase, vascular changes and hypertension. Curr Hypertens Rep 2001;3:139–144.

20 Soifer SJ, Morin FC III, Kaslow DC, Heymann MA. The developmental effects of prostaglandin D2 on the pulmonary and systemic circulations in the newborn lamb. J Dev Physiol 1983;5:237–250.

21 Jiallard S, Larrue B, Deruelle P *et al.* Effects of phosphodiesterase 5 inhibitor on pulmonary vascular reactivity in the fetal lamb. Ann Thorac Surg 2006;81:935–942.

22 Fukumoto Y, Matoba T, Ito A *et al.* Acute vasodilator effects of a Rho-kinase inhibitor, fasudil, in patients with severe pulmonary hypertension. Heart 2005;91:391–392.

23 Wong J, Fineman JR, Heymann. The role of endothelin and endothelin subtypes in regulation of fetal pulmonary vascular tone. Pediatr Res 1994;35:664–670.

24 Ivy DD, Parker TA, Ziegler JW *et al.* Prolonged endothelin A receptor blockade attenuates chronic pulmonary hypertension in the ovine fetus. J Clin Invest 1997;99: 1179–1186.

25 Ivy DD, Parker TA, Kinsella JP, Abman SH. Endothelin A receptor blockade decreases pulmonary vascular resistance in premature lambs with hyaline membrane disease. Pediatr Res 1998;44:175–180.

26 Waypa GB, Chandel NS, Schumacker PT. Model for hypoxic pulmonary vasoconstriction involving mitochondrial oxygen sensing. Circ Res 2001;88:1259–1266.

27 Kinsella JP, Parker TA, Davis JM, Abman SH. Superoxide dismutase improves gas exchange and pulmonary hemodynamics in premature lambs. Am J Respir Crit Care Med 2005;172:745–749.

28 Abman SH, Accurso FJ. Acute effects of partial compression of ductus arteriosus on fetal pulmonary circulation. Am J Physiol 1989;257:H626–H634.

29 Levin DL, Hyman AI, Heymann MA, Rudolph AM. Fetal hypertension and the development of increased pulmonary vascular smooth muscle: a possible mechanism for persistent pulmonary hypertension of the newborn infant. J Pediatr 1978;92:265–269.

30 Ardran GM, Dawes GS, Prichard MML, Reynolds SRM, Wyatt DG. The effect of ventilation of the foetal lungs upon the pulmonary circulation. J Physiol 1952;118: 12–22.

31 Cassin S, Dawes GS, Mott JC, Ross BB, Strang LB. The vascular resistance of the foetal and newly ventilated lung of the lamb. J Physiol 1964;171:61–79.

32 Lauer RM, Evans JA, Aoki H, Kittle CF. Factors controlling pulmonary vascular resistance in fetal lambs. J Pediatr 1965;67:568–577.

33 Teitel DF, Iwamoto HS, Rudolph AM. Changes in the pulmonary circulation during birth-related events. Pediatr Res 1990;27:372–378.

34 Leffler CW, Hessler JR, Terragno NA. Ventilation-induced release of prostaglandinlike material from fetal lungs. Am J Physiol 1980;238:H282–H286.

35 Velvis H, Moore P, Heymann MA. Prostaglandin inhibition prevents the fall in pulmonary vascular resistance as a result of rhythmic distension of the lungs in fetal lambs. Pediatr Res 1991;30:52–58.

36 Moore P, Velvis H, Fineman JR, Soifer SJ, Heymann MA. EDRF inhibition attenuates the increase in pulmonary blood flow due to oxygen ventilation in fetal lambs. J Appl Physiol 1992;73:2151–2157.

37 Ivy DD, Lee DS, Rairigh RL, Parker TA, Abman SH. Endothelin B receptor blockade attenuates pulmonary vasodilation in oxygen-ventilated fetal lambs. Biol Neonate 2004;86:155–159.

38 Post J, Hume J, Archer S, Weir EK. Direct role for potassium channel inhibition in hypoxic pulmonary vasoconstriction. Am J Physiol 1992;262:C882–C890.

39 Archer SL, Wu XC, Thébaud B *et al.* Preferential expression and function of voltage-gated, O_2-sensitive K^+ channels in resistance pulmonary arteries explains regional heterogeneity in hypoxic pulmonary vasoconstriction: ionic diversity in smooth muscle cells. Circ Res 2004;95:308–318.

40 Staub NC, Storey WF. Relation between morphological and physiological events in lung studied by rapid freezing. J Appl Physiol 1962;17:381–390.

41 Haworth SG, Hall SM, Chew M, Allen K. Thinning of fetal pulmonary arterial wall and postnatal remodelling: ultrastructural studies on the respiratory unit arteries of the pig. Virchows Arch A Pathol Anat Histopathol 1987;411:161–171.

42 Hassoun PM, Thappa V, Landman JA, Fanburg BL. Endothelin 1: mitogenic activity on pulmonary artery smooth muscle cells and release from hypoxic endothelial cells. Proc Soc Exp Biol Med 1992;199: 165–170.

43 Danilowicz DA, Rudolph AM, Hoffman JIE, Heymann MA. Physiologic pressure differences between main and branch pulmonary arteries in infants. Circulation 1972;45:410–419.

44 Holm P, Lisca J, Clozel M, Franco-Cereceda F. The endothelin antagonist bosentan: hemodynamic effects during normoxia and hypoxic pulmonary hypertension in pigs. J Thorac Cardiovasc Surg 1996;112:890–897.

45 Ruan Z, Koizumi T, Sakai A, Ishizaki T, Wang Z. Endogenous nitric oxide and pulmonary circulation response to hypoxia in high-altitude adapted Tibetan sheep. Eur J Appl Physiol 2004;93:190–195.

46 Palmer LA, Semenza GL, Stoler MH, Johns RA. Hypoxia induces type II NOS gene expression in pulmonary artery endothelial cells via HIF-1. Am J Physiol 1998;274: L212–L219.

47 Rudolph AM, Auld PA, Golinko RJ, Paul MH. Pulmonary vascular adjustments in the neonatal period. Pediatrics 1961;28:28–34.

48 Durmowicz AG, Stenmark KR. Mechanisms of structural remodeling in chronic pulmonary hypertension. Pediatr Rev 1999;20:e91–e102.

49 Stenmark KR, Fagan KA, Frid MG. Hypoxia-induced pulmonary vascular remodeling: cellular and molecular mechanisms. Circ Res 2006;99:675–691.

50 Rabinovitch M, Konstam MA, Gamble WJ *et al.* Changes in pulmonary blood flow affect vascular response to chronic hypoxia in rats. Circ Res 1983;52:432–441.

51 Rabinovitch M. EVE and beyond, retro and prospective insights. Am J Physiol 1999;277:5–12.

52 Reddy VM, Wong J, Liddicoat JR, Johengen M, Chang R, Fineman JR. (1996) Altered endothelium-dependent responses in lambs with pulmonary hypertension and increased pulmonary blood flow. Am J Physiol 271, H562–H570.

53 Steinhorn, RH, Fineman JR. (1999) The pathophysiology of pulmonary hypertension in congenital heart disease. Artificial Organs 23, 970–974.

54 Fratz S, Geiger R, Kresse H, Roemer G, Henning M, Sebening W, Hess J. (2003) Pulmonary blood pressure, not flow, is associated with net endothelin-1 production in the lungs of patients with congenital heart disease and normal pulmonary vascular resistance. J Thorac Cardiovasc Surg 126, 1724–1729.

55 Adatia I, Haworth SG. (1993) Circulating endothelin in children with congenital heart disease. Brit Heart J 69, 233–236.

56 Rudoiph AM, Neuhauser EBD, Golinko RJ, Auld PAM. (1961) Effects of pneumonectomy on pulmonary circulation in adult and young animals. Circ Res 9, 856–861.

57 Wagenvoort CA, Wagenvoort N, Vogel JH. (1969) The pulmonary vasculature in cattle at an altitude of 1,600 metres with and without one-sided pulmonary arterial ligation. J Comp Pathol 79, 517–523.

58 Vogel JH, McNamara DG, Blount SG Jr. (1967) Role of hypoxia in determining pulmonary vascular resistance in infants with ventricular septal defects Am J Cardiol 20, 346–349.

59 Heath D, Edwards JE. (1958) The pathology of hypertensive pulmonary vascular disease; a description of six grades of strudtural changes in the pulmonary arteries with special reference to congenital cardiac septal defects. Circulation 18, 533–547.

60 Fry DL. (2002) Arterial intimal-medial permeability and Coevolving structural responses to defined shear-stress exposures. Am J Physiol Heart Circ Physiol 283, H2341–H2355.

61 Deng Z, Morse JH, Slager SL, Cuervo N, Moore KJ, Venetos G, Kalachikov S, Cayanis E, Fischer SG, Barst RJ, Hodge SE, Knowles JA. (2000) Familial primary pulmonary hypertension (gene PPH1) is caused by mutations in the bone morphogenetic protein receptor-II gene. Am J Hum Gen 67, 737–744.

62 Morse JH. (2002) Bone Morphogenetic Protein Receptor 2 Mutations in Pulmonary Hypertension. Chest 121, 50S–53S.

63 Roberts KE, McElroy JJ, Wong WPK, Yen E, Widlitz A, Barst RJ, Knowles JA, Morse JH. (2004) BMPR2 mutations in pulmonary arterial hypertension with congenital heart disease. Eur Respir J 24, 371–374.

64. Rudolph AM, Paul MH, Sommer LS, Nadas AS. (1958) Effects of tolazoline hydrochloride (priscoline) on circulatory dynamics of patients with pulmonary hypertension. Am Heart J 55, 424–432.

65 Wimmer M, Schlemmer M. (1992) Long-term hemodynamic effects of nifedipine on congenital heart disease with Eisenmenger's mechanism in children. Cardiovasc Drugs Ther. 6, 183–186.

66 Galiè N, Beghetti M, Gatzoulis MA, Granton J, Berger RM, Lauer A, Chiossi E, Landzberg M. (2006) Bosentan Randomized Trial of Endothelin Antagonist Therapy-5 (BREATHE-5) Investigators. Bosentan therapy in patients with Eisenmenger syndrome: a multicenter, double-blind, randomized, placebo-controlled study. Circulation. 114, 48–54.

67 Rosenzweig EB, Kerstein D, Barst RJ. (1999) Long-term prostacyclin for pulmonary hypertension with associated with congenital heart defects. Circulation 99, 1858–65.

68 Baquero H, Soliz A, Neira F, Venegas ME, Sola A. (2006) Oral sildenafil in infants with persistent pulmonary hypertension of the newborn: a pilot randomized blinded study. Pediatrics. 117, 1077–1083.

69 Badesch DB, Abman SH, Simonneau G, Rubin LJ, McLaughlin W. Medical therapy for pulmonary arterial hypertension: updated ACCP evidence-based clinical practice guidelines. Chest. 2007 131, 917–28.

CHAPTER 6

The ductus arteriosus and persistent patency of the ductus arteriosus

Patent ductus arteriosus is considered to be one of the more common types of congenital cardiovascular malformations. Various studies report an incidence of 5.3–11.0% (median 7.1%) of all congenital cardiac lesions [1]. Based on an estimated incidence of congenital cardiovascular malformations of 0.8%, the incidence of patent ductus arteriosus in the population is about 0.06%. However, these numbers do not include the occurrence of patent ductus in preterm infants. The incidence in these infants depends on gestational age and is discussed below. Also, since the introduction of echocardiography and Doppler flow studies, the presence of a small patent ductus can occasionally be diagnosed even though no clinical manifestations are evident. The term *silent patent ductus arteriosus* has been used to describe these malformations. The incidence of silent ductuses is not known, but it has been estimated that as many as 0.1–0.2% of the population may be affected [2]. This would suggest that patent ductus arteriosus is about three times more common than currently estimated.

Ductus arteriosus in the fetus

The ductus arteriosus is a large channel normally present in the mammalian fetus. It develops from the distal portion of the embryonic sixth branchial arch by about the sixth week of embryonic development in the human. Normally, the ductus arteriosus develops from the left sixth arch and extends from the pulmonary trunk to the left-sided descending aorta. In the fetus, the ductus is about the same diameter as the descending aorta; in the human fetus at term this is about 10 mm. The main pulmonary trunk arising from the right ventricle leads into the ductus arteriosus, and in the fetus the left and right pulmonary arteries appear to arise as branches from the major pulmonary–ductus arteriosus trunk (Figure 6.1). The ductus arteriosus connects with the aorta just beyond the arch, about 5–10 mm distal to the origin of the left subclavian artery.

Morphological features

The morphology of the ductus differs from the adjacent main pulmonary artery and aorta. The walls of the aorta and pulmonary artery, which are about the same thickness as that of the ductus, are mainly composed of circumferentially arranged elastic fibers. The medial layer of the ductus arteriosus largely consists of smooth muscle, which is arranged circumferentially in the outer layers and longitudinally in the inner layers. It has been suggested that some of the smooth muscle is arranged spirally. Contraction of the smooth muscle would thus result not only in narrowing of the lumen but also in shortening of the ductus. The outer layer of the smooth muscle is interspersed with numerous, small, thin-walled vasa vasorum, but the inner layers are avascular. The medial layer is separated from the intima by a well-formed internal elastic lamina. The intimal layer is thin during most of the gestational period, but prior to birth the intima thickens and the internal elastic lamina begins to show some fragmentation.

Congenital Diseases of the Heart, 3rd edition. By A. Rudolph
 ISBN: 9781405162456

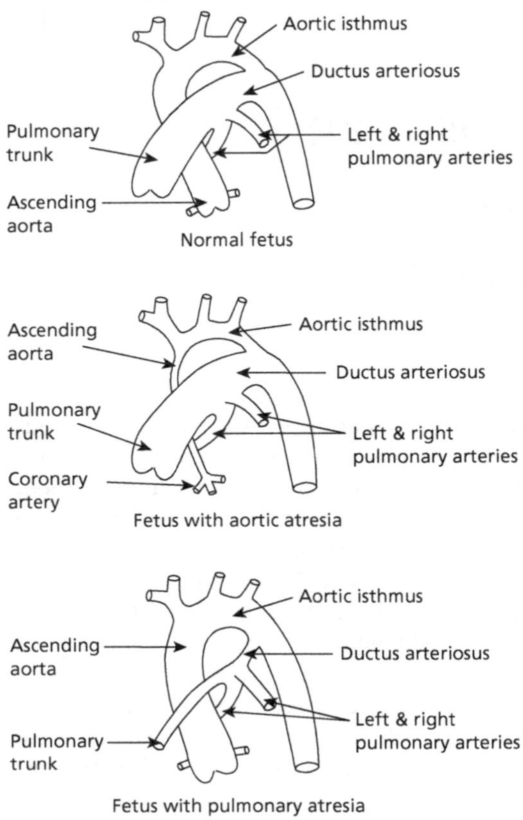

Figure 6.1 Relationships and sizes of the ductus arteriosus and of the aorta, pulmonary trunk and pulmonary arteries in a normal fetus, a fetus with aortic atresia, and a fetus with pulmonary atresia.

Function

In the fetus, the ductus arteriosus carries a major proportion of total or combined ventricular output (CVO) from the right ventricle to the descending aorta. Studies in fetal lambs have shown that the right ventricle ejects about 66% of CVO and that 80–90% of this blood traverses the ductus arteriosus (see Figure 1.6, p. 7). Thus, about 55–60% of CVO passes from the pulmonary trunk to the descending aorta through the ductus arteriosus in fetal lambs. The blood passing across the ductus is pulmonary arterial blood that has a Po_2 of about 18 mmHg in the fetal lamb, compared with an ascending aortic blood Po_2 of about 26 mmHg. There is normally no pressure difference across the ductus, between the pulmonary trunk and the descending aorta, during most of gestation in the lamb. However, during the 10–15 days prior to term, a small pressure gradient of 5–8 mmHg is frequently noted to develop in chronically instrumented fetuses.

In the human fetus, measurements of the proportion of CVO and of right ventricular output flowing across the ductus arteriosus show considerable variation. Mielke and Benda [3] reported that about 45% of CVO passed through the ductus. This is only moderately lower than the proportion of CVO passing through the ductus in the lamb. However, in their studies pulmonary blood flow was considerably lower than that reported by others in human fetuses. In other studies in human fetuses, right ventricular output was about 55% of CVO and pulmonary blood flow represented about 25% of CVO [4,5]. Therefore, based on these measurements, only about 30% of CVO passes across the ductus arteriosus in the human, as compared with almost 60% in the lamb fetus.

It is interesting to speculate on the function of the ductus in the fetal circulation. In the fetus, gas exchange occurs in the placenta and not in the lungs. There is thus need for only a small amount of blood in the lungs for nutritional and metabolic needs. The ductus diverts blood away from the lungs and to the descending aorta and umbilical–placental circulation. Shunting of blood away from the lungs could be effected by increasing right-to-left flow across the foramen ovale to the left atrium and left ventricle. If this did occur, the right ventricle would receive less volume and this could interfere with its development. The other advantage of the ductus is that it distributes blood of relatively low oxygen saturation to the descending aorta and to the placenta for oxygenation. This, in association with the preferential streaming of well-oxygenated blood from the ductus venosus across the foramen ovale, facilitates the separation of oxygen contents in ascending and descending aortic blood (see Chapter 1).

The ductus arteriosus is widely patent in the fetus and it was proposed that it is kept open passively by the pressure in the lumen. However, during the latter weeks of gestation in the lamb, the ductus does constrict with mechanical manipulation and studies on isolated strips or rings of ductus arteriosus have shown that the fetal ductus is capable of responding to numerous constrictor agents.

The question has been considered whether patency of the ductus is maintained in the fetus by active vasodilatation and whether closure after birth is due to removal of vasodilator stimuli, or to active vasoconstriction. The factors that have been considered as agents that maintain patency of the ductus arteriosus in the fetus include exposure to low Po_2, circulating or locally produced prostaglandins, local nitric oxide (NO) production, and circulating adenosine. Factors that have been proposed as vasoactive agents causing postnatal constriction include oxygen, endothelin-1, norepinephrine, acetylcholine, and bradykinin.

Postnatal closure of the ductus arteriosus

In small animals such as the rat, rabbit and guinea pig, the ductus closes rapidly after birth. However, in calves and foals, as well as full-term human infants, based on the ability to auscultate a murmur, it has been assumed that the ductus arteriosus is functionally open for about 12–15 hours after birth. Because murmurs may be the result of many flow disturbances, this assumption is questionable. Sequential studies by ultrasound have shown the presence of bidirectional shunting through the ductus for several hours after birth, followed by a small left-to-left shunt [6]. In 25 infants first examined 2–7 hours after birth, there was bidirectional flow in 19 and six had flows only in a left-to-right direction. In only 3 of the 19 infants with bidirectional flow was it noted on the second examination, at 12, 18, and 24 hours postnatally. Absence of any shunt, indicating complete functional closure, was first noted at 8 hours after birth. Functional closure was noted in 44% of the infants by 24 hours and 88% by 48 hours; no shunt was detected by 72 hours after birth.

These shunting patterns are related to the changes in pulmonary vascular resistance. In the early neonatal period, when pulmonary vascular resistance is still somewhat elevated and pulmonary arterial pressure still relatively high, some right-to-left shunt persists. This shunt occurs during systole, when the kinetic energy generated during ventricular systole carries blood through the main pulmonary artery and the ductus to the descending aorta. During diastole, blood flows from the aorta to the pulmonary artery, because pulmonary vascular resistance is lower than systemic vascular resistance. When pulmonary vascular resistance and pulmonary arterial pressure fall further, only a left-to-right shunt occurs as long as the ductus is still open. During this period of functional closure, the ductus is still responsive to changes in Po_2. Inhalation of gas with reduced oxygen (15–16%) increases pulmonary vascular resistance and possibly dilates the ductus and results in right-to-left shunting from the pulmonary artery to the aorta.

After the ductus has constricted fully and no lumen is detected, it is much more resistant to relaxation. The ductus appears to behave like the umbilical artery; this has been likened to the action of the so-called "catch" muscle in the clam, which can be readily relaxed when partially constricted but requires a much more potent stimulus to release when fully constricted. Constriction of the ductus is frequently ineffective in preterm infants and patency often persists for a longer period after birth. The more immature the infant, the greater the likelihood that the ductus will not close normally after birth. It thus also commonly reopens after initial partial closure (see below).

As mentioned above, the intimal layer gradually thickens over the latter part of gestation, but after birth the thickening increases rapidly and mounds of intima form that greatly decrease the size of the lumen. Associated with the disruption of the internal elastic lamina, smooth muscle cells migrate into the intimal mounds, as do endothelial cells. Potentially at this stage, if the smooth muscle relaxes, the ductus could reopen, so further changes must occur to close the ductus permanently. Studies by Clyman *et al.* [7] in the baboon have shown that constriction of the ductus induces severe hypoxia in the inner portion of the wall. Vasa vasorum provide blood flow and oxygen supply only to the adventitia. The intima and media receive oxygen supply from blood flowing through the lumen. However, when the ductus constricts, the wall is thickened and because oxygen diffuses only into the intima and inner layers of the media, the central medial layer becomes hypoxic. Constriction of the ductus reduces the Po_2 of the inner muscle layer to 5 mmHg or less on the first day, and by the fifth day it falls to less than 0.3 mmHg. This severe hypoxia results in cell destruction with fibrous replacement, and appears to be necessary to permanently seal the ductus. The process of constriction appears to start initially at the pulmonary arterial end of the ductus and progresses to the aortic end. A small projection from the descending aorta may be seen for several weeks after birth, particularly well demonstrated by angiography, at the site where the ductus is attached. This has been termed the ductus ampulla or bulb.

Permanent closure of the ductus is usually complete within 5–7 days in most infants but may not occur for up to 21 days.

Regulation of the ductus arteriosus

Role of oxygen

As mentioned above, the lumen of the ductus is perfused by blood with a Po_2 of about 18 mmHg in the fetal lamb. The vasa vasorum appear to receive blood from branches of the coronary arteries and possibly from intercostal arteries; this blood has a Po_2 of about 26 mmHg. Because arterial Po_2 increases to 90–100 mmHg after birth, the role of the increased level of oxygen in causing ductus closure has been considered. Since Kennedy and Clark [8] showed that oxygen constricts the ductus arteriosus, numerous investigators have confirmed its important role in studies of isolated ductus rings or strips, in isolated perfused ductus preparations, as well as in intact fetal lambs. The isolated ductus arteriosus is completely relaxed when the Po_2 in a fluid bath is between 20 and 35 mmHg. Increasing or decreasing the Po_2 from this range results in constriction of the ductus derived from mature fetal lambs (Figure 6.2) [9]. With increasing Po_2, the ductus constricts at levels of 40–50 mmHg and is intensely constricted at a Po_2 of 120–150 mmHg. When Po_2 is reduced below 15 mmHg, mild constriction is noted, and at 5–8 mmHg the degree of constriction is almost as great as the maximal constriction with raised Po_2.

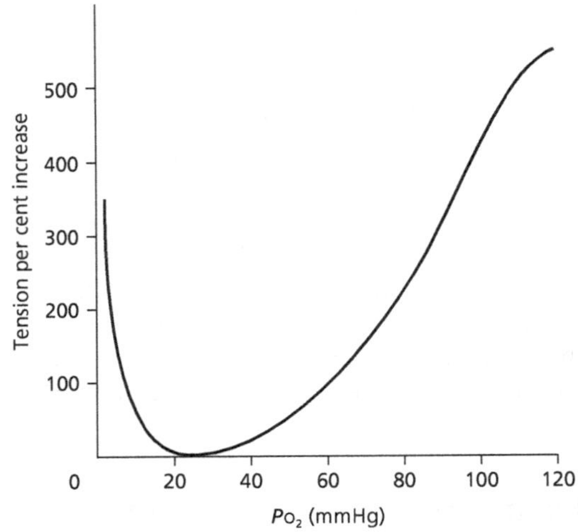

Figure 6.2 Effect of changing Po_2 in the bath fluid on the tension of a ductus arteriosus ring derived from a mature fetal lamb.

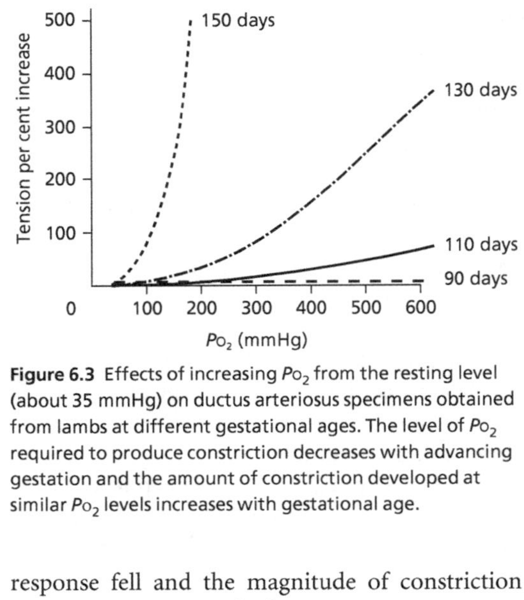

Figure 6.3 Effects of increasing Po_2 from the resting level (about 35 mmHg) on ductus arteriosus specimens obtained from lambs at different gestational ages. The level of Po_2 required to produce constriction decreases with advancing gestation and the amount of constriction developed at similar Po_2 levels increases with gestational age.

The response of the ductus arteriosus to oxygen is related to fetal gestational age. In studies of perfused fetal lamb ductus preparations, the ductus did not constrict even when Po_2 was raised to > 500 mmHg in lambs less than 80 days' gestation (term gestation in the lamb is 147–150 days). Responsiveness increased with advancing gestation; the initial level of Po_2 required to elicit a response fell and the magnitude of constriction increased (Figure 6.3) [10].

The lack of response of the immature ductus to oxygen is not entirely due to inability of the muscle to contract, because it does constrict in response to calcium and other agents, such as acetylcholine. The mechanism by which oxygen constricts the ductus has not yet been defined. The possibility that oxygen has a direct effect on the smooth muscle cells has been considered. Fay *et al.* [11] showed that the integrity of the cytochrome oxidase system is necessary for oxygen to produce ductus constriction, and Coceani *et al.* [12] has proposed that a cytochrome P450 hemoprotein located in the smooth muscle cell membrane is the receptor for the effects of oxygen. It was suggested that oxygen depolarizes the membrane, resulting in calcium influx, which induces contraction. Recently, it was suggested that oxygen-sensitive K^+ channels in the smooth muscle cell membrane could be involved in the ductus response to oxygen and that these channels are developmentally regulated. It is proposed that inhibition of oxygen-sensitive, voltage-gated K^+ channels depolarizes the ductus arteriosus smooth muscle cell, inducing activation of the voltage-sensitive L-type calcium channel; this stimulates influx of calcium that initiates constriction.

In a very interesting study, the preterm rabbit ductus arteriosus was found to contract poorly in response to oxygen; the ductus smooth muscle cells showed a diminished oxygen-sensitive K^+ current. Gene transfer of oxygen-sensitive K^+ channels to the preterm rabbit ductus induced a constrictor response to oxygen. Furthermore, transfer of the channels to human ductus smooth muscle enhanced constriction to oxygen exposure [13]. The poor response of the ductus arteriosus in preterm animals and infants could be related to the fact that oxygen-sensitive K^+ channels are not yet well developed and thus the constrictor response is weak or absent, depending on gestational age.

The Rho kinase system, which has recently been shown to be actively involved in constriction of the pulmonary vasculature (see Chapter 5), is now also thought to be an important contributor to maintaining oxygen-induced constriction of the ductus arteriosus. In studies on ductus arteriosus smooth muscle cells derived from term rabbit fetuses, oxygen activated the Rho kinase system and increased Rho kinase expression and induced sustained constriction. This response could be inhibited by the Rho kinase inhibitor fasudil. Studies of ductus arteriosus tissue derived from human infants with hypoplastic left heart syndrome at the time of surgery showed the same responses as the term rabbit ductus [14]. This raises the interesting possibility that Rho kinase inhibitors could be an additional means of inhibiting constriction of the ductus arteriosus after birth in infants with congenital cardiovascular malformations in whom survival is dependent on patency of the ductus.

Another concept that has been proposed suggests that oxygen results in the release of endothelin-1, reported by Coceani *et al.* [15] to be a potent constrictor of the ductus. However, blockade of endothelin receptors did not completely prevent the constrictor response to oxygen of the lamb ductus arteriosus in either isolated ductus tissue or the animal model [16]. It is possible that endothelin does contribute to the constrictor effect of oxygen and modification of potassium channel activity, although endothelin levels do not increase rapidly enough to account for the constriction of the ductus occurring after birth.

Role of prostaglandins

Prostaglandins are produced by the tissues of the wall of the ductus arteriosus in considerable amounts. The enzyme cyclooxygenase (COX) synthesizes prostaglandins from arachidonic acid. Two isoforms of the enzyme are now known to occur. The COX-1 isoform is present in most tissues and seems to be responsible for synthesis of prostaglandins; the COX-2 isoform is predominantly involved in the responses to inflammation. It was generally assumed that COX-1 is responsible for production of prostaglandin by the ductus. However, COX-2 is expressed in the ductus, and inhibition of COX-2 activity also constricts both the isolated ductus and the ductus in the intact fetal lamb [17]. Thus both isoforms are involved in prostaglandin production by the ductus and inhibition of either will cause ductus constriction. The relative importance of each isoform is yet to be assessed. The ductus synthesizes prostaglandin $(PG)E_2$ and PGI_2 (prostacyclin). Both prostaglandins relax ductus arteriosus smooth muscle. Although more PGI_2 is produced than PGE_2, ductus tone is probably regulated largely by the action of PGE_2, because isolated ductus rings are about 1000 times more sensitive to PGE_2 than to PGI_2 [18]. The sensitivity of the ductus to PGE_2 is so great that it has been proposed that circulating PGE_2 may have an important role in maintaining ductus patency *in utero*. Blood concentrations of PGE_2 are considerably higher in fetal lambs than in the mother. After birth PGE_2 concentrations fall rapidly and reach adult levels within about 3 hours

[19]. PGE_2 is metabolized in the lung and if lung disease or hypoxic pulmonary vasoconstriction reduces pulmonary blood flow, the fall in PGE_2 concentrations could be delayed. In early studies of the effect of PGE_2 on the ductus, it was thought that it had a relaxant effect on the ductus only in a low Po_2 environment; subsequently it was shown that it relaxed the ductus even at high Po_2, although the response was less sensitive [20]. PGE_2 has a more important role in ductus relaxation in the immature than the term fetus. Not only is more prostaglandin produced by the immature ductus but it is also more sensitive to the relaxant effect of PGE_2.

The production of prostaglandins can be reduced by administration of nonsteroidal antiinflammatory agents, which inhibit the cyclooxygenase enzyme. Most of these agents inhibit both COX-1 and COX-2, but specific inhibitors of COX-2 are also available. Indomethacin, a potent inhibitor, constricts the ductus both *in vitro* and *in vivo*. The constriction is not the result of an oxygen effect, because the constriction produced by indomethacin is accentuated by increasing Po_2 [21]. In the lamb, the relative contributions of indomethacin and oxygen to constriction change with gestational age. In the immature fetus, the magnitude of constriction with indomethacin is greater than that of oxygen, whereas in the term fetus oxygen is more effective in causing constriction. These findings have been interpreted to indicate that in the immature fetus, the ductus is more sensitive to the effects of dilator prostaglandins and that the sensitivity decreases with advancing gestational age. The mechanisms responsible for this reduction in sensitivity of the ductus to prostaglandin inhibition have not been fully resolved, but one possible factor is the effect of cortisol. Clyman *et al.* [22] administered cortisol to immature lamb fetuses *in utero* and found that the responses of the ductus to indomethacin and oxygen became similar to those of the normal mature fetus. In the lamb fetus, blood cortisol concentrations gradually increase from about 120 days' gestation and this could account for the change in ductus responsiveness to indomethacin and oxygen. Further evidence supporting the effect of cortisol in maturing the response of the ductus is the decrease in the incidence of patent ductus arteriosus in prematurely born human and animal newborns whose mothers had received antenatal corticosteroids.

Role of nitric oxide

Nitric oxide (NO) is a vasodilator in most organ circulations, including the lung. It is produced locally in endothelial cells from L-arginine by the action of nitric oxide synthase (eNOS). The likelihood that NO is active in vascular structures has been assessed by observing the presence of the synthase and also by examining the vasoconstrictor response to inhibitors of NO production. The ductus arteriosus has been shown to express eNOS in the endothelial cells lining the ductus as well as in the vasa vasorum. Also the inhibitor N-ω-nitro-L-arginine (L-NNA) does not affect the ductus at low Po_2, but produces constriction of the ductus arteriosus in fetal lambs only when Po_2 is high [23]. The relative roles of PGE_2 and NO in maintaining dilatation of the ductus have not been resolved. It is apparent that they act independently, because after inducing constriction by one inhibitor, the other agent results in further constriction. The relative sensitivities of the ductus to PGE_2 and NO may change with gestational age. In the rat, the ductus is more sensitive to PGE_2 than to NO in very late gestation, but in earlier gestation it is more sensitive to NO [24]. These gestational differences in relative sensitivities should be evaluated in other species.

Role of adenosine

Adenosine produces relaxation of the isolated ductus arteriosus and inhibits the constrictor response to oxygen. It has been proposed that adenosine may contribute to maintaining patency of the ductus prenatally [25]. Circulating adenosine concentrations are high in the fetus and fall rapidly after birth in the lamb [26] and this could explain postnatal constriction of the ductus. No information is available regarding the relative effects of adenosine, PGE_2 and NO, nor of possible interrelationships between their effects.

Role of other vasoactive agents

Acetylcholine, bradykinin, and norepinephrine have all been shown to produce constriction of the isolated ductus arteriosus. They all enhance the constrictor response to oxygen. However, none of these agents are essential for ductus constriction and selective blockade of each agent does not inhibit the constrictor response to oxygen. Norepinephrine could have some role in regulating ductus tone *in utero*, because numerous sympathetic nerve endings have been demonstrated in the media of the lamb ductus. Cholinergic nerves have not been observed in the media but have been detected in the adventitia. It is generally thought that these agents do not have a significant role in influencing the ductus, but their importance has not yet been defined.

Whether these mechanisms, or possibly others concerned with muscle contraction, are fully developed in the premature animal requires further study. We also do not know whether the ductus, which may be underdeveloped in infants with pulmonary atresia, responds normally to oxygen. Although Po_2 increase appears to be the most important mechanism responsible for ductus arteriosus closure, other factors must be operative because in infants with congenital heart disease in whom Po_2 may be maintained at levels below 40 mmHg after birth the ductus arteriosus may still close. It is not known what these factors are.

Ductus arteriosus in congenital heart disease

From a consideration of the course of the circulation in various congenital malformations, it is apparent that the volumes of blood carried by the ductus may be altered markedly. These possible changes are discussed in detail in the chapters on specific abnormalities, but a brief review is presented here.

Normally, the ductus arteriosus in the fetal lamb transmits about 55–60% of CVO from the pulmonary artery to the aorta. It joins the aorta at an obtuse inferior angle (see Figure 6.1) presumably because flow is directed down to the descending aorta. If aortic atresia or aortic isthmus interruption were present and if CVO were to be maintained, a much larger proportion of the output would have to flow through the ductus; in fact, with aortic atresia, the total output (excluding pulmonary flow) would cross the ductus. Thus, assuming that pulmonary blood flow represents about 20% of CVO in the human fetus, about 80% of CVO would be carried by the ductus, which could be considerably wider than normal. However, in the fetus with aortic atresia, there is complete admixture of systemic venous and umbilical venous blood in the right atrium, so that the blood entering the pulmonary artery and passing through the ductus arteriosus would have a higher than normal oxygen saturation and this could induce some degree of constriction of the ductus. The potential effects of these changes on pulmonary blood flow and the foramen ovale at different periods of gestation are discussed in detail in Chapter 5.

In the fetus with tricuspid or pulmonary atresia, no blood would be ejected from the right ventricle into the pulmonary artery. Blood will flow from the aorta through the ductus to the pulmonary arteries. Pulmonary blood flow is a relatively small proportion of CVO (about 10% in the lamb and probably about 20% in the human). The ductus may be quite narrow and underdeveloped and, because blood flows from the aorta to the pulmonary artery, the connection of the ductus with the aorta has an acute inferior angle (see Figure 6.1). In addition, because all systemic venous, umbilical venous, and pulmonary venous blood mixes in the left atrium, blood entering the aorta would have a somewhat lower oxygen saturation than normal for ascending aortic blood. However, this blood, which passes through the ductus arteriosus, has a higher oxygen saturation than the blood that passes from the pulmonary artery through the ductus in the normal fetus. This could result in some constriction of the ductus, particularly in later gestation, and possibly interfere with development of the pulmonary arteries (see Chapter 5 for detailed discussion).

In the presence of aortopulmonary transposition with no ventricular communication, the pulmonary artery receives blood ejected by the left ventricle. In the fetus, pulmonary arterial oxygen saturation would be considerably higher than normal and this could lower pulmonary vascular resistance and increase pulmonary blood flow. This may result in elevation of left atrial pressure and decreased size of the foramen ovale. Also, ductus arteriosus constriction may result, with elevation of pulmonary arterial pressure, possibly resulting in excessive development of pulmonary vascular smooth muscle and persistent pulmonary arterial hypertension postnatally (see Chapter 18 for detailed discussion).

The ductus arteriosus frequently does not close normally after birth in the presence of a number of congenital cardiac lesions. In infants with cyanotic lesions such as pulmonary or tricuspid atresia and aortopulmonary transposition, arterial Po_2 may remain at or only slightly above fetal levels after birth. If Po_2 does not rise above about 35 mmHg, the oxygen stimulus to constriction of the ductus would be greatly reduced; this could explain the prolongation of patency after birth. However, even if arterial Po_2 does remain at low levels after birth, the ductus does tend to constrict over a few days and may restrict pulmonary flow in infants in whom blood flow to the lungs is ductus dependent. Possibly ductus morphology is not normal, but we do not know what factors are responsible for the delayed closure of the ductus in these circumstances.

Infants with left-sided obstructive lesions may also have prolonged postnatal patency of the ductus. With anomalies such as severe aortic stenosis, aortic atresia, and interrupted aortic arch, blood flows from the pulmonary artery to the aorta after birth to provide some or all of systemic blood flow. In these infants, arterial Po_2 increases significantly after birth and may reach normal or near-normal postnatal levels, yet the ductus remains open. One factor that may have a role is that the ductus is exposed to the oxygen saturation of pulmonary arterial blood after birth, rather than to the high saturation of aortic blood and this may deter constriction. In these infants, pulmonary arterial pressure remains elevated after birth and the high pressure and relatively high flow through the ductus arteriosus is probably responsible for maintaining its patency. However, it is not known why the ductus constricts even though the pressure and flow are maintained.

Ductus arteriosus at high altitude and with hypoxia

There is considerable evidence indicating that the incidence of persistent patency of the ductus arteriosus in individuals born, and continuing to live, at high altitudes is greater than in those born at or near sea level. The incidence of patent ductus arteriosus increases slightly at altitudes above 3000 m and definitely above altitudes of 4000 m [27]. According to Peñaloza, the incidence at 4500–5000 m altitude is about 30 times greater than that at sea level [28]. The ductus may remain patent in newborn infants with hypoxemia due to lung disease. The patency of the ductus can be explained by lack of an adequate oxygen stimulus to cause constriction. However, this cannot be the only factor involved because, of all the people born at the same high altitude, only a small proportion have persistent patency of the ductus after birth.

We do not know whether the ductus will constrict in individuals born at high altitude if arterial Po_2 is raised later in life. I have observed several mature infants with lung disease in whom the ductus, which was patent for several weeks (in one infant for 3 months), closed spontaneously. However, there is no knowledge as to whether, or for how long, the ductus arteriosus retains its normal musculature after birth if it is kept patent by hypoxia or whether it retains its ability to respond to changes in oxygen environment.

Ductus arteriosus in premature infants

In premature infants, it has long been recognized that the ductus arteriosus may remain patent after birth beyond the time of normal closure in mature infants. Powell [29] suggested that the ductus may close at the time of normally expected full-term gestation, but this has not been corroborated. However, if the infants survive, the ductus closes spontaneously within days to several weeks. The more premature the infant, the higher the incidence, and more than 80% of infants weighing less than 750 g have patency of the ductus arteriosus beyond the third day after birth. This incidence has been modified by use of antenatal corticosteroid therapy. Recently, it has become evident that the ductus may constrict and appear to be clinically closed within a few days after birth, but then reopens. This is most likely to occur in very small preterm infants.

Mechanisms for ductus arteriosus patency

The cause of the high incidence of patent ductus arteriosus in premature infants has been the subject of much conjecture. It was previously suggested that premature infants are not able to achieve normal postnatal blood Po_2 levels and that the oxygen stimulus to constriction is inadequate. However, with assisted ventilation, Po_2 can be raised to levels even above usual postnatal values and this has not reduced the incidence of patency. Based on observations that the wall thickness of the ductus increases with gestational age, the possibility was considered that the smooth muscle is not adequate to achieve effective constriction in the immature fetus. This concept does not seem likely, because the immature ductus can be actively contracted by potassium. As mentioned above, the immature ductus has a high threshold of response to oxygen (see Figure 6.3). The isolated perfused ductus of the very immature lamb shows little constrictor response to Po_2 levels well above those normally achieved after birth. It is possible that the ductus does not constrict in the premature infant even though arterial Po_2 levels are achieved that are normal for, and effective in constricting the ductus in, a mature infant.

The immature ductus arteriosus is very sensitive to the relaxant effect of PGE_2 and it has been proposed that abnormally high concentrations of circulating PGE_2 may be responsible for maintaining ductus patency in the preterm infant. Clyman *et al.* [19] showed that PGE_2 concentrations in the lamb fell to normal adult levels within about 3 hours after birth. The concept has been proposed that premature infants have persistently high circulating levels of PGE_2 that maintain ductus patency. PGE_2 is metabolized almost completely in one pass through the lung in the adult, but the immature lung does not completely metabolize PGE_2 and this, as well as the frequent association of lung disease in preterm infants, could account for higher levels of PGE_2. Although high concentrations of plasma PGE have been detected in premature infants as long as 2–4 weeks after birth, results concerning the relationship to patent ductus are inconsistent. Lucas and Mitchell [30] found high levels of PGE_2 in a group of infants with patent ductus arteriosus, but others have found elevated PGE_2 concentrations in many infants with respiratory distress syndrome but only some of these infants had patency of the ductus [31]. It is thus possible that persistently high concentrations of PGE_2 may maintain patency of the ductus, but other factors also appear to be involved.

It has been proposed that persistent patency of the ductus arteriosus may be determined by the effectiveness of the initial closure [7]. The mature ductus constricts to completely close the lumen. This creates the characteristic intimal mounds and the severe hypoxia in the media that initiates the process of permanent closure (see Chapter 6). The fully constricted ductus is no longer responsive to changes in Po_2 or to PGE_2. However, the preterm ductus does not constrict sufficiently to obliterate the lumen and the intimal mounds are not as well developed. Flow of blood through the lumen continues to provide some oxygen to the media and the hypoxic changes in the media do not develop. The ductus that still has even a narrow lumen is more responsive to PGE_2 and other agents. It is thus possible that the ductus arteriosus in the premature infant may be constricted after birth, but subsequent exposure to a relaxing agent may result in widening of the lumen. The possible role of NO in affecting closure of the ductus in premature infants should be considered. In a study of the ductus in premature baboon infants, Clyman *et al.* [7] found that the number of cells containing eNOS increased in association with an increase in the vasa vasorum. He suggests that the ductus smooth muscle may be relaxed by NO production locally and that patency of the ductus is now maintained by NO rather than PGE_2. Based on these observations, the effect of administration of indomethacin alone or together with an NO inhibitor (L-NNA) was examined [32]. In the premature baboon, indomethacin alone did not produce complete obstruction of the ductus lumen, whereas the combined treatment resulted in complete closure with morphological changes typical of those in the mature ductus. This raises the interesting prospect that use of NO inhibitors could be effective in constricting the ductus in infants in whom indomethacin has not been effective in inducing or maintaining closure (see Chapter 6).

Hemodynamic considerations

Prior to birth, blood flows through the ductus arteriosus from the pulmonary artery to the aorta. Postnatally, closure of the ductus and decrease in pulmonary vascular resistance permit pulmonary arterial pressure to fall. If the ductus remains widely patent after birth, the pressures in the aorta and pulmonary artery will be equal as a result of the large communication. Blood flow through the ductus will be determined by the relationship between the systemic and pulmonary vascular resistances. A fall in pulmonary vascular resistance associated with ventilation will be associated with a left-to-right shunt through the ductus arteriosus and, with the same size of the ductus, the lower the pulmonary vascular resistance, the larger the shunt. It was proposed that pulmonary vascular resistance falls more rapidly in the premature compared with the mature infant because the resistance vessels in the lungs have a less developed smooth muscle medial layer. More recent studies have not confirmed this finding, but there is evidence to indicate that the pulmonary vasculature in immature lambs has less capacity to constrict in response to various stimuli. It is thus possible that pulmonary vascular resistance does fall more rapidly in preterm infants, because premature vessels do not maintain the same tone as mature vessels. Respiratory distress syndrome, which commonly occurs in premature infants, may delay the fall in pulmonary vascular resistance because alveolar hypoxia associated with the lung disease may maintain pulmonary vasoconstriction in some parts of the lung. Treatment of premature infants with pulmonary surfactant reduces the incidence and severity of respiratory distress syndrome and enhances left-to-right shunting through the ductus arteriosus [33].

Blood shunted through the ductus into the pulmonary artery returns to the left atrium and left ventricle. To provide adequate systemic blood flow, the left ventricle must increase its output. Thus, if 33% of the blood ejected by the left ventricle shunts through the ductus, left ventricular output would have to increase 1.5 times to maintain the same systemic blood flow. If 50% of left ventricular output were shunted, left ventricular output would have to double to maintain systemic blood flow. Left ventricular output normally increases after birth and the left-to-right shunt places a further load on the ventricle. If left ventricular performance can increase to eject the higher volume, systemic blood flow will be maintained. It was proposed that the fetal heart is unable to increase its output above resting levels even though end-diastolic pressure, or preload, is increased (see Chapter 1). Therefore the ability of the left ventricle to increase its output adequately to compensate for the left-to-right shunt was questioned. However, both in experimental studies in immature lambs by Clyman *et al.* and in observations in preterm infants it is apparent that the ventricle is capable of increasing its output when the ductus arteriosus is patent [34]. However, there is a limit to the magnitude of shunt that can be tolerated without compromising systemic blood flow. In the mature infant, systemic blood flow may be maintained with left-to-right shunts of as much as 75% of ventricular output, whereas in Clyman's studies in immature lambs systemic blood flow was inadequate with shunts greater than 50% of left ventricular output. The flow to the peripheral circulation (muscles and skin) fell, as did flow to the kidneys and gastrointestinal tract. The decrease in gastrointestinal flow has been incriminated as a contributing factor in causing necrotizing enterocolitis, which is not unusual in premature infants. In studies in human infants, necrotizing enterocolitis is associated with presence of patency of the ductus arteriosus and early closure of the ductus reduces the incidence of the disorder.

An additional factor that may contribute to inadequate perfusion of organs is the low arterial diastolic pressure frequently noted in preterm infants and which results from the left-to-right shunt through the ductus arteriosus into the low resistance pulmonary circulation. The organ most susceptible to the low diastolic pressure in the aorta is the heart, because the major blood flow to the myocardium occurs during diastole. Myocardial blood flow may be compromised not only by a decrease in aortic diastolic pressure but also by the increase in left ventricular end-diastolic pressure resulting from the large volume returning to the left atrium and ventricle associated with the ductus shunt. Thus myocardial oxygen supply could be compromised, particularly since oxygen requirements would be increased with the work to maintain the high output; interference in oxygen supply could result in failure of the ventricle to increase output to meet the requirements of the systemic circulation.

The increase in left ventricular output is the result of a decrease in afterload on the left ventricle resulting from the patent ductus. The preload on the ventricle also increases in association with the increased volume returning to the ventricle. Left ventricular end-diastolic pressure increases and left atrial and pulmonary venous pressures increase. Left atrial pressure usually does not reach very high levels, but in the preterm infant the permeability of the capillaries may be greater than in mature infants and thus pulmonary edema may develop, even at relatively low pulmonary venous pressures. Plasma albumin concentrations are usually relatively low in premature infants and the resultant lower plasma colloidal osmotic pressure would facilitate the development of pulmonary edema. An additional factor that may contribute to pulmonary edema formation is the fact that the size of the pulmonary vascular bed is not yet fully developed in the immature infant. Thus greater flow would occur through each vessel and this, combined with the elevation of pulmonary arterial and venous pressures, may result in edema formation.

Another manifestation of inadequate systemic blood flow is the observation by Evans [35] that superior vena cava (SVC) blood flow is often reduced in preterm infants, especially in the more immature fetuses. About one-third of preterm infants born before 30 weeks' gestation were found to have low SVC blood flow, which was often associated with adverse consequences such as cerebral intraventricular hemorrhage and neurodevelopmental delay [36]. A major factor responsible for the low SVC flow was the large left-to-right shunt through the ductus arteriosus. The low SVC flow in these infants was most frequently observed within the first 12 hours after birth, flows gradually approaching normal values by 24–48 hours. There was a poor correlation between SVC flow and measured arterial blood pressure or pulse pressure.

The observation that SVC flow is most likely to be low during the first 12 hours and improves by 24–48 hours after birth raises interesting questions about the mechanisms involved. The finding suggests that either left ventricular output does not change (but the proportion shunted through the ductus decreases) or that left ventricular output is increased. A decrease in the shunt could result from constriction of the ductus, or from an increase in pulmonary vascular resistance. Although it is well known that the ductus arteriosus is often patent for at least several days postnatally, the degree of constriction at various periods after birth could vary. Constriction of the ductus may be delayed to a greater extent in some infants, possibly because adequate oxygenation of arterial blood is not achieved. It might be expected that, if this were so, pulmonary venous blood may not be well oxygenated and this might interfere with the fall in pulmonary vascular resistance and thus reduce the magnitude of the shunt. Both the pulmonary circulation and the ductus are less sensitive to increase in oxygen content in earlier gestation, but the relationship of the response to specific changes in oxygenation at various periods of gestation may differ. Another possible mechanism for delayed constriction of the ductus may be that PGE_2 concentrations remain elevated in some infants during the early postnatal period and interfere with constriction; a gradual reduction in plasma levels over 12–24 hours may permit some degree of constriction and thus improve systemic blood flow.

The other possible explanation for the increase in systemic blood flow beyond the first 12 hours postnatally is that left ventricular performance improves and is thus capable of providing a higher output to compensate for the shunt. One of the factors responsible for increased left ventricular performance after birth in the mature lamb is increased sympathoadrenal activity [37]. The possibility that the preterm infant does not show the usual increase in plasma catecholamine concentrations noted in mature infants at the time of delivery could account for an early lack of enhancement in left ventricular performance, but a delayed increased catecholamine secretion could result in later improvement. This is not likely because norepinephrine concentrations in umbilical cord blood of preterm and term infants at the time of delivery are not significantly different and epinephrine concentrations are higher in the preterm infants [38]. Various catecholamines have been administered to preterm infants, usually as therapy for hypotension, with variable effects. Although dobutamine produced modest increases of SVC flow and dopamine increased blood pressure, almost half of infants under 30 weeks' gestation failed to respond at all [39]. Thus it is unlikely that low catecholamine concentrations soon after birth are responsible for reduced ventricular performance.

The possibility that the left ventricle does not respond adequately to catecholamines in the preterm infant has been considered. Based on the observations that some infants who do not respond adequately to catecholamines following cardiac surgery demonstrate an increase in cardiac output with administration of phosphodiesterase inhibitors, a trial of milrinone in preterm infants with low SVC flow has been instituted [40]. Preliminary results do not appear to be encouraging.

Serum concentrations of cortisol in umbilical cord blood of preterm compared with mature infants are low and the levels progressively increase with gestational age [41]. Cortisol has been administered to preterm infants with blood pressure considered lower than normal, even after infusion of catecholamines. Blood pressure was raised by cortisol; whether the effect was due to increased responsiveness of the peripheral circulation to catecholamines, or to a cardiac effect, has not been ascertained [42]. The effect of cortisol on systemic blood flow has not been assessed.

In studies in adult dogs, introduction of a large aortopulmonary shunt resulted in acute left ventricular failure, but if the animals were permitted to become adapted to a somewhat smaller shunt, they were soon able to tolerate the large shunt [43]. This adaptation is the result of myocardial hypertrophy that enhances left ventricular performance. It is possible that the ventricle of the preterm infant is capable of increasing myocyte mass rapidly after birth and this allows the ventricle to provide a higher output within 24–48 hours. Although it may seem that this is a short time for myocardial mass to increase, it is not an unreasonable hypothesis: in fetal lambs in which aortic obstruction was induced, left ventricular mass increased rapidly [44].

Clinical manifestations

The term "symptomatic ductus arteriosus" is frequently used to indicate that the infant has clinical manifestations of a patent ductus. This term distinguishes these patients from those who have only ultrasound evidence of a patent ductus arteriosus. The manifestations in these infants include presence of a cardiac murmur, increased precordial cardiac pulsatility, and bounding pulse due to increased pulse pressure. The term is unfortunate, because many of these infants do not have symptoms relating to ductus patency. The "symptoms" are the hemodynamic consequences of patency of the ductus, but evidence of pulmonary edema or cardiac failure may not develop.

The clinical features of patent ductus arteriosus vary with gestational age and thus the weight of the infant at the time of birth. Infants weighing 1500–1750 g may have mild respiratory distress syndrome, which usually resolves within a few days. It is estimated that about 20% of these infants develop a patent ductus arteriosus. After 3–10 days, when the infant appears to be well, a grade 2–3/6 systolic murmur is heard at the upper left sternal border or below the left clavicle, occupying about half of systole. The second heart sound may be somewhat accentuated in the pulmonary area. The murmur becomes somewhat louder and more prolonged, and occasionally extends beyond the second sound into early diastole. The pulses develop a bounding character due to the widening pulse pressure, and on occasion a third heart sound is noted at the apex. The precordial impulse becomes hyperactive due to the increased volume load on the left ventricle. Associated with these developments, the baby usually shows a slight increase in respiratory rate and effort. However, this may be the only symptom, and after 2–3 weeks the murmur becomes softer, the pulses less prominent, and within a few days no clinical evidence of patency of the ductus is present.

However, some infants develop more serious symptoms in association with the appearance of the murmur and widening pulse pressure. Respiration becomes more rapid and labored, and rales may be heard in the lung bases. Episodes of apnea may develop. The liver does not usually become enlarged. The electrocardiogram is not helpful and shows the degree of right ventricular hypertrophy normal for a premature infant. Chest radiography usually shows that the heart size is only slightly increased and pulmonary vascular markings may be prominent. Ultrasound examination shows moderate enlargement of the left atrium and left ventricle and the ductus is seen to be patent, but the diameter is usually less than half the aortic diameter. Doppler study shows only left-to-right shunting through the ductus. Most of the infants in this group respond well to conventional treatment of cardiac failure but infrequently surgical closure of the ductus may be necessary. This can be accomplished either by administration of prostaglandin synthesis inhibitors or, if necessary, by surgery. If closure of the ductus is not necessary to relieve symptoms, it frequently closes spontaneously within several weeks.

Infants weighing 1000–1500 g frequently have moderate to severe respiratory distress syndrome from birth. The respiratory distress may begin to improve after 2–3 days and then, either early or after a short latent period of 1–2 days, a change in ventilatory requirements signifies the possibility that the ductus arteriosus is open. The level of continuous positive airway pressure may have to be increased and inspiratory rate or pressures may have to be higher. The concentration of oxygen in inspired air may have to be increased to maintain arterial blood $P\text{O}_2$ levels. In addition a rise in arterial blood $P\text{CO}_2$ levels often occurs in association with the development of a patent ductus arteriosus. About 40–50% of infants in this weight range have persistent patency of the ductus. Because the ductus-related manifestations tend to be closely related to the features of respiratory distress syndrome, it is difficult to decide whether the recrudescence is due to the lung disease or is the result of a patent ductus arteriosus. The classical clinical features that are described include a systolic murmur at the upper left sternal border, bounding pulses due to a wide pulse pressure, and increased precordial activity resulting from the large volume load. However, these findings are quite variable; a murmur may not be audible, the pulse pressure may not be increased, and pulses may be weak. Increased precordial activity is difficult to assess in an infant with a thin chest wall. Hepatomegaly is not an important manifestation. The liver can be felt in most premature infants, and some degree of enlargement may occur, but it is not a striking finding. Findings on auscultation of the chest are difficult to evaluate because of the associated lung disease. Although rales may be heard posteriorly in both lungs, the signs of airway obstruction are more common.

Chest radiography is difficult to interpret, because the lungs show the changes of respiratory distress syndrome and it is difficult to assess whether the pulmonary vascular markings are increased. The heart may be moderately enlarged, but because the infants are usually intubated and maintained with continuous increased positive end-tidal pressure and positive pressure ventilation, the heart size may be normal. Ultrasound examination reveals enlargement of the left atrium and ventricle and active ventricular contraction. The size of the left atrium relative to the diameter of the ascending aorta as measured on an M-mode examination is a useful indicator of the size of the left-to-right shunt [45]; normally, this ratio is 0.7–0.9. If it is increased to more than 1.1, this indicates that there is a significant left-to-right shunt, and a ratio of 1.3 signifies a very large shunt. The ductus arteriosus can be imaged and its diameter estimated. Doppler examination shows left-to-right shunting. The flow pattern in the descending aorta beyond the ductus is often useful in estimating the magnitude of the shunt. With increasing ductus left-to-right shunt, the magnitude of forward flow during diastole decreases and with large shunts diastolic retrograde flow becomes evident. Retrograde flow in the descending aorta during diastole has been associated with feeding intolerance in premature infants with patent ductus arteriosus; this has been attributed to impaired splanchnic blood flow.

Infants weighing less than 1000 g frequently have severe respiratory distress from birth, unless the mother has received antenatal steroid treatment or the infant has received surfactant therapy. The ductus arteriosus remains patent in 80% or more of the infants who have received surfactant. Respiratory distress usually requires continuous positive pressure and assisted ventilation. The first evidence of a ductus left-to-right shunt may appear within 2–3 days after birth and includes increasing arterial $P\text{CO}_2$ and increasing ventilatory pressures and rate. There is often no obvious interval between the presentation of the features of hyaline membrane and those associated with patency of the ductus. It is difficult to assess whether the problems are related to continuation of the pulmonary pathology alone or whether the patent ductus is contributing to the symptoms. As in the other two groups, the development of bounding pulses or a wide pulse pressure on an umbilical arterial pressure tracing is helpful. However, the majority of these infants have low systolic and diastolic pressures and thus the pulse pressure is not wide [46]. The precordial impulse may be increased, but this is often difficult to assess in the infant being ventilated with high positive pressures. A systolic murmur may be heard, but absence of a murmur is not unusual in this group. Hepatomegaly is not a striking feature.

The electrocardiogram usually shows a pattern of right ventricular hypertrophy of a degree normal for a newborn infant. Occasionally, ST segment depression and flattening or inversion of T waves in the left precordial leads are noted. Chest radiography is of no value in differentiating between the lung disease and a patent ductus arteriosus. The lungs usually show severe changes of respiratory distress syndrome and the vasculature is not clearly visible. The heart may be mildly to moderately enlarged. In these infants, manifestations of left ventricular failure and pulmonary edema often occur with only a mild degree of cardiomegaly. The echocardiographic findings are similar to those mentioned above for infants weighing 1000–1500 g. In these infants, the ductus arteriosus may be imaged and seen to be widely patent. In the early postnatal hours, the left-to-right shunt may not be very large because pulmonary vascular resistance is elevated as the result of poor ventilation and alveolar hypoxia, but as ventilation improves a large shunt becomes manifest. In these infants the left atrium/aortic diameter ratio will not be greatly increased in the early phase but increases as left-to-right shunt develops.

Complications of patent ductus arteriosus in the premature infant

Several complications have been ascribed to the presence of a patent ductus arteriosus. These associations have been confirmed by documenting a decrease in their incidence in infants in whom the ductus has been closed early, or before the onset of symptoms. Prophylactic treatment of premature infants with pulmonary surfactant increases the incidence of patent ductus arteriosus [47]. Closure of the ductus arteriosus reduces the risk of pulmonary hemorrhage. Intolerance of enteral feeding and necrotizing enterocolitis are frequently noted in premature infants. As mentioned above, the incidence of these conditions appears to be associated with the decrease in gastrointestinal blood flow; this has been observed in premature lambs with patent ductus arteriosus [48]. The incidence of necrotizing enterocolitis is reduced significantly in infants in whom the ductus has been closed [49].

Infants with a widely patent ductus arteriosus have elevated pulmonary arterial pressure, and if a large left-to-right shunt is present, left atrial and pulmonary venous pressures are increased. This results in increased transudation of fluid into the lung tissues and alveoli. In the preterm infant, the pulmonary capillaries appear to be more permeable than in mature infants. Plasma proteins may enter the air sacs and interfere with surfactant function, thus reducing lung compliance. To achieve adequate oxygenation, it is necessary to increase mean airway pressures and to raise inspired oxygen concentration. It has been proposed that these factors may contribute to the development of lung damage and to the subsequent occurrence of chronic lung disease or bronchopulmonary dysplasia. Early closure of the ductus arteriosus significantly reduces the risks of bronchopulmonary dysplasia.

Therapeutic considerations

The approach to management of patent ductus arteriosus in the premature infant was changed dramatically in the mid 1970s, when it was shown that administration of prostaglandin synthesis inhibitors closed the ductus in about 80% of premature infants in whom it was demonstrated to be patent [50]. Prior to this, management was similar to that of cardiac failure in infants, with the use of digoxin and diuretic agents. The use of digoxin involved considerable risk of toxicity, because the tendency was to increase dosage in an attempt to achieve an effect without inducing toxicity. It was administered in doses similar to those recommended for mature infants: 40–50 μg/kg as a digitalizing dose over about 24 hours followed by a maintenance dose of one-quarter to one-third of the digitalizing dose every 24 hours. It was soon appreciated that toxic effects, especially heart block, were quite common. This, it was realized, was due to the reduced renal elimination of digoxin in the premature infant. The recommended dose was then reduced to about 25–30 μg/kg as a digitalizing dose. However, considerable questions were raised about whether digoxin was effective in relieving symptoms, and in many centers the use of digoxin for treatment of patent ductus arteriosus in the premature infant was abandoned.

Diuretic therapy proved to be very useful in improving pulmonary edema. The agent most commonly recommended was furosemide (Lasix), given parenterally in doses of 1 mg/kg two to four times daily. It is important, particularly in these premature infants, to check serum electrolytes before and after giving diuretics, because severe degrees of hyponatremia and hypokalemia can be induced. If furosemide is used over extended periods, hypocalcemia may develop. Furthermore, as a result of the increased urinary excretion of calcium, renal calculi may develop in infants maintained on high doses of furosemide for many weeks.

If the infant did not respond to medical management, the only option was to close the ductus surgically. This was done with some reluctance because, at that time, the risks of thoracotomy on small preterm infants were considerable. However, with experience, the mortality was reduced to a very low rate. After ligation of the ductus, the infants usually improved rapidly with a decrease in end-expiratory pressure requirement, a reduction in the percentage of inspired oxygen necessary to maintain adequate arterial $P\text{O}_2$, and a fall in arterial $P\text{CO}_2$.

Inhibition of prostaglandin synthesis

Indomethacin is the prostaglandin synthesis inhibitor that was first used and is still generally recommended. In the early studies with indomethacin, it was found to be effective in closing the ductus arteriosus, in various reports, in about 75–90% of infants. However, the relative numbers of infants of less than 1000 g that are now being encountered have increased. Consequently, the incidence of patent ductus arteriosus in infants born at a younger gestational age is higher; of infants born before 30 weeks' gestation who develop severe respiratory distress, 80% or more have a patent ductus arteriosus demonstrated by ultrasound. However, only about half of these infants develop the classic clinical manifestations of patent ductus arteriosus. Indomethacin is more effective in closing the ductus arteriosus in infants of greater gestational age; the younger the gestational age at birth, the less effective is indomethacin in inducing permanent closure of the ductus. The ductus may be constricted by indomethacin initially, but often reopens within 2–3 days.

Initially, indomethacin was administered when the ductus was considered to be "symptomatic," as indicated by the presence of a murmur, increased precordial activity, bounding pulses, and deterioration in respiratory status. Many infants were therefore not treated until 7 days or more after birth. As mentioned above, the ductus can often be demonstrated to be patent by ultrasound study in the absence of clinical manifestations, particularly in very preterm infants. Mahony *et al.* [51] studied the effectiveness of administering indomethacin prophylactically before manifestation of the clinical features of patent ductus arteriosus in preterm infants with birth weights of less than 1700 g. In those above 1000 g, there was no significant difference in the clinical features of those given indomethacin compared with those given placebo. However, in the smaller infants, 80% of those given placebo developed large ductus shunts. Prophylactic indomethacin greatly reduced the incidence of large shunts and reduced the need for surgical ligation.

Based on these studies, it would seem desirable to treat premature infants prophylactically with indomethacin rather than wait for the clinical manifestations of patent ductus arteriosus. However, this would result in a large number of infants being treated unnecessarily, because the ductus would have closed spontaneously. If indomethacin had no undesirable effects, this would not be of great concern. However, indomethacin does have potential adverse effects. When administered by intravenous injection, it frequently causes hypertension. It also results in decreased gastrointestinal perfusion; this could contribute to the development of necrotizing enterocolitis, although there is no clinical evidence of increased incidence of this condition after indomethacin administration. The drug decreases renal blood flow and urinary output and may induce a rise in plasma creatinine concentrations. In addition, it interferes with platelet function and could increase any bleeding tendency. Indomethacin reduces cerebral blood flow and oxygen supply, but in experimental studies in fetal lambs it did not significantly affect cerebral oxygen consumption [52]. Also no adverse cerebral effects have been observed in clinical studies.

Despite the effect of prophylactic therapy with indomethacin in closing the ductus, it offers no advantage compared with treatment when the ductus becomes clinically manifest, with regard to the incidence of chronic lung disease or to survival

[53]. The recommendations regarding timing of indomethacin therapy vary considerably. Some delay treatment until clinical manifestations of the patent ductus arteriosus appear. Others consider that prophylactic therapy during the first 24–48 hours after birth is indicated. It seems reasonable to recommend early treatment (during the first 24 hours) in those infants most likely to develop clinical evidence of patency, namely infants with birth weights less than 1000 g.

If a prostaglandin synthesis inhibitor that had fewer side effects than indomethacin could be identified, perhaps its early administration would be more generally favorable. In view of the adverse effects of indomethacin, another prostaglandin synthesis inhibitor, ibuprofen, was recommended, because it appeared to have no adverse effect on renal blood flow. Several studies have compared the effects of ibuprofen and indomethacin. In an analysis in a Cochrane review, the conclusions were that, with the use of ibuprofen, there was indeed less reduction of urine output compared with indomethacin. Apart from this there was no statistically significant difference in the occurrence of intraventricular hemorrhage or necrotizing enterocolitis, but there was possibly a higher incidence of chronic lung disease in the infants receiving ibuprofen. Both drugs were equally effective in achieving ductus closure. The conclusion was that there is no current indication to change the recommendation to use indomethacin [54].

The regimen of treatment with indomethacin varies somewhat in different institutions. The lyophilized preparation is administered by intravenous infusion over 20–30 min. This relatively slow rate of administration is used because it avoids the marked systemic arterial hypertension that often follows rapid intravenous injection. The drug is usually administered in two or three doses. The recommended first dose is 0.2 mg/kg at all postnatal ages and at all gestational ages. The second dose is given after 12 hours, but the dose depends on postnatal age and birth weight. Beyond 7 days, the second dose is also 0.2 mg/kg for infants of all weights. However, infants with birth weights of less than 1250 g are given only 0.1 mg/kg during the first postnatal week. The difference in dosage is based on the change in plasma clearance of indomethacin. At 7 days postnatally, the half-life is 21 hours, but on the first day it is 71 hours. Thus the plasma concentration may be maintained at high levels over a prolonged period during the first week. The third dose is given 36 hours after the first dose in the same amount as the second dose. In one report, a single dose of indomethacin given on the first postnatal day was effective in closing the ductus. This requires confirmation.

The current recommendation in most centers is to administer indomethacin for three doses over a 36-hour period. However, in small premature infants, the ductus may reopen within several days, after apparently having closed initially. This could be related to the fact that plasma prostaglandin concentrations gradually rise again within about a week after cessation of therapy. It has therefore been proposed by some that indomethacin should be administered over a more prolonged period of 5–7 days with a daily dose of 0.1 mg/kg. However, a Cochrane review in 2007 concluded that prolonged indomethacin therapy did not appear to improve important outcomes, such as failure of the ductus to close, intraventricular hemorrhage, chronic lung disease, or mortality [55]. Although the effect of indomethacin on the kidney is somewhat reduced by prolonged therapy, there is a significant increase in the incidence of necrotizing enterocolitis. The authors concluded that a prolonged course of indomethacin cannot be recommended for the routine treatment of patent ductus arteriosus in preterm infants.

Contraindications to the use of indomethacin include necrotizing enterocolitis, overt bleeding, and increased plasma creatinine concentrations.

Nitric oxide inhibitors

As mentioned above, infants born very prematurely are less likely to respond to prostaglandin synthesis inhibitors and are also more likely to experience reopening of the ductus after initial constriction by indomethacin. Because it is possible that patency of the ductus after birth may be maintained by NO activity, a trial of the use of inhibitors of NO production has been instituted [56]. Infants with gestational ages below 28 weeks were initially given the usual regimen of indomethacin therapy. Those who still had persistent left-to-right shunts by ultrasound were divided into two groups: 38 infants received a second course of indomethacin therapy and ductus closure was achieved in 42%; 12 infants received an NOS inhibitor, *N*(G)-monomethyl-L-arginine, in addition to a second course of indomethacin and ductus closure was successful in 92%. Thus NOS inhibitors could be a useful addition to indomethacin for treating patent ductus in preterm infants, but at present it cannot be recommended because it has significant adverse effects, particularly systemic arterial hypertension as well as a rise in serum creatinine concentrations.

Surgery

In early experience with surgical ligation of the ductus arteriosus in premature infants, there was considerable mortality, partly because the procedure was delayed until the infant had severe cardiorespiratory distress and partly because of lack of experience with managing preterm infants after thoracotomy. The procedure can now be performed with few postoperative complications and low mortality. In many centers the surgery is performed in the neonatal intensive care facility; this offers the advantage of not having to transport small infants who are being mechanically ventilated, and also avoids many of the difficulties of maintaining body temperature that often arise in the operating room.

Because of the small size of the infant, it is necessary to make a relatively large chest incision and to retract ribs extensively to obtain access with conventional surgical instruments and techniques. Recently, successful ligation of the ductus arteriosus using video-assisted thoracoscopy has been reported [57]. There was no operative mortality. This procedure avoids the large chest incisions and could also be readily performed in the neonatal unit. It will very likely become standard practice after surgeons gain more experience with the technique.

Persistent patency of the ductus arteriosus: the abnormal ductus

If the ductus arteriosus is exposed to the normal oxygen stimulus after birth, and the infant is not premature, failure of the normal constriction is probably related to some biochemical or structural abnormality. Little is known about the factors that may occasion such abnormalities, but there is a high incidence of patent ductus arteriosus in infants who have been infected with rubella virus *in utero*. The rubella virus appears to have a predilection for the ductus and the adjacent pulmonary trunk and pulmonary arteries. The walls of the vessels show hyaline degeneration and fibrosis with persistent patency of the ductus and stenosis of the left or right pulmonary artery, or both, at their origin. Often, the main pulmonary artery is involved, so that it too is narrowed between the ductus and the pulmonary valve. Apart from this specific infection, little is known about the failure of the ductus to close. Histological studies have not been revealing, mainly showing some collagen fibers in the wall with some elastic tissue, but this may be a secondary replacement process. An interesting observation has been made by Patterson and Detweiler [58], who used inbreeding to create a line of dogs with a better than 80% incidence of persistent patent ductus arteriosus. Examination of the ductus of these fetal puppies has shown some replacement of normal muscle, explaining the lack of constriction. The reason for this anomaly has not been explained. Patent ductus arteriosus has been known to occur on a hereditary basis, and I have encountered two families in which patent ductus arteriosus occurred in the females of three generations.

Patent ductus arteriosus may occur in association with other lesions, such as aortic coarctation or stenosis, ventricular septal defect, atrial septal defect, and endocardial cushion defects. The ductus arteriosus may be the only means of maintaining pulmonary blood flow after birth in infants with right-sided obstructive lesions, such as tricuspid or pulmonary atresia. It may also provide total systemic blood flow in infants with aortic atresia, and blood flow to the lower portion of the body in patients with aortic arch interruption. The role of the ductus in these other congenital lesions is discussed in the relevant chapters.

Hemodynamic considerations

The circulatory consequences of persistent patency of the ductus arteriosus after birth are related to the size of the ductus, the relationship between pulmonary and systemic vascular resistance, and the performance of the myocardium.

Small to moderate-sized ductus arteriosus

If the ductus arteriosus is narrow, pulmonary arterial pressure will fall as pulmonary vascular resistance falls after birth, and an increasing left-to-right shunt, related to the drop in pulmonary vascular resistance, will develop. Depending on the magnitude of the shunt, systemic arterial diastolic pressure may fall and pulse pressure widens (Figure 6.4). Pulmonary blood flow increases and the venous return to the left atrium increases. Left ventricular filling is increased and stroke volume is increased in association with an increase in left ventricular end-diastolic pressure and left atrial pressure. Usually, left ventricular output increases sufficiently to provide an adequate systemic blood flow despite the left-to-right shunt. If systemic arterial diastolic pressure falls, peripheral vascular resistance may decrease in an attempt to achieve adequate peripheral flow. In most of these infants, no evidence of serious cardiac failure occurs; there may be tachycardia, some tachypnea, and mild increase of respiratory effort, but the infant is usually not in severe distress.

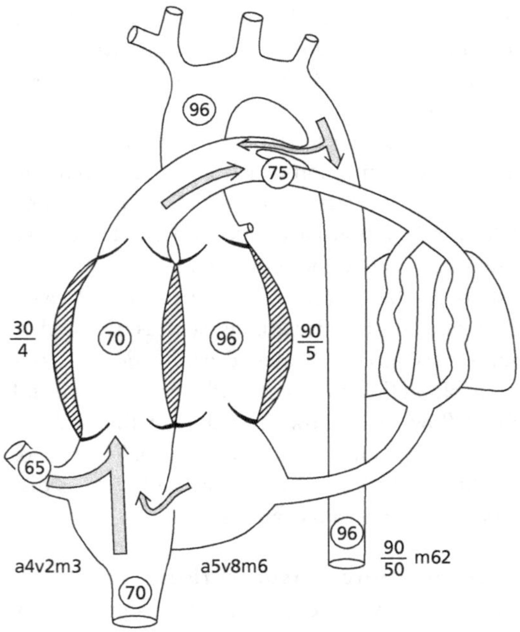

Figure 6.4 Small patent ductus arteriosus: course of the circulation, oxygen saturations (circled), and pressures in the heart and great vessels in an infant postnatally. m, mean pressure.

Patients with a small patent ductus arteriosus usually do not show any serious hemodynamic consequences beyond infancy; there is little risk of the development of pulmonary vascular changes or of exercise limitation in later life. There is a risk that infective endocarditis may develop.

Large ductus arteriosus

When the ductus is very large, pressures between the aorta and the pulmonary artery will remain equal after birth, and the patterns of flow are determined primarily by the relationship between pulmonary and systemic vascular resistance. Immediately after birth, the rise in systemic vascular resistance and the fall in pulmonary vascular resistance associated with ventilation of the lungs create some degree of left-to-right shunting. During the neonatal period and early infancy, it is not at all unusual for bidirectional shunting through the ductus to occur. This probably is related to the fact that with ventricular systole, the right ventricle ejects in a stream directed through the main pulmonary artery to the ductus and thus some pulmonary arterial blood may pass into the descending aorta in early systole, because systolic pressures are nearly equal. This kinetic effect may be aided by the fact that the aortic stream during systole is channeled around the arch to the descending aorta and may create a Bernoulli effect at the ductus orifice. The left-to-right shunt occurs predominantly during diastole.

Pulmonary vascular resistance falls after birth but, as has been mentioned, the presence of a large systemic–pulmonary communication may retard normal maturation of the pulmonary vessels after birth. Thus, the decrease may be prolonged over several weeks. This is associated with an increasing left-to-right shunt, widening of pulse pressure, and increased pulmonary circulation, with a large volume overload of the left ventricle. Left ventricular end-diastolic pressure increases, as do left atrial and pulmonary venous pressures. Left ventricular failure with pulmonary edema first supervenes, possibly followed by right ventricular failure; usually, the manifestations of cardiac failure appear within 3–8 weeks after birth but may occur earlier (Figure 6.5).

In many infants with a large patent ductus arteriosus and elevated left atrial pressure, a left-to-right shunt, often of large magnitude, occurs at the

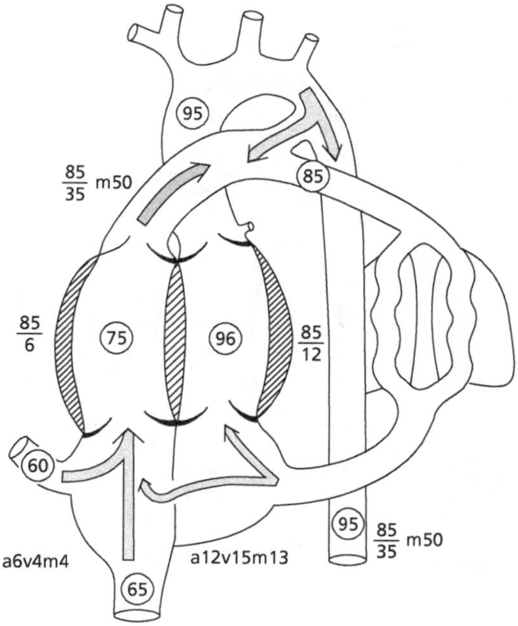

Figure 6.5 Large patent ductus arteriosus: course of the circulation, oxygen saturations (circled), and pressures in the heart and great vessels in an infant 3 months after birth. m, mean pressure.

atrial level. In most of these babies there is a large pressure difference between the left and right atrium, and after the ductus has been closed the shunt disappears. The shunt is due to stretching of the atrial septum because of left atrial enlargement, with resultant incompetence of the foramen ovale, or possibly due to herniation of the lower margin of the foramen ovale under the crista dividens into the right atrium.

The development of cardiac failure in infants with a large patent ductus is related not only to the pulmonary vascular resistance decrease but also to the ability of the left ventricle to handle the increased volume load. As mentioned above, the left ventricle of the immature fetal lamb is capable of increasing its output in response to increased preload resulting from increased pulmonary venous return associated with expansion of the lung after birth [34]. Furthermore, it can increase its output to maintain an adequate systemic blood flow if about 50% of its output is shunted through the ductus arteriosus. If a greater proportion is shunted, systemic blood flow falls and left ventricular failure develops.

The more mature the infant and the longer after birth that the increased volume load is presented to the myocardium, the greater the likelihood that it will tolerate the increased volume load without failing. An important factor is the development of hypertrophy in response to an increased workload; if there is a rapid decline in pulmonary vascular resistance, with rapid development of the volume load on the ventricle, failure may develop because there is inadequate time for hypertrophy. With more gradual evolution of the changes there may be an opportunity for adequate hypertrophy to occur to allow the ventricle to handle the load.

An additional factor that could be important in determining the ability of the left ventricle to increase its output in infants with patent ductus arteriosus is the adequacy of coronary blood flow. Relatively little myocardial blood flow to the left ventricular myocardium occurs during systole, because intramyocardial pressure is as high as aortic pressure. Coronary blood flow to the left ventricular myocardium occurs predominantly during diastole. The perfusion pressure providing coronary blood flow is determined by the difference between aortic diastolic pressure and the diastolic pressure in the ventricular chamber. In the infant with patent ductus arteriosus, aortic diastolic pressure is reduced and left ventricular diastolic pressure is increased, so that there is a marked reduction in the pressure difference. Furthermore, with increased heart rate and some degree of prolongation of left ventricular systolic ejection time, the total duration of diastole over a unit of time may be reduced. Coronary flow may therefore be reduced severely in a situation in which increased oxygen requirements are necessary for the increased ventricular work, and coronary blood flow and oxygen delivery may be compromised, particularly to the subendocardial region of the myocardium. These factors may account for the development of ST segment depression and T-wave flattening or inversion in the left precordial leads in the electrocardiogram.

An additional factor that may contribute to reduction in oxygen supply to the myocardium is the physiological fall in hemoglobin concentration after birth. In the normal infant, hemoglobin concentration falls to about 10–11 g/dL by 8–10 weeks after birth. The decrease in hemoglobin level will accentuate the reduction of oxygen supply to the myocardium. Also systemic blood flow has to be increased to meet tissue oxygen requirements, with a resultant increased demand on the left ventricle.

Extramyocardial factors are important in determining the clinical manifestations of cardiac failure. These are discussed extensively in Chapter 7. Other conditions that may stimulate demands for increased systemic blood flow are infection and increased environmental temperature. The introduction of these added stresses to an infant who otherwise is tolerating an increased volume load reasonably well may precipitate the onset of left ventricular failure.

In view of the importance of pulmonary vascular resistance in determining the subsequent hemodynamic events, conditions that maintain a high pulmonary vascular resistance after birth may prevent the development of left ventricular failure or allay its severity. Infants born and continuing to live at high altitude do not have the same incidence or severity of heart failure as those born at sea level. Also, an infant with a large ductus arteriosus who is not in any serious difficulty may conceivably develop cardiac failure within a relatively short time (days to weeks) on descending from altitude to sea level, because pulmonary vascular resistance falls quite rapidly. We have also had experience with infants who have had lung disease and a large patent ductus arteriosus who have developed left-sided heart failure after the lung disease has been treated and hypoxia relieved.

If the infant survives the cardiac failure, there is usually a gradual improvement in clinical manifestations, related to the development of increasing pulmonary vascular resistance. The evolution of these changes is discussed in detail in Chapter 5. Associated with the increasing pulmonary vascular resistance there is a decrease in left-to-right shunt; when the pulmonary vascular changes become severe enough to raise pulmonary vascular resistance above systemic levels, right-to-left shunt develops. The shunted systemic venous blood flows predominantly to the descending aorta, thus resulting in an oxygen saturation difference between the upper and lower parts of the body (Figure 6.6). If

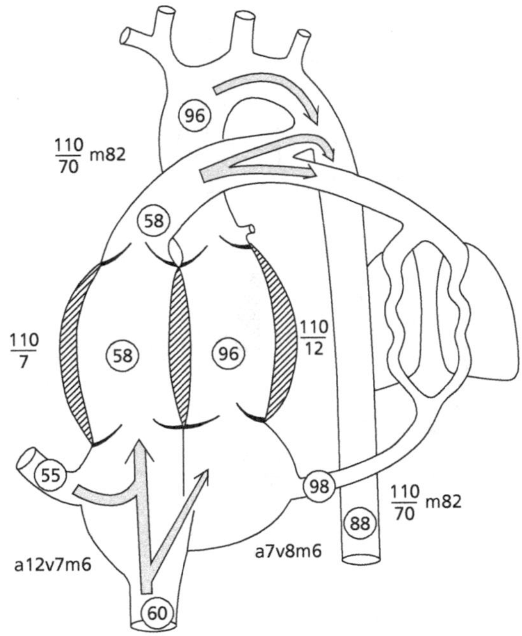

Figure 6.6 Large patent ductus arteriosus with markedly increased pulmonary vascular resistance: course of the circulation, oxygen saturations (circled), and pressures in an adult. m, mean pressure.

pulmonary vascular resistance is moderately elevated, right-to-left shunt and cyanosis of the lower body may be mild at rest, but increase with exertion. With further increases of pulmonary vascular resistance, cyanosis becomes persistent. With a relatively fixed pulmonary vascular resistance, changes in systemic vascular resistance will greatly influence the clinical manifestations. With exertion, for example, systemic vascular resistance falls and there is increased right-to-left shunt. The consequences of the development of severe pulmonary vascular obstruction are described in Chapter 5.

Clinical manifestations

Small ductus arteriosus

The patient with a small ductus arteriosus usually has no symptoms referable to the cardiovascular system and also has normal development. Blood pressure is usually normal if the shunt is small, but with somewhat larger shunts pulse pressure may increase. Cardiac activity and pulsations are normal, but mild left ventricular hyperactivity may be noted. The first and second heart sounds are normal. The only significant finding is the presence of a continuous murmur in the left infraclavicular area, along the upper left sternal border. The murmur varies greatly in character. It usually starts shortly after the first sound and extends beyond the second sound, but usually ends in mid-diastole. It tends to have peak accentuation at the second sound. With a small patent ductus, the murmur does not usually have the rough or "rocky" quality described with larger ductuses. The murmur may be heard better in some postures than in others, and frequently varies with respiration, increasing in intensity with expiration.

"Silent" ductus arteriosus

Since the introduction of ultrasound techniques, particularly Doppler flow studies, it has been recognized that a small ductus arteriosus detectable by ultrasound may not result in the typical clinical features of a patent ductus arteriosus. In some of these individuals, a soft grade 1–2/6 continuous murmur may be heard in the infraclavicular area intermittently; in others, only a grade 1–2/6 systolic murmur may be evident. Occasionally, no murmur is audible. There are also no other clinical manifestations to suggest the diagnosis.

In the individual with a small patent ductus arteriosus, the electrocardiogram is usually normal, but may show a modest increase in the height of the R wave in left precordial leads and prominent S waves in the right precordial leads. Chest radiography is also usually normal, but may reveal mild increase in pulmonary arterial markings and slight increase in left ventricular size.

Moderate-sized patent ductus arteriosus

This usually presents the so-called classic clinical picture of patent ductus arteriosus. The infant may appear well but may, often in retrospect, have had some tachypnea. Weight gain may be slow. By about 8–10 weeks after birth, evidence of left ventricular failure may appear. The infant is irritable, feeds poorly, becomes breathless or "tired" with feeding, and perspires excessively, particularly in relation to feeding. Increasing tachypnea and dyspnea develop. The pulse is rapid and bounding in quality and pulse pressure is increased. The heart is enlarged and there is hyperactivity of the left ventricle. The first sound is accentuated at the apex, and the pulmonary second sound, which may not be heard well at the upper left sternal border as it may be masked by the murmur, is usually moderately increased in intensity. There is a typical "machinery" murmur, a continuous murmur starting shortly after the first sound, reaching maximal accentuation at the second sound, and then declining in intensity to end in mid to late diastole. The murmur has an irregular intensity and a low frequency, often with very rough components; it is heard best at the upper left sternal border. A prominent third sound, and usually a short mid-diastolic murmur of low frequency, are heard at the apex, associated with the increased diastolic flow across the mitral valve. Rales may be heard at the lung bases. Hepatomegaly of varying degree is usually noted.

These infants may survive the cardiac failure without therapy and gradually, presumably due to the development of left ventricular hypertrophy, show improvement. They may be at some risk of developing pulmonary vascular changes in late adolescence, but certainly do not have the same risks as those with large ductuses. They are often poorly developed, have limitation of exercise tolerance, and perspire excessively.

The electrocardiogram in infancy shows an increase in left ventricular forces and also, in the first 6 months or so, evidence of increased right ventricular forces. Beyond infancy there are predominantly increased left forces, with tall R waves in leads V5 and V6, but T waves are usually not inverted. A broad bifid P wave in standard leads I and II may reflect left atrial enlargement.

Chest radiography shows an enlarged heart with predominant left ventricular prominence. The left atrium is large; the main pulmonary artery segment is prominent and the pulmonary vascular markings are increased. The ascending aorta and aortic knob are usually well seen, because they are enlarged due to the increased volume they conduct.

Large patent ductus arteriosus

When the ductus arteriosus is very large, the clinical picture described for the moderate-sized ductus is exaggerated. Evidence of cardiac failure may present somewhat earlier, often within 3–6 weeks after birth, and is more severe. The pulses are bounding, with a wide pulse pressure. The cardiac impulse is prominent, both left and right ventricles being hyperactive. The first sound is loud at the apex and the second sound is accentuated at the upper left sternal border. A loud continuous murmur with features similar to those described above for the moderate-sized ductus is usually heard. However, only a systolic murmur of grade 2–4/6 intensity, often peaking in late systole, may be heard. Although the characteristic extension of the murmur into mid-diastole may be absent, on careful auscultation extension of the murmur beyond the second sound into early diastole may be appreciated. Rarely, a murmur may not be audible at the upper left sternal border. A prominent low frequency mid-diastolic flow rumble is usually audible at the apex. It may not be evident when the infant is in cardiac failure and has marked tachycardia, but with slowing it becomes obvious. Evidence of cardiac failure, such as pulmonary rales and hepatomegaly, occurs to varying degrees.

The electrocardiogram usually shows biventricular hypertrophy and often a broad bifid P wave, and chest radiography shows features similar to those mentioned above. The heart may be more strikingly enlarged and evidence of pulmonary edema may be present.

These infants are at risk of succumbing to cardiac failure if not treated. They may show response to treatment for failure initially, but often mild failure persists, growth is slow, and infections may aggravate the manifestations of cardiac failure. If the lesion is not corrected, the infant has persistent sweating, increased respiratory rate and effort, and growth failure. The enlarged left and right ventricles result in anterior bulging of the sternum and costal cartilages. Over a varying period ranging from 3 to 6 months or more, the manifestations of cardiac failure improve, related to a gradual increase in pulmonary vascular resistance and reduction in the magnitude of left-to-right shunt (see Chapter 5). The degree of sweating and the respiratory distress decreases, and appetite and weight gain increase. The heart becomes smaller and cardiac activity decreases. The mid-diastolic apical murmur gradually disappears and the pulmonary second sound becomes louder. The continuous murmur at the upper left sternal border may become less harsh and the diastolic component may become shorter in duration. On chest radiography, the heart size decreases and right ventricular enlargement becomes more evident. The central pulmonary arteries become very prominent, but the peripheral vascular markings become less evident. The electrocardiogram may show evidence of increasing right ventricular hypertrophy.

The time course of subsequent changes varies, depending on the rate of progression of the pulmonary vascular changes. As pulmonary vascular resistance increases there is a further lessening of symptoms of cardiac failure, the heart size decreases, left ventricular activity decreases, and the right ventricular impulse becomes dominant. The second pulmonary sound remains accentuated but becomes narrower. The diastolic component may disappear and later the systolic component may become shorter and softer. The apical mid-diastolic flow murmur also disappears.

In the late stages of the development of high pulmonary vascular resistance, pulmonary valve insufficiency may develop and manifest as a decrescendo diastolic murmur immediately following the second sound in the pulmonary area. Cyanosis begins to appear, usually with exertion, and is seen first only in the lower extremities. The differential cyanosis may become marked with exertion and later at rest. Clubbing of the toes, but not of the fingers, may become manifest. The pulmonary vascular resistance may increase toward the latter part of the first year, but progression may be slow. Evidence of markedly elevated pulmonary vascular resistance may become manifest within 2–3 years, but may be delayed to adolescence or early adult life. Pulmonary vascular obstructive changes occur at an early age in patients with patent ductus arteriosus living at high altitude.

The electrocardiogram shows a progressive reduction in left-sided and an increase in right ventricular forces. Chest radiography shows increasing right ventricular dominance, a very large main pulmonary artery and large hilar vessels, with progressive decrease or "pruning" of the peripheral lung vessels.

Patent ductus arteriosus associated with other left-to-right shunt lesions

Although patent ductus arteriosus with left-to-right shunt occurs as an isolated lesion in most patients, occasionally a ventricular septal defect, atrioventricular septal defect, or atrial septal defect is associated. The presence of the loud continuous murmur of the patent ductus arteriosus may mask the presence of an additional defect. Thus the murmur of atrial septal defect will not be evident and the separate murmur created by a ventricular septal defect may not be appreciated. In patients with a large patent ductus arteriosus and markedly increased pulmonary vascular resistance, an associated ventricular septal defect or atrioventricular septal defect may not be suspected clinically, because often there are no signs indicating the presence of the additional lesion.

Investigations

Ultrasound

In the early experience with ultrasound, the ductus arteriosus was not directly visualized, the technique providing information about the physiological consequences of the ductus left-to-right shunt. Left-to-right shunting at the ventricular level and/or mitral regurgitation could also result in the finding of left atrial and left ventricular dilation, with the left atrial diameter exceeding the diameter of the aortic root by a ratio greater than 1.1–1.3 and thus there was often uncertainty about the presence of the lesion. Two-dimensional echocardiography increased the sensitivity of echocardiography in finding ventricular septal defects, congenital malformations of the mitral valve and chordae, and direct visualization of the ductus arteriosus. The addition of color flow Doppler mapping has made it possible to detect even very small patent ductuses. Although the ductus may be visualized by two-dimensional and color flow Doppler ultrasound imaging, it is often difficult to image the ductus along its whole course and thus the narrowest diameter may not be evident. Apart from detecting patency of the ductus, other features to be clarified are the presence of associated lesions, estimation of the magnitude of the left-to-right shunt, and estimation of pulmonary arterial pressure.

A careful examination should be carried out to exclude other lesions. As mentioned above, it is often difficult to detect the presence of other left-to-right shunt lesions by clinical examination, so the ultrasound study should exclude ventricular septal defect, atrioventricular septal defect, and atrial septal defect. In the infant with a large patent ductus, the left atrium may be dilated and, associated with the high pressure, the atrial septum may bulge into the right atrium. The foramen ovale may be stretched and Doppler examination may detect a left-to-right shunt. In addition, pulmonary and aortic stenosis should be excluded, because clinical evidence of these lesions may be masked by a loud murmur of patent ductus arteriosus. Because patent ductus arteriosus is not infrequently associated with aortic coarctation, this should also be excluded.

A large-diameter ductus does not necessarily imply the presence of a large left-to-right shunt, because the shunting will be determined by the level of pulmonary vascular resistance. Ultrasound evidence of a large shunt includes enlargement of the left atrium and a large hyperdynamic left ventricle. A useful indicator of the magnitude of the left-to-right shunt is the pattern of flow in the descending aorta at the level of the diaphragm as assessed by Doppler flow study. Normally there is forward flow throughout diastole, but with increasing size of the left-to-right shunt, the forward flow decreases and, with large shunts, retrograde flow is evident in diastole. It is often difficult to calculate pulmonary blood flow by continuous flow Doppler because of turbulence resulting from the flow through the ductus into the pulmonary artery. Measurement of flow across the tricuspid valve provides an estimate of systemic blood flow and measurement of flow across the mitral valve provides an estimate of pulmonary blood flow.

The velocity of the jet in the ductus has been used to estimate the pressure gradient between the aorta and pulmonary artery in order to assess pulmonary arterial pressure. However, it may be unreliable if the ductus is long or tortuous. If pulmonary valve insufficiency is detected, the velocity of the regurgitant jet may provide an estimate of pulmonary arterial diastolic pressure.

Cardiac catheterization

Prior to the introduction of ultrasound techniques, cardiac catheterization and angiocardiography were performed for the purposes of confirming the diagnosis of patent ductus arteriosus, excluding other lesions, and calculating pulmonary vascular resistance. Ultrasound examination made it possible to confirm the diagnosis and to exclude other lesions, so that catheterization was performed to assess pulmonary vascular resistance and its response to pulmonary vasodilators. Recently, however, catheterization procedures are again being performed to close the ductus by transcatheter techniques.

Catheter manipulation

Using the groin approach, the venous catheter can almost invariably be passed through the ductus arteriosus from the pulmonary artery into the aorta. When the ductus arteriosus is large, the catheter usually passes preferentially through the ductus and considerable manipulation is required to pass the catheter into the branch pulmonary arteries. Occasionally, in the patient with a very small ductus, it may not be possible to pass the catheter through it. Typically, the catheter passes into the descending aorta, but rarely it may pass proximally into the arch and enter one or other carotid artery. If the latter does occur, it is important to exclude the possibility that the catheter has entered the carotid vessel from the ascending aorta, by passing from the pulmonary artery through an aortopulmonary septal defect. The exact nature of the lesion can be recognized by performing an angiogram with the catheter positioned in the aorta just beyond the ductus. If the venous catheter cannot be manipulated through the ductus, a catheter passed retrogradely from the femoral artery can usually be passed readily through the ductus into the pulmonary artery. An angiogram done in the aorta in the region of the attachment of the ductus arteriosus clearly demonstrates the lesion.

Oxygen saturation data

In small infants, particularly those with a large patent ductus, a left-to-right shunt at the atrial level is not infrequent. The oxygen saturation in SVC blood may be reduced to 50–60% if the infant is in cardiac failure. A rise of saturation of 10–15% and by as much as 20% at the atrial level is not unusual when the foramen ovale is stretched. The magnitude of the left-to-right shunt through the ductus may not be appreciated, because the atrial shunt may increase the oxygen saturation of right ventricular blood to such a high level that, even with a large ductus shunt, pulmonary arterial oxygen saturation is only slightly higher.

In the absence of an atrial left-to-right shunt, the increase in saturation is noted at the pulmonary arterial level. In some patients with a large ductus arteriosus, an increase in oxygen saturation may be noted in the right ventricular infundibular region, below the valve, due to pulmonary regurgitation. It is not usually possible to obtain a sample that is truly representative of mixed pulmonary arterial blood. Blood samples obtained in the main pulmonary artery may show considerable variation in oxygen saturation depending on whether the sample is obtained close to the ductus or in the stream ejected by the right ventricle. Oxygen saturation in the left pulmonary artery tends to be higher than that in the right pulmonary artery, because blood shunted through the ductus passes preferentially into the left side. When pulmonary vascular resistance is high, no increase in oxygen saturation on the right side of the heart may be detected.

Oxygen saturation in the left atrium and ventricle and in the aorta is usually normal. However, in small infants with cardiac failure, pulmonary edema may interfere with oxygenation in the lungs and the arterial saturation may be reduced to 90–92%. The oxygen saturation in the ascending aorta and the innominate or left carotid artery is usually normal in older infants and children. In infants with large defects, the oxygen saturation in the descending aorta or its branches may be reduced by up to 5–8% compared with the ascending aorta due to bidirectional shunting. In patients with increased pulmonary vascular resistance and large right-to-left shunts, a large reduction in oxygen saturation in the descending aorta is evident. Oxygen saturation in the left subclavian artery may be similar to that in the ascending aorta, but it may be somewhat reduced by retrograde flow of some blood shunted right to left through the ductus.

With a small patent ductus, the left-to-right shunt may be insignificant and may not be recognized on the basis of oxygen saturation data, but this should not exclude the diagnosis. An angiogram performed in the aorta will confirm the diagnosis.

Pressures

With a small patent ductus arteriosus, all vascular pressures are normal. With moderate-sized defects, right ventricular and pulmonary arterial systolic pressures are usually moderately elevated to about 35–65 mmHg; right ventricular end-diastolic pressure is normal or slightly increased. Pulmonary arterial diastolic and mean pressures are also moderately elevated, with mean pressures of 20–40 mmHg. Left atrial mean pressure is mildly to moderately elevated to 6–12 mmHg and the *v* wave is prominent. Left ventricular systolic pressure is normal and left ventricular end-diastolic pressure is slightly to moderately increased. Aortic diastolic pressure is reduced to a variable degree and pulse pressure is increased.

With large defects, right ventricular and pulmonary arterial systolic pressures are equal to those in the systemic circulation. Pulmonary arterial diastolic pressure may be relatively low at 25–40 mmHg. Aortic diastolic pressure is low and may be reduced to the same level as pulmonary arterial diastolic pressure. Left atrial mean pressure may be increased to 10–15 mmHg and left ventricular end-diastolic pressure may be raised to 15–20 mmHg. Occasionally, patients with very large left-to-right shunts demonstrate a systolic pressure difference between the left ventricle and ascending aorta at the site of the aortic valve. The gradient varies from 10 to 25 mmHg, but has been as high as 60 mmHg. It is due to a relative stenosis related to the high flow across the aortic valve. The aortic valve appears normal by both ultrasound and angiography, and after closure of the ductus the gradient disappears. When pulmonary vascular resistance increases, aortic diastolic pressure increases, as does pulmonary arterial diastolic and mean pressure. Simultaneous pressures measured in the aorta and pulmonary artery may show identical systolic and diastolic levels.

Blood flows

In view of the difficulty in obtaining a good mixed pulmonary arterial sample for oxygen analysis, calculations of pulmonary blood flow by the Fick method are often unreliable. Systemic blood flow can usually be measured, unless there is right-to-left shunt through the ductus, in which case calculations are unreliable because oxygen saturations in the ascending and descending aorta differ. Systemic blood flow is often reduced in infants with a large ductus arteriosus and cardiac failure.

Vascular resistances

Calculations of pulmonary vascular resistance may be unreliable, in view of the problems in measuring pulmonary blood flows. In early infancy, with large ductuses, the calculated resistances are usually somewhat increased, in the range of 3–5 units/m^2. If pulmonary vascular changes develop, the vascular resistance increases. Occasionally this begins to occur in the latter part of the first year, but may not develop for several years. In patients living at high altitudes, marked increases in pulmonary vascular resistance may occur at an early age. Systemic vascular resistance is usually normal, but may be increased in the infant with cardiac failure.

Angiocardiography

The size and site of origin of a patent ductus from the aorta and some indication of the magnitude of left-to-right shunt can be obtained from an angiogram performed in the aorta just distal to the arch at the origin of the ductus or just distal to it. It is usually best visualized in the lateral projection. In the presence of a small patent ductus arteriosus there often is a bulge in the aorta, the ductus ampulla, at the site of origin of the ductus. The small ductus arises from the apex of the ampulla and courses to the pulmonary artery. A jet of contrast medium may be seen to enter the pulmonary artery from the ductus. With large left-to-right shunts through the ductus, the ascending aorta is dilated.

Differential diagnosis

Large patent ductus arteriosus in the infant in cardiac failure

Several lesions may simulate a large ductus arteriosus because they may cause cardiac failure in infancy and are associated with a wide pulse pressure. Many of these are often also associated with loud murmurs that extend into diastole, including:

- aortopulmonary septal defect;
- truncus arteriosus communis;
- systemic arteriovenous fistula;
- aortic–left ventricular tunnel;
- aortic insufficiency with or without a ventricular septal defect;
- sequestration of the lung;
- coronary arteriovenous fistula.

Conditions that may cause a systolic and diastolic murmur but which are not associated with a wide pulse pressure include pulmonary arteriovenous fistula and tetralogy of Fallot with absent pulmonary valve. Examination by ultrasound, including Doppler flow studies, will usually readily differentiate between the lesions.

The clinical features of the rare aortopulmonary septal defect are indistinguishable from those of patent ductus arteriosus. Turbulence is noted in the main pulmonary artery on Doppler examination, but it is important to identify whether flow into the pulmonary artery is from the descending aorta, as with patent ductus arteriosus, of from the ascending aorta. Truncus arteriosus may present with many of the features of patent ductus arteriosus. Usually the infant has mild cyanosis, but with a large pulmonary blood flow, cyanosis may be so mild that it is not appreciated. With truncus arteriosus and very large pulmonary blood flows, the peripheral pulse pressure may not be very wide, because systolic pressure may be low. The murmur of truncus arteriosus is usually systolic, but may be continuous and is often heard in both sides of the chest. If truncus valve regurgitation is present, an early decrescendo diastolic murmur may be heard. A systemic arteriovenous fistula between the subclavian artery and vein may cause cardiac failure in infancy and be associated with wide pulse pressure and a continuous murmur. The murmur is more prominent below the outer end of the clavicle, rather than at the upper left sternal border, as with a ductus arteriosus. The murmurs of aortic–left ventricular tunnel or aortic insufficiency with ventricular septal defect are characterized by back and forth timing, rather than continuous, as with a patent ductus arteriosus. The systolic component does not usually extend to the second sound, so that there is a gap between the systolic and diastolic components of the murmur. With patent ductus the systolic murmur is crescendic to the second sound and continues into the diastolic component. A sequestered lobe of the lung may be supplied by a large artery from the descending aorta; high flow may result in cardiac failure. The murmur is often continuous but is located in the lower chest and is usually most prominent posteriorly. Coronary arteriovenous fistulae do not usually present with cardiac failure in infancy, but a large shunt may cause a wide pulse pressure and a continuous murmur, which is most commonly heard along the lower right sternal border.

Tetralogy of Fallot with absent pulmonary valve may present with a loud murmur, which may be confused with, but is not typical of, patent ductus murmur. The murmur has been described as "see-saw" in character, as discussed above. Pulmonary arteriovenous fistulae may present with continuous murmurs; these are usually best heard in the periphery of the lungs and cyanosis of varying degree is evident.

Small patent ductus arteriosus

The lesions that may be considered are mainly those producing continuous murmurs at the upper left sternal border or left infraclavicular area, including coronary arteriovenous fistula, anomalous origin of the left coronary artery from the pulmonary artery, intercostal arteriovenous fistula, peripheral pulmonary stenosis, venous hum, and pulmonary arteriovenous fistula. The distinction is readily made by ultrasound examination.

Principles of management

The approach is different in the preterm infant versus the mature infant and child. Management in the infant and child is usually based on the size of the ductus. No specific criteria have been developed to define what is large, medium or small, but often the size is based on the degree of elevation of pulmonary arterial pressure and the magnitude of the left-to-right shunt. Thus if systolic pressure in the pulmonary artery is above 40–50 mmHg, the ductus is considered to be large; if systolic pressure is normal or not above 25–30 mmHg, the ductus is considered to be small. If the ratio of pulmonary to systemic blood flow is greater than 2:1, the shunt is thought to be large; a ratio of less than 1.5:1 indicates a small shunt. The size of the ductus arteriosus, an estimate of the volume overload on the left ventricle, and information about pulmonary arterial pressure can usually be provided by ultrasound examination.

Patent ductus arteriosus in the premature infant

Treatment is discussed in the section 'Complications of patent ductus arteriosus in the premature infant' above.

Large patent ductus arteriosus

During infancy

If the infant with a large patent ductus develops cardiac failure, diuretic therapy should be instituted. If the infant does not respond rapidly to treatment, the ductus should be closed by surgery. If the failure responds and the infant is free of symptoms, two possible approaches can be considered. Surgical closure may be performed without delay, although it is now being suggested by some that if the cardiac failure is well controlled, it may be reasonable to observe the infant until the age of 6–8 months, at which time transcatheter closure may be feasible. Currently, transcatheter closure is not usually recommended in infants weighing less than about 5 kg. However, successful procedures have been reported in a few small infants, and this could become routine as more experience is gained and better devices developed (see Chapter 6).

It is widely accepted practice to close the ductus arteriosus either with a device or by surgery if the infant has had cardiac failure, even if it has responded to medical therapy. This seems reasonable if the child is not thriving or if pulmonary arterial pressure is elevated. However, if there is no evidence of cardiac failure, the infant is growing well, and pulmonary arterial pressure is only slightly increased, it might be justified to delay closing the ductus. Spontaneous closure of the ductus may occur during the first year, but the incidence of closure during this period is not defined.

Beyond infancy

If the ductus diameter is large and pulmonary arterial systolic pressure is elevated above about 30 mmHg, closure is indicated because there is the risk of development of pulmonary vascular changes with progressive increase in pulmonary vascular resistance. Beyond infancy, closure may still occur, at an estimated rate of 0.6% per year [59]. It is not known, however, what the incidence of closure is with ductuses of different size. Beyond early infancy, cardiac failure is rare before the age of 20–30 or even 40 years; right heart failure may then develop as a result of progressive pulmonary vascular disease. The main risk before that time is considered to be the development of infective endocarditis. This is discussed below.

Large patent ductus arteriosus with increased pulmonary vascular resistance

Patients of this type should no longer be encountered, because they should have been treated in infancy. In the child who has markedly increased pulmonary vascular resistance with right-to-left shunt, surgical closure of the ductus is not generally advised, as many of these patients do not survive the procedure because systemic blood flow is compromised; also acute right heart failure may ensue. An approach that might be considered is to treat the patient with a pulmonary vasodilator drug such as bosentan, sildenafil, or intravenous PGI_2 for several months (see Chapter 5) in an attempt to reduce pulmonary vascular resistance prior to attempting ductus closure.

It is in the patient with moderately increased pulmonary vascular resistance (8–12 units/m^2) that the decision is difficult. If pulmonary vascular resistance falls considerably with a pulmonary vasodilator such as tolazoline, PGI_2 or NO, closure of the ductus should be performed. If the patient has been living at high altitude, it is advisable to observe whether the pulmonary vascular resistance falls after living near sea level. If it does fall significantly, surgery is advised.

Often, however, there is no good basis on which to decide whether surgery should be performed. Some patients with this level of resistance survive surgery and show improvement in the pulmonary circulation. Others, however, show a progressive increase in pulmonary vascular resistance after the ductus has been closed and usually do not survive long. We do not know what determines the outcome, and the decision whether or not to recommend closure of the ductus is very difficult. All these patients should be treated with pulmonary vasodilator drugs after closure of the ductus. Possibly this will improve the long-term expectancy.

Moderate-sized, small, and silent ductus arteriosus

Decisions regarding management of a patent ductus arteriosus are determined by its potential adverse effects. The main concerns are cardiac failure, pulmonary vascular obstructive disease, left ventricular myocardial damage, and infective endocarditis (endovasculitis). As mentioned above, there is general agreement that the ductus should be closed if acute cardiac failure is present and response to medical therapy is inadequate. Also, if pulmonary arterial pressure is elevated to above half of systemic arterial pressure, the ductus should be closed to try to avoid pulmonary vascular abnormalities.

Left ventricular myocardium

Concern has been raised that a moderate-sized left-to-right shunt places a chronic volume load on the left ventricle and this could induce myocardial hypertrophy and also fibrosis, resulting in myocardial failure after many years. As Campbell reported, beyond infancy, cardiac failure is rare in patients with patent ductus arteriosus before the age of 30 or even 40 years [59]. Based on this information, most pediatric cardiologists recommend that the ductus should be closed if there is a moderate left-to-right shunt and/or if there is cardiomegaly noted in chest radiography or ultrasound examination, in order to prevent possible damage to the left ventricular myocardium. There are several questions regarding this reasoning. Campbell's report was based on purely clinical observation and there is no information regarding the size of the left-to-right shunt and volume overload. It is possible that all those individuals who developed cardiac failure had very large shunts and possibly some had early coronary artery disease. A recent report on the natural history of ventricular septal defect suggests that the risks of myocardial damage related to a moderate left-to-right shunt have been overstated [60].

Follow-up of patients with ventricular septal defect with moderate left-to-right shunts and evidence of left ventricular enlargement showed no progression over at least 2 years, but rather a decrease in heart size and no echocardiographic evidence of left ventricular dysfunction. It may not be appropriate to compare patients with patent ductus arteriosus with those with ventricular septal defect, because ventricular septal defects are probably more likely to become smaller over time. Furthermore, the study does not resolve the issue whether exposure to a moderately increased volume load for decades may have adverse effects on the left ventricular myocardium. However, there is little convincing evidence that a moderate increase in volume load on the left ventricle from a left-to-right shunt has significant adverse effects on the myocardium. The issue needs to be examined by prospective studies.

Without further information, it is difficult to make specific recommendations about whether to close a patent ductus arteriosus to avoid the possible risk of left ventricular failure in later life. Pediatric cardiologists have generally regarded a shunt as being large if the ratio of pulmonary to systemic blood flow is greater than 2:1, but this is arbitrary. A ratio greater than 2:1 has often been used as a basis for recommending closure of the ductus. As mentioned above, it is often difficult to measure pulmonary blood flow reliably even by catheterization, because oxygen contents of the right and left pulmonary artery may differ. Also, measurement of flows by ultrasound is not reliable.

Currently, my view is that a patient who has a mild to moderate shunt based on clinical examination, but with no symptoms, should be studied by ultrasound to assess left ventricular size and performance and then should be reevaluated at 1–2 year intervals. If there are progressive changes in the ventricle or if symptoms develop, the ductus should be closed.

Issues of infective endocarditis

Until recently, it was recommended that all patients with a patent ductus arteriosus should receive antibiotic prophylaxis for infective endocarditis [61]. With the advent of ultrasound examination, and especially Doppler flow study, increasing numbers of individuals are being identified who have no clinical evidence of a patent ductus arteriosus but in whom a very small patent ductus is detected. This is referred to as silent patent ductus arteriosus (see Chapter 6). Questions have been raised about the necessity for recommending antibiotic prophylaxis in these individuals. Although infective endocarditis has been reported in patients with small patent ductus arteriosus, the necessity for prophylaxis in the individual with a silent patent ductus has to be considered. If it is decided that prophylaxis is indicated, this raises the issue of whether ultrasound studies should be performed in the whole population in order to detect whether an individual has a silent patent ductus arteriosus.

Endocarditis certainly occurs with patent ductus arteriosus, but the incidence has been controversial.

In 1968, Campbell [59] estimated that almost half the deaths related to patent ductus arteriosus could be related to infective endocarditis. However, about 20 years later, the incidence appeared to have fallen dramatically [62]. Although it is possible that the decrease in incidence is related to introduction of prophylactic antibiotic therapy, this does not seem likely in view of the current concept that antibiotic prophylaxis is not very effective in preventing infective endocarditis. It could be the result of improvements in dental hygiene or to a general reduction in the occurrence of infections in the population. There has also been great interest in the influence of ductus size on the incidence of infective endocarditis. Although infection has been reported in a patient with a silent ductus [63], this is exceedingly rare. In fact, in an adult population the diameter of the ductus arteriosus was less than 4.5 mm in 60%, but greater than 4.5 mm in all those who developed endocarditis [64].

There is increasing evidence that in recent years endocarditis is not an important complication in patients with patent ductus arteriosus, and certainly not in those with small ductuses. Thus in Sweden a review of almost 3 million deaths over the period 1960–1993 found that only two deaths could be attributed to infective endocarditis; both were in adults, one with Eisenmenger syndrome and in the other autopsy confirmation was not obtained [65]. These authors reviewed 207 children and adults with patent ductus over an aggregate of 1196 years at risk and did not encounter any instance of infective endocarditis.

The primary reason why pediatric cardiologists and pediatric cardiac surgeons recommended closing the ductus was to prevent the development of infective endocarditis. Also, because prophylactic therapy was strongly recommended, closure was advised to eliminate the need for repeated administration of antibiotics. However, the guidelines for prophylaxis of infective endocarditis have now changed and antibiotic prophylaxis is no longer recommended for patients with patent ductus arteriosus [66]. It is still the practice in most centers to close even small patent ductuses. It is justified on the basis that device closure has minimal risk and it is therefore advisable to close the ductus to prevent possible development of endocarditis. Some, but not all, recommend that even silent ductus arteriosus should be closed. With the overwhelming evidence that endocarditis is rare, and because it can be successfully treated in the rare event that it may occur, this approach is unreasonable. As stated by Sullivan [67], "the natural history of a small arterial duct with a negligible left-to-right shunt is not known with certainty, but the risk of endocarditis is vanishingly small."

Based on current information there appears to be diminishing justification for closing small to moderate-sized ductus arteriosus, even though it can be done with little risk and few complications.

Techniques for ductus arteriosus closure

Surgical closure of the ductus can be accomplished through a left thoracotomy without the use of cardiopulmonary bypass. In the early experience with surgery, following ligation of the vessel, occasionally a small residual shunt was detected. It therefore became the practice of most surgeons to divide the ductus and suture the two open ends. With a large ductus, this procedure entailed some risk of hemorrhage, particularly in small infants. Currently, it has become common practice to ligate the ductus in small infants. It is likely that instances of apparent recanalization were due to inadequate ligation of a large ductus. The procedure has very low morbidity and mortality. The complications that may result are recurrent laryngeal nerve palsy, because the left nerve is closely related to the ductus, and trauma to the thoracic duct, resulting in chylothorax. Recently, ligation of the ductus arteriosus has been successfully accomplished in infants using video-assisted thoracoscopic surgery through very small incisions in the chest [57].

Transcatheter closure of the ductus arteriosus was first accomplished by Portsmann *et al.* [68]. Their technique required an approach through both a femoral vein and artery and the use of very large catheters and was not widely accepted. Subsequently, Rashkind *et al.* [69] have developed a double-umbrella device. This consists of a stainless steel wire frame that is held open by a spring mechanism; covering the frame is polyurethane fabric. This device can be used to close ductuses up to 8 mm diameter. This device has been modified by Lock to allow closure of ductuses with diameters up to 12 mm. Several other devices have been developed. The Gianturco coil is a stainless steel spring coil onto which have been embedded fibers of various materials. The device is placed in its uncoiled state in a catheter and embolized into the patent ductus; they are preformed to create coils of 2–8 mm diameter. The advantage of this device is that it can be delivered through a very small catheter. The coil and the embedded fibers induce thrombosis that closes the ductus. An important disadvantage is that the coil may embolize into the pulmonary artery. Although it can usually be retrieved, this is not always possible. To overcome this problem, Cook has recently developed a retrievable coil system; the delivery wire remains attached to one end of the coil and is freed by a screw mechanism when the coil has been satisfactorily positioned. Another technique using a button device has been developed for transcatheter closure of the patent ductus arteriosus. More recently, another device called the Amplatzer ductus occluder has become available. It is constructed of Nitinol wire mesh and has a skirt on the aortic side to retain it in the ductus ampulla. When implanted, the device expands so that the wire is pushed against the ductus wall. Fabrics made of polyester induce thrombosis.

The largest experience has been gained with the use of Gianturco coils and the Rashkind double-umbrella device. After placement of the device, there may be a left-to-right shunt of varying size for a variable period. Complete closure is achieved in about half the patients soon after the procedure, but in some closure is not complete until 2–3 years after the procedure, and in a very small percentage complete closure may not be accomplished. There is currently some reluctance to use transcatheter approaches in the infant under the age of 2–3 months who has a large patent ductus. Also the technique has not been applied to closure of ductuses in premature infants.

Currently, most patients with patent ductus arteriosus can have successful closure by transcatheter techniques beyond early infancy with no mortality and very low morbidity. The advantages of this approach are that a thoracotomy is avoided and many procedures can be done on an outpatient basis. Apart from the risk of embolization of coils into the pulmonary artery, the other main concern is damage to the femoral artery if an approach is made through this vessel, particularly in small infants. Many centers therefore prefer to use a venous approach if at all possible.

One of the questions that has been raised is whether the foreign material in the aorta or pulmonary artery is a potential site for development of infective endocarditis. Frequently the end of a Gianturco coil projects into the aorta or pulmonary artery; whether this could be the site for thrombosis or infective endocarditis is yet to be resolved. In follow-up for several years, it does not appear that any difficulties have been observed, but further more extensive information is necessary. Occasional instances of partial obstruction of the left pulmonary artery and less frequently of the descending aorta have been observed.

In a number of patients, a second procedure has been necessary to effect closure of the ductus, because the first attempt did not achieve complete closure. Important unresolved issues include the indications and timing of a second procedure. Because closure after the initial procedure may be delayed for months or even 2–4 years, it is necessary to make a determination about if and when a second procedure should be performed. Rarely, a second procedure is required due to detection of mechanical hemolytic anemia secondary to a residual high-velocity shunt jet past the foreign body that was imbedded in the ductus arteriosus during the first procedure.

References

1 Hoffman JIE. In: Rudolph CD, Rudolph AM, Hostetter MK, Lister G, Siegel NJ, eds. Rudolph's Pediatrics. New York: McGraw-Hill, 2002: 1781.

2 Lloyd TR, Beekman RH III. Clinically silent patent ductus arteriosus [Letter]. Am Heart J 1994;127:1664–1665.

3 Mielke G, Benda N. Cardiac output and central distribution of blood flow in the human fetus. Circulation 2001;103:1662–1668.

4 Sutton MS, Groves A, MacNeill A, Sharland G, Allan L. Assessment of changes in blood flow through the lungs and foramen ovale in the normal human fetus with gestational age: a prospective Doppler echocardiographic study. Br Heart J 1994;71:232–237.

5 Rasanen J, Wood DC, Weiner S, Ludomirski A, Huhta JC. Role of the pulmonary circulation in the distribution of human fetal cardiac output during the second half of pregnancy. Circulation 1996;94:1068–1073.

6 Shiraishi H, Yanagisawa M. Bidirectional flow through the ductus arteriosus in normal newborns: evaluation by Doppler color flow imaging. Pediatr Cardiol 1991;12: 201–205.

7 Clyman RI, Chan CY, Mauray F *et al.* Permanent anatomic closure of the ductus arteriosus in newborn baboons: the roles of postnatal constriction, hypoxia, and gestation. Pediatr Res 1999;45:19–29.

8 Kennedy JA, Clark SL. Observations on the physiological reactions of the ductus arteriosus. Am J Physiol 1942;136: 140–144.

9 Oberhansli-Weiss I, Heymann MA, Rudolph AM, Melmon KL. The pattern and mechanisms of response of the ductus arteriosus and umbilical artery to oxygen. Pediatr Res 1972;6:693–700.

10 McMurphy DM, Heymann MA, Rudolph AM, Melmon KL. Developmental changes in constriction of the ductus arteriosus: responses to oxygen and vasoactive substances in the isolated ductus arteriosus of the fetal lamb. Pediatr Res 1972;6:231–238.

11 Fay FS, Nair P, Whalen WJ. Mechanism of oxygen induced contraction of ductus arteriosus. Adv Exp Med Biol 1977;78:123–134.

12 Coceani F, Hamilton NC, Labuc J, Olley PM. Cytochrome P450-linked monooxygenase: involvement in the lamb ductus arteriosus. Am J Physiol 1984;246:H640–H643.

13 Thébaud B, Michelakis ED, Wu XC *et al.* Oxygen-sensitive Kv channel gene transfer confers oxygen responsiveness to preterm rabbit and remodeled human ductus arteriosus: implications for infants with patent ductus arteriosus. Circulation 2004;110:1372–1379.

14 Kajimoto H, Hashimoto K, Bonnet SN *et al.* Oxygen activates the Rho/Rho-kinase pathway and induces RhoB and ROCK-1 expression in human and rabbit ductus arteriosus by increasing mitochondria-derived reactive oxygen species: a newly recognized mechanism for sustaining ductal constriction. Circulation 2007;115:1777–1788.

15 Coceani F, Kelsey L, Seidlitz E. Evidence for an effector role of endothelin in closure of the ductus arteriosus at birth. Can J Physiol Pharmacol 1992;70:1061–1064.

16 Coceani F, Kelsey L. Endothelin-1 release from lamb ductus arteriosus: relevance to postnatal closure of the vessel. Can J Physiol Pharmacol 1991;69:218–221.

17 Takahashi Y, Roman C, Chemtob S *et al.* Cyclooxygenase-2 inhibitors constrict the fetal lamb ductus arteriosus both in vitro and in vivo. Am J Physiol 2000;278:R1496–R1505.

18 Clyman RI, Mauray F, Roman C, Rudolph AM. PGE2 is a more potent vasodilator of the lamb ductus arteriosus than is either PGI2 or 6 keto PGF1alpha. Prostaglandins 1978;16:259–264.

19 Clyman RI, Mauray F, Roman C, Rudolph AM, Heymann MA. Circulating prostaglandin E2 concentrations and patent ductus arteriosus in fetal and neonatal lambs. J Pediatr 1980;97:455–461.

20 Clyman RI, Heymann MA, Rudolph AM. Ductus arteriosus responses to prostaglandin E1 at high and low oxygen concentrations. Prostaglandins 1977;13: 219–223.

21 Clyman RI, Mauray F, Heymann MA, Rudolph AM. Ductus arteriosus: developmental response to oxygen and indomethacin. Prostaglandins 1978;15:993–998.

22 Clyman RI, Mauray F, Roman C *et al.* Effects of antenatal glucocorticoid administration on ductus arteriosus of preterm lambs. Am J Physiol 1981;241:H415–H420.

23 Clyman RI, Waleh N, Black SM, Riemer RK, Mauray F, Chen YQ. Regulation of ductus arteriosus patency by nitric oxide in fetal lambs: the role of gestation, oxygen tension, and vasa vasorum. Pediatr Res 1998;43:633–644.

24 Momma K, Toyono M. The role of nitric oxide in dilating the fetal ductus arteriosus in rats. Pediatr Res 1999;46:311–315.

25 Mentzer RM Jr, Ely SW, Lasley RD, Mainwaring RD, Wright EM Jr, Berne RM. Hormonal role of adenosine in maintaining patency of the ductus arteriosus in fetal lambs. Ann Surg 1985;202:223–230.

26 Sawa R, Asakura H, Power GG. Changes in plasma adenosine during simulated birth of fetal sheep. J Appl Physiol 1991;70:1524–1528.

27 Alzamora-Castro V, Battilana G, Abigattas R, Sialer S. Patent ductus arteriosus and high altitude. Am J Cardiol 1960;5:761–763.

28 Penaloza D, Arias-Stella J, Sime F, Recavarren S, Marticorens E. The heart and pulmonary circulation in children at high altitudes. Physiological, anatomical and clinical observations. Pediatrics 1964;34:568–582.

29 Powell ML. Patent ductus arteriosus in premature infants. Med J Aust 1963;2:58–60.

30 Lucas A, Mitchell MD. Plasma-prostaglandins in preterm neonates before and after treatment for patient ductus arteriosus. Lancet 1978;ii:130–132.

31 Clyman RI, Brett C, Mauray F. Circulating prostaglandin E2 concentrations and incidence of patent ductus arteriosus in preterm infants with respiratory distress syndrome. Pediatrics 1980;66:725–729.

32 Seidner SR, Chen YQ, Oprysko PR *et al.* Combined prostaglandin and nitric oxide inhibition produces anatomic remodeling and closure of the ductus arteriosus in the premature newborn baboon. Pediatr Res 2001;50:365–373.

33 Shimada S, Kasai T, Konishi M, Fujiwara T. Effects of patent ductus arteriosus on left ventricular output and organ blood flows in preterm infants with respiratory distress syndrome treated with surfactant. J Pediatr 1994;125:270–277.

34 Clyman RI, Roman C, Heymann MA, Mauray F. How a patent ductus arteriosus effects the premature lamb's ability to handle additional volume loads. Pediatr Res 1987;22:531–535.
35 Evans M. Assessment and support of the preterm circulation. Early Hum Dev 2006;82:803–810.
36 Kluckow M, Evans NJ. Low superior vena cava flow and intraventricular haemorrhage in preterm infants. Arch Dis Child 2000;82:F188–F194.
37 Teitel DF, Sidi D, Chin T, Brett C, Heymann MA, Rudolph AM. Developmental changes in myocardial contractile reserve in the lamb. Pediatr Res 1985;19: 948–955.
38 Newnham JP, Marshall CL, Padbury JF, Lam RW, Hobel CJ, Fisher DA. Fetal catecholamine release with preterm delivery. Amer J Obstet Gynecol 1984;149:888–893.
39 Osborn DA, Kluckow M, Evans N. Randomised trial of dobutamine vs dopamine in preterm infants with low systemic blood flow. J Pediatr 2002;140:183–191.
40 Paradisis M, Evans N, Kluckow M, Osborn D, McLachlan AJ. Pilot study of milrinone for low systemic blood flow in very preterm infants. J Pediatr 2006;148:306–313.
41 Kari MA, Raivio KO, Stenman UH, Voutilainen R. Serum cortisol, dehydroepiandrosterone sulfate, and steroid-binding globulins in preterm neonates: effect of gestational age and dexamethasone therapy. Pediatr Res 1996;40:319–324.
42 Seri I, Tan R, Evans J. Cardiovascular effects of hydrocortisone in preterm infants with pressor resistant hypotension. Pediatrics 2001;107:1070–1074.
43 Rudolph AM, Scarpelli EM, Golinko RJ, Gootman N. Hemodynamic basis for clinical manifestations of patent ductus arteriosus. Am Heart J 1964;68:447–458.
44 Fishman NH, Hof RB, Rudolph AM. Models of congenital heart disease in fetal lambs. Circulation 1978;58: 354–364.
45 Silverman NH, Lewis AB, Heymann MA, Rudolph AM. Echocardiographic assessment of ductus arteriosus shunt in premature infants. Circulation 1974;50:821–825.
46 Evans N, Moorcraft J. Effect of patency of the ductus arteriosus on blood pressure in very preterm infants. Arch Dis Child 1992;67:1169–1173.
47 Clyman RI, Jobe A, Heymann M *et al.* Increased shunt through the patent ductus arteriosus after surfactant replacement therapy. J Pediatr 1982;100:101–107.
48 Clyman RI, Mauray F, Heymann MA, Roman C. Cardiovascular effects of patent ductus arteriosus in preterm lambs with respiratory distress. J Pediatr 1987;111:579–587.
49 Mosalli R, Alfaleh K. Prophylactic surgical ligation of patent ductus arteriosus for prevention of mortality and morbidity in extremely low birth weight infants. Cochrane Database Syst Rev 2008:23, CD006181.
50 Heymann MA, Rudolph AM, Silverman NH. Closure of the ductus arteriosus in premature infants by inhibition of prostaglandin synthesis. N Engl J Med 1976;295: 530–533.
51 Mahony L, Carnero V, Brett C, Heymann MA, Clyman RI. Prophylactic indomethacin therapy for patent ductus arteriosus in very-low-birth-weight infants. N Engl J Med 1982;306:506–510.
52 Van Bel F, Bartelds B, Teitel DF, Rudolph AM. Effect of indomethacin on cerebral blood flow and oxygenation in the normal and ventilated fetal lamb. Pediatr Res 1995;38:243–250.
53 Fowlie PW, Davis PG. Prophylactic indomethacin for preterm infants: a systematic review and meta-analysis. Arch Dis Child 2003;88:F464–F466.
54 Ohlsson A, Walia R, Shah S. Ibuprofen for the treatment of patent ductus arteriosus in preterm and/or low birth weight infants. Cochrane Database Syst Rev 2005;19: CD003481.
55 Herrera C, Holberton J, Davis P. Prolonged versus short course of indomethacin for the treatment of patent ductus arteriosus in preterm infants. Cochrane Database Syst Rev 2007;18:CD003480.
56 Keller RL, Tacy TA, Fields S, Ofenstein JP, Aranda JV, Clyman RI. Combined treatment with a nonselective nitric oxide synthase inhibitor (L-NMMA) and indomethacin increases ductus constriction in extremely premature newborns. Pediatr Res 2005;58:1216–1221.
57 Villa E, Vanden Eynden F, Le Bret E, Folliguet T, La Borde F. Paediatric video-assisted thoracoscopic clipping of patent ductus arteriosus: experience in more than 700 cases, Eur J Cardiothorac Surg 2004;25:387–393.
58 Patterson DF, Detweiler DK. Hereditary transmission of patent ductus arteriosus in the dog. Am Heart J 1967;74:289–290.
59 Campbell M. The natural history of patent ductus arteriosus. Heart 1968;30:4–13.
60 Kleinman CS, Tabibian M, Starc TJ, Hsu DT, Gersony WM. Spontaneous regression of left ventricular dilation in children with restrictive ventricular septal defects. J Pediatr 2007;150:583–586.
61 Dajani AS, Taubert KA, Wilson W *et al.* Prevention of bacterial endocarditis. Recommendations by the American Heart Association. Circulation 1997;96:358–366.
62 Awadallah SM, Kavey RE, Byrum CJ, Smith FC, Kveselis DA, Blackman MS. The changing pattern of infective endocarditis in childhood. Am J Cardiol 1991;68:90–94.
63 Balzer DT, Spray TL, McMullin D, Cottingham W, Canter CE. Endarteritis associated with a clinically silent patent ductus arteriosus. Am Heart J 1993;125: 1192–1193.
64 Schrader R, Kadel C. Persistierender Ductus arteriosus: istauch bei asymptomatischen Erwachsenen mit kleinem

Ductus und genngen Shunt ein Verschluss indiziert? Z Kardiol 1993;82:563–567.

65 Thilen U, Astrom-Olsson K. Does the risk of infective endarteritis justify routine patent ductus arteriosus closure? Eur Heart J 1997;18:503–506.

66 Wilson W, Taubert KA, Gewitz M *et al.* Prevention of infective endocarditis: guidelines from the American Heart Association: a guideline from the American Heart Association Rheumatic Fever, Endocarditis and Kawasaki Disease Committee, Council on Cardiovascular Disease in the Young, and the Council on Clinical Cardiology, Council on Cardiovascular Surgery and Anesthesia, and the Quality of Care and Outcomes Research Interdisciplinary Working Group. Circulation 2007;116:1736–1754.

67 Sullivan ID. Patent arterial duct: when should it be closed. Arch Dis Child 1998;78:285–287.

68 Portsmann W, Wierny L, Warneke H *et al.* Closure of the persistent ductus arteriosus: 62 cases treated without thoracotomy. Radiol Clin North Am 1971;9:203–218.

69 Rashkind WJ, Mullins CE, Hellenbrand WE, Tait MA. Non-surgical closure of patent ductus arteriosus: clinical application of the Rashkind PDA occluder system. Circulation 1987;75:583–592.

CHAPTER 7

Ventricular septal defect

The incidence of all congenital cardiovascular malformations is generally reported to be about 8 per 1000 births. Isolated ventricular septal defect is by far the most common lesion, comprising 20–30% of all patients in numerous publications. In most of these reports, the diagnoses were based on clinical assessment. With the advent of echocardiography and particularly of the use of color flow Doppler examination, it is now appreciated that many individuals have congenital cardiovascular malformations that are not readily recognized, or completely unrecognized, by clinical evaluation. The real incidence of ventricular septal defect is now known to be considerably higher than thought previously. Based on careful routine echocardiographic observations within 1 week of birth of over 1000 consecutively born neonates, more than 5% had defects in the muscular portion of the ventricular septum [1]. Furthermore, the actual incidence of ventricular septal defect is even higher, because many close spontaneously prior to birth. This was observed in nearly half of isolated ventricular septal defects in 26 fetuses [2]. Based on these reports, the incidence of ventricular septal defects, including fetuses, is about 10% of all pregnancies. In addition, the concepts regarding the incidence of congenital cardiovascular malformations require reconsideration.

As discussed below, many ventricular septal defects close spontaneously within the first few years after birth, so that the incidence reported in many series is underestimated. It also is of interest that ventricular septal defects are quite unusual in adults. Although this is partly related to the fact that some patients die in infancy, it is not the whole explanation and is probably accounted for by the spontaneous closure of the defects even some considerable time after infancy.

Ventricular septal defects also frequently occur as an integral part of other anomalies, among which are truncus arteriosus communis, tetralogy of Fallot, atrioventricular septal defects, double-outlet right ventricle, and aortopulmonary transposition. This chapter discusses only isolated ventricular septal defects; the importance of the defect in other complexes is discussed in the chapters relating to the specific lesions.

Morphological considerations

Ventricular septal defects vary greatly in location and in size. Although the more frequent types of anatomical defect are described, I would like to stress that the location of the defect does not appear to have any major influence on the physiological abnormalities, except insofar as adjacent structures may also be involved. However, the location of the defect may determine some of the clinical features and the likelihood of spontaneous closure and is of some importance surgically.

Numerous classifications of ventricular septal defect have been proposed. In my view, it is convenient to consider the defects in relation to the position in the ventricular septum when viewed from the right ventricle (Figure 7.1). The most common, comprising about 75% of all ventricular septal defects, is located in the mid-portion of the upper region of the septum and is related to the aortic valve. It has been called an infracristal or subaortic defect, or type II defect in Kirklin's classification. Recently, because it involves the trabecular portion of the septum, it has become common practice to use the term *perimembranous trabecular defect.* Spontaneous closure is likely in a relatively high

Congenital Diseases of the Heart, 3rd edition. By A. Rudolph
© 2009 Blackwell Publishing, ISBN: 9781405162456

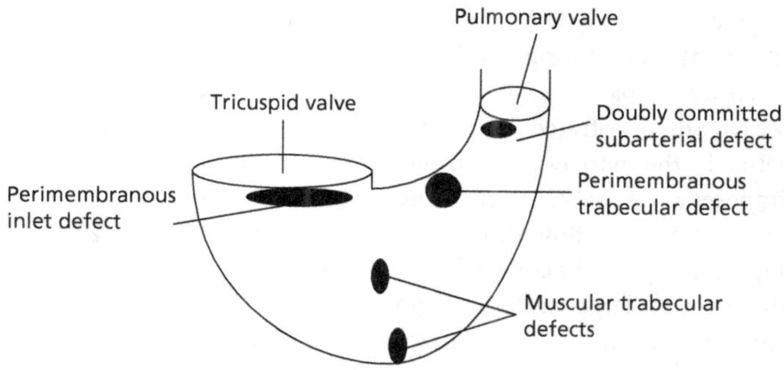

Figure 7.1 Location of various types of ventricular septal defect as viewed from the right ventricular aspect of the septum.

proportion of these defects. Spontaneous closure of defects is discussed below.

A defect in the anterior and superior portion of the septum is closely related to both the pulmonary and aortic valves. It has been called a supracristal or subpulmonary defect, or type I defect in Kirklin's classification. It is now usually referred to as a *perimembranous outlet defect* or, because it is adjacent to both the aortic and pulmonary valves, as a *doubly committed subarterial defect*. In this defect the support structure for the right coronary cusp may be disturbed, resulting in prolapse and sometimes aortic insufficiency. There is not always a correlation between the size of the defect and the severity of the insufficiency but, generally, small defects (< 4 mm diameter) are not usually associated with aortic insufficiency. These defects comprise about 5% of ventricular defects in the USA, but in Asian populations they are more common, accounting for about 25% of defects.

A defect in the posterior superior portion of the septum is adjacent to and beneath the septal leaflet of the tricuspid valve and has been called an atrioventricular canal defect or type III defect of Kirklin, but the more recent nomenclature is *perimembranous inlet defect*. These comprise about 5% of ventricular septal defects.

The fourth group, comprising about 10% of ventricular septal defects, includes those that are entirely within the muscular portion of the septum. They may be located anywhere in the muscular septum, as far down as the apex. They are often slit-like, especially when small, and may be difficult to identify at surgery or at autopsy, especially from the right side, because the opening may be hidden in the trabecular portion of the septum. These defects, which were termed muscular or type IV defects of Kirklin, are now referred to as *muscular trabecular defects*. They are the defects most likely to undergo spontaneous closure. These defects may be multiple, and when numerous fenestrations are present the term "Swiss cheese septum" has been applied; this type of defect is not as prone to close spontaneously as single defects. Multiple small ventricular septal defects may allow a large left-to-right shunt, because the total cross-sectional area of the defect is quite large.

Hemodynamic considerations

Fetal circulation with ventricular septal defect

The majority of infants born with ventricular septal defect, apart from those who have other genetic anomalies, are quite normally developed, so it appears that the defect does not have any significant effect on blood flow to the fetal organs or to the placenta. It is not known whether ventricular septal defects produce any significant alterations in the course of the fetal circulation. Right and left ventricular pressures, as well as aortic and pulmonary trunk pressures, are almost equal in the fetus. Also the atrial pressures and end-diastolic pressures in the ventricles are similar on the two sides of the heart. Therefore shunting patterns will be determined largely by the impedances of the aorta and pulmonary trunk. Most of the blood from the pulmonary trunk normally flows through the ductus arteriosus to the descending aorta, because pulmonary vascular resistance is high and placental vascular resistance relatively low. It might be expected that, in a fetus with a ventricular septal defect, some degree of shunting from the right to the left ventricle might occur during systole through the defect.

However, based on observations in fetal lambs, we have demonstrated that the aortic isthmus in the fetus is the narrowest portion of the aorta. It imposes a relatively high resistance to left ventricular ejection, and flow through it is quite low (see Figure 1.7, p. 7). In contrast, the ductus arteriosus diameter is large and the right ventricle ejects through it into the relatively low-resistance placental circulation. If a communication is created between the two circulations, blood is likely to flow from the circulation with high impedance to that of lower impedance. Based on these considerations, one would predict that, in the fetus with a ventricular septal defect, left-to-right ventricular shunting would be likely to occur during systole.

This concept is supported by echocardiographic and Doppler flow studies in a few human fetuses. Either no flow was observed in either direction through a ventricular septal defect, or left-to-right shunting was noted during systole in an occasional fetus. In some instances, a right-to-left shunt through the defect was observed during diastole. This latter observation is difficult to understand, but the most plausible explanation is that left-to-right shunting during systole results in more effective emptying so that during ventricular filling, a small amount of flow occurs from the right to the left ventricle.

Whatever flow pattern does occur, the magnitude of the shunt is not likely to be great. Because relatively small amounts of blood would be shunted to the ascending or descending aorta respectively, it would not be likely to alter the normal difference between the Po_2 of the upper and lower body greatly. A small decrease in the normal oxygen saturation difference between the ascending and descending aorta could occur. A small increase in oxygen saturation in pulmonary trunk blood may be present because the Po_2 of left ventricular blood is higher than that of right ventricular blood in the fetus (see Figure 1.5, p. 5). This would result in a slight increase in oxygen saturation of blood perfusing the lungs and in blood in the descending aorta (Figure 7.2).

The position of the defect possibly could influence the shunt depending on kinetics of blood flow. A large doubly committed subarterial or sub-

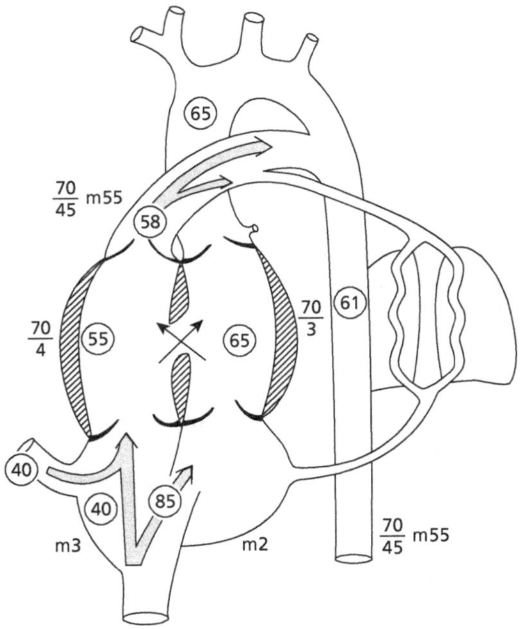

Figure 7.2 Large ventricular septal defect in the fetus: course of the circulation, oxygen saturations (circled), and pressures in the heart and great vessels during fetal life. m, mean pressure.

pulmonary ventricular septal defect could possibly be associated with a larger left-to-right shunt. During systole, blood ejected by the left ventricle could be directed preferentially through the defect into the pulmonary artery. An additional factor that may contribute to the shunting of blood away from the left ventricle through the subpulmonary defect is the presence of some degree of stenosis of the outflow tract of the left ventricle. Perimembranous defects are also occasionally associated with a shelf or ridge in the left ventricular outflow tract. Although this may not cause a significant gradient between the left ventricle and the aorta, it may further enhance the outflow resistance of the ventricle and increase the size of the left-to-right shunt.

If a larger left-to-right shunt did occur, the proportion of left ventricular output ejected into the ascending aorta would be reduced. This would have a significant effect on the volume of flow across the aortic isthmus to the descending aorta, and could result in narrowing of the isthmus in the fetus (Figure 7.3). This concept is discussed in detail in Chapter 12.

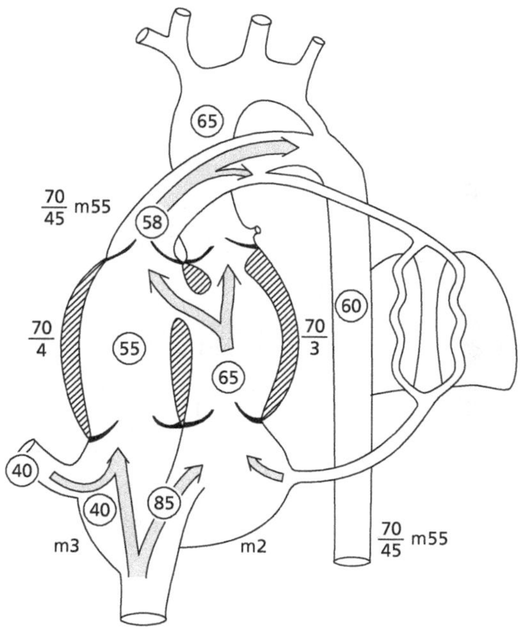

Figure 7.3 Large doubly committed subarterial ventricular septal defect with narrowing of subaortic region: course of the circulation, oxygen saturations (circled), and pressures in the heart and great vessels during fetal life. Note narrowing of the aortic isthmus. m, mean pressure.

The pattern of blood flow in the fetus with a left-to-right shunt will differ from that postnatally. After birth, blood shunted through a ventricular septal defect passes through the pulmonary circulation and returns to the left atrium and ventricle (see below). This enhances filling of the left ventricle and its output is increased as a result of increased pulmonary venous return. In the fetus, shunted blood ejected by the left ventricle enters the pulmonary artery and is then likely to flow through the ductus arteriosus, rather than through the pulmonary circulation, because fetal pulmonary vascular resistance is high. Pulmonary resistance could possibly be lowered slightly by the small increase in pulmonary arterial oxygen content resulting from the shunt (see Figure 7.3), but this effect is probably not significant. Thus, if left ventricular filling is not increased, the reduction of flow into the ascending aorta may further contribute to poor development of the aortic isthmus. If, associated with the left-to-right shunt, the left ventricle ejects a larger volume, end-systolic volume will be reduced and filling may be maintained to some extent by increased flow through the foramen ovale.

Postnatal circulatory adaptation

The hemodynamic effects of ventricular septal defects after birth are related largely to two factors: (i) the size of the defect and (ii) the relative outflow resistances of the right and left ventricles. The location of the defect is not of particular importance in determining the magnitude of the shunt or the clinical consequences. The postnatal changes in the relationship between pulmonary and systemic vascular resistances determine the direction and magnitude of shunting and the pressure and volume loads placed on the right and left ventricle, respectively.

Systemic vascular resistance is increased suddenly when clamping or constriction of the umbilical arteries eliminates the low-resistance umbilical–placental circulation. Pulmonary vascular resistance is decreased when the lungs are expanded by ventilation with air (see Chapter 5). In the hours immediately after birth, only a small left-to-right shunt occurs because pulmonary vascular resistance is still moderately elevated (Figure 7.4).

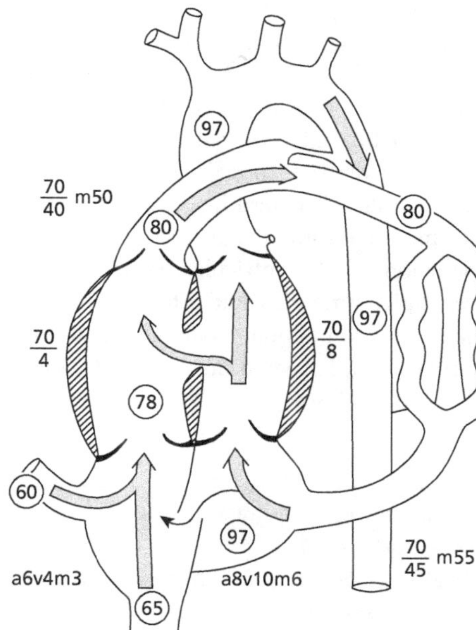

Figure 7.4 Large perimembranous ventricular septal defect in the immediate newborn period: course of the circulation, oxygen saturations (circled), and pressures in the heart and great vessels. m, mean pressure.

Large ventricular septal defect

With a large communication between two fluid-filled chambers, the pressures in the chambers are equal. Equalization of pressures is attained between the right and left ventricles with septal defects about the same diameter as the aortic orifice. In subsequent discussion ventricular septal defects of this size or larger are termed "large" or "nonrestrictive" defects. Under these circumstances of equal ejection pressure, the outflow resistance determines the volume ejected by each ventricle. This could be increased by associated obstructive lesions such as pulmonary stenosis on the right side, or aortic stenosis or coarctation of the aorta on the left side. In the absence of these associated anomalies, ejection into the systemic and pulmonary circulations is determined by their relative vascular resistances.

As pulmonary vascular resistance falls after birth, there is preferential flow to the lungs and, in addition to systemic venous return, the right ventricle and pulmonary artery receive blood that flows across the ventricular septal defect. The total pulmonary blood flow returns to the left atrium and the left ventricle (Figure 7.5). The left ventricle thus receives a larger volume during diastole, resulting in increased end-diastolic volume. The muscle fiber length is increased and based on the Frank–Starling mechanism, the left ventricle contracts more forcibly and its output is increased. The ability of the left ventricle to maintain an adequate systemic blood flow is determined by its myocardial performance and the magnitude of shunting. The proportion of left ventricular blood shunted influences the volume distributed to the systemic circulation. Thus to maintain systemic blood flow at its normal level, left ventricular output would have to change as follows.

- A 25% shunt would require a 1.33-fold increase in left ventricular output
- A 50% shunt would require a twofold increase in left ventricular output
- A 75% shunt would require a fourfold increase in left ventricular output
- An 80% shunt would require a fivefold increase in left ventricular output

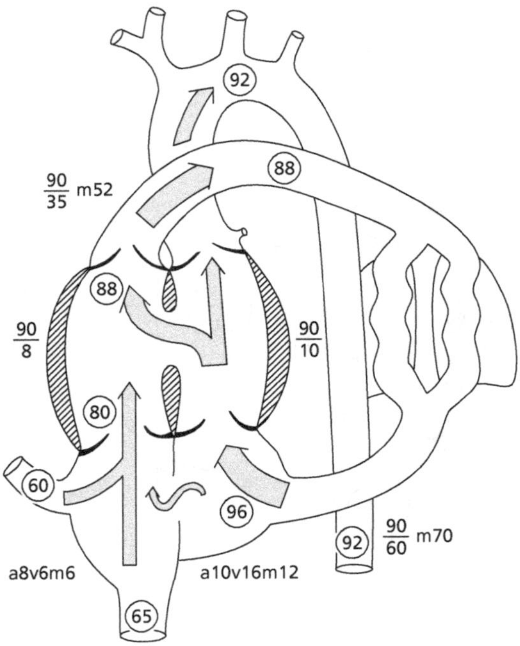

Figure 7.5 Large ventricular septal defect in an infant: course of the circulation, oxygen saturations (circled), and pressures in the heart and great vessels. Compared with Figure 7.4, there has been a decrease in pulmonary vascular resistance; left-to-right shunt and pulmonary blood flow have increased and left atrial pressure is raised. Left-to-right shunt also occurs across the stretched foramen ovale. m, mean pressure.

It has become common practice to indicate the magnitude of left-to-right shunting by using the ratio of pulmonary to systemic blood flow ($\dot{Q}p/\dot{Q}s$). Because pulmonary venous blood all returns to the left ventricle, pulmonary blood flow is represented by left ventricular output. Thus $\dot{Q}p/\dot{Q}s$ is 1.33:1 for a 25% shunt, 2:1 for a 50% shunt, and 4:1 for a 75% shunt. At $\dot{Q}p/\dot{Q}s$ ratios above about 4:1, left ventricular output has to increase enormously to maintain an adequate systemic blood flow. Small increases in the percentage shunt are associated with huge increases in $\dot{Q}p/\dot{Q}s$. Ratios above 4:1 are unusual, because the left ventricle is usually incapable of sustaining such large ejection volumes without developing failure.

The increased left atrial pressure and resultant enlargement may cause stretching of the atrial septum, with incompetence of the foramen ovale, and possible herniation of the lower margin of the fossa ovalis into the right atrium, resulting in secondary atrial left-to-right shunting (see Figure 7.5). The left-to-right shunt through the foramen ovale is usually small but sometimes is of considerable magnitude and may be important in modifying the clinical features. Unless there is a true atrial septal defect, the mean pressure in the left atrium exceeds that in the right atrium by several mmHg, indicating that the foramen ovale opening is still of limiting size.

It has been proposed that shunting of blood away from the left atrium may be of benefit in diverting blood from a failing left ventricle that is on the descending limb of its ventricular function curve. By reducing left ventricular volume loading and left ventricular end-diastolic pressure, a fall in left atrial and pulmonary venous pressures would ensue and lead to an improvement in pulmonary edema. However, infants with a large ventricular septal defect and a large atrial left-to-right shunt are usually symptomatic very early, and tend to have severe symptoms. This is related to the fact that the shunt at the atrial level does not permit left ventricular end-diastolic pressure to rise. Therefore, left ventricular output cannot be increased greatly, with the result that systemic blood flow cannot be maintained. The increased flow of blood into the right atrium would enter the right ventricle, placing an increased diastolic volume load on the right side. Because, with a large defect, pressure in the right ventricle is equal to that in the left ventricle, the right ventricle is confronted with a large increase in pressure and volume loading, and failure of this ventricle may dominate the clinical picture.

Effect of afterload on the left ventricle

An increase in afterload on the left ventricle may result from associated valvar or subvalvar aortic stenosis or from interruption or coarctation of the aorta. It may also occur if systemic vascular resistance is increased. The adverse effects of high systemic vascular resistance in these patients forms the basis for the use of afterload-reducing agents in their treatment (see Chapter 7).

An elevation in outflow resistance of the left ventricle will increase the magnitude of the left-to-right shunt, thereby aggravating the volume load on the ventricle; it will also tend to reduce systemic blood flow and increase the manifestations of cardiac failure. Systemic vascular resistance is increased as a result of α-adrenoceptor stimulation via the direct action of sympathetic nerves and by increased circulating catecholamine concentrations. Other mechanisms that tend to raise systemic vascular resistance in patients with large defects are increased angiotensin II and vasopressin concentrations (see Chapter 7).

The continued reduction in pulmonary vascular resistance over the first few weeks results in an increasing left-to-right shunt; this is accentuated to some extent by a modest increase in systemic vascular resistance. There is thus a progressive augmentation of pulmonary blood flow, pulmonary venous return, and left atrial and ventricular filling (see Figure 7.5). The high volume load on the left ventricle is associated with elevation of left ventricular end-diastolic, left atrial and pulmonary venous pressures, and pulmonary edema results from increased hydrostatic pressure. Ultimately, with the inability of the left ventricle to maintain the high stroke volume, systemic blood flow falls and circulatory shock develops.

Factors influencing the onset of cardiac failure

Pulmonary circulatory changes

The evolution of cardiac failure is very much dependent on the postnatal changes in the pulmonary circulation. On the basis of the maturational pattern observed in normal animals and infants, it would be expected that the volume overload on the left ventricle, with onset of failure, would occur within 1–2 weeks after birth. Because the pulmonary vascular changes and reduction in vascular resistance are delayed when pulmonary arterial hypertension persists (see Chapter 5), the onset of failure in mature infants born and living near sea level may be delayed until about 8–10 weeks after birth.

Effect of altitude

The rate of decline in pulmonary vascular resistance may be influenced by other factors, which may have a bearing on the patient with ventricular septal defect. These are discussed in detail in Chapter 5, but are mentioned briefly here in regard to their special role in this lesion. In babies born at high altitude, the lower inspired Po_2 results in hypoxia of variable degree, with consequent delay in the fall in pulmonary vascular resistance. At high altitudes of 4000 m, as in the Peruvian Andes, this effect is striking, and severe cardiac failure is unusual in infants with ventricular septal defect born into this environment. However, even at lower altitudes, such as at 1800 m in Denver, Colorado, there appears to be a lesser incidence, lesser severity, and later onset of heart failure in infants with ventricular septal defects. Similar effects may occur in infants with ventricular septal defect who have persistent chronic pulmonary disease after birth. It is also of interest that infants with Down syndrome and a large ventricular septal defect often have high pulmonary vascular resistance and do not present with cardiac failure. Whether this is due to their tendency to suffer frequent respiratory infections, which may cause variable degrees of hypoxia, or whether the pulmonary vasculature is abnormal in these infants has not been resolved.

Decreased alveolar ventilation

The advent of pulmonary edema may itself delay the fall in pulmonary vascular resistance. Accumulation of edematous fluid in the peribronchial tissues may cause compression of small bronchioles, with resulting hypoventilation and hypoxia in the lung segment involved. This could result in an interesting development, because the increased pulmonary vascular resistance related to the hypoxia could decrease the left-to-right shunt; venous return to the left atrium would be reduced and left atrial and pulmonary venous pressures would fall. An interesting balance may therefore develop between the magnitude of the shunt and the effects of pulmonary edema that may maintain the infant in a relatively stable state of chronic pulmonary edema and respiratory distress.

Infants with Down syndrome are prone to respiratory difficulty, which may interfere with adequate ventilation and delay the fall in pulmonary vascular resistance after birth. Furthermore, there is some evidence suggesting that the pulmonary vasculature may be abnormal in infants with Down syndrome, perhaps genetically related, and this would also tend to preserve a high pulmonary vascular resitance.

Prematurity

In premature infants with ventricular septal defects, the onset of cardiac failure is frequently noted within 1–2 weeks after birth. This is probably, at least in part, related to the fact that pulmonary vascular reactivity is not as well developed in the preterm infant (see Chapter 5) and thus pulmonary vascular resistance may not be sustained as in the mature infant. Furthermore, the likelihood of increased transudation of fluid from the capillaries into the alveoli is greater. Another important consideration in the preterm infant is the high level of oxygen consumption in relation to body weight, because the preterm infant has a high surface area relative to body weight. Therefore, the requirement for cardiac output to provide oxygen to the tissues is greater and a larger load would be placed on the left ventricle.

Metabolism and oxygen requirements

In serial studies in newborn lambs, Lister showed that cardiac output related to body weight fairly closely parallels changes in oxygen consumption [3]. Factors that increase oxygen consumption will therefore place a greater demand on the heart to provide a larger systemic blood flow to the tissues. Oxygen requirements may be increased by several mechanisms in the infant with a ventricular septal defect.

Body and environmental temperature

The optimal ambient temperature at which oxygen consumption is lowest is 32–33°C. Surface cooling results in increased metabolism to maintain body temperature; this increases oxygen consumption. Environmental temperatures above the optimal, as well as fevers resulting from infection, also raise oxygen consumption. Infants who have a defect with no manifest failure, or who have had cardiac failure well controlled by therapy, frequently develop failure when an infection is superimposed.

Sympathoadrenal stimulation

Stimulation of the sympathetic nervous system results from distension of the cardiac chambers and from baroreflex stimulation if cardiac output is reduced and arterial pressure falls; plasma catecholamine concentrations also increase. Enhanced catecholamine activity has been demonstrated in infants with cardiac failure by observation of high excretion rates of vanillylmandelic acid in the urine [4]. Sympathoadrenal stimulation increases metabolic activity, largely through β-adrenoceptors, and thus increases oxygen consumption and cardiac output requirements.

Increased respiratory effort

In the normal infant breathing quietly, the oxygen consumption attributable to respiratory activity is quite low. However, the infant with a large left-to-right shunt has both tachypnea and dyspnea, and this considerably increases oxygen consumption requirements for the increased work of breathing. Increased left atrial and pulmonary venous pressures may increase pulmonary interstitial fluid and greatly increase the work of breathing, so that oxygen consumption may increase several fold as a result.

Anxiety

Oxygen consumption may be increased considerably in the anxious child. Not only is there increased sympathetic nervous and catecholamine activity, but restlessness creates increased physical activity and this, as well as the effort of crying, may increase oxygen consumption markedly.

Hemoglobin concentration

The amount of hemoglobin determines the oxygen content of blood. Therefore, to provide the same amount of oxygen to the tissues, a higher cardiac output would be required with a lower hemoglobin concentration (see Chapter 3). Normally, newborn infants have an average hemoglobin concentration of 15–17 g/dL. Red cell production is depressed for 6–8 weeks after birth, and hemoglobin concentration falls to about 11 g/dL by 8 weeks. This fall in hemoglobin concentration does not affect oxygen supply in the normal infant, but it may be an important contributing factor to the development of cardiac failure in an infant who has increased metabolic activity and a left ventricle already overburdened with the increased output due to left-to-right shunting. This may also explain the manifestation of cardiac failure at 6–8 weeks after birth.

The importance of the decreased hemoglobin concentration in influencing the onset of cardiac failure has been well demonstrated by Lister *et al.* [5] in infants with ventricular septal defect with large left-to-right shunts. Hemoglobin concentration was increased by an isovolumic exchange transfusion to avoid changes in blood volume. This resulted in a fall in systemic and pulmonary blood flow and a marked decrease in the left-to-right shunt. Systemic oxygen transport did not change, despite the fall in systemic flow.

In the preterm infant, hemoglobin concentration falls to even lower values. By about 8 weeks it drops to about 9.5 g/dL in infants with birth weights of 1500–2000 g, to 9.0 g/dL in those with birth weights of 1000–1500 g, and even lower in smaller infants. Thus the preterm infant with a ventricular septal defect would be even more susceptible to cardiac failure as a result of the fall in hemoglobin concentration.

Type of hemoglobin

At birth, about 75% of hemoglobin is of the fetal type in the mature infant. This is gradually replaced by adult hemoglobin with postnatal hematopoiesis, and by 4 months only about 20% of hemoglobin is of fetal type. The high concentration of fetal hemoglobin reduces the P_{50} of blood and this limits the amount of oxygen extracted at the tissue site (see Chapter 3). Therefore, for the same oxygen consumption by the tissues, a higher cardiac output is required. It is fortunate for the infant that the amount of fetal hemoglobin falls as total hemoglobin concentration falls, because this compensates to some extent. However, because the fall in fetal hemoglobin concentration is the result of production of new red cells with adult hemoglobin, at 6–8 weeks after birth when hemoglobin concentration reaches its lowest postnatal level, about 40–60% of hemoglobin is still of the fetal type.

The preterm infant is born with higher concentrations of fetal hemoglobin, and this may be a more important consideration in the onset of failure in the presence of a ventricular septal defect than in the mature infant.

It has been shown in piglets that replacement of hemoglobin with a low P_{50} by hemoglobin with a high P_{50} reduces cardiac output: cardiac output was inversely related to hemoglobin P_{50} [6]. Furthermore, reducing the proportion of fetal hemoglobin in infants with cardiac failure by exchange transfusion with adult blood results in considerable clinical improvement [5].

Factors involved in manifestations of failure

In adults, cardiac failure is most commonly associated with disturbances in heart muscle function, so that a decrease in ventricular output is an early manifestation. In infants and children with congenital heart lesions, the myocardium is usually normal until late in the course of the syndrome of failure. Ventricular output is initially normal and may, with shunt lesions, be markedly increased. The term "cardiac failure" is not really appropriate, because the heart is maintaining not only a normal but often an increased output. In left-to-right shunt lesions such as ventricular septal defect and patent ductus arteriosus, the demands on the left ventricle to maintain normal systemic blood flow are not remarkable with shunt proportions of up to about 60% (see Chapter 7). With shunt percentages larger than this, the $\dot{Q}p/\dot{Q}s$ ratio or left ventricular output has to increase dramatically for small increases in the proportion of output shunted. It is usually at these levels of shunt that the heart is unable to maintain an output adequate to provide normal systemic blood flow. The clinical manifestations of what we now designate cardiac failure may appear well before this occurs, and are due to a combination of neurohormonal events and pulmonary circulatory changes.

Neurohormonal changes

Increase in volume of the heart and great vessels stimulates stretch receptors in the walls of the atria and veins. This results in sympathetic stimulation that exerts its effects directly through the nervous system and also by influencing several hormonal functions. Plasma catecholamine concentrations are increased in infants with large shunts [6]. The direct effects of sympathetic nerve stimulation are not separable from those of circulating catecholamines.

Increased activity of sympathetic cholinergic fibers accounts for the sweating that is a common manifestation in infants with cardiac failure. Stimulation of α-adrenoceptors in the splanchnic, renal, and peripheral circulations causes vasoconstriction and increases systemic vascular resistance. Constriction of skin vessels causes pallor. Renal vasoconstriction results in a fall in renal blood flow and this may contribute to sodium retention because a reduced glomerular filtration rate interferes with sodium excretion.

The increased catecholamine secretion may also be a factor in the increased metabolism and oxygen consumption (see Chapter 7). Glucose metabolism may also be altered in these infants. Hait has described suppression of insulin response to an oral glucose load in infants in cardiac failure associated with large left-to-right shunts [7]. Often there is also resting hyperglycemia and an abnormally high response, similar to a diabetic curve, after an oral glucose load. This could interfere with tissue deposition of carbohydrates. The high catecholamine secretion could induce the altered handling of glucose; this could also explain the low insulin levels, because α-adrenergic stimulation depresses insulin secretion by the pancreatic islets.

Stimulation of β-adrenoceptors in the myocardium causes tachycardia and enhances myocardial contractility. However, β-adrenoceptors become downgraded over time, so that myocardial responses to catecholamine or sympathetic stimulation are somewhat blunted.

Sympathetic and catecholamine activity stimulates renin secretion from the juxtaglomerular cells in the kidney. Renin acts on angiotensinogen, an α_2-globulin synthesized by the liver, to produce angiotensin I. This decapeptide is acted on by angiotensin-converting enzyme (ACE) synthesized by pulmonary vascular endothelium to produce angiotensin II, the active octapeptide, which is a potent vasoconstrictor.

Plasma aldosterone concentrations are increased in infants with cardiac failure. This is probably largely due to stimulation of the adrenal glands by angiotensin II, but if hepatic blood flow is reduced as a result of failure, disturbed aldosterone clearance may also contribute to the high levels. Aldosterone is an important contributor to the sodium retention that is a prominent feature of cardiac failure.

Arginine vasopressin (AVP) concentration in plasma may also be raised in infants in cardiac failure. The most likely mechanism for increased AVP concentrations is baroreceptor stimulation resulting from a decrease in cardiac output. AVP enhances water retention by the kidney and this, together with the sodium retention, further contributes to increased plasma and tissue fluid volumes.

It is apparent that these neurohormonal mechanisms may result in many of the manifestations of cardiac failure in patients with left-to-right shunts, before there is any reduction in cardiac output.

Pulmonary edema

Pulmonary blood volume is increased in the presence of a left-to-right shunt because pulmonary arterial and venous diameters are larger than normal. Pulmonary arterial diameter will be increased markedly if pulmonary arterial pressure is raised, as with a large ventricular septal defect. If left atrial and pulmonary venous pressures are elevated, pulmonary venous distension occurs. This increase in vascular volume in the thorax, in association with an increase in heart size associated with the large volume load, may result in increased ventilatory effort, mainly tachypnea but also some dyspnea.

If left ventricular end-diastolic pressure is considerably increased as the result of a large left-to-right shunt, left atrial and pulmonary venous pressures are elevated and this may cause increased fluid transudation with interstitial accumulation of fluid in the lungs, resulting in dyspnea. The level of left atrial pressure at which significant fluid accumulation occurs in the lung is probably lower in preterm than in mature infants. This is related to the fact that plasma oncotic pressure is low because albumin concentrations are low in preterm infants. As a result, at similar hydrostatic pressure, the pulmonary capillaries allow greater diffusion in the preterm compared with the mature lamb [8].

Pulmonary vessel morphology

The postnatal development of the pulmonary circulation and the effects of congenital heart lesions on the pulmonary vessels postnatally are discussed in Chapter 5. Pulmonary vascular resistance does not fall to normal levels after birth in infants with large ventricular septal defects. It drops to levels of 3–4 units/m^2 over the first 3–6 months compared with the normal decrease to 1–2 units/m^2. There may then be a fairly stable period for a varying length of time. The elevated pulmonary vascular resistance is largely due to retention of the thick smooth muscle medial layer during the first 6–12 months after birth. There is then progressive replacement of the muscle with collagen, and fibrosis of the media becomes increasingly evident. The time course of these changes in the medial layer is quite variable: smooth muscle may be dominant for many years; the fibrotic changes gradually increase and later predominate.

In addition to the medial changes there is gradual proliferation of the intimal layer. Often the changes affect only a portion of the lumen and are eccentric, but eventually become severe enough to markedly decrease lumen size. The intimal changes also vary in the rate they develop, both in regard to time and to the vessels involved. They may be present in only relatively few vessels in the first year or two, but changes gradually progress with regard to the severity and number of vessels involved. Sometimes extensive changes are seen by 3–4 years, but may be delayed for 10–15 years. The cause of this marked variation in progression of pulmonary vascular changes is not known. However, if the pulmonary vessels are exposed to very high pressures, such as in infants with large ventricular septal defects associated with coarctation of the aorta, left and right ventricular sysyolic pressure may be 120–160 mmHg. Pulmonary vessel changes are observed very early and progress rapidly. The mechanisms that may be involved in causing the pulmonary vascular abnormalities in congenital heart disease are discussed in Chapter 5.

As pulmonary vascular resistance increases, the left-to-right shunt, pulmonary blood flow, and venous return to the left atrium diminish. Left atrial and left ventricular end-diastolic pressures fall and left-sided failure improves (Figure 7.6). This usually starts to occur in the latter half of the first year, and during the second year manifestations of cardiac failure have typically improved. As pulmonary vascular resistance progresses to the point at which it exceeds systemic vascular resistance, right-to-left shunting of blood across the defect occurs, first mainly during exercise, because of the associated fall in systemic vascular resistance. Later, right-to-left shunt occurs at rest, with persistent cyanosis. Ultimately, there is a marked fall in pulmonary blood flow, with persistent hypoxemia. Right ventricular failure finally supervenes. The development of pulmonary vascular obstructive disease is discussed in Chapter 5.

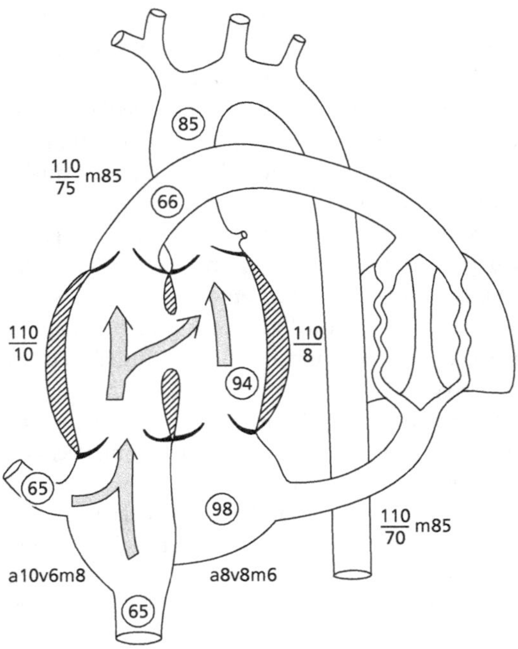

Figure 7.6 Large ventricular septal defect with markedly increased pulmonary vascular resistance: course of the circulation, oxygen saturations (circled), and pressures in the heart and great vessels. Note that right-to-left shunt has developed across the ventricular septal defect. m, mean pressure.

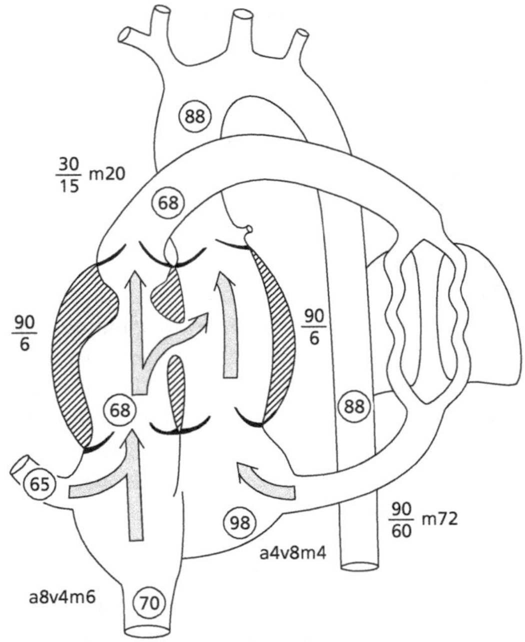

Figure 7.7 Large ventricular septal defect with development of right ventricular infundibular stenosis: course of the circulation, oxygen saturations (circled), and pressures in the heart and great vessels. Muscular hypertrophy of the infundibulum has increased right ventricular outflow resistance, resulting in a right-to-left shunt through the defect. m, mean pressure.

Effect of associated lesions

Left ventricular outflow obstruction

As mentioned above, outflow obstruction of the left ventricle will exaggerate the size of the left-to-right shunt and thus contribute to the early onset of cardiac failure. This occurs with lesions such as aortic stenosis (Chapter 10), aortic arch interruption, and aortic coarctation (Chapter 12).

Right ventricular outflow obstruction

Hypertrophy of muscle in the right ventricular infundibulum develops in some patients with ventricular septal defect, particularly those with perimembranous trabecular defects. There may be no clinical evidence of obstruction to right ventricular outflow at birth, but over a variable period, with a variable time of onset, muscular hypertrophy results in narrowing of the outflow tract (Figure 7.7). With the increasing resistance to right ventricular ejection, the left-to-right shunt decreases. With severe muscle hypertrophy, shunt may occur from the right to the left ventricle and aorta, usually first during exercise. Cyanosis occurs, first intermittent and later persistent. Clinical manifestations similar to those of tetralogy of Fallot result (see Chapter 14). The development of infundibular hypertrophy is one of the factors that may account for improvement of cardiac failure in an infant with a large ventricular septal defect.

Although the clinical manifestations of infundibular stenosis are not evident in many infants with ventricular septal defect who develop outflow obstruction, it is not unusual to find that cardiac catheterization records a small systolic pressure gradient of 10–25 mmHg across the outflow tract. More recently, narrowing of the outflow tract with only a small pressure gradient has been observed by ultrasound. Progression to severe stenosis has been documented by both ultrasound and catheterization.

Aortic insufficiency

Aortic insufficiency is most likely to develop in patients with doubly committed subarterial defects, but has been noted with other defects. The support structure for the right coronary cusp is deficient. Initially, during infancy and early childhood, no functional insufficiency may be present, although the cusp may be prolapsed; progressive regurgitation may develop. This is potentially a serious complication because if there is already a large left-to-right shunt through the defect, the regurgitation places an additional volume load on the left ventricle and progressive failure may occur (Figure 7.8).

It has been suggested that there may be kinetic factors involved in the production of aortic valve prolapse, based on the high velocity of flow through the ventricular septal defect. This hypothesis proposes that the flow of blood across the ventricular septal defect results in a Bernoulli type of effect on the aortic cusp immediately related to the defect, pulling it into the ventricle and over the course of time resulting in prolapse and insufficiency. This hypothesis seems unlikely, because the major left-to-right shunt through a ventricular septal defect occurs during systole. At this time the aortic valve cusps would be pushed up away from the annulus by the stream of blood being ejected into the aorta, and would be unlikely to be affected by the stream crossing the defect.

Small ventricular septal defect

Ventricular septal defects vary in size from the large defects described above to very small openings, and a spectrum of all sizes occurs. For convenience, I now discuss the opposite extreme: small defects. Small defects are most frequently located in the muscular portion of the septum but may occur elsewhere. Since they do not permit equalization of pressures between the ventricles, after birth the pulmonary arterial pressure falls when the ductus arteriosus closes. Maturation of the pulmonary circulation proceeds in its usual time course, or may be slightly delayed. Associated with the fall in pulmonary vascular resistance, left-to-right shunt occurs across the defect, resulting in a small to moderate increase in pulmonary blood flow (Figure 7.9).

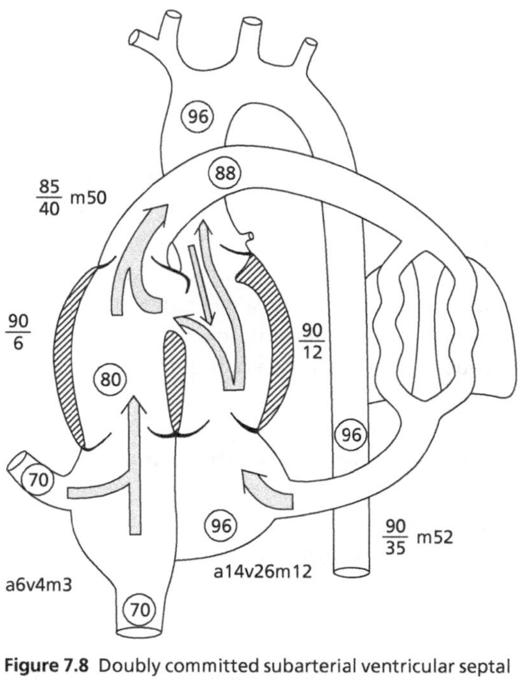

Figure 7.8 Doubly committed subarterial ventricular septal defect with secondary aortic insufficiency: course of the circulation, oxygen saturations (circled), and pressures in the heart and great vessels. m, mean pressure.

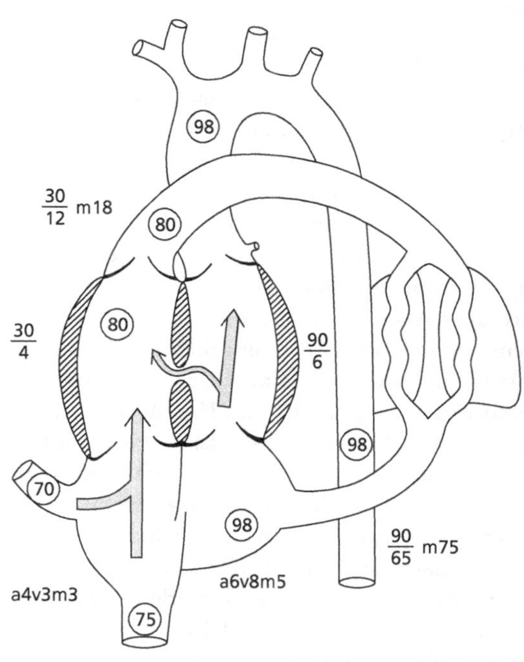

Figure 7.9 Small ventricular septal defect in infancy: course of the circulation, oxygen saturations (circled), and pressures in the heart and great vessels. m, mean pressure.

However, the size of the shunt is limited by the size of the defect. Shunting occurs almost entirely during ventricular systole. The left-to-right shunt is usually less than 50% of left ventricular output, with a ratio of pulmonary to systemic blood flow of less than 2:1.

Because the increase in pulmonary blood flow is not great, there is only a small increased volume load on the left ventricle. Pulmonary arterial and right ventricular pressures may be increased slightly but left-sided pressures are usually normal and cardiac failure does not occur. There is almost no risk of developing pulmonary vascular obstructive changes. A very high percentage of small ventricular septal defects close during the first 2 years after birth, but closure may be delayed until later (see below).

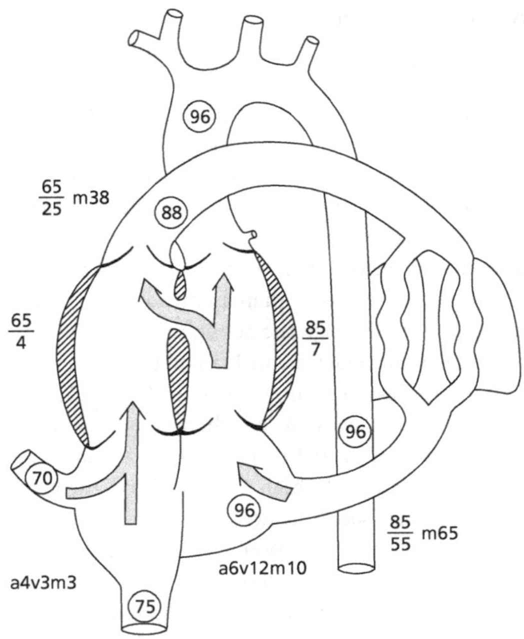

Figure 7.10 Medium-sized ventricular septal defect in infancy: course of the circulation, oxygen saturations (circled), and pressures in the heart and great vessels. m, mean pressure.

Medium-sized ventricular septal defect

The hemodynamic changes with these defects vary; they may tend toward those with nonrestrictive ventricular septal defects or to the small muscular defects, depending on their size. Following closure of the ductus arteriosus, right ventricular and pulmonary arterial systolic pressures fall but do not reach normal levels (Figure 7.10). As pulmonary vascular resistance falls, an increasing left-to-right shunt develops. Left ventricular end-diastolic and left atrial pressures increase, and if the shunt is large, left ventricular failure develops. It is usually not as severe as with the large defects and is controlled more readily by medical management. The course varies with the size of the defect and the degree of pulmonary arterial and right ventricular hypertension. In those patients with pulmonary arterial systolic pressures greater than 50% of systemic arterial systolic pressure, there is a significant risk of pulmonary vascular changes similar to those occurring with large defects. The measured pulmonary vascular resistance falls to high normal levels in infancy and, unless the defect becomes smaller, only gradually rises over the ensuing years. These individuals may have a relatively stable hemodynamic and clinical picture for several years, with a persistent moderate left-to-right shunt and moderate pulmonary arterial hypertension with mild, or no, cardiac failure.

When pulmonary arterial and right ventricular systolic pressures are less than 50% of systemic arterial systolic pressure, a moderate or large left-to-right shunt develops, with possible cardiac failure. The failure is usually controlled easily and these patients may maintain this relatively stable hemodynamic status for many months. Pulmonary vascular resistance usually does not increase after the initial fall after birth, but there is a small risk for it to increase progressively. There is a tendency for these defects to become smaller over time, with improvement in symptoms; the incidence of spontaneous closure of the defect is quite high in these patients.

Spontaneous closure of ventricular septal defects

Spontaneous closure of ventricular septal defects has long been recognized from clinical examination. In a large number of patients who had serial cardiac catheterization, we documented spontaneous closure of about 30% of all defects diagnosed in infancy, during the first 2 years after birth [9]. More recently, a high incidence of closure has been confirmed by repeat echocardiographic studies.

The actual incidence of closure is not known, and the reported rate varies in different series, depending on age at first diagnosis and on diagnostic acumen. As mentioned above, many defects not diagnosed clinically become apparent by color flow Doppler examination. The fact that ventricular septal defects are encountered infrequently either clinically or in routine autopsy series in adults, especially considering their relatively high frequency in childhood, suggests that most defects close spontaneously, because few people die of ventricular septal defects beyond infancy. Because, as mentioned above, the actual incidence of ventricular septal defects in the fetus is probably much higher than previously considered, the incidence of spontaneous closure must exceed 75%. We do not know what factors are responsible for closure. It is quite clear, though, that small or medium-sized defects are much more likely to close, as are defects located in the muscular portion of the septum. In several studies of ventricular septal defect first diagnosed in infancy, spontaneous closure within the first year was documented in 75–85% of muscular defects, but in only 25% of perimembranous defects [10,11]. As mentioned above, almost 50% of muscular defects detected in fetuses close spontaneously. Little information is available regarding the likelihood for doubly committed subarterial defects to close spontaneously, although it has generally been thought that it is small. This was confirmed in a report from Japan of 742 patients with this defect, where closure could be documented in only about 4% by annual ultrasound studies [12].

There are several different mechanisms by which a ventricular septal defect may close. Perhaps the most frequent is by growth and hypertrophy of the muscular portion of the septum around the defect. Muscular septal defects are usually ovoid in infancy, but later in life they are slit-like. As the heart grows, the septum enlarges more in apex to base than in anteroposterior wall dimension. This would tend to elongate the defect. The septum also increases in thickness and force of contraction. These factors would all lead to a reduction in defect size, particularly during systole, when most of the left-to-right shunt occurs. When only a thin narrow slit remains, closure may occur. Occasionally, small defects of this type may be seen at autopsy in individuals who no longer had evidence of a ventricular septal defect by clinical and catheterization studies. This corroborates the fact that functional systolic closure may occur with muscle defects.

A possible mechanism that has been proposed is that subacute bacterial endocarditis, which is not clinically apparent but which is cured by treatment given for a nonspecific infection, may be responsible for closure. If the infection develops at the rim of the defect, the septal leaflet of the tricuspid valve may be involved and become adherent to the defect in the healing process. If the cusp itself becomes involved in the infectious process, it may be damaged and perforated, resulting in a communication between the left ventricle and the right atrium. It is interesting that a high incidence of subacute bacterial endocarditis has been reported in patients with left ventricular to right atrial shunts [13]. It seems highly unlikely, however, that what is usually considered as inadequate therapy for bacterial endocarditis could successfully resolve the infection. It is quite possible that these represent patients who had ventricular septal defects, developed subacute bacterial endocarditis, and then the left ventricular to right atrial shunt.

Another mechanism that has been suggested for tricuspid leaflet apposition is through the negative pressure effect exerted by a high-velocity stream flowing through the defect. If the defect is not large, the high velocity of the left-to-right shunt during systole, if directed appropriately, may create a negative pressure immediately beyond the defect under the valve cusp and thus tend to attract it to the margin of the defect. It is conceivable that over a prolonged period the cusp may become adherent to the upper margin of the defect, decreasing its size.

Frequently, closure is associated with the development of a so-called ventricular septal aneurysm. Several mechanisms have been proposed to account for these aneurysms. It appears that involvement of tricuspid valve tissue adjacent to the defect is the most usual mechanism. Adherence of the septal leaflet of the tricuspid valve creates a membranous structure over the defect, and presents as an aneurysmal formation, and eventually may result in complete closure of the defect.

A ventricular defect may also become smaller by gradual proliferation of the tissues around its margins, with encroachment on the orifice. This type of closure occurs mainly in defects of the membranous portion of the septum but can also occur in the muscular septum. The process is probably initiated by intimal proliferation along the rim of the defect; ultimately, even large defects may close almost completely. Evidence of this type of closure has been found at autopsy; the margins of the defect can be seen, and the original opening is seen to be filled by a membrane, in the center of which a small hole still persists, surrounded by a thick rolled edge. This type of closure is not infrequently associated with the development of aneurysms of the ventricular septum.

Most aneurysms are fairly small, flat, conical projections of a thin membrane arising from the margin of the septal defect and bulging about 1–2 cm into the right ventricle. A small opening is usually present at the apex, allowing a small left-to-right shunt. Although most ventricular septal aneurysms do not cause any difficulties, complications may occur, even as late as adult life. They may result in tricuspid regurgitation, probably when the valve is involved in forming the aneurysm. Infective endocarditis has been reported as a late complication, but it probably occurs in those individuals in whom a left-to-right shunt is still present. The length of the aneurysms varies greatly; rarely they may extend a considerable distance into the right ventricle and may reach the infundibular region and have been reported to cause some degree of obstruction of the right ventricular outflow tract. The late development of aortic valve prolapse has been noted in association with ventricular septal aneurysms, but the mechanism responsible for the development has not been determined.

It is also possible that a doubly committed subarterial defect may be functionally closed by prolapse of an aortic cusp over the defect orifice. Subsequent prolapse of the cusp through the defect could result in severe aortic regurgitation through the defect into the right ventricle.

Clinical features

The clinical manifestations of ventricular septal defect cover a wide spectrum. They are related to the hemodynamic changes and the associated lesions and range from detection of a cardiac murmur with no other symptoms or signs to severe and life-threatening cardiac failure in infancy. As in the section on hemodynamic disturbances, the clinical features are presented in relation to the size of the defect.

Large ventricular septal defect

The infant with a large defect has no manifestations in the immediate postnatal period. Apart from a moderate increase in respiratory rate to 50–60/min and a tachycardia to 140–160/min, the infant may appear to be doing quite well. After a variable period of 1–7 days after birth, a systolic murmur becomes evident along the lower left sternal border. The onset of the murmur may be delayed for a longer period in infants with very large defects or if pulmonary vascular resistance is maintained at high levels because of associated pulmonary disease. The second heart sound is loud in the pulmonary area and usually narrowly split. During the second to eighth weeks, the infant develops increasing respiratory distress. This is often first evident during feeding, when the baby becomes tired and has to stop sucking because of the effort of respiration. Infants take only small volumes at each feeding and become hungry and irritable within a short period. Their total daily intake is small and this contributes to their failure to thrive. Growth in body length is less delayed than increase in weight; also head circumference is not interfered with in early infancy, but if the manifestations of failure continue for months, head growth may also be delayed. Excessive perspiration is noted, particularly around the forehead and the back of the neck. It occurs most prominently with feeding, and the mother also notes that the sheet under the head is constantly moist. Respiratory symptoms become progressively worse and lower sternal retractions may be noted; the infant becomes progressively more distressed. Generalized pallor due to peripheral vasoconstriction is noted and mild cyanosis may occur. The progression of symptoms varies; some infants may develop severe cardiac failure within 4–6 weeks after birth, whereas in others moderate symptoms may persist for 2–3 months.

Early in the course, physical examination reveals increased respiratory rate and effort, and the skin is clammy. Heart rate is increased to 140–160/min and the pulses are weak. Pulse pressure tends to be reduced. Chest auscultation does not reveal any findings initially, but as cardiac failure progresses, rales may be heard at the lung bases and air entry may be decreased. Associated with this progression, respiratory rate may increase to 60–80/min or more and substernal retractions are common. Initially the liver is not significantly enlarged, even though respiratory effort may be greatly increased, but progressively it does enlarge and the edge may reach the level of the umbilicus or lower. Deformity of the chest is unusual in the first 2–3 months after birth, even with very large ventricular septal defects. However, if the large left-to-right shunt and cardiac failure persist, bulging of the lower sternum and adjacent ribs frequently develops by 5–6 months. The sternal prominence does not usually occur in infants with large left-to-right shunts and only mildly elevated right ventricular pressures. It is noted in those who have a large volume load on the right ventricle as well as an elevation of pressure, indicative of a nonrestrictive defect.

The precordium becomes more active as the magnitude of the left-to-right shunt increases. The impulse is diffuse, involving the left and right ventricles. The cardiac apex is displaced outside the left mid-clavicular line as the heart enlarges and occasionally a systolic thrill is palpable over the precordium. The first heart sound is usually normal or soft and the second sound is accentuated in the pulmonary area at the upper left sternal edge; it is well split, but it is difficult to define the degree of splitting at the rapid heart rates present in these infants. A systolic murmur is almost invariably present. Soon after birth, the murmur may be of grade 2–3/6 intensity, is of medium frequency, and may extend only about halfway through systole. It is usually best heard along the lower left sternal border, but in some infants with a doubly committed subarterial defect, the murmur may be more prominent along the upper left sternal edge. As the left-to-right shunt increases, the murmur becomes louder and somewhat harsher, extends throughout the whole of systole, radiates to the whole precordium, and may be heard all over the chest. Its contour is one of even intensity throughout the whole of systole. A third heart sound or a short mid-diastolic low-frequency murmur is often noted at the apex, but may not be identified because of the tachycardia. The apical mid-diastolic murmur reflects a relative mitral stenosis due to increased flow through a normal-sized mitral valve; it is usually heard only when the ratio of pulmonary to systemic blood flow is about 2:1 or greater.

If the baby is not treated, pulmonary edema becomes progressively more severe, systemic blood flow falls, resulting in weak pulses and pallor, and death may ensue. Treatment with digoxin, diuretics and possibly afterload reducers usually results in rapid improvement of the manifestations of failure. Respiratory rate and degree of distress improve, the liver becomes smaller, heart rate decreases, and pulse volume increases. With improvement in cardiac contraction, precordial hyperactivity may increase. This, together with slowing of the heart rate, makes the systolic murmur more prominent and the apical mid-diastolic murmur becomes longer and more evident.

If the infant survives and acute symptoms improve, the subsequent course is one of persistent dyspnea, sweating, poor feeding with failure to thrive, and susceptibility to repeated respiratory infections. Cardiac failure may become much more severe with infection.

Improvement in symptoms

Symptoms of cardiac failure often slowly begin to improve spontaneously with no change in therapy. This may occur within weeks after onset of the severe symptoms, or several months later, by 5–10 months of age. This improvement may be related to several mechanisms, such as decrease in size of the ventricular septal defect, increase in pulmonary vascular resistance, or development of right ventricular outflow obstruction due to hypertrophy of muscle in the infundibular region. The clinical features of each of these mechanisms are presented, but patients should be followed carefully by ultrasound study.

Each of these developments results in a decrease in left-to-right shunt and pulmonary blood flow. Thus, cardiac activity decreases, the heart becomes smaller, and the apical diastolic murmur becomes softer. It is important to differentiate between the mechanisms resulting in this improvement. If the defect is closing, the second sound becomes softer and the murmur becomes higher in frequency and shorter in duration; if closure is complete, the murmur disappears. If a ventricular septal aneurysm develops, an early systolic click may be heard at the left sternal border.

If pulmonary vascular resistance is increasing, the second pulmonary sound continues to be very loud and also becomes narrower. The left ventricular impulse becomes less prominent and right ventricular pulsation increases. Frequently there is bulging of the lower sternum. These findings increase progressively and there may be a period of good health for several years. The systolic murmur gradually decreases in intensity and duration, and eventually cyanosis occurs with exertion. The features of severe pulmonary vascular obstruction, decreasing exercise tolerance, increasing cyanosis, hemoptysis, and right heart failure eventually develop (see Chapter 5). These changes may occur by 5–10 years of age, but in most patients are not evident before the late teens. In many individuals, though, they may be delayed to the late twenties and survival into the thirties may occur. When pulmonary vascular obstruction is marked there is no hyperactivity of the cardiac impulse, but a prominent right ventricular pulsation may be noted. The second sound is loud and narrow in the pulmonary area and sometimes there is an early diastolic decrescendo murmur reflecting pulmonary valve incompetence. Systolic murmurs may be absent or soft and short.

If infundibular hypertrophy develops, there is also a decrease in evidence of left-to-right shunt. The intensity of the second sound in the pulmonary area decreases, and often a systolic murmur of more crescendo–decrescendo character, stenotic in quality, becomes evident at the upper left sternal border in addition to the ventricular septal defect murmur. The stenosis may become severe enough to result in shunt reversal with cyanosis, first on exercise only, then persistent, and also other features of Fallot tetralogy such as exercise limitation may ensue (see Chapter 14).

Small ventricular septal defect

As mentioned above, a small defect may be considered one in which the left-to-right shunt is less than 50% of left ventricular output and pulmonary arterial pressure is not elevated. An infant with a small defect is usually asymptomatic, but within 2–8 weeks after birth, moderate tachypnea and tachycardia may develop; this is more likely to occur in association with an infection. The infant usually has normal weight gain and development.

Precordial activity may be increased somewhat, but no clinical cardiomegaly is evident. A systolic murmur is usually audible within the first week; it is of grade 2–4/6 intensity, of medium frequency, and maximal along the lower left sternal border. The murmur may extend through the whole of systole, but may occupy only the first half to two-thirds of systole. The shorter murmurs also tend to be of higher frequency. Spontaneous closure occurs in a high proportion of small defects; this is associated with a decrease in intensity and duration and increase in frequency of the murmur. Within 2 months to 2 years, the murmur may not be detectable, but it may persist throughout childhood. An apical diastolic murmur is not usually heard with a small defect.

Medium-sized ventricular septal defect

Infants with these defects are asymptomatic at birth. Within 2–8 weeks after birth, symptoms may appear. There is a spectrum of severity of symptoms, depending on the size of the defect. With larger defects, tachypnea and dyspnea, excessive perspiration, poor feeding, and failure to thrive become manifest, as described above for large defects. The infant is often anxious and fussy, takes frequent small feedings, and has poor weight gain. Rales may be heard at the lung bases, and hepatomegaly may be present. The precordium is hyperactive, and both left and right ventricular impulses are increased. The cardiac apex is displaced outside the left mid-clavicular line. The first heart sound is usually soft and often obscured by the systolic murmur, which is evident within 2–3 days after birth, increases in amplitude to grade 3–5/6, and becomes holosystolic. The murmur is best heard at the lower left sternal border and is usually well heard in the xiphoid region; it radiates throughout the precordium and frequently is distributed to both left and right chest. The second sound is split and is moderately accentuated in the pulmonary area, along the upper left parasternal edge. A third heart sound, often followed by a short mid-diastolic low-frequency murmur, is heard at the apex.

The infant usually improves rapidly with diuretic therapy and digoxin; respiratory rate and effort improve, liver size decreases, and heart rate slows. However, the cardiac findings do not change significantly. If the size of the defect does not decrease, and even though manifestations of cardiac failure have improved, tachypnea and poor feeding persist and the infant continues to thrive poorly; weight gain suffers more than growth in length, and head circumference may not increase normally. With decrease in defect size, development of increasing pulmonary vascular resistance, or right ventricular outflow obstruction, the course is similar to that described above for large ventricular septal defects.

With the smaller defects, the clinical features are similar to those described above for small ventricular septal defects. However, there may be some tachypnea and increased perspiration and the infant may gain weight slowly. The second sound is of normal or slightly increased intensity. A grade 3–5/6 systolic murmur extending through two-thirds or the whole of systole is heard along the left sternal border, and a short apical mid-diastolic murmur may be audible. These infants usually develop quite well and do not usually require any therapy. Most of these infants develop spontaneous closure of the defect. However, some continue to thrive poorly, even though clinical assessment suggests that the ratio of pulmonary to systemic blood flow is only about 2:1.

Aortic valve prolapse and regurgitation

Aortic valve involvement is most likely to be associated with doubly committed subarterial defects. As mentioned above, with these defects the systolic murmur may be best heard at the upper left sternal border. Prolapse of the valve support mechanism is not associated with clinical manifestations, and it may become marked without being recognized. Insufficiency of the valve is associated with development of an early high-frequency diastolic murmur, starting immediately after the second heart sound, along the left sternal border. With progression of the aortic regurgitation, the murmur becomes louder and longer, left ventricular hyperactivity increases, and the pulse pressure increases with the fall in diastolic arterial pressure.

Investigations

Electrocardiography

In general, the electrocardiogram reflects the increased volume and pressure loads on the respective ventricles. In patients with small ventricular septal defects, it is usually quite normal. With medium-sized defects there often is some mild increase in left ventricular precordial voltages. With large defects there is usually right axis deviation and increase in right and left ventricular voltages reflecting combined hypertrophy. As the defect becomes smaller, right forces diminish first. If pulmonary vascular resistance increases, left forces begin to decrease and right ventricular hypertrophy becomes more prominent. Similar changes occur if infundibular obstruction of the right ventricle develops. A number of patients with moderate-sized defects have a ventricular axis in the 0–30° range. The reason for this is not clear but it could be related to the position of the defect.

Radiographic features

The chest radiograph may be quite normal in the infant and child with a small defect. With a large defect, the heart is enlarged and both left and right ventricles are prominent. The main pulmonary artery is enlarged and the pulmonary arteries are prominent, extending out to the periphery of the lungs. The left atrium is also enlarged, and if failure is present the lung fields may be hazy, particularly in the hilar region, due to pulmonary edema. When pulmonary vascular resistance increases there is often anterior bulging of the sternum. Right ventricular enlargement becomes more prominent whereas the left ventricle decreases in size. The main pulmonary artery becomes very large and there is enlargement of the main pulmonary arteries in the hilum, but the peripheral pulmonary arteries are much less prominent and, later, the vascular markings in the periphery of the lung are decreased.

Echocardiography

Prior to the availability of echocardiography and Doppler flow studies, cardiac catheterization and angiography were frequently performed in patients with suspected ventricular septal defect to confirm the diagnosis, exclude associated lesions, and assess the size and location of the defect. In addition pulmonary arterial pressure was measured and the magnitude of left-to-right shunt and of pulmonary vascular resistance was calculated. Most of this information can now be deduced from ultrasound examination. In fact, echocardiography, including color flow Doppler examination, is more reliable than cardiac catheterization in detecting the presence of small ventricular septal defects.

An ultrasound study should be directed at specifically answering several questions.

- What is the size and location of the defect?
- Are there multiple defects?
- Are there any associated cardiovascular anomalies?
- What is the magnitude of the pulmonary to systemic blood flow ratio?
- What is the pressure in the right ventricle and pulmonary artery?
- What is the size of the left ventricle?
- What is the performance of the left ventricle?
- What are the relationships between the papillary muscles and chordal attachments and the ventricular septal defect?

The size and location of the defect and the possible presence of additional defects or other lesions can be evaluated by both echocardiography and color flow mapping. The pulmonary and systemic blood flows can be measured with a reasonable degree of reliability by obtaining the cross-sectional area of the aorta and pulmonary artery just beyond the valves and recording the aortic and pulmonary arterial velocity profiles. Recording the maximal velocity of the shunt by Doppler methods allows estimation of the systolic pressure gradient across the defect. By subtracting this value from the measured arterial systolic blood pressure, it is possible to obtain an estimate of right ventricular pressure. This helps to determine whether the defect is restrictive or not and, in the absence of right ventricular outflow obstruction, provides an estimate of pulmonary arterial systolic pressure. In many instances a small amount of tricuspid regurgitation can be detected by the Doppler method. If present, it provides another means of estimating right ventricular pressure from the velocity of the regurgitant jet.

Cardiac catheterization

Although cardiac catheterization and angiocardiography were frequently used to confirm the diagnosis, exclude associated lesions, and assess hemodynamic features in infants and children with clinically diagnosed ventricular septal defects, the procedures are performed much less often since echocardiographic evaluation has become increasingly reliable. In recent years, many centers are not subjecting patients with ventricular septal defect to catheterization prior to surgery unless a specific indication is identified. Usually this is to assess pulmonary vascular resistance and its response to pulmonary vasodilator agents. Transcatheter techniques are being applied with increasing frequency to close ventricular septal defects and these procedures are discussed below.

Oxygen saturation data

In patients with a small ventricular septal defect there usually is a modest increase in oxygen saturation at the right ventricular level. This may vary between 5 and 20%, but with very small shunts there may be no detectable increase in oxygen saturation of statistical significance, despite the clinical observation of a murmur and echocardiographic demonstration of a small defect. The oxygen saturation increase is often small in blood samples obtained just beyond the tricuspid valve or at the right ventricular apex and may be more prominent in the infundibular region. A small additional rise may be noted in the pulmonary artery. In patients with doubly committed subarterial defects there may be only a small increase in oxygen saturation in the body of the ventricle, and the major increase is noted in the main pulmonary artery because of streaming of the shunted blood across the pulmonary valve. With large defects and large left-to-right shunts, oxygen saturation in the pulmonary artery may reach 85–90% and it is in these cases that it is difficult to exclude an additional patent ductus arteriosus on the basis of oxygen saturation data.

In some patients, particularly in infants with cardiac failure, in addition to an increase in oxygen saturation at the ventricular level, an increase is noted in the right atrium. This may be only 5–10% above superior vena cava levels, but on occasion it is much larger, on the order of 20% or more. It is then necessary to distinguish between three possibilities: an atrial septal defect alone, with streaming of shunted blood through the tricuspid valve, which creates a further rise in right ventricular oxygen saturation; a ventricular septal defect with tricuspid regurgitation; and the presence of both an atrial and a ventricular septal defect. Infants with a large ventricular septal defect and left atrial hypertension and enlargement often develop an atrial left-to-right shunt as a result of stretching and incompetence of the foramen ovale. Any of the conditions mentioned above that may reduce the magnitude of the left-to-right shunt will decrease the rise in oxygen saturation at the level of the right ventricle.

Pulmonary venous and left atrial blood usually shows normal oxygen saturation and blood gases, but in infants in cardiac failure oxygen saturation is often reduced to 90–92%. $P\text{CO}_2$ may be mildly increased to 45–50 mmHg, with a small decrease in pH to about 7.30. The systemic arterial oxygen saturation is usually normal, but when failure occurs, systemic arterial blood shows the same findings as in left atrial blood. When pulmonary vascular resistance increases, systemic arterial oxygen saturation falls, the level depending on the degree of pulmonary vascular obstruction. In these cases, oxygen saturations in the left atrium and body of the left ventricle are usually normal, and the right-to-left shunt is detectable by the lower aortic or peripheral arterial oxygen saturation and $P\text{O}_2$. When pulmonary and systemic vascular resistances are fairly balanced, the oxygen saturation may be noted to fall during exercise or with peripheral vasodilator agents.

Pressures

In patients with small ventricular septal defects, intravascular pressures are usually normal. With medium-sized defects, there is an increase in right ventricular systolic pressure to 30–50 mmHg, but end-diastolic pressure is usually normal. Systolic pressure in the pulmonary artery is elevated to the same level as in the right ventricle but diastolic pressure may be only slightly elevated and pulse pressure in the pulmonary artery is increased. The mean pressure is elevated to 20–30 mmHg. Left atrial pressure is often mildly increased to mean levels of 6–10 mmHg and there is a prominent *v* wave. Left ventricular end-diastolic pressure is raised to 8–15 mmHg and systolic pressure is normal, as is systemic arterial pressure.

With large defects, right atrial pressure may be increased slightly whereas left atrial mean pressure is usually raised to 10–15 mmHg or sometimes even more. In preterm infants, however, left atrial mean pressure is usually not above 10–12 mmHg, even when there is clinical evidence of pulmonary edema. There is a mean pressure difference of variable degree, sometimes as high as 8–15 mmHg, between the left and right atrium. Pulmonary venous mean pressure is often 3–4 mmHg higher than mean pressure in the left atrium. This could be due to high flow through the relatively small pulmonary vein, but could possibly be the result of some constriction of muscle at the junction between the pulmonary vein and left atrium.

Systolic pressures in the right ventricle and pulmonary artery are equal to those in the left ventricle and the systemic arteries. The magnitude of left and right ventricular systolic pressures is of value in assessing the size of the defect. If they are always identical, the defect is unrestrictive and must be very large, i.e., greater than the diameter of the aortic annulus. If right ventricular and either left ventricular or aortic pressure are measured simultaneously, induction of ectopic beats by advancing the catheter against the wall of the right ventricle will show that, with unrestrictive defects, the systolic pressures do not separate, either during ectopic beats or in the postectopic potentiated beat. If the defect is smaller, systolic pressures may be equal, but when ectopic beats are induced there is a separation, usually with left ventricular pressure exceeding right ventricular pressure. Similar separation of systolic pressure may be noted when pulmonary vasodilatation is induced and systolic pressures in the right ventricle and pulmonary artery fall below those in the left ventricle and aorta.

When there is a large left-to-right shunt, pulmonary arterial diastolic pressure is relatively low, often in the range of 20–30 mmHg. The diastolic and mean pressures in the pulmonary artery are contrasted with the normal aortic diastolic and mean pressures, so that even though systolic pressures are identical there may be a mean pressure difference of 10–25 mmHg between the aorta and the pulmonary artery. When systolic pressure in the pulmonary artery is close to that in the systemic arteries, low pulmonary arterial diastolic and mean pressures are indicative of a relatively low pulmonary vascular resistance (see Chapter 5), although unusually could be due to the presence of pulmonary valve insufficiency.

In some infants with large left-to-right shunts there is a systolic pressure drop of up to about

25 mmHg across the pulmonary valve. This may disappear when the flow is reduced by closure of the defect or development of pulmonary vascular disease, and is probably functionally produced by the high flow. Also, during early infancy, there may be a pressure difference of up to 25 mmHg systolic and 15 mmHg mean between the main pulmonary artery and the left and right branches. This may be related to the persistence of the fetal pattern of origin of the branch arteries from the main pulmonary trunk; the high pulmonary blood flow accentuates the small pressure difference noted in normal infants (see Chapter 5).

As pulmonary vascular resistance increases, left atrial and left ventricular end-diastolic pressures fall and the diastolic pressure in the pulmonary artery increases. With severe pulmonary vascular obstruction, aortic and pulmonary arterial pressures are almost identical, mean and diastolic as well as systolic levels.

When right ventricular infundibular stenosis develops, there is a systolic pressure drop across the hypertrophied muscle area and pulmonary arterial pressures are lower. Left atrial and left ventricular end-diastolic pressures also fall as the magnitude of the left-to-right shunt decreases. With aortic insufficiency, the systemic arterial diastolic pressure falls and left ventricular end-diastolic and left atrial pressures rise.

Blood flows

Systemic blood flow is usually normal, except in infants in severe failure. The level of pulmonary blood flow depends on the magnitude of the left-to-right shunt. At high levels of pulmonary blood flow, the actual level of flow calculated by the Fick method may be inaccurate, in view of the small arteriovenous differences across the pulmonary circulation (see Chapter 4). Also, when there is a bidirectional shunt, calculation of flows and shunts is likely to be unreliable.

Vascular resistances

Systemic vascular resistance is usually normal but may be increased in patients in cardiac failure. Pulmonary vascular resistance is normal in the presence of a small ventricular septal defect. In patients with large ventricular septal defects, pulmonary vascular resistance is either mildly or moderately increased in infants living at sea level, but it increases with advancing age. In interpreting pulmonary vascular resistance and its changes, it is necessary to take into account the reliability of the pressure and flow data used in the calculation, as well as the actual levels of pressure and flow, particularly left atrial pressure (see Chapter 4). The response of pulmonary vascular resistance to oxygen and pulmonary vasodilator agents has been considered important in making recommendations for surgery in patients with ventricular septal defect and high resting pulmonary vascular resistance. This is discussed in the section on management.

Cineangiography

Demonstration of the defect by angiography has become less important because echocardiography and Doppler flow examinations are very effective in defining the defects by noninvasive techniques. A detailed study of patients with ventricular septal defect includes a biplane angiographic study with a left ventricular contrast injection to define the location and size of the defect. The defect is best defined when the image intensifier and X-ray tube are positioned so as to provide a fairly steep left anterior oblique projection (70°) with cranial angulation of about 25°. Defects of the inlet septum are better visualized in a less steep left anterior oblique projection (about 25°) and more cranial angulation (about 50°).

In patients with small defects, the left ventricular cavity is normal in size and configuration. A small jet of contrast medium is seen to pass through the defect and may be located either low in the muscular septum or just below the aortic valve. With doubly committed subarterial defects, the jet of contrast medium may be seen to enter the infundibulum just below the pulmonary valve and stream almost directly into the pulmonary artery.

Ventricular septal aneurysms are usually seen as small conical projections from the left ventricle, a little below the aortic valve. A small jet of contrast medium passes from the apex of the aneurysm into the right ventricle.

With large defects and large shunts, the left ventricular cavity is enlarged and there is an increase in its ejection fraction. If there is failure, the residual volume of the ventricle is increased. The shunt can be seen to cross the defect as a wide stream of contrast medium. It is important to carefully observe whether there is a single large defect or whether there is diffuse shunting through various sites in the septum, as the latter may indicate multiple small defects. If ventricular ectopic beats occur during the injection, some degree of mitral regurgitation is frequently noted.

The size of the right ventricle is usually normal or slightly large with small defects, but is enlarged with large defects. A right ventricular injection may show some contrast medium crossing the defect and entering the left ventricle and aorta when a large defect with purely physiological left-to-right shunt is present. This right-to-left shunt is probably due to the elevation of right ventricular pressure during the injection, with momentary shunting. Also, if ventricular ectopic beats occur during the injection, commonly some degree of right-to-left shunt and tricuspid regurgitation are seen.

In the presence of large shunts, the main pulmonary artery is enlarged and the pulmonary vessels are prominent in the hilum and the peripheral lung fields. The left atrium is also dilated. In the recirculation phase, contrast medium may be seen to pass into the right atrium in the presence of an atrial left-to-right shunt. Left and right ventricular angiograms are also helpful in distinguishing an atrial left-to-right shunt in addition to the ventricular shunt or demonstrating significant tricuspid regurgitation when there is an increase in oxygen saturation at the right atrial level.

When pulmonary vascular resistance increases, left ventricular size and ejection fraction decrease. The most striking development is that the proximal pulmonary arteries become very prominent and there is a reduction in the number of small vessels in the periphery. The hilar pulmonary arteries become tortuous and there appears to be a sharp pruning of the peripheral vessels, the so-called "tree in winter" appearance.

If aortic valve insufficiency is suspected, a supravalvar aortic injection should be made by retrograde arterial passage of a catheter; this will demonstrate its presence. An injection through the venous catheter passed across the aortic valve via the defect may not be reliable, as some regurgitation may result from the presence of the catheter across the valve. It is recommended that an aortogram be performed in all patients with doubly committed subarterial defects, because of the tendency for aortic insufficiency to develop in this type of defect. Prolapse of the sinus on Valsalva associated with origin of the right coronary artery may be noted before any functional aortic insufficiency is apparent.

In patients developing outflow tract obstruction, a right ventricular angiogram shows hypertrophy of muscle in the outflow tract. The infundibular region narrows considerably during systole but may be quite wide in diastole. On occasion, a localized rim of narrowing in the lower region of the infundibulum is noted, with a distinct chamber between the stenotic segment and the pulmonary valve.

In patients with left ventricular to right atrial shunts, the angiogram done in the left ventricle shows contrast medium passing directly from the left ventricle to the right atrium, often as a systolic jet.

Differential diagnosis

The wide range of clinical manifestations and complicating lesions associated with ventricular septal defects can result in confusion with many other cardiac malformations. In this section, only a brief discussion of the diagnoses to be considered with each of the major clinical syndromes is presented.

Small ventricular septal defect

Because the only important manifestation of this lesion is a systolic murmur, conditions that should be differentiated are functional murmurs such as a pulmonary ejection murmur and a Still murmur, mild pulmonary stenosis, mild aortic valvar stenosis, and idiopathic hypertrophic subaortic stenosis. The pulmonary ejection murmur is best heard at the upper left sternal border, is usually of somewhat higher frequency than a ventricular septal defect murmur, and has a crescendo–decrescendo contour. In pulmonary stenosis the murmur is heard best at the upper left rather than lower left sternal border; it is more ejection in character and radiates to the left clavicle. There is often a prominent ejection click and the second sound is well split. Chest radiography may be helpful in showing post-stenotic dilatation of the main pulmonary artery.

In aortic valvar stenosis, the murmur is also ejection in quality, is most prominent at the upper right sternal border, and radiates to the neck. In infants, however, the murmur of aortic stenosis may be well heard at the mid-left sternal border and may be readily confused with ventricular septal defect. A systolic ejection click is also often heard in patients with aortic stenosis. When a ventricular septal aneurysm is present, the late systolic sound could be confused with a systolic ejection click, although it occurs later in systole. Chest radiography in aortic valvar stenosis may be helpful in showing post-stenotic dilation of the ascending aorta.

Idiopathic hypertrophic subaortic stenosis is associated with a systolic murmur along the lower left sternal border, with some radiation to the upper right chest. Although these patients usually have evidence of marked left ventricular hypertrophy with ST- and T-wave changes when the lesion is severe, in the earlier stages of the disease only an increase in left ventricular precordial voltages may be noted and the differential may be difficult by clinical means.

Large ventricular septal defect

In infancy, large ventricular septal defects must be differentiated from any lesion producing a large left-to-right shunt with cardiac failure. This includes patent ductus arteriosus; atrioventricular septal defect; other lesions in which ventricular septal defect is part of a complex, such as double-outlet right ventricle of the Taussig–Bing variety; aortopulmonary transposition with large ventricular septal defect; truncus arteriosus communis; and tricuspid atresia with large ventricular septal defect. Although there are many clinical, radiographic, and electrocardiographic guides that assist in making a differential diagnosis, the specific diagnosis can rarely be made with assurance; detailed echocardiography with Doppler flow studies, and if necessary cardiac catheterization and angiocardiographic studies, should be done.

Several clinical features are particularly helpful. A continuous murmur at the upper left sternal border or in the subclavicular area suggests a patent ductus arteriosus, but it is important to recognize that this lesion may be associated with a ventricular septal defect. A continuous murmur may also be heard with truncus arteriosus. With both these lesions, pulses may be bounding because of the wide pulse pressure. Cyanosis of moderate degree suggests truncus arteriosus, transposition with ventricular septal defect, Taussig–Bing anomaly, or tricuspid atresia with a large ventricular septal defect. However, mild cyanosis may occur in an infant with an isolated ventricular septal defect who has severe failure with pulmonary congestion and edema. Weak pulses or lower blood pressure in the lower as compared with the upper extremities, suggesting the presence of aortic arch obstruction, is often associated with Taussig–Bing anomaly or atrioventricular canal defect, but may indicate the association of aortic arch interruption or aortic coarctation with a ventricular septal defect.

Left axis deviation on the electrocardiogram occurs with atrioventricular canal defects and tricuspid atresia with ventricular septal defect, and may be noted occasionally in Taussig–Bing anomaly.

Medium-sized ventricular septal defect

The lesions with which a medium-sized defect is most likely to be confused include endocardial cushion defect, mitral insufficiency, and left ventricular to right atrial shunt. In endocardial cushion defects there is often increased activity of the left ventricle due to mitral regurgitation and of the right ventricle due to atrial shunting. There may also be a harsh systolic murmur and a mid-diastolic murmur at the apex. The electrocardiogram is most helpful in that there is left axis deviation with a counterclockwise loop in the frontal plane in endocardial cushion lesions. However, since there is sometimes an axis of 0–30° in some patients with ventricular septal defects, confusion may arise.

In patients with mitral insufficiency, the increased left ventricular hyperactivity, the systolic murmur, and mid-diastolic low-frequency murmur at the apex may create some confusion. The murmur of mitral insufficiency is more prominent at the apex and radiates to the axilla. In left ventricular to right atrial shunt, the murmur radiates well to the right side of the sternum but otherwise the clinical features are similar. The diagnoses are clearly distinguished by ultrasound studies.

Ventricular septal defect with aortic insufficiency

This lesion may be difficult to differentiate from lesions that produce a loud, rough, continuous murmur or a loud systolic and diastolic murmur at the upper left sternal border and a wide pulse pressure. The lesions to be considered include large patent ductus arteriosus, sinus of Valsalva fistula, aortic stenosis and insufficiency, large coronary arteriovenous fistula, and truncus arteriosus communis. It is rarely possible to be positive about the diagnosis from the clinical, radiographic, and electrocardiographic features. Ultrasound and, if necessary, catheterization and angiographic studies are necessary. Aortography may be crucial in making a diagnosis.

Ventricular septal defect with markedly increased pulmonary vascular resistance

These patients present with features similar to those noted in all patients with systemic–pulmonary communications and pulmonary vascular obstructive disease, often referred to as Eisenmenger complex or Eisenmenger syndrome. Thus, patients with pulmonary vascular obstruction associated with patent ductus arteriosus, endocardial cushion defect, atrial septal defect, aortopulmonary transposition with ventricular septal defect, and similar lesions all have similar clinical features. Echocardiography with Doppler flow studies and, if necessary, cardiac catheterization and angiography are necessary to differentiate the lesions.

Principles of management

The approach to management of patients with ventricular septal defect has undergone considerable change since the natural history of the lesion has become apparent. The important features that have emerged are as follows: (i) most small defects close spontaneously; (ii) many large defects tend to decrease in size; (iii) pulmonary vascular changes may begin to develop within 6–12 months and often are quite advanced by 2–3 years after birth in infants with large defects; and (iv) patients with doubly committed subarterial defects are prone to develop aortic insufficiency.

In making decisions regarding management, several questions should be raised.

1 *What is the size of the defect?* The size of the defect can be assessed clinically from the loudness of the second sound and the character of the murmur. A loud second sound at the upper left sternal border indicates that pulmonary arterial and therefore right ventricular pressure is elevated, suggesting that the defect is large. A systolic murmur that does not extend through the whole of systole, but occupies only the first half to two-thirds, suggests that the defect is quite small. Most of these defects have proven by echocardiography to be 3 mm or less in diameter. This is, of course, not the case in the early newborn period, or in the older infant or child who has pulmonary arterial hypertension. The size as well as the location of the defect can usually be defined by echocardiography.

2 *What is the magnitude of the left-to-right shunt?* The magnitude of the left-to-right shunt is evaluated clinically from the degree of precordial hyperactivity and the presence of an apical diastolic murmur. A large left-to-right shunt is associated with a forceful left as well as right ventricular impulse. A middiastolic murmur at the apex usually signifies that the shunt is large enough to result in a pulmonary to systemic blood flow ratio of 2:1 or greater.

3 *Are there manifestations of "cardiac failure"?* Cardiac failure is evidenced by a history of sweating, increased respiratory rate and effort, and failure to thrive. On examination, there is tachypnea and dyspnea, tachycardia, and usually hepatomegaly.

4 *What is the location of the defect?* It is difficult to define the location of the defect clinically. However, if the systolic murmur is heard maximally at the upper left sternal border, rather than in the usual location of the mid to lower left sternal border, a doubly committed subarterial defect should be suspected. Also, if an early diastolic murmur suggesting aortic insufficiency is heard, this would suggest that the defect is of the subarterial type.

5 *What is the pulmonary arterial pressure?* Pulmonary arterial pressure and resistance can be assessed clinically from the second sound. An accentuated second sound signifies pulmonary arterial hypertension. If the sound is well split, pulmonary vascular resistance is probably not markedly increased, but a narrow or single accentuated sound indicates that pulmonary vascular resistance is greatly elevated.

Ventricular septal defects in infancy

Large defects

Infants with large defects and severe cardiac failure should be treated immediately with diuretics and possibly catecholamines such as dobutamine or dopamine. If the baby is having severe respiratory distress and is anxious and irritable, administration of morphine sulfate subcutaneously in a dose of 0.05–0.1 mg/kg is often helpful. It is desirable to administer the initial dose of diuretic (most commonly furosemide) intravenously or intramuscularly. Although it can be given intramuscularly, this is not recommended because it is extremely painful. Digitalis, most commonly administered intravenously as digoxin, was given routinely to these infants. However, recent evidence indicates that it is of little value, and currently its use is not recommended. If there is no improvement or pulmonary edema progresses despite the use of diuretics, intravenous infusion of catecholamine inotropic agents such as dopamine or dobutamine is currently widely recommended. Dopamine should not be infused at rates above about 5 μg/kg per min, because at higher doses it exerts significant α-adrenoceptor stimulation; the resultant increase in afterload may limit the increase in cardiac output achieved by lower doses. Recently, the use of catecholamine infusions has been questioned in treatment of preterm infants with systemic hypotension because there is no convincing evidence that this therapy alters the outcome (see Chapter 6). Whether it is beneficial in the treatment of infants with cardiac failure remains to be evaluated. Other cardiac inotropic agents, such as milrinone, have also been used in the treatment of acute cardiac failure, but their effectiveness has still to be evaluated.

As in any infant with cardiac failure, an ultrasound study should be performed on an urgent basis to define the lesion. It is important to do a careful and complete examination and if a large ventricular septal defect is identified, associated lesions such as atrioventricular canal defect, patent ductus arteriosus, coarctation of the aorta and other lesions should be excluded. If the diagnosis of an isolated ventricular septal defect is confirmed, the size and location of the defect and the number of defects should be defined. It is distinctly unusual that a defect in the muscular septum induces cardiac failure but if there are multiple defects in the muscular septum, the left-to-right shunt may be large and induce failure. Cardiac failure in infancy is most often associated with a perimembranous defect but occasionally with a subarterial defect.

If cardiac failure has developed in an infant with a ventricular septal defect without a precipitating cause such as infection, the likelihood that spontaneous closure will occur is quite small, particularly if the defect is of the perimembranous type. Also, even if the infant responds rapidly to medical therapy, mild manifestations of failure often persist, such as sweating, tachypnea and poor feeding and the infant fails to thrive. Closure of the defect is recommended in these infants (see below). If, for some reason, it is decided not to proceed with closure of the defect, it is very important to follow the baby carefully to evaluate the possible development of increasing pulmonary vascular resistance.

Small defects

The newborn infant with a murmur who is suspected on clinical diagnosis to have a small ventricular septal defect, who has no cardiovascular symptoms, no evidence of a large shunt or of pulmonary arterial hypertension, and in whom no other lesions are suspected may be followed without obtaining additional studies. The parents should be counseled to seek medical advice if the infant shows respiratory difficulty or sweating, or tires with feeding, and the infant reassessed at about 10 weeks of age to ensure that cardiac failure has not developed. If the murmur persists but the baby is asymptomatic and developing normally, the parents should be reassured that the lesion is not affecting heart function.

There is some controversy regarding performance of echocardiographic studies. Some advise that a study be done in early infancy to make a positive diagnosis. My opinion is that many unnecessary studies may be done, because the murmur, whether due to a tiny ventricular septal defect or some other mechanism, often disappears. I recommend the echocardiographic study be done about a year after birth if the murmur is still present. Because, as mentioned above, more than 75% of small ventricular septal defects will have closed by then, a large number of procedures can be avoided. Ultrasound studies are also not always infallible; occasionally a small defect is not evident by echocardiography or color flow Doppler studies on one occasion but is detected subsequently.

If the murmur disappears and there is no evidence of a defect on ultrasound, no further follow-up is necessary. If a bulging ventricular septal aneurysm develops with closure of the defect, the child is followed every 2–3 years. The reason for the long-term supervision is that, although highly unlikely, the aneurysm may increase in size and cause obstruction to right ventricular outflow (see above). Failure of the defect to close during infancy creates a dilemma.

Medium-sized defects

Infants with medium-sized defects who have clinical evidence of large shunts and moderate pulmonary hypertension should be studied by echocardiography to confirm the diagnosis, exclude lesions such as patent ductus arteriosus, aortic coarctation or double outlet right ventricle, and to attempt to assess right ventricular and pulmonary arterial pressures. This is done by measuring the velocity of a tricuspid regurgitant jet or of the jet across the defect.

If there is evidence of mild cardiac failure with cardiomegaly, or of obvious cardiac failure, the infant should be treated with diuretics. Usually the response is rapid, with improvement in respiration, decrease in liver size, lessening of sweating, and increased weight gain. If improvement occurs, it is reasonable to follow the infant in the hope that the defect will close spontaneously. The issues to be considered in the follow-up are (i) whether the cardiac failure improves; (ii) the concern that infection may cause recurrence of cardiac failure; (iii) the possibility that pulmonary vascular changes may occur; (iv) poor physical development; and (v) the size and location of the defect.

If cardiac failure does not improve considerably, addition of afterload-reducing drugs such as ACE inhibitors, peripheral α-adrenoceptor inhibitors, or calcium channel blockers may be considered; in general, these promote only limited additional improvement. Calcium channel blockers should not be given to young infants with cardiac failure because acute cardiovascular collapse has occurred after their administration. The decision then has to be made whether closure of the defect should be recommended. This will depend on the morbidity and mortality of the procedure in young infants in the center where the surgery is to be performed. If low, surgical closure should be recommended; if relatively high, it may be preferable to tolerate a modest degree of failure and continue with medical management, with the possibility that clinical improvement will occur gradually due to decrease in size of the defect.

Not infrequently in an infant with a medium-sized ventricular septal defect with cardiac failure who has had a satisfactory response to therapy, cardiac failure may recur in association with an infection. This is most common with respiratory infection, a common cause of which in infants is respiratory syncytial virus (RSV). All infants with ventricular septal defect and moderate to large shunts should receive prophylactic immunization against RSV by monthly palivizumab injections during the RSV season. The infant who is infected may become acutely ill, but it is unthinkable to consider surgery during the time of acute respiratory infection. Medical treatment should be continued and diuretic dosage should be increased during this period. The addition of an afterload reducer may also be considered. Infections should be treated aggressively with antibiotic or antiviral agents as indicated. Although it has previously been reported that RSV infections are associated with a very high mortality in infants with cardiac lesions, this is not our recent experience. This is probably because more aggressive treatment of failure is instituted, and the management of the respiratory infection has improved. However, use of prophylactic immunization is strongly recommended.

Pulmonary vascular changes are unlikely to develop to a significant degree in infants less than 6 months of age with isolated ventricular septal defects. Furthermore, with medium-sized defects, in which pulmonary arterial pressure is usually less than half systemic arterial pressure, the likelihood that significant pulmonary vascular endothelial proliferative and obstructive changes will develop within the first 2–3 years of life is quite small. Therefore, if it is possible to assess right ventricular and pulmonary arterial systolic pressure from the ultrasound study and they are estimated to be less than systemic arterial pressure, it is reasonable to follow the infant's progress with little concern for pulmonary vascular pathology. If the pressures are deemed to be greater than half the systemic arterial levels, the infant should be followed carefully, with repeat ultrasound studies within 3 months to assess the progress of pulmonary arterial pressure. If it is evident that it remains elevated, consideration should be given to closing the defect. If at any stage of the evaluation pulmonary arterial pressure can not be gauged definitively by ultrasound study, cardiac catheterization is indicated to accurately assess the hemodynamic status and pulmonary vascular resistance.

Some infants with medium-sized defects show mild respiratory symptoms, and some whose symptoms improve with therapy fail to thrive. Usually weight gain is affected more than height. This often occurs despite what is considered to be a normal caloric intake for an infant. As mentioned above, this is probably the result of increased metabolic rate. Measurement of oxygen consumption shows a value high for the infant's weight and body surface area, and catecholamine turnover is increased [4]. Associated conditions, including chromosomal defects, that may account for the poor physical development should be excluded. These infants should be assessed at 2–3 monthly intervals to determine whether they are growing. If weight follows the low percentile and is not falling further, it is reasonable to follow the infant; often, as the defect size decreases, weight gain improves. However, if weight percentile shows a downward trend, closure of the defect should be considered. In most infants with ventricular septal defect, head circumference is normal and increases normally with age. Occasionally, however, an infant who is not growing normally also shows a reduction in head growth. It has been suggested that this may be an indication for surgery, although there is no evidence that defect closure improves head circumferential growth. It is likely that factors other than the ventricular septal defect are responsible.

Surgery for ventricular septal defect

If cardiac failure persists or improvement is only modest, closure of the defect should be considered. It is desirable to close the defect with a device placed by an interventional cardiac catheterization procedure. However, although this has been accomplished successfully in older children with small or medium-sized defects, the procedure has been performed in only a small number of infants; it is still very difficult technically and has considerable complications, such as device embolization, arrhythmias, particularly complete heart block, and possible aortic valve damage. Currently, therefore, surgery is generally recommended in infants.

The decision regarding surgery, and the type of surgery, must be made on the basis of the relative risk in individual centers. In many centers, the risk of surgical closure of ventricular septal defects of most types is quite low, even in small preterm infants, so this is the procedure recommended. An exception to this recommendation is the presence of multiple defects. Because the inner wall of the right ventricle is heavily trabeculated, location of multiple defects may be very difficult. The procedure may be only partially successful and failure often persists. Also, the mortality of surgery to close multiple defects is higher than with single defect closure.

If the estimated risks are greater than 5%, the decision may be made to continue to manage the failure by medical measures until the infant is somewhat larger and the risks lower. The problem with this approach is that even if it is possible to achieve some improvement of cardiac failure, the infant usually grows very slowly, so surgery may be delayed for many months if the surgeon requests that the infant achieve a specified weight. An additional concern is that if the defect does not decrease in size, there is the risk that pulmonary vascular resistance may increase; significant increases in resistance have been observed within 6–9 months after birth.

A second surgical approach in the infant with cardiac failure is banding of the pulmonary artery. This procedure is now rarely performed for ventricular septal defect; it is recommended by some in infants who have multiple defects, because complete closure is frequently difficult to accomplish surgically. This procedure is designed to increase the outflow resistance of the right ventricle, thereby decreasing the left-to-right shunt and left ventricular end-diastolic and left atrial pressures. The main difficulty concerning pulmonary artery banding is that there are no specific guidelines for the surgeon as to what degree of narrowing to produce. The main pulmonary artery is constricted by various means; the ideal constriction is one that will reduce pulmonary blood flow enough to overcome cardiac failure but not severe enough to result in a right-to-left shunt.

Measurement of blood flow is not practicable at surgery, and pressure measurements have been used to give some indication of the adequacy of constriction. Usually the pulmonary artery is constricted to about 30–50% of its original diameter. Systolic pressure in the pulmonary artery is at systemic levels before operation, and the objective of the procedure is to band the main pulmonary artery sufficiently tightly to produce a systolic pressure of about 25–30 mmHg beyond the constriction. If the constriction is too tight there is enlargement of the right ventricle, cardiac slowing, and cyanosis and the band must be loosened immediately. If an adequate constriction is produced, the heart is noted to decrease in size and become less active and the anesthesiologist notices that pulmonary compliance increases. One of the main problems with the procedure is that even though the constriction may be perfect with the chest open and the baby anesthetized and ventilated by positive-pressure breathing, following closure of the chest and recovery there will be an alteration in both systemic and pulmonary vascular resistances. The banding then may be found to be inadequate or too severe. On the whole, it is really rather surprising that so many infants do improve and continue to do well for several years after banding. However, some infants with inadequate constriction show only moderate improvement in failure but can be controlled with medical measures reasonably well. Others develop cyanosis fairly soon, although failure is improved. A further problem is that with growth of the infant and increasing cardiac output, the band, which is a fixed constriction, becomes too tight and increasing cyanosis with hypoxemia and decreased exercise tolerance occur after a variable period.

The child with pulmonary arterial banding develops a loud systolic murmur at the upper left sternal border, which radiates to both lungs; some extension into diastole may occur. The second sound becomes widely split, with both components being well heard. When these patients are studied by cardiac catheterization, pulmonary arterial pressures are quite characteristic. In the segment between the pulmonary artery and the band, systolic pressure is equal to that in the right ventricle but the diastolic pressure is very low, often only slightly higher than right ventricular end-diastolic pressure, even though no pulmonary valve insufficiency is noted. This pressure tracing is characteristic of supravalvar stenosis of the aorta and pulmonary artery in general.

At some stage, the child should be subjected to closure of the ventricular septal defect, and the presence of the band complicates the subsequent repair, since it must be removed. In some instances, removal of the band allows the pulmonary artery to assume an adequate diameter, but it may be necessary to open the constricted fibrosed segment and reconstruct the vessel. If the child is not in any significant failure and has only mild cyanosis, operation may be delayed for 4–5 years; sometimes, however, earlier repair is necessary. Although it is unusual, occasionally the ventricular septal defect may decrease in size spontaneously, so that pressure in the right ventricle exceeds that in the left ventricle due to the obstructed outflow. In view of these difficulties with the banding procedure there has been an increasing reluctance to recommend it.

Ventricular septal defects beyond infancy

Large defects

It is becoming increasingly uncommon to encounter children beyond 1 year of age who have large ventricular septal defects, because most are closed surgically during infancy. However, some children are seen who have not had adequate medical care. There is the risk of progressive increase in pulmonary vascular resistance with age, and this becomes an important consideration regarding closure of the defect. Although it is unusual to encounter very high pulmonary vascular resistances before the age of 3–4 years in children living at sea level, high values may be noted occasionally. In patients living at altitudes above about 1550 m, pulmonary vascular resistance may be markedly increased at considerably earlier ages, as a result of the synergistic effects of increased pulmonary blood flow, elevated pulmonary arterial pressure, and relative hypoxia. As mentioned in Chapter 5, closure of the defect in patients with high pulmonary vascular resistance may not be well tolerated. Acute right ventricular failure with low cardiac output and shock may develop. If pulmonary vascular resistance does not fall after closure of the defect, chronic right ventricular failure may ensue.

The level of pulmonary vascular resistance at rest, breathing room air, at which it is generally considered that risk of closure is relatively low is about 8 mmHg/L per min per m^2 (resistance units). At levels above about 12 resistance units, closure of the defect is usually contraindicated. In the range 8–12 resistance units, the risks are very high. Cardiac catheterization is indicated in all children with suspected large defects to assess pulmonary vascular resistance and to evaluate its response to 100% oxygen inhalation and pulmonary vasodilators. Children with a high resting pulmonary vascular resistance that responds to these measures may tolerate closure of the defect quite well.

In all children with high pulmonary vascular resistance, the risks of surgery are greater; careful monitoring should be instituted in the postoperative period and ventilation and oxygenation should be carefully regulated, because pulmonary arterial pressure is very labile, and hypoxia may result in sudden and dramatic changes in resistance. Use of pulmonary vascular dilators is indicated to try to reduce pulmonary vascular resistance.

There is little to offer children with very high pulmonary vascular resistance. Vasodilator therapy, as discussed in Chapter 5, may improve functional capacity and prevent or delay progressive pulmonary vascular changes. When resistance is very high and not reactive, and the patient begins to become symptomatic, a remaining option is to perform a lung transplant and close the defect. Although immediate survival from this procedure seems promising, the long-term survival rates are still uncertain.

Medium-sized defects

This group of patients includes those infants who had large defects that have become smaller with age and those who have medium-sized defects that have not changed from infancy. If pulmonary arterial systolic pressure is 50–75% of systemic arterial systolic pressure, there is a definite risk of development of pulmonary vascular disease. However, this does not usually occur to a serious degree until beyond the age of 4 or 5 years. It is therefore reasonable to delay closing the defect until the age when interventional catheterization techniques seem feasible. However, the child should be observed to ensure that pulmonary vascular changes are not occurring. If there is any concern, the defect should be closed surgically.

If pulmonary arterial systolic pressure is less than 50% of systemic systolic pressure, the risk of developing pulmonary vascular disease is low, but there is a risk for infective endocarditis in association with the defect. Prophylactic antibiotic therapy was previously advised for all patients with ventricular septal defect of any size, but in June 2007 the recommendations were modified and now prophylaxis is not recommended for infective endocarditis [14].

The decision has to be made regarding if and when the defect should be closed. If defect size is decreasing on ultrasound examination, it is reasonable to delay surgery for many years. I have observed a patient in whom defect closure was documented as late as 17 years of age. One of the main concerns regarding patients with ventricular septal defect with moderate-sized left-to-right shunts is that the prolonged increased volume load on the left ventricle could result in myocardial damage with progressive dilation, including an increase in collagen formation, and that this could interfere with myocardial performance. This rationale has prompted the recommendation for closure of the defect even in the absence of symptoms. In a recent study, Kleinman *et al.* [15] followed 33 children with moderate left-to-right shunts with left ventricular dilation for a range of 2.8–22 years. In most of these patients, left ventricular end-diastolic dimension decreased over time; in only two was there a small increase. Thus in the majority of these individuals, surgical or device closure of the defect is contraindicated.

Small defects

Small defects do not impose any significant volume overload on the heart and are not associated with pulmonary vascular complications. There is a risk for the development of infective endocarditis, but this appears to be low with small defects.

Currently, closure of small defects is not usually advised. Possibly opinions may change if defects can be closed by interventional techniques with minimal risk and sequelae, but there seems to be little compelling reason to close a small ventricular septal defect at any age.

Doubly committed subarterial defects

The risks of pulmonary vascular disease and subacute bacterial endocarditis are similar in these defects to those in other ventricular septal defects, but there appears to be a much higher incidence of the development of aortic insufficiency in these patients. In view of this, some have advised closure of medium-sized and even small supracristal defects by 3–4 years of age, especially if ultrasound examination shows prolapse of the aortic annulus or a cusp, even in the absence of any obvious insufficiency. It was thought that this may prevent the onset of aortic insufficiency. However, there is considerable controversy regarding the likelihood for aortic insufficiency to develop. In a large study in Hong Kong, over a mean follow-up time of 8.6 years, aortic valve prolapse developed in 78%, and almost 80% of these developed aortic insufficiency. It was recommended that all defects with a diameter greater than 5 mm should be closed, but the risk seemed to be less with smaller defects [16]. There is disagreement about the relationship of size of the defect and the development of prolapse of the aortic cusp. Some suggest it is more likely to occur with small defects [17] but others consider closure of small defects is not indicated unless there is already evidence of prolapse [18].

Transcatheter closure of ventricular septal defects

Various devices have been developed to attempt to close ventricular septal defects by transcatheter techniques. Considerable success has been reported, but there is a relatively high risk of complications, many serious. The main devices currently being tested are the CardioSEAL and a modification STARFlex, and the Amplatzer device. The CardioSEAL device is a double umbrella with Nitinol metal arms attached to Dacron fabric. A modification, the STARFlex device, has a self-centering mechanism to aid in placement of the device. The Amplatzer Muscular VSD Occluder consists of two disks made of self-expanding Nitinol; it has been modified for closure of perimembranous defects. There are numerous reports of successful closure of both muscular and perimembranous defects with very low mortality. However, complications are frequent; most are transient, but some persist. Device embolization, vascular complications, and rhythm abnormalities are noted in about 15% of patients. The most serious problem is the development of complete heart block; this may occur during the procedure, but has developed at a later date. In a report from the European VSD Registry, transcatheter devices were placed in 430 patients with ventricular septal defect, of which 364 were Amplatzer devices. Procedures were successful in 95%, but complications included device embolization, aortic regurgitation, tricuspid regurgitation, and rhythm disturbances. One patient died and complete heart block developed in 16 patients, 10 of whom required pacemakers.

As mentioned above, the procedure is technically difficult in infants and has not been generally performed below the age of 3–4 years. It is in this age group that closure is predominantly indicated for relief of cardiac failure. A major concern is that, as the procedure is gaining acceptance, the indications for closing small to medium-sized defects will be relaxed and many patients not now considered candidates for surgical closure will be subjected to transcatheter closure unnecessarily.

References

1 Roguin N, Du ZD, Barak M, Nasser N, Hershkowitz S, Milgram E. High prevalence of muscular ventricular septal defect in neonates. J Am Coll Cardiol 1995;26: 1545–1548.

2 Paladini D, Palmieri S, Lamberti A, Teodoro A, Martinelli P, Nappi C. Characterization and natural history of ventricular septal defects in the fetus. Ultrasound Obstet Gynecol 2000;16:118–122.

3 Lister G, Walter TK, Versmold HT, Dallman PR, Rudolph AM. Oxygen delivery in lambs: cardiovascular and hematologic development. Am J Physiol 1979;237: H668–675.

4 Lees MH. Catecholamine metabolite excretion of infants with heart failure. J Pediatr 1966;69:259–265.

5 Lister G, Hellenbrand WE, Kleinman CS, Talner NS. Physiologic effects of increasing hemoglobin concentration in left-to-right shunting in infants with ventricular septal defects. N Engl J Med 1982;306:502–506.

6 Teisseire BP, Ropars C, Vallez MO, Herigault RA, Nicolau C. Physiological effects of high-P50 erythrocyte transfusion on piglets. J Appl Physiol 1985;58:1810–1817.

7 Hait G, Corpus M, Lamarre FR, Yuan SH, Kypson J, Cheng G. Alteration of glucose and insulin metabolism in congenital heart disease. Circulation 1972;46:333–346

8 Bland RD, Carlton DP, Scheerer RG, Cummings JJ, Chapman DL. Lung fluid balance in lambs before and after premature birth. J Clin Invest 1989;84:568–576.
9 Hoffman JI, Rudolph AM. The natural history of ventricular septal defects in infancy. Am J Cardiol 1965; 16:634–653.
10 Lin MH, Wang NK, Hung KL, Shen CT. Spontaneous closure of ventricular septal defects in the first year of life. J Formos Med Assoc 2001;100:539–542.
11 Hiraishi S, Agata Y, Nowatari M *et al.* Incidence and natural course of trabecular ventricular septal defect: two-dimensional echocardiography and color Doppler flow imaging study. J Pediatr 1992;120:409–415.
12 Tomita H, Arakaki Y, Yagihara T, Echigo S. Incidence of spontaneous closure of outlet ventricular septal defect. Jpn Circ J 2001;65:364–366.
13 Mellins RB, Cheng G, Ellis K, Jameson AG, Malm JR, Blumenthal S. Ventricular septal defect with shunt from left ventricle to right atrium. Bacterial endocarditis as a complication. Br Heart J 1964;26:584–591.
14 Wilson W, Taubert KA, Gewitz M *et al.* Prevention of infective endocarditis: guidelines from the American Heart Association: a guideline from the American Heart Association Rheumatic Fever, Endocarditis, and Kawasaki Disease Committee, Council on Cardiovascular Disease in the Young, and the Council on Clinical Cardiology, Council on Cardiovascular Surgery and Anesthesia, and the Quality of Care and Outcomes Research Interdisciplinary Working Group. Circulation 2007;116:1736–1754.
15 Kleinman CS, Tabbian M, Starc TJ, Hsu DT, Gersony WM. Spontaneous regression of left ventricular dilation in children with restrictive ventricular septal defects. J Pediatr 2007;150:583–586.
16 Lun K, Li H, Leung MP *et al.* Analysis of indications for surgical closure of subarterial ventricular septal defect without associated aortic cusp prolapse and aortic regurgitation. Am J Cardiol 2001;87:1266–1270.
17 Hernández Morales G, Vázquez Antona CA, Muñoz Castellanos L *et al.* Aortic valve complications associated with subarterial infundibular ventricular septal defect. Echocardiograpic follow-up. Rev Esp Cardiol 2002;55: 936–942.
18 Bütter A, Duncan W, Weatherdon D, Hosking M, Cornel G. Aortic cusp prolapse in ventricular septal defect and its association with aortic regurgitation: appropriate timing of surgical repair and outcomes. Can J Cardiol 1998;14: 833–840.

8

CHAPTER 8

Atrial septal defect and partial anomalous drainage of the pulmonary veins

In this chapter, interatrial communications that do not involve development of the septum primum and the endocardial cushions are discussed. These communications occur in three main sites:

1 in the central portion of the atrial septum in the position of the foramen ovale, termed *fossa ovalis or secundum defects*;

2 in the region of the junction of the superior vena cava (SVC) and right atrium, termed *sinus venosus defects*;

3 between the left atrium and the coronary sinus at its ostium into the right atrium, termed *unroofing of the coronary sinus.*

Defects of the atrial septum associated with abnormal development of the septum primum and the endocardial cushions are presented in Chapter 9.

In this chapter, only isolated atrial septal defects are discussed. Interatrial communications are common in association with other defects and may be crucial for survival. Thus in patients with tricuspid or pulmonary atresia, or with total anomalous pulmonary venous return, the interatrial opening is essential for blood flow into the left atrium and ventricle to maintain systemic blood flow. In the presence of mitral atresia and hypoplastic left ventricle, an interatrial communication is the only pathway for pulmonary venous blood to return to the right side of the heart. In infants with aortopulmonary transposition, in the absence of a ventricular septal defect, an interatrial communication may allow bidirectional flow adequate to permit survival.

Congenital Diseases of the Heart, 3rd edition. By A. Rudolph
 ISBN: 9781405162456

An atrial defect is not uncommonly associated with aortic coarctation, aortic stenosis, patent ductus arteriosus, or ventricular septal defect in infants and may complicate the clinical features of these lesions.

I have included a section on partial anomalous drainage of the pulmonary veins because the hemodynamic changes and clinical manifestations of this anomaly and atrial septal defects are almost identical. In fact, atrial septal defects are found in association with all but a rare case of partial pulmonary venous drainage anomaly, and these are the instances in which the right pulmonary veins drain into the inferior vena cava (IVC).

Interatrial communications, other than patent foramen ovale, comprise about 7–8% of all congenital cardiac defects; about two-thirds of these are fossa ovalis or sinus venosus defects. Atrial septal defect is a feature of two conditions inherited in an autosomal dominant manner. Holt–Oram syndrome includes upper limb bony abnormalities such as absent radius bones and prolonged atrioventricular conduction; the other is a syndrome of atrial septal defect with prolonged atrioventricular conduction without bony anomalies. Partial anomalous pulmonary venous drainage has been noted in about 10% of the reported cases, but it is of interest that it is not commonly associated with atrial defects of the endocardial cushion type, including ostium primum defect and common atrium.

Morphological and embryological considerations

Separation of the two atria commences when the septum primum grows into the common chamber from the posterosuperior portion of the wall and moves toward the atrioventricular junction, where the developing endocardial cushions are separating the atria and the ventricles. The lower part of the septum primum is completed by fusion with endocardial cushion tissue, but prior to the complete closure of the septum primum, a number of fenestrations develop in its mid-portion, thus maintaining a continuing communication between the atria. A second septum, the septum secundum, then develops in the posterosuperior region of the atrial wall, just to the right of the septum primum and it too grows inward to the atrioventricular junction. It has a semilunar edge that is concave anteroinferiorly and this margin only partly covers the central hole in the septum primum; it forms the crista dividens of the fetal heart.

Atrial septal defects of the so-called secundum type usually occur in the region of the fossa ovalis, i.e., anterior to the rim of the crista dividens. They could be due to either an excessively large central hole in the septum primum or to inadequate development of the septum secundum. Although these disturbances may be primarily local developmental defects, the possibility that hemodynamic changes in flow patterns from the SVC and IVC may influence atrial septal development during fetal life should be considered. Since SVC blood is directed into the tricuspid valve and a considerable proportion of IVC return passes through the foramen ovale, it is possible that a decrease in SVC or an increase in IVC flow could influence the size of the normal fetal atrial opening. The defects vary greatly in size. A small opening beneath the limbus of the fossa ovalis region represents persistence of the foramen ovale. Large openings may extend anteroinferiorly to the atrioventricular valve region or posteriorly and superiorly to the SVC or IVC entry. However, there is always a rim of septum present along the anteroinferior margin, which is the endocardial cushion contribution to the atrial septum. Sometimes two or even more openings may be found in the fossa ovalis region, with strands of septal tissue separating them.

Patency of the foramen ovale persists through childhood into adult life in about 25% of the population. The opening, not more than a few millimeters in size, is the result of incomplete sealing of the septum secundum to the septum primum. The septum secundum usually completely covers the defect from the right side and, because after birth left atrial pressure is higher than right atrial pressure, the opening is functionally closed by apposition of the two septa. However, when right atrial pressure is increased, shunting from the right to left atrium may occur through the opening.

Incompetence of the foramen ovale occurs quite frequently in infants. If the foramen is examined, it is often noted, even in apparently normal hearts, that the limbus of the fossa does not completely cover the opening when it is apposed to the membranous valve-like portion, and a small opening is evident. In some infants who have left atrial enlargement due to associated lesions, such as aortic stenosis, patent ductus arteriosus or ventricular septal defect, the septum bulges into the right atrium and an orifice of variable size results due to stretching of the normal foramen. Occasionally, when the membranous portion of the valve of the foramen is redundant, it has been seen to herniate through the foramen, resulting in an opening of considerable size.

The embryological basis for partial anomalous pulmonary venous connection to the systemic venous system is obscure. It has been suggested that it is due to partial premature obliteration of the common pulmonary vein at a time when there is still a communication through channels of pulmonary and systemic venous systems and that one or more of these channels persist. The pulmonary veins from the right lung usually connect with portions of the systemic venous system derived from the right cardinal system, namely the SVC and IVC and the right atrium. The left veins connect with elements of the left cardinal system, the coronary sinus and the left innominate vein, but this is not always the case. The majority of patients with anomalous pulmonary venous drainage have associated atrial septal defects of the fossa ovalis type. In the unusual instances in which the atrial septum is intact, the most frequent abnormality is drainage of the right pulmonary veins to the IVC. This has been termed the vena cava–bronchovascular syndrome or *scimitar syndrome*. The right lower lobe vein or all the right pulmonary veins drain into the IVC just above or below the diaphragm. This syndrome is characterized by associated hypoplasia of the right lung and often an arterial supply to the lower lobe by an artery arising from the abdominal aorta and passing through the diaphragm to the lung (sequestration of the lower lobe).

The development of sinus venosus defects is even more difficult to explain. These defects are located in the posterosuperior portion of the atrial septum and may even extend into the SVC. Developmentally, they probably should not, strictly speaking, be considered atrial septal defects, because they are not related to abnormalities of the septum primum or secundum. A possible mechanism for their development has been proposed. As the right lung grows, the upper right pulmonary vein becomes apposed to the surface of the SVC and the walls of these two venous structures fuse in this region, forming a membrane that is continuous with the atrial septum. If, for some unexplained reason, this membrane degenerates, a connection between the right upper pulmonary vein and the SVC would develop. With further growth, this may enlarge and thus appear to extend into the upper posterior portion of the atrial septum. The location of the sinus venosus defect is such that on looking into it from the right atrium and the SVC, the right pulmonary vein can be seen directly related to the opening. In some instances, the lower margin appears to project forward so that the SVC seems to be overriding the defect.

Coronary sinus defects result from either failure of development, or resorption, of the common thin wall separating the coronary sinus and the left atrium. They may involve a portion, or the whole, of this wall. These defects are also termed "unroofing of the coronary sinus" and are frequently associated with a persistent left SVC, which drains into the coronary sinus.

Hemodynamic considerations

Fetal circulation

Since normally there is a large communication between the two atria in the fetus, it is unlikely that an additional developmental atrial septal abnormality would profoundly affect the fetal circulation. The main effects that may result are that flow patterns of SVC and IVC returns may be modified. Normally, in the lamb fetus, IVC blood is split into two streams over the crista dividens as it enters the atria. One stream, comprising about 40% of the total and consisting mainly of well-oxygenated ductus venosus blood, passes directly into the left atrium; the remainder passes into the right atrium. It is possible that if there were a larger than normal central defect of the septum primum, more ductus venosus blood could enter the left atrium, increasing the blood oxygen content of the left ventricle as well as the ascending aorta. The right ventricle would receive less ductus venosus blood, and relatively more SVC and distal IVC blood. Right ventricular and pulmonary arterial Po_2 would therefore be reduced somewhat. Because descending aortic blood is derived from the pulmonary artery through the ductus arteriosus, its oxygen content could be slightly reduced and there would be a wider than normal oxygen content difference between ascending and descending aortic blood. If the reduction in Po_2 of blood moving to the lungs is great enough, it could perhaps maintain a higher pulmonary vascular resistance and stimulate greater than normal development of pulmonary vascular smooth muscle.

However, if the defect was related to inadequate development of the septum secundum, with a high crista dividens not related to the IVC, or if the defect were of the sinus venosus type, the effect on venous flow patterns might be quite different. The effect of the crista dividens in deflecting IVC flow into the left atrium could be lost or reduced, and in sinus venosus defects there may indeed be preferential flow of SVC blood into the left atrium. The normal separation between left and right atrial Po_2 and therefore of ascending and descending aortic Po_2 would be reduced. The somewhat higher than normal Po_2 in blood distributed to the lungs could possibly achieve a lower than normal pulmonary vascular resistance and effect a reduction in development of the smooth muscle layer in the pulmonary arterioles (see Chapter 5). Apparently any changes of this type do not materially affect fetal development, because most newborn infants with atrial septal defects are physically normal in relation to gestational age.

Partial anomalous pulmonary venous drainage probably does not have any significant influence on the fetal circulation. Because pulmonary blood flow in the fetus is quite low, comprising only 8–10% of combined ventricular output in the fetal lamb, the drainage of one or two veins to the systemic venous system would provide only 2–3% of combined ventricular output, a relatively insignificant amount. In the human fetus, in which pulmonary blood flow constitutes up to 25% of combined ventricular output, each pulmonary vein would carry only about 6–7% of combined ventricular output.

Postnatal circulation

Normal and abnormal foramen ovale

Dramatic changes in the flow and pressure relationships of the major veins and left and right atria occur after birth. IVC flow is markedly reduced by elimination of umbilical venous return. Ventilation of the lungs with air results in a marked increase in flow through the lungs and in pulmonary venous return to the left atrium. Before birth, the pressure in the vena cava and the right atrium exceeds that in the left atrium. With the change in flow patterns after birth there is a reversal of pressure relationships, the mean left atrial pressure being about 1–2 mmHg higher than right atrial pressure. This small pressure difference is adequate to close the foramen ovale functionally by pressing the membranous valve against the upper portion of the septum. A contributory factor to closure of the foramen is the reduction in velocity of the stream from the ductus venosus through the IVC passing to the left of the crista dividens during fetal life because umbilical venous return is disrupted.

In the immediate postnatal period, before the lungs are fully expanded, there is a period of several hours during which blood may shunt from the right to the left atrium, since the atrial pressures are still similar and may be altered by many factors. This shunt may be phasic in nature, occurring particularly during atrial systole, since the *a* wave in the right atrium is higher than that in the left atrium after birth. In most normal infants, the atrial right-to-left shunt is not evident after a few hours, based on measurements of systemic arterial Po_2. However, there are many factors that may result in recurrence of the right-to-left shunt. Crying or breath-holding may increase pulmonary vascular resistance, resulting in a rise in right ventricular and right atrial pressure and shunting across the foramen ovale. A common cause of shunting in infancy is pulmonary disease, particularly idiopathic respiratory distress syndrome. The hypoxia associated with inadequate alveolar ventilation produces pulmonary vasoconstriction, which may be accentuated by metabolic acidemia. The resulting pulmonary arterial and right ventricular hypertension and increased right ventricular end-diastolic and right atrial pressures produce right-to-left atrial shunts that may be quite large, as much as 50% or more of systemic venous return. Similar effects of hypoxia on pulmonary vessels after birth occur in infants born at high altitude, and often they have atrial left-to-right shunting for a longer period after birth than those at sea level.

The foramen ovale usually becomes anatomically sealed within about 2–3 months after birth, but it may be patent for a longer time, and a small opening persists in 15–25% of individuals into adult life. It is of interest that in individuals who have cardiac lesions that produce a persistent increase in left atrial pressure in childhood or adolescence, the foramen ovale is rarely patent.

In many congenital cardiac defects, survival after birth depends on persistent patency of the foramen ovale. Thus in those conditions associated with obstruction to the right side of the heart, such as tricuspid atresia or pulmonary atresia with intact ventricular septum, the foramen ovale is necessary to provide systemic blood flow. This is also the manner by which systemic flow is provided in total anomalous pulmonary venous drainage. The foramen ovale is also important in aortopulmonary transposition and mitral atresia. The role of the foramen ovale is discussed in the chapters describing these lesions.

Although the frequency of right-to-left shunt through the foramen ovale after birth has been well recognized, the occurrence of left-to-right shunts through the foramen ovale after birth has not been fully appreciated. In a number of infants without any evidence of congenital heart lesions, but studied by cardiac catheterization and angiography for various reasons, left-to-right shunt through the foramen ovale was demonstrated [1]. The shunts were considerable, with ratios of pulmonary to systemic flow as high as 2:1 during infancy. However, within several months, the shunts decreased and could not be detected by 18–24 months. It is likely that the foramen ovale is incompetent because the inferior septum primum flap does not fully seal at the upper margin against the crista dividens. These infants do not have any symptoms directly related to the incompetent foramen ovale, but some pulmonary ejection murmurs could be related to the increased pulmonary blood flow. The fate of the foramen ovale in these children is not known. The incompetent foramen ovale in the otherwise normal circulation probably becomes smaller as the child grows and it may eventually close. It is also possible, however, that these individuals continue to have small openings of the foramen ovale throughout life.

This shunting of blood through the foramen ovale in the absence of a true atrial septal defect is exaggerated in many infants who have lesions that result in left atrial pressure elevation, such as patent ductus arteriosus, ventricular septal defect, aortic coarctation, and aortic stenosis. Considering the mechanism by which the foramen is closed normally, one might expect that this would favor early and effective closure. The shunt through the foramen ovale in these infants may be enormous, producing pulmonary to systemic flow ratios of 3:1 or greater. The foramen ovale is stretched by bulging of the atrial septum associated with left atrial enlargement, and thus it becomes incompetent. There thus appears to be a spectrum of competence of the foramen ovale (Figure 8.1). In some infants, the valve of the foramen reaches well beyond the crista dividens and it is always competent after

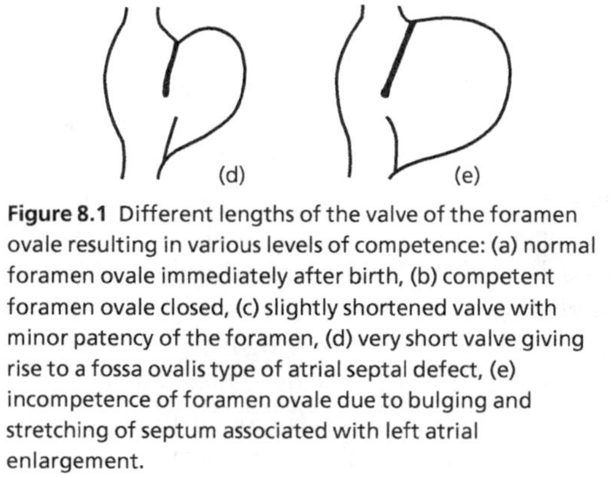

Figure 8.1 Different lengths of the valve of the foramen ovale resulting in various levels of competence: (a) normal foramen ovale immediately after birth, (b) competent foramen ovale closed, (c) slightly shortened valve with minor patency of the foramen, (d) very short valve giving rise to a fossa ovalis type of atrial septal defect, (e) incompetence of foramen ovale due to bulging and stretching of septum associated with left atrial enlargement.

birth. In others, there is apposition of the two septa, with only a small degree of overlap, so that when the atrial septum is stretched by left atrial hypertension there is separation with incompetence. Atrial left-to-right shunts have been shown to disappear in infants after closure of a ventricular septal defect or a patent ductus arteriosus.

Atrial septal defect

When there is a communication between the atria, the circulatory changes after birth favor alteration of the prenatal right-to-left flow to a left-to-right shunt. The magnitude of the left-to-right shunt will be determined by the size of the communication and the relative outflow resistances from the atria into the respective ventricles or inflow resistances of the ventricles.

The size of the defect that will permit a large atrial shunt is greater than with defects of the ventricular septum or aortopulmonary communications. The atria are low-pressure chambers, and the pressure differences between the left and right sides are considerably lower than those encountered in the ejection portion of the heart. Large atrial septal defects may be considered as those that have a diameter equal to or greater than that of the mitral valve. If the defect is large, it is nonrestrictive and pressures between the atria are similar. Mean as well as phasic pressures are almost equal, although left atrial pressure is slightly higher than right atrial pressure throughout most of the cardiac cycle. Because atrial filling pressures are similar, flow through the mitral and tricuspid valves and the magnitude and direction of shunt will be related to the relative inflow resistances of the left and right ventricles.

The concept that the inflow into the ventricles is determined by the distensibility (compliance) of the chamber, and that this is related to muscle thickness, has been widely accepted. This hypothesis has been used to explain the fact that infants with atrial septal defect rarely have any symptoms and, in fact, often do not show the usual clinical features encountered in older children. It has been suggested that because left and right ventricular muscle masses are similar postnatally, they have equal compliances and therefore no atrial shunt occurs. Soon after birth, the left ventricular myocardium grows rapidly and wall thickness increases, resulting in a change in compliance over a period of several months. Because pulmonary vascular resistance and right ventricular pressure fall, the right ventricular myocardium does not grow as rapidly as the left ventricular muscle after birth, the wall of the right ventricle becomes thinner than that of the left, and its compliance becomes relatively higher. The left-to-right shunt, it is postulated, parallels these changes in relative muscle mass. It has been difficult to explain, on the basis of this hypothesis alone, the fact that in catheterization studies, infants with equal or almost equal left and right atrial pressures have shown large atrial left-to-right shunts within a few days after birth.

The presence of the shunt within a few hours after birth can be explained by the changes in pulmonary and systemic vascular resistances. The volume of blood ejected by a ventricle is related to the preload (end-diastolic volume), myocardial contractility, and afterload (outflow resistance). The preload is determined by the filling pressure (end-diastolic and atrial pressures) and by the compliance of the ventricular wall. Myocardial contractility will not be discussed further at this stage, as it can be assumed that the two ventricles are under similar sympathetic and catecholamine stimulation and are being influenced similarly by other factors affecting the muscle. Afterload, or outflow resistance, is dependent on changes in pulmonary and systemic vascular resistances. In the presence of a large atrial defect, atrial pressures are almost equal and thus filling pressures are equal. If it is assumed that the compliances of the two ventricles are equal after birth, they will be filled to the same extent and thus preload is similar. With ventricular systole, the pulmonary and systemic vascular resistances determine the stroke volume. In the immediate postnatal period, with resistances nearly equal, the volumes ejected would be the same and the end-systolic or residual volume would also be the same. No atrial shunt of significance would occur. When pulmonary vascular resistance falls below systemic vascular resistance, the stroke volume of the right ventricle will exceed that of the left and the residual volume and therefore pressure at the end of systole will be lower in the right ventricle. If left and right atrial pressures are equal, the pressure difference between atria and ventricles will be greater on the right side, so more blood will flow into that ventricle. Progressive decline in right ventricular afterload as pulmonary vascular resistance falls will result in an increasing stroke volume, smaller residual volume, and augmented filling from the right and also the left atrium, with the development of an increasing left-to-right shunt. The continuing increase in systemic vascular resistance that gradually occurs after the immediate rapid rise at birth will accentuate the difference in afterloads and thus the left-to-right shunt. The left-to-right shunt in atrial septal defect may thus be considered a *dependent shunt*, in that it is dependent on changes in pulmonary and systemic vascular resistances.

The fall in pulmonary vascular resistance follows the normal pattern seen after birth. Since there are no ventricular or aortopulmonary communications, high pulmonary arterial pressure is not maintained. It is possible that the increased flow that occurs as the result of the left-to-right shunt could have some effect in retarding the maturational change in the pulmonary vessels but, if so, it is not striking. As the pulmonary arterial and right ventricular pressures fall, the right ventricular muscle thins relative to the left. This is not due to actual atrophy or loss of mass but to the rapid increase in left ventricular mass, whereas right ventricular mass is stationary. After about 10–14 days, growth of both ventricles is relatively proportionate. This relative decrease in right ventricular muscle may also result in greater compliance of the right ventricle relative to the left, allowing it to distend more at the same filling pressure, thus increasing the preload, the fiber length of the right ventricular myocardium, and further increasing its stroke volume.

The points in the above discussion regarding the development of shunting in patients with atrial septal defects are graphically demonstrated in Figure 8.2, which shows two pressure–volume (i.e., compliance) curves. The solid line shows an arbitrary pressure–volume curve of both the left and right ventricles at about 2–5 days after birth; they are superimposed, since right and left ventricular mass is similar. With ejection against different afterloads, the left ventricle has a smaller stroke volume than the right, and right ventricular end-systolic pressure (RES) is lower than left ventricular end-systolic pressure (LES). In this example, the stroke volume of the right ventricle (RSV_1) is

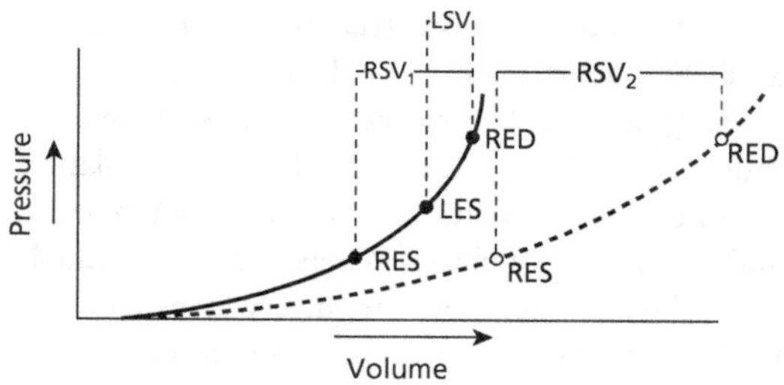

Figure 8.2 Effects of changes in stroke volumes of left and right ventricles associated with changes in pulmonary vascular resistance and with changes in compliance of the respective ventricles after birth in the presence of an atrial septal defect. Detailed description is given in the text.

2.5 times that of the left ventricle (LSV). When the right ventricular wall becomes relatively thinner than the left, the compliance curve moves to the right, as shown by the broken curve. At the same end-diastolic pressure (RED) the ventricle is now much more distended because of the higher compliance. With systole, if both the right and left ventricular end-systolic pressures are the same as with the early curve, the stroke volume of the right ventricle (RSV_2) will be five times that of the left.

The relationship of systemic and pulmonary vascular resistances is important not only in the development of shunting postnatally but also in later life. The effects of vascular resistance changes on shunting patterns have been shown clearly by Douglas *et al.* [2] in adult dogs with surgically created atrial septal defects. A reduction in systemic vascular resistance or a rise in pulmonary vascular resistance decreases left-to-right shunt. Similarly, right ventricular outflow obstruction by pulmonary stenosis will decrease left-to-right shunting and, if severe enough, could precipitate right-to-left shunt across the atrial septal defect. Also, left-sided obstructive lesions, such as aortic stenosis and aortic coarctation, may aggravate the left-to-right shunt.

The effect of atrial shunting on the circulation is to markedly increase blood flow returning to the right atrium and ventricle (Figure 8.3). With large defects, they both enlarge considerably, as do the pulmonary arteries; pulmonary venous and left atrial return also increases greatly. The right ventricle usually tolerates the extra volume load quite well, since it is handling a large volume at low ejection pressures. Occasionally, cardiac failure

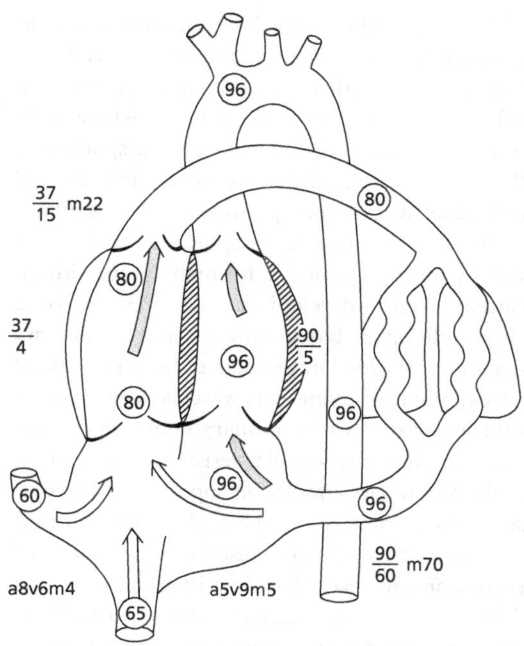

Figure 8.3 Atrial septal defect with moderate left-to-right shunt: course of the circulation, oxygen saturations (circled), and pressures in the heart and great vessels. m, mean pressure.

develops in infancy, but this is quite unusual, and the possibility exists that it is precipitated by such complicating factors as hypoxia or infections involving the myocardium. We have noted an interesting occurrence of a high hematocrit in several newborn infants with atrial septal defect who developed cardiac failure. Whether the atrial left-to-right shunt played a part is difficult to say, as failure occurs in infants with high hematocrit without atrial left-to-right shunts. However, if the high viscosity resulting from the high hematocrit effectively increases the pulmonary and systemic vascular resistances, the left-to-right shunt would still occur but the right ventricle, now confronted with a combined pressure and volume load, may fail.

If infants with atrial septal defects develop pulmonary disease with a high pulmonary vascular resistance due to hypoxia, the left-to-right shunt decreases in magnitude, and right-to-left shunt may occur with resultant cyanosis. Episodic cyanosis may also be seen with crying or breath-holding, presumably due to the effect on pulmonary vascular resistance.

The large volume of blood entering the right ventricle results in dilation and also in prolongation of right ventricular systole, as compared with left ventricular systole, throughout the whole of the respiratory cycle. This results in wide splitting of the second sound, which does not, as in the normal individual, narrow on expiration (see Chapter 8).

The large volume loads appear to be handled well by the right ventricle for many years without cardiac failure developing. The presence of a large pulmonary blood flow without pulmonary hypertension does not produce the same risk of development of pulmonary vascular disease as in ventricular or aortopulmonary communications. In fact, pulmonary vascular resistance is quite low, as the pulmonary circulation appears to dilate passively to accommodate the high flow. The pulmonary vascular smooth muscle undergoes normal regression. However, there is a risk to the patient of development of secondary vascular changes. These are rather slow to develop and are variable in different individuals. It is uncommon to find marked changes before the age of 15–25 years, and most often they are delayed even longer. Rarely, however, pulmonary vascular disease is marked by 8–10 years of age, but it is difficult to determine whether these are patients with primary pulmonary hypertension who coincidentally also have an atrial septal defect. It is also possible that these patients are genetically prone to develop pulmonary vascular disease (see Chapter 5).

In patients with atrial septal defect who develop pulmonary vascular changes, the first manifestations are those of intimal proliferation, which may be patchy. This is followed by gradual occlusion of the lumens of the small vessels, and some degree of thrombosis occurs on the occluded area, with organization and fibrosis. The changes are probably initiated by the shear forces induced by the high-velocity flow on the endothelial lining of the small vessels, occurring over many years (see Chapter 5). When pulmonary vascular resistance begins to increase, left-to-right shunting is decreased and right ventricular and pulmonary arterial pressures increase; there is progressive pulmonary arterial hypertension and the shunt becomes reversed to right to left, with development of cyanosis, and death occurs from heart failure or pulmonary hemorrhage.

When patients with atrial septal defect reach adult life, apart from the risk of developing pulmonary vascular disease, the main cause of deterioration is atrial arrhythmia, particularly fibrillation or flutter and probably due to atrial enlargement, and right heart failure. When these individuals reach the age when coronary artery disease or systemic hypertension produces interference in left ventricular function, they do not develop evidence of left heart failure but rather that of right heart failure. The high end-diastolic pressure in the left ventricle results in left atrial pressure elevation; this is transmitted to the right atrium and congestion of the systemic rather than the pulmonary venous system is manifested.

Patterns of shunting

Effects of respiration

Respiration influences the pattern of shunting across atrial septal defects. During inspiration, venous return to the right atrium increases as a result of the development of a larger intrathoracic negative pressure. Venous return from the pulmonary veins to the left atrium falls because the volume of blood in pulmonary vessels is greater. Thus during inspiration there is a decrease in the left-to-right shunt across the defect and a small right-to-left shunt might occur in this phase of the respiratory cycle. During expiration, with the increase in intrathoracic pressure, systemic venous return to the right atrium decreases; also, pulmonary venous return to the left atrium increases. These events result in an increase in left-to-right and a decrease in right-to-left shunt through the defect.

Effect of cardiac cycle

The changes in shunting patterns during the cardiac cycle have been examined by cineangiography, as well as ultrasound techniques [3]. The maximal left-to-right shunt occurs during ventricular systole, particularly in late systole, at the time of the peak of the *v* wave. This coincides with the time of greatest difference between left and right atrial pressures. A small right-to-left shunt may occur at the beginning of ventricular diastole; this is probably the result of the rapid systemic venous flow into the atrium at this time, with passage of some IVC blood across the defect. A small right-to-left shunt may occur at the onset of ventricular contraction.

Pattern of blood flow

Dye dilution studies, with selective injection of dye into the right and left pulmonary arteries, have shown that in fossa ovalis defects there is greater shunting from the right pulmonary veins than from the left [4]. As much as 80% of the right pulmonary arterial flow may be shunted across the defect as compared with only 20–40% of left pulmonary flow. This seems to be related to the location of the defect in the septum, as this difference is not noted in patients with defects located low in the septum in association with atrioventricular septal defects. With sinus venosus defects, almost all the drainage of the upper right pulmonary veins may cross the defect directly to the right atrium or SVC, because the pulmonary vein entry is closely related to the defect.

Although significant right-to-left shunts do not occur with atrial septal defects unless right ventricular outflow resistance rises, small right-to-left shunts have been detected by indicator dilution techniques, and this has been confirmed by ultrasound studies. These are noted most commonly in patients with sinus venosus defects, in whom there may be right-to-left shunts from the SVC, since the defect is so closely related to this vessel and streaming may occur directly into the left atrium. These shunts are usually small, but on rare occasions may be of consequence and reduce systemic arterial oxygen saturation slightly. In patients with fossa ovalis defects, small right-to-left shunts may be noted from the IVC across the defect. Most often these are detected in infants or young children. They can be exaggerated by suddenly increasing venous return from the IVC and can be demonstrated by a number of physiological maneuvers of the circulation. If systemic arterial oxygen saturation is continuously monitored by an ear oximeter, rapid changes can be detected. In patients with large atrial septal defects, a Valsalva maneuver causes a drop in systemic arterial oxygen saturation within 3–4 s after the release. This is due to peripheral venous pooling; with release, there is a sudden increase in IVC return, with a small right-to-left shunt. In some individuals, a small fall in peripheral arterial oxygen saturation is also noted with exercise. This is probably due to a combination of two factors: the decrease in systemic vascular resistance favors filling of the left ventricle relative to the right, and the increased IVC return may increase flow across the defect because of the increased velocity of IVC flow.

Effect of posture

Shunting may also be affected by posture. In the erect position, right-to-left shunting is unusual, probably because pooling of blood in the lower limbs reduces IVC flow. However, right-to-left shunting may occur in the recumbent position, associated with the increased IVC flow.

The changes in shunting patterns help explain the fact that most patients with atrial septal defects have good exercise tolerance. During exercise, the relatively greater decrease in systemic vascular resistance would favor emptying of the left ventricle during systole. Since left ventricular end-systolic volume is lower, preferential filling of the left ventricle would occur, with less left-to-right shunt across the defect. Pulmonary vascular resistance, which is already very low, would not change and thus right ventricular emptying would not be significantly influenced by afterload changes. The increased venous return to the right atrium would compete with the flow across the defect during right ventricular filling and so total left-to-right shunt would be reduced and systemic blood flow well maintained.

Partial anomalous pulmonary venous drainage

After birth, pulmonary venous return increases as pulmonary vascular resistance falls. There is thus a direct relationship between the magnitude of the pulmonary venous return to the systemic circulation, which is effectively a left-to-right shunt, and the drop in pulmonary vascular resistance. The magnitude of shunt occurring immediately after birth directly through each anomalous pulmonary vein is not very large, and it is related to the number of abnormally connected veins. However, the flow through each vein is considerably higher than what might be expected if only the normal venous drainage returned from the respective lobe of the lung. This is related to the fact that the veins are draining into the right atrium, in which, soon after birth, the pressure falls below that of the left atrium, so that the total resistance to flow from the pulmonary artery to the right atrium is lower. Also, in a manner similar to that described for the development of shunting in atrial septal defects, the decrease in end-systolic volume and pressure in the right ventricle associated with a decrease in pulmonary resistance after birth will accentuate the flow from the pulmonary veins draining into the right atrium. Since pulmonary arterial pressure is equal in the left and right sides, the magnitude of flow to the vein with anomalous drainage is related to differences in outflow resistance. Since most partial anomalous pulmonary venous drainage is associated with an atrial septal defect, it is difficult to assess how much left-to-right shunt is occurring through the veins as compared with the defect. In those cases in which there is a large associated atrial septal defect, the ratios of flow from the normal and abnormal pulmonary veins are probably not very different from usual, since left and right atrial pressures are equal. The abnormal hemodynamics and the subsequent course of these patients are similar to those described above for atrial septal defects.

Clinical features

The clinical presentation of patients with atrial septal defect depends on age, size of the defect, location of the defect, and presence of associated increase in pulmonary vascular resistance.

Atrial septal defects in infancy

Premature infants

Most preterm infants with atrial septal defect do not have symptoms. However, premature infants with a moderate-sized or large defect occasionally present with persistent respiratory distress and pulmonary edema. Usually these infants develop respiratory distress syndrome (hyaline membrane disease) within the first 2–3 days after birth; although they improve after several days, the respiratory distress may persist and the infant continues to be ventilator dependent. Prior to the introduction of ultrasound, cardiac catheterization revealed the presence of atrial septal defects in some preterm infants with persistent respiratory distress. The magnitude of the left-to-right shunts varied, with pulmonary to systemic blood flow ratios ranging from 1.5:1 to greater than 2.5:1. Yet even when the shunt was relatively small, closure of the defect resulted in rapid improvement of the respiratory symptoms, and it was possible to wean the infant off assisted ventilation. Because closure of an atrial septal defect has been so effective in some of these infants, it is strongly recommended that any infant with bronchopulmonary dysplasia with severe respiratory distress should have an echocardiogram to exclude the presence of an atrial defect with a left-to-right shunt.

The mechanism by which the atrial left-to-right shunt causes respiratory distress is not known. It appears that the symptoms are related to pulmonary edema, because diuretic agents such as furosemide produce some improvement. Similar clinical findings have been encountered with left-to-right shunts of similar magnitude associated with ventricular septal defect or patent ductus arteriosus. Possible mechanisms are discussed in Chapter 5.

There are no characteristic clinical findings, apart from the respiratory distress, to suggest the presence of an atrial septal defect in the premature infant. It is therefore important to perform echocardiography with Doppler flow studies in any preterm infant who requires assisted ventilation beyond the period when improvement from hyaline membrane disease would have been expected.

Mature infants

Most infants with atrial septal defect with or without partial anomalous pulmonary venous drainage are asymptomatic. In early infancy, mild cyanosis may be noted with crying, but it is difficult to distinguish this from the suffusion that may occur normally. Prior to the development of the left-to-right shunt, there are no clinical features indicating the presence of the defect. Thus the second sound is not widely split and no murmurs may be audible.

Large defects

Some infants with large defects with pulmonary to systemic blood flow ratios of about 2.5:1 or more may present with mild symptoms. They may show slow weight gain and usually at about 3–6 weeks after birth develop increased perspiration. They may also have an increased respiratory rate, but do not usually manifest dyspnea. The heart rate is usually increased to 140–160/min and the pulse volume is reduced. The liver is usually palpaple 2–3 cm below the right costal margin, but it is not firm.

The cardiac impulse is increased and maximal over the lower sternum and along the lower left sternal border. The first heart sound is accentuated, often markedly, at the lower left sternal border. This is probably related to the tricuspid leaflets being opened maximally by the high flow; marked distension of the right ventricle causes forceful contraction and the widely open leaflets snap shut, causing the prominent sound. The second sound is of normal or moderately increased intensity and is widely split during expiration as well as inspiration. A grade 2–3/6 systolic ejection murmur of medium frequency is audible most prominently at the upper left sternal border, but radiation may occur into both lung fields. It is not known why some individuals with large atrial septal defects develop these features relatively early in infancy. If the defect is not closed, the infants usually show no progression of symptoms but do not thrive. The main concern is that if untreated they may have permanent limitation of growth. However, this is open to question. The features associated with the defect with advancing age are discussed below.

Medium-sized and small defects

Medium-sized and small atrial septal defects do not cause symptoms during infancy and early childhood. Often they are not diagnosed until later in life, because the only manifestations are a soft murmur and possibly an abnormal second sound.

Atrial septal defects beyond infancy

This lesion is not uncommonly overlooked in infancy and early childhood because many clinicians do not appreciate the fixed splitting of the second sound, and interpret the murmur as a functional pulmonary ejection murmur. Atrial septal defects do not usually cause symptoms during childhood. Children with large defects may have poor physical development and frequently have both heights and weights in the lower percentiles. Most children have normal exercise tolerance, but occasionally a child with a large left-to-right shunt may have some limitation.

The pulse volume is usually normal but may be decreased. The liver is usually of normal size. With larger shunts, the heart is clinically enlarged and cardiac pulsation is increased over the lower sternum, indicating volume overloading of the right ventricle. In children with thin chest walls, pulsation may also be noted over the upper left sternal border, due to increased activity of the right ventricular outflow region. When the shunt is small, the heart size and pulsations are normal.

The first heart sound is often accentuated at the lower left sternal border with large shunts, but is of normal intensity with moderate-sized or small shunts. The second heart sound is typically widely split and fails to show the usual respiratory variation in splitting. Both aortic and pulmonary components are of normal intensity at the upper left sternal border. Normally, the pulmonary component of the second sound is heard shortly after the aortic component during expiration, so the sound is narrowly split. Inspiration induces greater venous return to the right atrium, resulting in increased right ventricular stroke volume and prolongation of systolic ejection. This causes a greater degree of separation of the two components of the second sound (wide splitting). With large atrial shunts there is a continuously high flow into the right atrium and ventricle and thus the second sound is widely split in all phases of respiration. In children with smaller shunts, the second sound may be split only moderately or not at all during expiration, depending on the size of the shunt. The degree of splitting of the second sound may be influenced by other factors; with faster heart rates and lower stroke volumes, and increased respiratory rates, splitting of the sound may be less evident.

A systolic ejection murmur, crescendo–decrescendo in character, is usually heard at the upper left sternal border and probably originates from the large flow across the pulmonary valve. In large shunts, it is of grade 2–3/6 intensity, of medium to high frequency, occupies most of systole, and may radiate to the lungs. With small shunts it is softer and may not extend beyond the first half or two-thirds of systole. A prominent third heart sound is often present at the lower left sternal border. Usually, with moderate-sized to large shunts, a grade 1–3/6 short low-frequency diastolic murmur is heard at the lower left sternal border. It starts shortly after the second sound, at the usual timing of the third sound and has been described as "scratchy" in character. This murmur is thought to originate from the tricuspid valve as a result of the high flow across a normal-sized valve, creating functional tricuspid stenosis.

The majority of children, even those with large defects, appear healthy and do not experience any symptoms relating to the cardiac lesion. Unlike ventricular septal defects, most of which tend to become smaller with advancing age, atrial septal defects usually grow in proportion with heart size, and there is evidence suggesting some defects may become relatively larger as age increases. However, as mentioned above, some left-to-right shunts decease in size with growth. The main concerns in individuals with atrial septal defects are (i) the development of pulmonary vascular disease, (ii) occurrence of atrial arrhythmias, (iii) onset of cardiac failure, (iv) possible cryptogenic stroke, and (v) possible migraine.

Pulmonary vascular disease

The association of pulmonary vascular disease with atrial septal defect is unusual during childhood. It has been conjectured that other factors may be involved in the rare infant or child in whom it does occur. The presence of an atrial septal defect with a high pulmonary blood flow would probably contribute to progression of the pulmonary vascular lesions. In children living at high altitudes, the incidence of increased pulmonary vascular resistance with atrial septal defect is considerably higher than in those at sea level. The incidence of pulmonary hypertension with elevated pulmonary vascular resistance increases with advancing age, but significant pulmonary vascular disease is unusual before the age of 25–30 years. Even beyond this age, a high pulmonary vascular resistance is encountered in only 5–10% of patients. The development of pulmonary vascular disease is related to the altitude at which individuals with atrial septal defect reside. Even at altitudes above about 1220 m (4000 feet), elevated pulmonary vascular resistance is more frequent and occurs at earlier ages. Females are twice as likely as males to develop pulmonary vascular changes. Pregnancy in an individual with atrial septal defect and high pulmonary vascular resistance is associated with high mortality. The pulmonary vascular changes associated with high pulmonary blood flow are discussed in Chapter 5.

Elevation of pulmonary vascular resistance increases afterload on the right ventricle and thus limits systolic emptying. This reduces inflow into the ventricle during diastole and thus decreases the left-to-right shunt. Pulmonary arterial and right ventricular pressures increase, resulting in right ventricular hypertrophy, which may reduce compliance of the ventricle and thus further decrease the left-to-right shunt. The right ventricular volume load is thus reduced and the impulse is less evident. Also, the pulmonary ejection murmur becomes softer and shorter and the diastolic murmur at the lower left sternal border disappears. Splitting of the second heart sound is reduced during both inspiration and expiration. However, the second (pulmonary) component of the second sound becomes accentuated. An early high-frequency murmur immediately following the pulmonary component of the second sound may appear because pulmonary valve insufficiency may result from pulmonary arterial hypertension. As pulmonary vascular resistance increases, right-to-left shunting through the defect may occur, with appearance of cyanosis, first only with exertion, and later continuously. Exercise tolerance is limited and right heart failure becomes increasingly severe. Pulmonary vascular changes, once evident, are usually rapidly progressive and patients rarely survive more than 18–24 months. Recently, these patients have been treated with long-term pulmonary vasodilator therapy, as with primary pulmonary hypertension. Preliminary observations suggest they do derive some benefit (see Chapter 5). Death may result from cardiac failure or other consequences of pulmonary vascular disease.

Atrial arrhythmias

Abnormal rhythms, particularly atrial fibrillation but also flutter and paroxysmal tachycardia, occur commonly in older patients with atrial septal defect, but are unusual in children and adolescents. They are probably related to the atrial enlargement that occurs in patients with large shunts. In various reports arrhythmias have been noted in about 15–50% of patients beyond the age of 20 years; the incidence increases with advancing age. Only 1–2% of individuals less than 20 years of age have atrial arrhythmias. However, sinus node dysfunction has been detected by electrophysiological studies in children with atrial septal defect; 40% or more of children above the age of 5 years had delayed sinus node recovery time after atrial pacing [5]. Although the cause of this is not known, it may contribute to the high incidence of arrhythmias in older patients. It is possible that sinus node dysfunction is more common in patients with sinus venosus defects.

Cardiac failure

As mentioned above, cardiac failure is unusual in children with atrial septal defects, even when left-to-right shunts are huge. It is encountered in patients beyond the age of 20 years who have large shunts, or in those with pulmonary vascular disease. Because the main increased load is on the right ventricle, right-sided failure occurs, with hepatomegaly, venous congestion, and fluid retention. In older adults who develop left ventricular dysfunction as a result of coronary artery disease or systemic hypertension, the presenting features of cardiac failure are predominantly those of right heart failure, because the high left atrial pressure is transmitted through the defect to the right atrium and systemic venous system. Development of mitral valve disease, as with rheumatic fever, may also increase left-to-right shunting through an atrial septal defect and result in right heart failure (Lutembacher syndrome).

Investigations

Electrocardiography

The P waves are usually normal in patients with atrial septal defect; however, in some with sinus venosus defects, the P-wave axis is displaced toward 0°. Atrioventricular conduction is normal but may be moderately prolonged with large defects. The QRS axis is usually deviated to the right with a mean frontal vector of +90° to +180°. In older children and adults, the electrical axis may be in the +70° to +90° range, particularly with smaller defects. There is right ventricular hypertrophy with a rather typical rsR′ or rSR′ in the right precordial leads, often incorrectly referred to as incomplete right bundle-branch block. The QRS complex may be slightly widened, but true right bundle-branch block is not a feature of atrial septal defect. There may be complete reversal of RS progression across the chest in the precordial leads; the S wave in V6 is often widened. In defects with small or medium shunts, left precordial leads usually show normal R waves. The R wave in the right precordial leads is rarely very tall and usually does not exceed 10–15 mm. With the development of pulmonary vascular disease, the right precordial R waves increase and the left decrease.

Chest radiography

Chest radiography shows a heart of variable size. In large shunt lesions, there is usually moderate enlargement, with some right atrial and right ventricular enlargement; the outflow region of the right ventricle is particularly evident in the oblique and lateral views. The main pulmonary artery is enlarged and the pulmonary vascular markings are increased, usually out to the peripheral lung fields. It is important to stress that although prominent pulmonary vascular markings are indicative of a large left-to-right shunt, it is possible to have large shunts with only slight to moderate prominence of the pulmonary vasculature. The lack of marked distension of the pulmonary arteries in the presence of large shunts can be explained on the basis of the very low pulmonary vascular resistance. The large stroke volume is easily accommodated at low pulmonary arterial pressure and there is also systolic flow through the pulmonary circulation without much expansion of the large vessels. I have encountered many adolescents who have torrential left-to-right shunts, in whom the pulmonary vasculature has been interpreted as "top normal" or "somewhat increased." When pulmonary vascular resistance increases, the main pulmonary artery and the hilar vessels increase in size and the peripheral markings are decreased. Enormous, almost aneurysmal, dilatation of the main and right and left pulmonary arteries may develop, with severe pulmonary vascular obstruction and marked diminution of peripheral vascular markings.

Echocardiography

Echocardiography is currently the preferred technique for confirming the presence of an atrial septal defect. The defect can be identified and its size and location may be defined. Depending on the size of the shunt, the right atrium and ventricle may be enlarged. With large left-to-right shunts, the enlarged right ventricle may result in diastolic displacement and paradoxical systolic motion of the ventricular septum. Color flow Doppler studies are very sensitive in detecting the flow patterns across the defect. Large left-to-right shunts are readily demonstrated, but even small left-to-right shunts across a patent foramen ovale may be detected. In addition phasic right-to-left shunting may be noted with either color flow Doppler or contrast echocardiography. Right-to-left shunting of SVC blood through a sinus venosus defect into the left atrium is clearly demonstrable by contrast echocardiography with an injection into an upper extremity vein.

The magnitude of pulmonary and systemic blood flows can be estimated from measurement by Doppler of blood flow velocity in the main pulmonary artery and ascending aorta and of their diameters to estimate cross-sectional areas. This permits calculation of the pulmonary to systemic blood flow ratio and the magnitude of the shunt.

The diagnosis of atrial septal defect with or without associated pulmonary venous drainage anomaly can usually be made clinically and confirmed by echocardiography without resorting to cardiac catheterization. Prior to the use of cardiopulmonary bypass for surgical repair of atrial septal defects, closure was attempted without visualization of the atrial cavity; it was important to document whether the pulmonary veins drained normally. Exposure of the interior of the atrium during cardiopulmonary bypass made it possible to visualize whether pulmonary veins were draining abnormally and to handle this appropriately. Recently, the use of devices to close atrial septal defects by transcatheter techniques has made the identification of drainage of pulmonary veins important.

Cardiac catheterization

Prior to the introduction of ultrasound techniques, cardiac catheterization was recommended in patients with suspected atrial septal defect for several reasons. It was performed to confirm the diagnosis, determine the magnitude of the left-to-right shunt, exclude the presence of associated defects, and assess pulmonary arterial pressure and pulmonary vascular resistance. Also, as mentioned above, it was performed to assess the possible association of partial abnormal pulmonary venous connection. Currently, ultrasound studies by qualified echocardiographers can, in most instances, resolve many of these issues. The main indication for cardiac catheterization is to assess pulmonary vascular resistance in those individuals in whom pulmonary hypertension is suspected. It may also be indicated if the pulmonary venous connections cannot be defined by ultrasound studies and transcatheter closure is being contemplated.

Approach and catheter manipulation

The groin approach is usually preferred, as it is much easier to manipulate the catheter through fossa ovalis defects from the IVC. In sinus venosus defects, the catheter can usually be passed easily through the defect from the groin approach, and it tends to enter the upper right pulmonary vein, which connects in close approximation to the defect. There may be some difficulty in manipulating the catheter into the body of the left atrium in patients with sinus venosus defects from the groin approach because the defect is high in the septum and a sharp angle is required to turn the catheter down toward the mitral valve.

When a right pulmonary vein drains into the IVC, the anomalous vein can usually be entered quite easily using the groin approach. Attempts should be made to pass the catheter into the right pulmonary veins to try to assess whether they are draining into the left or right atrium. When the oxygen saturation in the SVC is relatively high (greater than 75–80%), the possibility of pulmonary venous drainage of the upper right pulmonary vein should be considered and attempts made to enter it from the region of the cava–atrial junction. Also, the possibility should be entertained that one of the left pulmonary veins is draining into the left innominate vein either directly or through the vertical vein; the catheter should therefore be advanced to the left innominate vein and, if necessary, beyond. In order to complete the probing for anomalous pulmonary venous drainage, attempts should be made to pass the catheter into the coronary sinus to measure oxygen saturation and, if necessary, probe for pulmonary veins entering the coronary sinus.

If it is not possible to manipulate the catheter through a fossa ovalis defect from the groin approach, a sinus venosus defect or isolated anomalous pulmonary venous drainage should be considered. When a right pulmonary vein is entered from the atrium along the right heart border, it may be difficult to assess whether the catheter has passed across the defect into the pulmonary vein from the left atrium or whether it has passed directly into the vein from the right atrium. It has been suggested that this can be determined by rotating the catheter clockwise as it is withdrawn, and if it is the left atrium, this indicates that drainage is into the left atrium. However, this maneuver is not reliable, as the catheter, on withdrawal from a vein entering the right atrium, may flip through the defect into the left atrium. The differentiation usually has to be made by angiography.

Oxygen saturation data

Atrial septal defects and partial anomalous pulmonary venous drainage are characterized by an increase in oxygen saturation in the right atrium compared with the vena cava. Depending on the magnitude of the shunt, the increase may be 10–25%. It is difficult to obtain a reliable mixed venous sample because oxygen saturations in the SVC and IVC are different and their respective contributions to mixed venous return are not known. Also, the shunt at the atrial level does not permit collection of a truly representative SVC or IVC sample. It has been demonstrated by angiography that there is almost always some reflux of blood from the right atrium into the IVC, and even into the hepatic veins, in patients with atrial septal defect. Although there is also some reflux into the SVC, it is usually not as great nor does it usually extend as far into the vessel. However, this allows the atrial blood, more highly oxygenated because of the left-to-right shunt, to contaminate cava blood near the right atrium. Blood samples should therefore be obtained in the SVC just proximal to the innominate–jugular junction and also low down at the atrial junction, in order to be able to select the most reliable mixed venous sample. In the IVC, a sample above the hepatic vein entry is not reliable; a sample below the hepatic vein level should be obtained, but this is not usually representative of mixed IVC blood because of streaming of flows from different organs in this vessel (see Chapter 4).

When there is anomalous pulmonary venous drainage into the SVC, it is even more difficult to obtain a reasonably representative mixed venous sample. Often a very high oxygen saturation is found in a blood sample obtained in the SVC, since it may be obtained at the site of entry of the vein. When there is drainage of pulmonary veins into the left innominate system, a high oxygen saturation is measured in the SVC and the left innominate vein. It is important to consider this possibility when an oxygen saturation above 80% is obtained in the SVC. To exclude the possibility that the high oxygen saturation is merely due to anxiety with a high cardiac output and low arteriovenous oxygen difference, a sample should be obtained in the right jugular vein and right subclavian veins. If these show lower oxygen saturations than the caval and innominate samples, further exploration is indicated.

If the coronary sinus oxygen saturation is greater than 45–50%, the possibility should be considered that there is either a persistent left SVC or an anomalous pulmonary vein entering it. The catheter should be advanced further and usually it will enter a persistent left cava. If an anomalous pulmonary vein is draining into the coronary sinus, it may also be entered with the catheter.

There may be considerable variation in oxygen saturation in samples obtained from different regions of the right atrium, and there is frequently a further increase in oxygen saturation in the body of the right ventricle due to streaming of some of the shunted blood directly across the tricuspid valve. If there is a large left-to-right shunt, oxygen saturation levels may reach 90–92% in the right ventricle and the pulmonary artery. Because of this it is difficult to exclude the possibility of additional left-to-right shunts beyond the atrial level, as only small further additional increases in oxygen saturation would occur even with large shunts (see Chapter 4).

The oxygen saturations in the pulmonary veins, left atrium and ventricle, and systemic arteries are usually normal. However, in patients with very large pulmonary blood flows, these oxygen saturations may be slightly reduced to 94–95%, with a corresponding slight reduction in Po_2. It is suggested that this is due to a disturbance in ventilation–perfusion relationships; the very high pulmonary flow does not permit normal oxygen uptake when alveolar ventilation is normal. This may be even more important when a patient has been sedated and ventilation is somewhat reduced. As mentioned above, small right-to-left shunts may be present in patients with atrial septal defects, particularly sinus venosus defects, and in these cases oxygen saturation in the left atrium is slightly lower than that in the pulmonary veins. Po_2 measurements are more likely to demonstrate the difference at these high saturation levels. When pulmonary vascular resistance increases, greater right-to-left shunts occur and left atrial and systemic arterial oxygen saturations and Po_2 may be reduced considerably.

Pressures

The right atrial pressure tracing is normal in small defects, but with large defects there is usually a change in the pressure contour, with a deep *x* descent after the *a* wave and a prominent *v* wave; *a* and *v* waves are usually equal in height, in contrast to the higher *a* wave seen in the right atrium normally. The mean pressure and *a* and *v* wave levels are not elevated. With large defects, the left and right atrial mean pressures are equal, as are the phasic pressures.

The pulmonary venous pressures of veins draining to the left atrium are normal, showing a dominant *v* wave. It is of interest that an anomalous pulmonary vein does not assume the pressure characteristics of the right atrium. A dominant *v* wave is noted in the peripheral portion of the vein, as is seen normally, but just a short distance from its entry into the systemic venous system, the contour becomes more characteristic of that in the right atrium.

Right ventricular and pulmonary arterial systolic pressures are often slightly elevated to 35–40 mmHg in infants under 1 year, but beyond this age pressures are usually in the 25–30 mmHg range. In all age groups, systolic pressure differences of up to 15–30 mmHg may be noted between the right ventricle and pulmonary artery. This systolic pressure difference, which usually disappears after closure of the defect, is thought to be due to the large flow across the pulmonary valve. Pulmonary arterial diastolic and mean pressures are usually in the normal range, but slight increases in pulmonary arterial mean pressure to 20–25 mmHg may occur. In infants in particular, but also in older children on occasion, a systolic pressure difference of up to 10–15 mmHg may be noted between the main and branch pulmonary arteries, with a mean pressure change of up to 5–8 mmHg. This is also thought to be related to high flow across the junction of the branches of the pulmonary arteries with the trunk; it is an exaggeration of the pressure differences observed in many normal infants after birth (see Chapter 5). In view of these pressure gradients, which are encountered quite commonly, it is important to use pressures obtained in the branch pulmonary arteries in calculating pulmonary vascular resistance, if any significant pressure difference exists.

When pulmonary vascular resistance begins to increase, the pulmonary arterial and right ventricular systolic pressures rise. The pulmonary arterial pressure may actually exceed systemic arterial pressure when severe pulmonary vascular changes occur. Right ventricular end-diastolic pressure increases and right atrial pressure rises as cardiac failure progresses.

Pressures in the left atrium are usually normal, but in large defects mean pressure may be slightly reduced and the contours in the two atria are similar. Left ventricular and systemic arterial pressures are normal.

Blood flows and shunts

The measurement of blood flows by the Fick method is particularly unreliable in patients with atrial septal defects. Usually systemic blood flow is in the normal range, but calculations of flow may not be accurate because of the difficulty in obtaining a reliable mixed venous blood sample. Calculation of pulmonary blood flow is reasonably reliable when the flow is not very large. However, when pulmonary flow is markedly increased by a large left-to-right shunt, actual blood flow measurements may be erroneous. Pulmonary arteriovenous oxygen difference may be low because pulmonary arterial oxygen saturation is high and pulmonary venous oxygen somewhat reduced. When the arteriovenous oxygen difference is small, minor inaccuracies in measurement of arterial or venous oxygen levels can result in large differences in flow calculation (see Chapter 4). Thus, with the unreliability of both pulmonary and systemic blood flows, the calculation of left-to-right shunt and estimation of pulmonary to systemic flow ratios may also be inaccurate.

Vascular resistances

Systemic vascular resistance is usually normal in patients with atrial septal defects. Pulmonary vascular resistance is low in the majority of patients with atrial defects or anomalous pulmonary venous drainage. Actual resistance levels are often as low as 0.8–1 units/m^2, suggesting that the pulmonary vessels are widely dilated. In fact, if the pulmonary vascular resistance is greater than 3.0 units/m^2, a figure considered normal in most individuals, it should be regarded with suspicion in a patient with atrial septal defect as being indicative of early pulmonary vascular intimal disease. As pulmonary intimal disease progresses, pulmonary vascular resistance may rise to extremely high levels of greater than 20 units/m^2.

Indicator dilution studies

Dye dilution curves were previously used extensively to determine whether anomalous pulmonary venous drainage was associated with an atrial septal defect, but are rarely used now because the connections of the pulmonary veins can usually be defined by echocardiography, or by angiography during cardiac catheterization.

Angiocardiography

Angiograms are most helpful in assessing whether pulmonary veins that have been entered by the catheter are connected to the right or the left atrium. An injection of contrast medium into the vein may show it clearly draining directly into the right atrium, as there will be no filling of the left atrium. If it enters the left atrium there may be some confusion, as the right atrium fills through the atrial septal defect and very little may flow directly into the left atrium from the specific vein. The atrial septal defect may be demonstrated by a left atrial injection and is visualized best in the oblique rather than the direct anteroposterior and lateral views. An atrial left-to-right shunt can also be detected after an injection of contrast medium is made into the right ventricle or the pulmonary artery. When the contrast medium returns from the lungs to the left atrium, the atrial septum is seen to be poorly defined, in comparison with the usual sharp border noted, and filling of the right atrium is also seen.

In infants with large atrial left-to-right shunts and pulmonary arterial hypertension, the possibility of an associated ventricular septal defect or patent ductus arteriosus should be seriously considered and can be readily excluded by left ventricular and aortic angiograms.

Whenever drainage of the right pulmonary veins into the IVC is diagnosed, an aortogram should always be done to demonstrate whether any part of the lung receives its arterial supply from the aorta.

Differential diagnosis

Usually it is not possible to determine from clinical examination whether the patient who has a large atrial left-to-right shunt has an atrial septal defect alone or whether there is associated partial anomalous pulmonary venous drainage. Although large atrial septal defects may be diagnosed readily with reasonable assurance by clinical examination, radiography, and electrocardiography, there are several situations that may be confusing clinically.

"Functional" murmurs

The systolic ejection murmur of atrial septal defect may be difficult to differentiate from a "functional" murmur, because the mechanism of its production, i.e., high-velocity flow across the pulmonary valve, is similar. The constancy of splitting of the second sound in atrial septal defect is helpful, but when the shunt is small and the pulmonary to systemic flow ratio is less than 2:1, the second sound may show respiratory variation, although it may not narrow to a single sound on expiration. In children old enough to cooperate, the performance of a Valsalva maneuver may be helpful in differentiation. Functional murmurs disappear instantaneously because venous return to the right atrium and ventricle is reduced immediately. However, murmurs of atrial septal defect usually persist for several beats after the onset of the Valsalva maneuver. Radiography may not be helpful, since the heart and pulmonary vessels may not appear abnormal in patients with small shunts. Similarly, with small-to-moderate shunts, the electrocardiogram may not be conclusive, as there may be right ventricular conduction delay and mild prominence of right ventricular forces in young children normally.

Usually there is adequate information to differentiate by clinical features, but echocardiography will help to exclude the presence of an atrial septal defect. Recently, with the use of color flow Doppler, it has been possible to detect a small left-to-right shunt through a tiny defect in the atrial septum; this is probably a patent foramen ovale. This has created an enigma with regard to management (see Chapter 8).

Mild pulmonary stenosis

This produces a systolic ejection murmur at the upper left sternal border and increased splitting of the second sound, features quite similar to those of atrial septal defect. There may also be a lower left sternal border impulse due to right ventricular hypertrophy. The presence of a systolic ejection click, almost always present in valvar pulmonary stenosis, is helpful, as this is heard rarely in patients with atrial septal defects. The second sound, although well split, shows the usual narrowing on expiration. Although the systolic murmur tends to be louder and harsher in pulmonary stenosis, there is considerable variation in the intensity and quality of the murmur. The presence of a mid-diastolic murmur at the lower left sternal border in patients with atrial septal defects is helpful in differentiation. The electrocardiogram is not helpful, because with mild pulmonary stenosis, right ventricular forces may be only modestly increased, as occurs with atrial septal defect. Chest radiography shows a prominent main pulmonary artery segment in both conditions, and prominence of the right ventricle may be seen in both lesions. However, peripheral pulmonary vascular markings will be increased in atrial septal defects if the shunt is moderate to large. The differential is readily made by echocardiography.

Ebstein anomaly

This lesion often produces clinical features similar to those of atrial septal defect, and cases of mild Ebstein anomaly and medium-sized atrial septal defect may be easily confused. Although many patients with Ebstein malformation exhibit mild cyanosis, it is not always present. In patients with Ebstein anomaly, examination reveals a right ventricular impulse at the lower left sternal border, and the second sound may also be widely split due to intraventricular conduction delay. A fourth heart sound, as well as a third sound or short mid-diastolic murmur at the lower left sternal border is often associated with Ebstein anomaly. Chest radiography may be helpful, because with Ebstein anomaly the right atrium and right ventricle are prominent, with no enlargement of the pulmonary artery segment. The electrocardiogram is also helpful, as it shows prominent P waves, often some prolongation of atrioventricular conduction, and also intraventricular conduction delay, sometimes with complete right bundle-branch block. Echocardiography will differentiate between the two lesions.

Atrioventricular septal defect and common atrium

The ostium primum type of atrioventricular septal defect is associated with a left-to-right shunt into the right atrium. The clinical features of ostium primum lesions and other atrial septal defects are similar, including the right ventricular impulse, widely split second sound, mid-diastolic murmur at the lower left sternal border, and similar chest radiographic features. In ostium primum defects, there may be an additional systolic murmur, usually decrescendo in contour, at the apex or lower left sternal border, due to the mitral valve lesion. There may also be a left as well as a right ventricular impulse. The electrocardiogram clearly differentiates the lesions because, in patients with ostium primum defect, with rare exceptions, it shows left axis deviation with counterclockwise rotation of the vector loop in the frontal plane. Ultrasound study usually defines the location of the atrial septal defect extending to the atrioventricular valve mechanism and may show mitral valve regurgitant flow.

Total anomalous pulmonary venous drainage

Drainage of all the pulmonary veins into the coronary sinus or the vertical vein may produce a clinical picture quite similar to that of a large atrial septal defect. The cyanosis may be minimal so that it is not appreciated. All the clinical features are otherwise identical, although a quadruple rhythm may be evident in patients with total anomalous pulmonary venous drainage. Chest radiography and electrocardiography may not help in differentiation. If the veins drain into the vertical vein, prominence of the superior mediastinum may be evident on the chest radiograph. The electrocardiogram usually shows more prominent right ventricular forces in patients with total anomalous pulmonary venous drainage. An echocardiogram differentiates between the two lesions. The abnormal pulmonary venous connections can usually be defined and right-to-left shunting of blood through the atrial septal defect is seen, rather than the left-to-right shunt, as occurs with atrial septal defect. Even at cardiac catheterization, confusion may arise, particularly when the pulmonary veins all drain into the coronary sinus, because the large increase in oxygen saturation at the right atrial level may suggest the diagnosis of atrial septal defect.

Principles of management

Atrial septal defects rarely produce symptoms during infancy or childhood. Closure of defects is generally recommended if they are large because it is believed that this reduces or eliminates the risk for developing pulmonary vascular disease, cardiac failure, and atrial arrhythmias in later life. Unlike most other congenital heart lesions, atrial septal defect is not associated with a significant risk of infective endocarditis. Consequently, although prophylactic antibiotic therapy was recommended for those with congenital cardiac lesions until recently, it was not recommended for atrial septal defect.

Premature infants with atrial septal defect

As mentioned above, occasionally a preterm infant with cardiorespiratory distress who does not respond to usual therapeutic measures is found by ultrasound examination to have a left-to-right shunt through an atrial septal defect. Estimation of the magnitude of the left-to-right shunt has revealed that even relatively small shunts, with pulmonary to systemic blood flow ratios of 1.5–1.7, may contribute to the respiratory distress. Closure of the defect is therefore indicated. Currently this procedure has to be done surgically, because transcatheter interventional techniques have not yet been developed for preterm infants. Closure of the defect usually results in rapid improvement of respiratory distress and the infant can be weaned from assisted respiration.

The decision to recommend surgical closure of the defect will depend on the expertise of the neonatologists and the cardiovascular surgeon. Surgeons experienced with cardiac surgery on small infants can perform the procedure with little risk. If the surgeon has had little experience with infants, it may be preferable to persevere with diuretic therapy in the hope that the respiratory symptoms will improve.

Large atrial septal defects in infancy

Generally, a large atrial septal defect has arbitrarily been defined as one associated with a pulmonary to systemic blood flow ratio greater than 2:1. Most infants with large atrial septal defects do not have symptoms. An occasional infant has mild to moderate cardiac failure at 2–6 months after birth. As mentioned above, this may be related to the normal postnatal fall in hemoglobin concentration, or to respiratory or gastrointestinal infection. The failure should be treated with diuretic therapy. If improvement does not result, closure of the defect should not be contemplated before treating associated anemia or infection. Rarely, cardiac failure may persist despite all these measures, in which case closure of the defect may be recommended. Currently, this may have to be accomplished surgically, but techniques for transcatheter closure are being modified to make them applicable to closure of defects in infants.

In a recent report, closure was accomplished with an Amplatzer occluder in 14 of 15 infants aged 2 weeks to 11 months. In 11 it was performed percutaneously and in three by a transatrial approach through a thoracotomy [6]. In those centers where the procedure is not yet being performed in infants, it is preferable to delay closure of the defect if the infant does not have persistent uncontrollable cardiac failure.

Occasionally an infant with a large atrial septal defect fails to thrive. Weight gain may be slow and height may be in the lower percentile. Closure of the defect has been recommended in many of these infants, but it has not always been successful in improving the child's development. Caution should be exercised in recommending closure of the defect in these infants and other possible causes for the failure to thrive should be considered. Thus if the infant has associated genetic abnormalities or chronic infection, it is probable that these are responsible for the failure to thrive rather than the atrial septal defect. Experience has shown that closure of the defect does not improve growth in most of these infants. If other causes for failure to thrive have been carefully excluded, closure of the defect may result in rapid weight gain.

Increased pulmonary vascular resistance is rarely associated with atrial septal defect in infancy beyond the neonatal period. In those infants in whom it has occurred, the difficult decision had to be made whether to recommend closure of the defect. Closure of the defect may have no influence on progression of the pulmonary vascular disease; therefore closure is probably not indicated if pulmonary vascular resistance is greater than 8 units/m^2. As mentioned above, the possibility of a genetic association with pulmonary hypertension should be considered.

Large atrial septal defects in children

The current view is that an atrial septal defect with a large left-to-right shunt causing a pulmonary to systemic blood flow ratio of 2.0 or more should be closed. In long-term observations, it has been noted that the potential for development of high pulmonary vascular resistance is greatly reduced or abolished. Also the future risk of cardiac failure is eliminated. Whether surgical closure of defects reduces the incidence of future atrial arrhythmias is less certain.

Prior to the early 1980s, all closures of atrial septal defects were performed surgically. In 1974 King and Mills [7] developed a device that could be used to close atrial septal defects without surgery. Later, a prosthetic device that could be manipulated through a catheter was developed by Rashkind. It consisted of a disk of polyurethane supported by radiating metal struts. The device was folded into the catheter, which was passed through the defect; it was delivered on the left atrial side of the septum and withdrawn against the septum where it was held by hooks. Although several defects were closed successfully, serious complications requiring immediate surgery occurred in the initial series of patients. Subsequently several modifications have been developed. A so-called double clamshell device was designed by Lock; it consisted of two square pieces of polyester fabric, each with four struts radiating from the center. The device was delivered through a catheter so that one of the squares opened on the left atrial side and the other on the right atrial side of the defect. The device could be placed successfully, but almost 50% of patients had residual shunts, usually of small magnitude. A major concern was that the metal struts fractured in a number of the prostheses and although no serious complications developed, it was considered desirable to remove them.

Since these early experiences, several modifications of either a single-membrane or double-membrane prosthesis have undergone clinical evaluation. These include a modified version of the double clamshell, known as the CardioSEAL clamshell device. Other devices in various stages of clinical trial are the Sideris "buttoned" device, the Das-Angel Wings atrial septal occlusion device, the Monodisk, and the Amplatzer septal defect occluder. In some the struts have been eliminated by use of a flexible Nitinol or stainless steel metal frame or weave. In Germany, a device known as the Babic atrial septal defect occlusion system (ASDOS) has undergone testing. Placement requires a complex procedure of establishing a venoarterial loop from the femoral vein through the defect to the femoral artery.

Successful closure of atrial septal defects has been accomplished in carefully selected patients. Many patients have had small residual left-to-right shunts during the first few months after insertion of the device, but the tendency is for these to disappear. There has been essentially no mortality, but complications have been encountered. During or occasionally following the procedure, the device has been dislodged and has had to be retrieved surgically. Rare episodes of cerebral embolism with stroke have occurred. Some devices have moved away from the center of the defect resulting in reestablishment of a shunt. A concern related specifically to the Amplatzer atrial septal occluder is the development of erosion and perforation of the upper margin of the left or right atrium; this has at times extended into the aortic root with resultant pericardial tamponade.

These prostheses are not suited for closure of all atrial septal defects. At present, only fossa ovalis defects are being closed with the devices. Current criteria for using the devices include the following.

- The patient should be large enough for the femoral vein to accommodate the inserting device.
- The defect should be small enough to be closed by the device (usually less than 21 mm stretched diameter, although the CardioSEAL device may be

used for 28–33 mm defects and recently an Amplatzer device has been developed to close defects with diameters of up to 34 mm).

- There must be adequate margins around the defect for the device to be firmly fixed in position with no opening around the edges.
- There must be an adequate rim of tissue to allow placement of the device without interfering with the atrioventricular valve mechanism.

Improvements in design and methods of delivery of the prostheses will undoubtedly permit their use in smaller patients and with greater success and fewer complications.

As mentioned above, it is important to exclude the presence of associated abnormal pulmonary venous connections, because device closure will not correct the left-to-right shunt through pulmonary veins draining into the systemic veins or right atrium. It is therefore important to identify the connections of all the pulmonary veins either by ultrasound prior to the procedure or at the time of cardiac catheterization before inserting the prosthesis. In the event that one or more pulmonary veins are abnormally connected, surgery to close the defect and correct pulmonary venous drainage is indicated.

Surgery is still recommended for closure of sinus venosus defects and coronary sinus defects, because current devices are not suitable for their closure.

Large atrial septal defects in adolescents and adults

Large atrial septal defects first encountered in adolescents should be treated in the same manner as those in children, i.e., they should be closed. Controversy has arisen regarding the management of adults with atrial septal defects. Several reports have recommended closure of atrial septal defects in adults because many have experienced decreased exercise tolerance and, as discussed above, the incidence of elevated pulmonary vascular resistance has been thought to increase as individuals reach the second and third decades. Most patients were reported to experience improved performance after closure of the defect.

A series of patients from the Hammersmith Hospital in London in whom atrial septal defects were first diagnosed after the age of 25 years were followed for 25 years. No difference was observed in symptoms, in the incidence of pulmonary vascular disease, or of new arrhythmias in those in whom the defect was not closed as compared with those in whom it was closed. Furthermore, neither group developed progressive pulmonary vascular disease [8].

Unfortunately, in many reports of the course of patients with atrial septal defects, the size of the defect and the left-to-right shunt has not been considered in relation to the development of symptoms and complications. More detailed natural history studies of children and adults are therefore indicated to determine whether it is important to close atrial septal defects.

Small atrial septal defects

Apart from premature infants, children with atrial septal defects with left-to-right shunts with a pulmonary to systemic blood flow ratio less than 2.0 do not have symptoms. The practice of most cardiologists had been to follow these patients and not recommend surgical closure. This was based on the fact that surgery entailed some risk, and that as many as 50% of patients developed atrial arrhythmias either soon or some months after surgery. In recent years, the risks of surgery performed by capable cardiac surgeons have become exceedingly small and improvements in technique have significantly reduced the postoperative incidence of arrhythmias. Current practice recommends closure of the defect when the pulmonary to systemic blood flow ratio is 1.5–2.0, but not when the ratio is below 1.5.

However, as techniques and prostheses for closing atrial septal defects by transcatheter approach are improving, it is likely that closure of defects with even smaller left-to-right shunts will be recommended. Whether this is appropriate is questionable: it depends on the risks imposed by the presence of the defect. As stated above, individuals with atrial septal defects are not at risk for infective endocarditis; the potential risks are for development of pulmonary vascular disease, cardiac failure, and arrhythmias. Unfortunately, we do not know the risks of developing these complications with defects of different size. It is likely that patients with large defects are more prone, but whether a patient with a pulmonary to systemic blood flow ratio of 1.5–2.0 will ever suffer any of these events is not known. Without this information, our decisions are arbitrary. The one justification (or excuse) for closing the defect is to prevent future stroke resulting from right-to-left embolization through the defect (see Chapter 8).

Patent foramen ovale

Based on autopsy reports, up to 25% of adults are thought to have a patent foramen ovale, which is not associated with symptoms. These have not been recognized, except during cardiac catheterization, when a catheter has been manipulated through the foramen, or otherwise at autopsy. Recently, color flow Doppler studies have demonstrated small left-to-right shunts through atrial openings that are very small and which are assumed to be patent foramina ovale. At present, it is not recommended that these be closed. Recently, however, the possibility that patent foramen ovale may be associated with the development of cerebral stroke in some individuals, and of migraine, has been proposed. This issue is discussed below. Closure of the foramen ovale is being performed in some individuals with recurrent stroke, but there is concern that the foreign material of the device may attract some risk. Attempts have been made to close the foramen by percutaneous approach without using a device. This has been achieved successfully in 27 of 35 patients by means of radiofrequency [9].

Sinus venosus defects

Currently, sinus venosus defects are not amenable to closure by transcatheter techniques and are closed surgically. Although the sinoatrial node is usually located on the right side of the SVC–right atrial junction, the artery to the node may be closely related to the defect. Because damage to the arterial supply could result in atrial arrhythmias, including sick sinus syndrome, there is concern that closure of the defect could impose this risk. The experience of many centers is that there is a significantly greater risk of postoperative arrhythmia after closure of sinus venosus defects as compared with any other type of defect. However, in other centers there does not appear to be any difference in the incidence of postoperative arrhythmia, dependent on the location of the defect. This is probably related to differences in surgical technique.

Coronary sinus defects

These defects also cannot currently be closed by transcatheter techniques. Many of these defects are associated with drainage of the left SVC into the coronary sinus. It is important to define whether this anomaly is present by ultrasound. At the time of surgery, the left SVC can be ligated if there is adequate collateral communication of the left SVC system to the right side. However, if ligation of the vein at the time of surgery results in distension and marked increase in venous pressure, it should be anastomosed to the right atrium to avoid postoperative venous engorgement.

Atrial septal defect with pulmonary arterial hypertension

The presence of pulmonary arterial hypertension and increased pulmonary vascular resistance significantly increases the risk of surgical closure of the defect. Closure of defects when pulmonary vascular resistance is 15 units/m^2 is associated with a high immediate mortality or progression of pulmonary vascular disease and it is therefore not recommended in these patients. Pulmonary vascular resistance of 8–15 units/m^2 is associated with a mortality of as high as 50% if the defect is closed, whereas the mortality is about 10% when resistance is 4–8 units/m^2. It is very difficult to decide whether to recommend closure of the defect when pulmonary vascular resistance is elevated. I would not recommend closure if pulmonary vascular resistance is 12 units/m^2 or greater, and would quote a high mortality for those with pulmonary vascular resistance in the 8–12 units/m^2 range.

There is little experience with closure of defects by transcatheter techniques when pulmonary vascular resistance is increased. It is possible that the immediate risks following closure may be less than after surgery, because the concerns of further increasing pulmonary vascular resistance due to ventilatory disturbances associated with thoracotomy could be avoided. In recent years, more effective pulmonary vasodilator agents have become available (see Chapter 5). A trial of these agents to assess their effectiveness in reducing pulmonary vascular resistance prior to attempting to close the defect is indicated. If pulmonary vascular resistance is reduced, the procedure would be less risky.

Administration of pulmonary vasodilators after the closure has been accomplished could help to prevent or delay progression of the pulmonary vascular disease.

Postoperative atrial arrhythmias

Several reports have suggested that atrial arrhythmias are less frequent in patients who have had atrial septal defect closure than in those in whom closure has not been accomplished. However, a substantial number of children who have had surgical closure of the defect develop postoperative atrial arrhythmias. This may occur soon after surgery, but has developed months or years later. In various series, the incidence has been as high as 30–50%, but in some centers there appears to be a much lower incidence. This has suggested that surgical techniques may be important in determining the development of arrhythmia, and modification of techniques has reduced the incidence in some centers. Paroxysmal atrial tachycardia and atrial flutter or fibrillation are the usual dysrhythmias, but bradycardia/tachycardia syndromes have occurred and some patients have required pacemaker insertion.

Surgery in adolescents or adults has not been successful in significantly reducing the incidence of arrhythmias. If an older patient already has an arrhythmia, surgical closure of the defect will more often than not fail to abolish the arrhythmia. As mentioned above, in the Hammersmith Hospital report, there was no difference in the incidence of the onset of arrhythmia in adults who had surgery as compared with those who had not.

The incidence of postprocedure arrhythmias following closure of defects by transcatheter techniques has not yet been evaluated, but hopefully, by avoiding atrial incisions and damage to the sinus node, the incidence of arrhythmias will be reduced considerably.

Patent foramen ovale and cryptogenic stroke

In about 40% of patients the cause of stroke is cryptogenic (i.e., not known); most of these individuals are less than 50 years of age. In studies of cryptogenic stroke patients, a patent foramen ovale has been detected in 44–66% compared with 9–27% in patients with a known cause of stroke [10]. The recurrence rate for stroke has been reported to be 2–15% within 4 years, despite treatment with anticoagulant or antiplatelet drugs. The presence of a patent foramen ovale increases the incidence of recurrent events fivefold [11]. Closure of the patent foramen ovale by surgery or device significantly reduced the risk of recurrent stroke in some studies, especially if it was associated with an atrial septal aneurysm [12]. In others, results were marginal. Currently, it is generally agreed that if recurrent episodes of stroke have occurred despite the use of warfarin prophylaxis, the foramen ovale should be closed by a device. However, whether the defect should be closed after a first episode of cryptogenic stroke is controversial. At present, therefore, closure of the foramen ovale to prevent possible occurrence of stroke is not recommended.

Patent foramen ovale and migraine

The possible association of patent foramen ovale with migraine was proposed after it was noted that 70% of individuals who had closure of the foramen after a cryptogenic stroke found that migraine they had experienced prior to the stroke disappeared; the other 30% of individuals showed considerable improvement. This was particularly likely in those who had migraine with associated aura, but not in others. In a study of patients with migraine by Domitrz *et al.* [13], 54% of those with migraine and aura had a patent foramen ovale, whereas it was patent in only 25% of controls and 25% of migraine patients with no aura. Several trials are currently in progress to assess the effectiveness of device closure of patent foramen ovale in relieving migraine with aura. One study did show some benefit, but the results were more modest than had been anticipated [14]. The mechanism by which patent foramen ovale may account for the occurrence of migraine is not clear. It has been proposed that the foramen permits passage of some chemical, which is usually modified or destroyed in the lung, into the systemic circulation [15].

Although it is possible that closure of a patent foramen ovale may be indicated for treatment of severe migraine with aura, the effectiveness of the procedure requires a great deal more confirmation before it can be recommended routinely.

References

1 Hoffman JIE, Rudolph AM, Danilowicz D. Left to right atrial shunts in infants. Am J Cardiol 1972;30:868–875.

2 Douglas JE, Rembert JC, Sealy WC, Greenfield JC. Factors affecting shunting in experimental atrial septal defect in dogs. Circ Res 1969;24:493–505.

3 Levin AR, Spach MS, Boineau JP, Canent RV Jr, Capp MP, Jewett PH. Atrial pressure–flow dynamics in atrial septal defects (secundum type). Circulation 1968;37: 476–488.

4 Weidman WH, Swan HJ, Dushane JW, Wood EH. A hemodynamic study of atrial septal defect and associated anomalies involving the atrial septum. J Lab Clin Med 1957;50:165–185.

5 Bolens M, Friedli B. Sinus node function and conduction system before and after surgery for secundum atrial septal defect: an electrophysiologic study. Am J Cardiol 1984;53:1415–1420.

6 Diab KA, Cao QLK, Bacha EA, Hijazi ZM. Device closure of atrial septal defects with the Amplatzer septal occluder: safety and outcome in infants. J Thorac Cardiovasc Surg 2007;134:960–966.

7 King TD, Mills NL. Nonoperative closure of atrial septal defects. Surgery 1974;75:383–388.

8 Shah D, Azhar M, Oakley CM, Cleland JG, Nihoyannopoulos P. Natural history of secundum atrial septal defect in adults after medical or surgical treatment: a historical prospective study. Br Heart J 1994;71:219–223.

9 Sievert H, Fischer E, Heinisch C, Majunke N, Roemer A, Wunderlich N. Transcatheter closure of patent foramen ovale without an implant: initial clinical experience. Circulation 2007;116:1701–1706.

10 Sievert H, Taaffe M. Patent foramen ovale: the jury is still out. Eur Heart J 2004;25:361–362.

11 Di Tullio M, Sacco RL, Venketasubramanian N, Sherman D, Mohr JP, Homma S. Comparison of diagnostic techniques for the detection of a patent foramen ovale in stroke patients. Stroke 1993;24:1020–1024.

12 Mas J-L, Arquizan C, Lamy C *et al.* Patent Foramen Ovale and Atrial Septal Aneurysm Study Group. N Eng J Med 2001;345:1740–1746.

13 Domitrz I, Mieszkowskii J, Kaminska A. Relationship beween migraine and patent foramen ovale: a study of 121 patients with migraine. Headache 2007;47:1311–1318.

14 Schwerzmann M, Nedeltchev K, Meier B. Patent foramen ovale closure: a new therapy for migraine. Catheter Cardiovasc Interv 2007;69:277–284.

15 Tobis JM, Azarbal B. Does patent foramen ovale promote cryptogenic stroke and migraine headache? Tex Heart Inst J 2005;32:362–365.

CHAPTER 9

Atrioventricular septal defect

Atrioventricular septal defects are lesions that result from arrested or abnormal embryological development of the endocardial cushions in the primitive atrioventricular canal. They have also been termed atrioventricular canal defects and endocardial cushion defects. They have been classified as partial, or incomplete, defects and complete or common atrioventricular septal defects. The most important defining feature is that in incomplete defects, the common atrioventricular orifice is separated into two complete atrioventricular orifices that form distinct mitral and tricuspid openings, with attachment of both valves to the upper margin of the ventricular septum. In complete atrioventricular septal defects, the atrioventricular orifice is not fully divided, so that a variable distance separates the upper margin of the ventricular septum from the level of the common atrioventricular valve annulus.

Atrioventricular septal defects may occur as isolated lesions in otherwise normally developed infants and children. However, they are often encountered when other congenital anomalies are present. They are the most common of all congenital heart lesions in individuals with trisomy 21 syndrome (Down syndrome). In a study in the UK, almost 40% of fetuses with atrioventricular septal defect had trisomy 21 and 10% had other chromosomal anomalies. In this report, 12% of the fetuses had right atrial isomerism and 20% had left atrial isomerism [1]. In another study about 40% of fetuses with atrioventricular septal defect had left or right isomerism [2]. Almost all patients, if not all, with the asplenia syndrome have atrioventricular septal defect, and a high percentage of patients with polysplenia syndrome have this anomaly. Fetuses with left atrial isomerism are more likely to have associated complete heart block and left ventricular outflow obstruction. These fetuses with left atrial isomerism and atrioventricular septal defect have a relatively high mortality *in utero*, thus accounting for the much lower incidence postnatally [3]. The spectrum of atrioventricular septal defect in the fetus is quite different to that observed postnatally. Between 70 and 80% of patients with complete atrioventricular septal defect have been found to have trisomy 21 [4,5]. The prenatal and postnatal differences in the association of Down syndrome with atrioventricular septal defect is probably explained by a greater mortality *in utero* of those with isomerism, especially left atrial isomerism. About half of individuals with Ellis–van Creveld syndrome have congenital heart disease, and one of the common lesions is common atrium, considered to be one form of atrioventricular septal defect.

There are, not uncommonly, other lesions associated with atrioventricular septal defects: pulmonary stenosis of varying severity may occur; in infants, a patent ductus arteriosus is quite frequent; aortic isthmus narrowing, sometimes severe, may occur, and this is often associated with outflow obstruction of the left ventricle. When the atrioventricular defect is part of an asplenia or polysplenia syndrome, the other features of these syndromes, such as aortopulmonary transposition, pulmonary venous drainage anomalies and, in the asplenia syndrome, pulmonary stenosis, are usually associated.

In this chapter I consider atrioventricular septal defects predominantly in regard to the functional disturbances of the circulation and also outline the various anatomical derangements that have important surgical implications.

Congenital Diseases of the Heart, 3rd edition. By A. Rudolph
 ISBN: 9781405162456

Morphological and embryological considerations

The primitive atrioventricular canal is separated into atria and ventricles by the development of projections of the endomyocardial jelly at the atrioventricular junction. These develop into the atrioventricular valves and also contribute to the closure of the atrial septum and the ventricular septum (Figure 9.1). The larger and more important of these projections have been termed *endocardial cushions*, but are truly endomyocardial cushions, and are located in the anterior and posterior portions of the canal. Two other cushions form on the left and right sides, the so-called lateral cushions, but these are much smaller and less important in development of atrioventricular valve function.

The anterior (or superior) and posterior (or inferior) cushions grow in toward the center and become convex toward the atria. They join, first in the midline, to produce separate left and right atrioventricular orifices (see Figure 9.1). The cushions develop bulges on either side of the midline, which develop into the valve cusps. On the left side, the left portions of the anterior and posterior cushions join to form the septal leaflet of the mitral valve; with subsequent rotation of the ventricles, this cusp assumes a relatively anterior position. The formation of the tricuspid valve is more complex. The anterior leaflet is formed partly from endomyocardial jelly in the region of the anterior and right lateral cushion origin. The anterior cushion itself contributes only minimally to the anterior leaflet, and the medial portion of this leaflet, as well as the medial papillary muscle and chordae tendineae, are derived from the conotruncal septum. The right side of the posterior endocardial cushion contributes to the medial tricuspid valve leaflet and also completes the closure of the most posterior portion of the membranous ventricular septum. The lower edge of the septum primum, which separates the atria, fuses with the center of the anterior and posterior endocardial cushions, and as they grow toward each other and fuse, the orifice at the lower margin of the septum primum is sealed. As this process of closure of the interatrial septum proceeds, a series of foramina develop in the central portion of the septum primum to maintain communication between the atria.

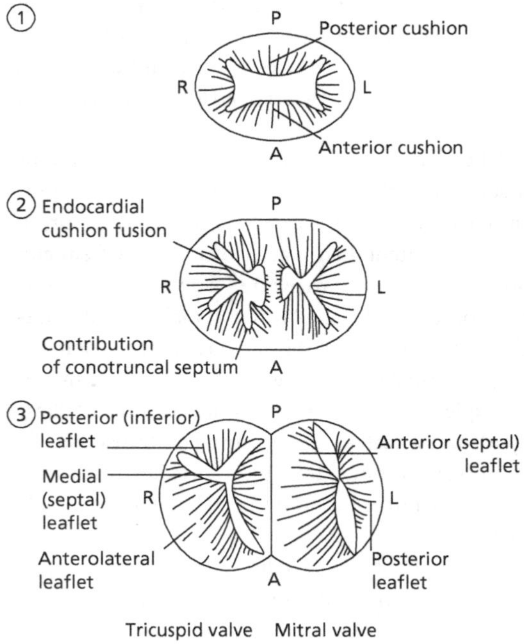

Figure 9.1 Stages in the development of tricuspid and mitral valves from primitive endocardial cushions.

Atrioventricular septal defects vary greatly in the type of anatomical disturbance and in severity, depending on which cushions are predominantly involved and the adequacy of their development. Since the cushions contribute to the development of the mitral and tricuspid valves and the atrial and ventricular septa, several different combinations of atrioventricular valve lesions and septal defects may occur. Classification into complete and partial or incomplete forms is convenient, as the partial forms are less likely to present with difficulties *in utero* or during infancy and are unlikely to present with residual atrioventricular valve insufficiency following surgery.

Partial atrioventricular canal defects are characterized by the development of almost complete central fusion of the anterior and posterior cushions, so that the annuli of the mitral and tricuspid valves are well formed. The most common complex of this type is the ostium primum defect, in which there is failure of fusion of the left portions of the anterior and posterior endocardial cushions, so that there is a cleft or separation in the anterior mitral valve leaflet (Figure 9.2). Associated with this is a defect of the central lower portion of the

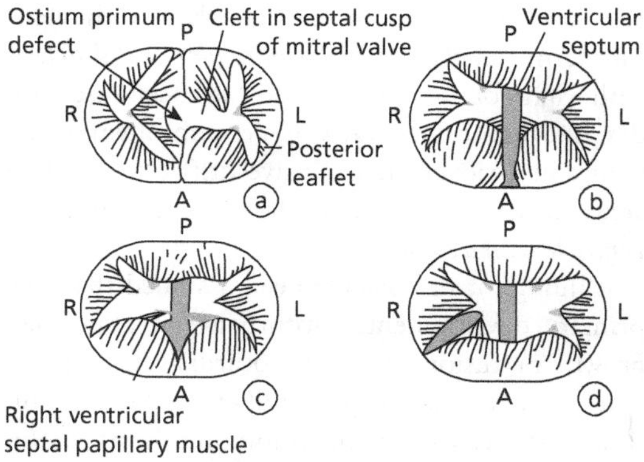

Figure 9.2 The atrioventricular valves in different types of atrioventricular septal defects. (a) Ostium primum defect or partial atrioventricular septal defect with cleft in anterior or septal leaflet of the mitral valve. (b) Complete atrioventricular septal defect with separation of anterior endocardial cushion into distinct mitral and tricuspid portions with chordae attached to upper portion of ventricular septum. (c) Complete atrioventricular septal defect with only partial separation of anterior cushion, and chordae extending from mitral component across ventricular septal defect to right ventricular papillary muscle. (d) Complete atrioventricular septal defect with no separation of anterior and posterior cushions.

atrial septum bordering on the mitral and tricuspid valve rings; the size of this defect is variable, but is usually large. Because the mitral valve and atrial septal defects border on the upper edge of the ventricular septum, a small rim of the ventricular septum is lacking. Although the tricuspid valve is usually normal, there may be a cleft of the medial leaflet.

A second partial defect, which is not always considered to be an atrioventricular septal defect, is the complex of ventricular septal defect with a cleft of the medial leaflet of the tricuspid valve. This lesion probably results from abnormal development of the right side of the posterior endocardial cushion, which contributes to the formation of the medial cusp and completes the closure of the ventricular septum. Probably not all instances of ventricular septal defect and tricuspid valve cleft are due to cushion defects; some may be primary ventricular septal defects, with adherence of the tricuspid valve to the rim of the defect and perforation of the cusp (see Chapter 7). The association of ventricular septal defect with mitral valve cleft may be another partial form of the defect, but it is not as common as the ostium primum defect.

Complete, or common, atrioventricular canal defects are typified by the absence of the development of separate mitral and tricuspid valve rings. This is due to failure of fusion of the central portions of the anterior and posterior endocardial cushions. In all these lesions there is a defect of the central lower portion of the atrial septum adjacent to the atrioventricular orifice, a ventricular septal defect in the posterior portion of the septum, and abnormalities in the development of the mitral and tricuspid valves. The atrial septal defect is usually quite large, but the size of the ventricular septal defect varies from a small defect of the upper posterior portion of the septum to very large communications. In general, the size of the ventricular septal defect is related to the stage of development of the cushions; the more primitive the cushion formation, the larger the defect, but this is not always the case.

Based largely on considerations for potential surgical correction, Rastelli *et al.* [6] have classified the complete atrioventricular septal defects into three main groups. These probably also coincide with the stage of cushion development. In all forms of common canal defects, the posterior endocardial cushion has failed to develop adequately. It is usually rather short, has firm rolled edges, and is not very mobile. However, the development of the anterior cushion appears to be more important in delineating the stage of embryological maturation and the functional status of the atrioventricular valves. In the embryologically most advanced form of development (Rastelli type A), the anterior cushion is partly separated into left (mitral valve) and right (tricuspid valve) portions. The lateral free margins of these leaflets are attached by chordae to the lateral portions of the respective ventricles; the medial margins are attached by short chordae to the upper portion of the ventricular septum (see Figure 9.2). In Rastelli type A there is minimal bridging of the anterosuperior leaflet across the atrioventricular canal. Most patients with Down syndrome and atrioventricular septal defect have the Rastelli type A form of atrioventricular valve anomaly.

In the moderately advanced Rastelli type B, the anterior cushion is also fairly well separated into right and left portions. However, whereas the right side is appropriately attached by chordae, the medial edge of the left (mitral) segment is attached by long chordae tendineae, which cross the upper border of the ventricular septum to a papillary muscle on the right ventricular side of the septum. There is thus a moderate degree of bridging of the anterosuperior leaflet across the atrioventricular orifice. An anterior cushion that has not separated into left and right segments characterizes the most primitive form of defect (Rastelli type C); there is a single anterior leaflet, common to the right and left sides, which is not attached to the ventricular septum. The lateral margins are attached to an anterior papillary muscle in each ventricle. This latter type of anomaly occurs only rarely as an isolated lesion and is encountered more commonly when there are other severe anomalies such as aortopulmonary transposition, double-outlet right ventricle, single ventricle, and pulmonary venous drainage anomalies. These complicated anomalies with the most severe form of atrioventricular septal defects are most common in asplenia and polysplenia syndromes. The Rastelli classification has largely been superseded by definition of the arrangement of individual leaflets and their attachments.

The abnormal development of the endocardial cushions creates additional morphological alterations. Normally, the mitral valve is on a slightly higher plane than the tricuspid valve, which is displaced toward the cardiac apex. There is a short segment of septal tissue that separates the left ventricle on its left, from the right atrium on its right side. With atrioventricular septal defect, the valves are at the same level and also somewhat lower than normal, so that there is a shorter distance between the valve and the apex of the heart. In addition, the left ventricular outflow tract and aorta are displaced. In the normal heart, the outflow tract is closely approximated to the anterior margins of the mitral and tricuspid valves, as is the aortic annulus. The presence of an atrioventricular septal defect results in anterior displacement of the outflow tract as well as anterior and superior displacement of the aortic valve. This produces the elongation and distortion of the left ventricular outflow tract referred to as "gooseneck" deformity.

In most patients with complete atrioventricular septal defects, the atrioventricular canal is positioned so that there is more or less equal opening into the left and right ventricles. Occasionally, in about 5% of patients, the atrioventricular orifice is committed predominantly to one or other ventricle, more commonly to the right than to the left. The term *unbalanced atrioventricular septal defect* with right or left dominance has been used to describe this occurrence. Major commitment of the common atrioventricular valve orifice to the left ventricle has been referred to as *double-inlet left ventricle with a common valve.*

Although it has usually been assumed that the primary developmental disturbance is abnormal growth or fusion of the endocardial cushions, I would like to raise the possibility that alteration of flow patterns within the embryonic heart could have a role in the production of cushion defects. If the flows from the superior vena cava (SVC) and inferior vena cava (IVC) are changed, the streaming patterns within the atria and the ventricles could be modified and thus result in preferential growth of an unusual type. A simple example of what could occur is that the secondary openings that develop in the central portion of the septum primum just prior to the sealing of the lower opening by fusion of the septum primum with the cushions, may be delayed or not occur at all. This may interfere with normal closure of the lower portion of the septum primum, because blood flow may still be directed through it. Persistent streaming of blood through this opening may also prevent normal union of the anterior and posterior cushions in this region, resulting in a cleft mitral valve cusp.

Atrioventricular septal defects of various degrees of severity are common in heterotaxias with right or left atrial isomerism (asplenia and polysplenia syndromes), and although they could be due to primary disturbances of intracardiac development, abnormalities of flow could be contributory. Abnormal systemic, hepatic, pulmonary, and coronary venous return, commonly present in these patients, could result in alterations of venous flow patterns and intracardiac streaming. Almost all patients with right atrial, and about half of those with left atrial, isomerism have a complete atrioventricular septal defect [7].

Hemodynamic disturbances

General considerations

The hemodynamic disturbances associated with atrioventricular septal defects are not well understood. On the basis of the anatomical abnormalities, patients with endocardial cushion defects may be expected to demonstrate one or more of the following disturbances: shunting across the atrial septal defect, shunting through the ventricular septal defect, mitral regurgitation, and tricuspid regurgitation. However, it is of considerable interest that there is not always a clear relationship between the functional circulatory changes and the morphological anomalies apparent at autopsy. I propose first to discuss the major circulatory disturbances that occur and then to indicate how these alter the circulation in the fetus, the adaptations after birth, and later development of the circulation.

Patterns of shunting

Shunting through the atrial septal and ventricular septal components of the defect are subject to the same factors that influence shunting through an atrial septal defect (see Chapter 8) and a ventricular septal defect (see Chapter 7). Thus, the direction of shunt is determined by the relationship between the outflow resistance (afterload) of the left and right ventricles. When pulmonary vascular resistance is high, or when pulmonary stenosis is present, the shunt is right to left, so that systemic arterial oxygen saturation is reduced and cyanosis occurs. When pulmonary vascular resistance is lower than systemic resistance, left-to-right shunt develops, and the magnitude of the shunt is related to the ratio of pulmonary and systemic vascular resistances. This type of left-to-right shunt may be termed *dependent shunting*, because it is dependent on the changes in pulmonary vascular resistance.

Another type of shunting commonly present in endocardial cushion defects is *obligatory shunting* (see Chapter 5). The left-to-right shunt occurs from a high-pressure to a low-pressure chamber, namely from the left ventricle to the right atrium. This may occur from the left ventricle through the common atrioventricular canal of the complete defect directly into the right atrium. In the partial form of the defect, left ventricular blood may pass through a cleft anterior leaflet of the mitral valve and across the ostium primum defect into the right atrium. Less commonly, the shunt travels through a ventricular septal defect and across a tricuspid valve cleft into the right atrium.

The pattern of left-to-right shunting cannot be clearly correlated with the anatomical derangement. In some instances of ostium primum defect, the shunt almost exclusively is from the left atrium to the right atrium, and these behave like atrial septal defects of the secundum type; in others, there is considerable left ventricular to right atrial shunting. In the complete forms of atrioventricular canal there may be separate atrial and ventricular left-to-right shunts, mainly atrial with small ventricular shunts, or large left ventricular to right atrial shunts.

It is also apparent that when there is an obligatory left-to-right shunt, it would be possible for a right-to-left shunt to be present simultaneously if pulmonary vascular resistance were higher than systemic resistance. As mentioned below, if the ductus arteriosus is still patent and pulmonary vascular resistance is elevated, even though a large obligatory left-to-right shunt from the left ventricle to the right atrium is present, right-to-left shunting through the ductus may occur.

Atrioventricular valve function

The degree of effective closure of the atrioventricular valves is crucial in determining the physiological disturbance in patients with atrioventricular septal defects. In this group of lesions the relationship between structure and function may not be predictable. It is surprising that, with an obvious cleft in the anterior leaflet of the mitral valve continuing into an ostium primum atrial septal defect, there may be no mitral regurgitation detectable clinically or by echocardiography or angiography. Also, in patients with common atrioventricular canal lesions, even though there is a communication between the four cardiac chambers, only minimal degrees of regurgitation may be demonstrable.

When atrioventricular valve insufficiency is present in ostium primum defects, the mitral valve is usually involved. The morphology of the region of the ostium primum and the anterior mitral valve leaflet cleft is such that direct streaming of blood may occur from the left ventricle through the cleft into the right atrium, producing an obligatory left-to-right shunt. In common atrioventricular canal, there may be a greater degree of regurgitation directly into the left atrium but, in most instances, valvar regurgitation is also manifested by an obligatory left ventricular to right atrial shunt. The presence of mitral valve dysfunction is most important in determining the clinical course of infants with cushion defects.

Tricuspid valve insufficiency is less frequent than mitral insufficiency. This may be due to the fact that the anterior and lateral cusps of the tricuspid valve are usually well formed, and a cleft of the medial leaflet may not be of much significance. Even when the medial leaflet is small and deformed, severe tricuspid insufficiency is not common. It has been stated that the prognosis is most grave in those patients with atrioventricular septal defects who have tricuspid insufficiency. This is probably related to the fact that a combination of mitral and tricuspid insufficiency, together with left-to-right shunting, imposes a very large volume load on the heart.

The adequacy of atrioventricular valve function in the face of actual anatomical defects or inadequate development seems difficult to explain. However, it is known that the ventricle shortens and the annulus becomes narrower during systole. Thus, although there may be a cleft in the valve apparent in the relaxed heart at autopsy, narrowing of the annulus during systole may permit apposition of the edges of the cleft, thus avoiding significant regurgitation. Even though the chordae tendineae are sometimes thicker and shorter than normal, there may not be enough retraction of the cusp to produce insufficiency, due to approximation of the apex and base of the ventricle during systole. While at autopsy, when the heart is relaxed, there is free communication between all four cardiac chambers, in complete atrioventricular canal defects adequate apposition of the anterior and posterior bridging leaflets during systole may produce effective valve function with no or only minimal regurgitation. Factors important in determining the adequacy of atrioventricular valve function are the degree of development of the leaflets, their mobility, and their attachments. A leaflet that is short, has thick rolled edges, and short thick chordae tendineae, which greatly limits its mobility, is hardly likely to permit effective function. The frequency of dysplastic common atrioventricular valve is more common in patients who do not have Down syndrome (22%) compared to those with Down syndrome (only 3%) [4].

Another factor that has received scant attention is the effect of changes in ventricular, and thus annulus, size (either by enlargement or growth) on atrioventricular valve function. It is well recognized that in individuals who have normally developed mitral or bicuspid valves, marked cardiomegaly may produce some degree of insufficiency. In the patient with endocardial cushion defects of the ostium primum type, enlargement of the left ventricle could separate the cleft in the anterior leaflet and thus precipitate or exaggerate the insufficiency. Once developed, the regurgitation would augment the volume loading of the left ventricle, thus further increasing ventricular size and the degree of insufficiency. When a common atrioventricular canal is present, enlargement of either the left or right ventricle could have an adverse effect on valve function. Thus, if a left-to-right shunt develops after birth and the shunt is mainly from the left to the right atrium, the increased volume presented to the right ventricle could produce right ventricular enlargement and tricuspid valve insufficiency. The regurgitant common valve could result in an obligatory left ventricular–right atrial shunt and also cause tricuspid insufficiency. This could exaggerate enlargement of both ventricles, resulting in progressive insufficiency. Left-to-right shunt through the ventricular septal defect would result in an increased volume load on the left ventricle, with left ventricular enlargement; this could cause or aggravate mitral insufficiency.

Normal growth of the heart could have similar effects on atrioventricular valve function. We do not know whether the abnormal valves grow in proportion to the rest of the heart. It is possible that a valve leaflet that is thickened and which has short thick chordae tendineae does not develop commensurate with the rest of the heart. Thus, with normal cardiac growth and annulus enlargement, valvar insufficiency could become manifest or be aggravated.

Atrioventricular septal defect with right ventricular outflow obstruction

Common atrioventricular canal is not infrequently associated with severe pulmonary stenosis, particularly in those patients with Down syndrome. Tetralogy of Fallot is associated with about 5% of patients with complete atrioventricular septal defect [8]. Tetralogy of Fallot with atrioventricular septal defect is not discussed in detail in this section. It produces hemodynamic disturbances and presents with clinical features similar to those of pulmonary stenosis with ventricular septal defect (tetralogy of Fallot). If the right ventricular outflow tract is significantly obstructed, right-to-left shunting through either the atrial defect or the ventricular septal defect, or both occurs. The differential diagnosis is discussed in Chapter 14. It is of interest that significant degrees of atrioventricular valve insufficiency are not common in patients with endocardial cushion defect and pulmonary stenosis. This can probably be explained by the fact that the low pulmonary blood flow resulting from pulmonary stenosis decreases venous return to the left atrium and ventricle, thus averting the development of left ventricular enlargement. This could permit atrioventricular valve function to be maintained for a longer period.

Left ventricular outflow obstruction

As mentioned above, narrowing of the outflow tract of the left ventricle is usually present in patients with atrioventricular septal defects due to anterior displacement of the outflow tract and aorta and superior displacement of the aortic valve. This produces the so-called gooseneck deformity. However, this is not usually associated with functionally significant obstruction to left ventricular outflow. The left ventricular outflow tract tends to be narrowest in the subaortic region in patients with Rastelli type A morphology. Outflow obstruction may result from abnormal position and attachment of the left side of the anterior endocardial cushion. Normally, the edge of the cusp is attached to the anterior papillary muscle of the left ventricle. When the mitral portion of the common anterior cushion is attached either to the upper margin of the ventricular septum or across to the right ventricular papillary muscle, the leaflet may encroach on the outflow region of the left ventricle. Left ventricular outflow obstruction may also be caused by a fibrous ridge in the subaortic region. The most severe forms of obstruction to left ventricular outflow are associated with those patients who have an unbalanced commitment of the atrioventricular valve with right ventricular dominance. The left ventricle is also small in these individuals.

Fetal physiology

Atrioventricular septal defects may significantly affect fetal circulatory function. It is not unusual to find these malformations in stillbirths, particularly if there are other noncardiac anomalies, but whether the cardiac lesion was primarily instrumental in causing fetal death is not known; it is possible that other fetoplacental factors are involved. However, fetal hydrops, probably indicative of fetal cardiac failure, has been reported in fetuses with atrioventricular septal defect, in which atrioventricular valve regurgitation has been a prominent feature.

Ostium primum defects probably do not produce any great alterations in the fetal circulation. If mitral valve function is normal, and this is a reasonable assumption because evidence of significant dysfunction is unusual in the newborn infant, the only effect could be some alteration in SVC and IVC flow patterns. Normally, almost all SVC blood is directed through the tricuspid valve to the right ventricle and only 2–3% of SVC return traverses the foramen ovale. In view of the close proximity of the ostium primum defect to the tricuspid valve, it is possible that a greater proportion of SVC blood with a low oxygen saturation may cross the atrial septum to the left atrium. This would tend to reduce the saturation in the ascending aorta and decrease the normal oxygen saturation difference between the ascending and descending aorta in the fetus. Also, there could be some increase in the Po_2 of blood ejected by the right ventricle, because some of the blood of lower Po_2 returning from the SVC would be shunted away from the right ventricle. This would increase the Po_2 of blood to the lungs, with a possible effect on pulmonary vascular smooth muscle development (see Chapter 5). Major redirection of caval flow patterns is improbable in ostium primum defects, so that it is unlikely that there is any significant effect on the fetal circulation. In the unusual circumstance of mitral valve insufficiency, the fetus may develop a large left ventricle and atrium and develop cardiac failure *in utero*, manifesting as hydrops.

In common atrioventricular canal lesions, modifications in intracardiac distribution of SVC blood similar to those described for ostium primum defects could occur. A large ventricular septal defect could be associated with some shunting of right ventricular blood into the ascending aorta through the defect. This combination of shunting of SVC blood across the atrial septum and of right

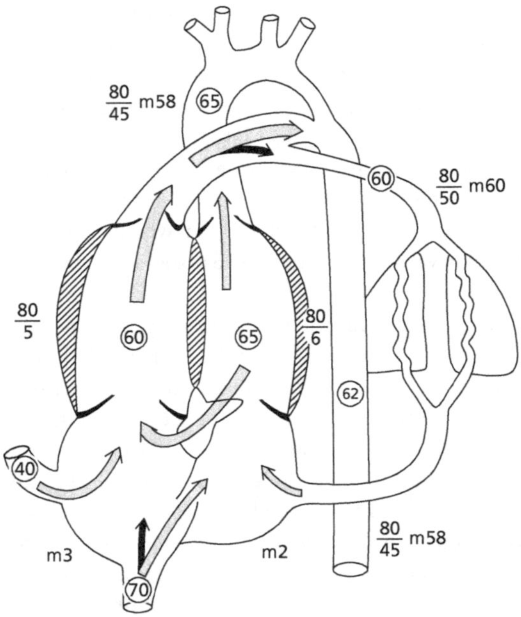

Figure 9.3 Atrioventricular septal defect with left ventricular to right atrial shunt in the fetus: course of the circulation, oxygen saturations (circled), and pressures in the heart and great vessels. m, mean pressure.

ventricular blood into the ascending aorta would have the same effect of decreasing the normal ascending–descending aortic Po_2 difference and increasing the Po_2 of blood perfusing the lungs.

If atrioventricular valve insufficiency were present in the fetus, important alterations in the circulation could develop. Figure 9.3 shows diagrammatically what could occur if the common atrioventricular valve were insufficient. The relative resistances of the pulmonary and systemic circulations would not influence the obligatory shunt that would develop, with blood being ejected from the left ventricle to the right atrium. The effect of this shunting would be to decrease the volume of left ventricular blood ejected into the aorta and provide an additional volume to the right atrium and the right ventricle. Furthermore, if there were some degree of left ventricular outflow obstruction, as is frequently present, flow into the ascending aorta would be even more compromised.

A decrease in ascending aortic flow from normal, even by a modest amount, could have a marked effect on aortic isthmus flow. In the human fetus, the left ventricle normally ejects about 45% of combined ventricular output (CVO), and about 35% of CVO is distributed to the coronary circulation, the head and neck, and the upper body. About 10% of CVO passes across the aortic isthmus to the descending aorta. If left ventricular output is reduced by as little as 5% of CVO, and normal blood flow is maintained to the upper body, flow across the isthmus would be reduced to 5% of CVO. This reduced flow across the isthmus may interfere with its development and result in narrowing or obstruction of the aortic isthmus, or in aortic coarctation (see Chapter 12).

The shunting of left ventricular blood, which has a relatively high Po_2 because it is derived from the IVC stream, will increase the Po_2 of blood in the right atrium, right ventricle, and pulmonary artery. Since the pulmonary arterioles of the fetus are quite sensitive to small changes in Po_2, the slightly higher Po_2 of blood perfusing the lungs would decrease pulmonary vasoconstriction and increase pulmonary blood flow. It is possible that the lesser degree of constriction of the pulmonary arterioles may retard the development of a thick medial muscle layer, so that a more rapid decrease in pulmonary vascular resistance may occur after birth (see Chapter 5).

If there is shunting of left ventricular blood into the right atrium and right ventricle, right ventricular output, as a proportion of CVO, would increase. Although some of this increased volume may pass through the lungs, there may also be an increased flow from the pulmonary trunk through the ductus arteriosus. This may increase the size of the ductus arteriosus.

Apparently major circulatory effects are not produced in the fetus, as most infants who do not have other congenital anomalies are well developed at birth. As discussed above, it is quite conceivable that atrioventricular valve function is not usually grossly impaired in the fetus because of the relatively small size of the ventricles.

Postnatal circulation

The adjustments of the circulation after birth may vary greatly in different infants. The hemodynamic abnormalities may be predominant atrial left-to-right shunt, predominant ventricular left-to-right shunt, or a combination of these.

Partial atrioventricular septal defects

Infants with ostium primum defect usually present the same hemodynamic features as those with atrial septal defects of the ostium secundum or fossa ovalis type. A detailed description of the adjustments after birth is presented in Chapter 8 and I review them briefly here. As pulmonary vascular resistance falls after birth, right ventricular afterload falls and right ventricular stroke volume increases and exceeds that of the left ventricle. The right ventricle fills preferentially and thus left-to-right shunting occurs through the atrial septal defect. With a further decrease in pulmonary vascular resistance and right ventricular pressure, the compliance of the right ventricle increases, thus enhancing its filling and increasing the left-to-right shunt.

Mitral insufficiency and left ventricular–right atrial shunting are not usually prominent features in infants with ostium primum defects. If present, in early infancy, mitral insufficiency results in a very large left ventricular to right atrial shunt with a large volume load on both the left and right ventricles and cardiac failure develops within weeks after birth. However, mitral valve dysfunction tends to increase progressively with advancing age, probably related to the effects of normal growth, as discussed above. Some patients do not ever develop mitral insufficiency and their course through adult life is similar to that of patients with ostium secundum types of atrial septal defects. Some degree of mitral insufficiency is frequently noted by 4–5 years of age. Blood is regurgitated through the mitral valve cleft into the left atrium or through the atrial septal defect into the right atrium. The left ventricle increases its stroke volume to maintain an adequate systemic arterial blood flow, resulting in left ventricular enlargement, which may then exaggerate mitral valve dysfunction. A progressive increase in mitral insufficiency and obligatory left-to-right shunt through the atrial septal defect will develop. The increasing volume of the left-to-right shunt places an excessive load on the right ventricle, eventually leading to combined left and right ventricular failure. Cardiac failure may occur at any age, but is most common after the age of 30 years.

Although cardiac failure is a sequel to the development of mitral regurgitation, it occurs more commonly in association with the onset of arrhythmias, particularly atrial fibrillation, which is also not usually manifest before the age of 30 years. As in atrial septal defects of the fossa ovalis type, development of pulmonary vascular disease is unusual with ostium primum defects; when it does occur, it does not usually appear before 20–30 years of age.

Complete atrioventricular septal defects

When the ventricular septal defect is large, the hemodynamic patterns are similar to those described for ventricular septal defects (see Chapter 7). With a large defect, pressures in the two ventricles are equal; as pulmonary vascular resistance falls after birth the left-to-right shunt and pulmonary blood flow increases. The increased pulmonary venous return is presented to the left atrium and ventricle. Blood shunted through the atrial septal defect presents an added volume load to the right ventricle, and since the right ventricular pressure is at systemic levels, it is subjected to an increased volume and pressure load, with a serious risk of failure. The increased venous return to the left ventricle increases its volume work and thus both left and right ventricular end-diastolic pressures and left and right atrial pressures increase. The left and right ventricular enlargement may increase the diameter of the atrioventricular annulus, thus producing or exaggerating atrioventricular valve insufficiency. The combination of atrial and ventricular left-to-right shunt with mitral and possibly tricuspid insufficiency results in a large volume load on both ventricles; severe and progressive cardiac failure ensues.

If the infant survives the cardiac failure, pulmonary vascular resistance increases, in a manner similar to that in patients with large ventricular septal defects (see Chapter 7). This results in a decrease in ventricular left-to-right shunting and volume loading of the left ventricle with clinical improvement. The decrease in left-to-right shunt may result in a reduction in atrioventricular insufficiency as ventricular size is reduced. With a further increase in pulmonary vascular resistance, right-to-left shunt develops across the ventricular septal defect and cyanosis occurs.

As with incomplete atrioventricular septal defects, obligatory shunts of large size are not common in the neonatal period (Figure 9.4). If a large obligatory left ventricular–right atrial shunt is

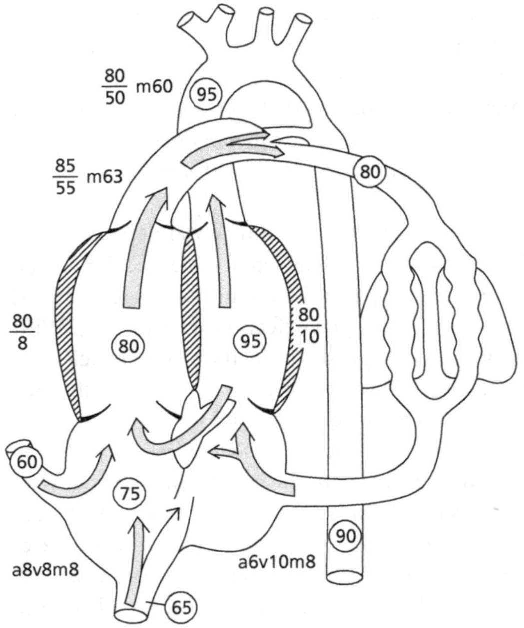

Figure 9.4 Atrioventricular septal defect with obligatory left ventricular to right atrial shunt in newborn infant: course of the circulation, oxygen saturations (circled), and pressures in the heart and great vessels. Note right-to-left shunt through the ductus arteriosus and narrowing of the aortic isthmus. m, mean pressure.

present, pulmonary blood flow is increased even though pulmonary vascular resistance may still be high, because shunting occurs from a high-pressure to a low-pressure chamber. The left-to-right shunt results in an increase in pulmonary blood flow in the early postnatal period. When this is presented to a pulmonary circulation in which there is still a considerable amount of smooth muscle in the arteriolar walls, pulmonary arterial hypertension persists (see Chapter 5).

The increased pulmonary blood flow and pulmonary arterial pressure interfere with the normal postnatal maturation of the pulmonary arterioles; the thick medial muscle layer is maintained and the fall in pulmonary vascular resistance is delayed. An interesting association may develop in some infants of an obligatory left-to-right shunt through the atrioventricular septal defect and simultaneous right-to-left shunting through the ductus arteriosus (see Figure 9.4). Pulmonary vascular resistance may be increased above systemic arterial resistance, and since shunting through the ductus arteriosus is dependent on this relationship, right-to-left shunting occurs. If intracardiac shunting is obligatory in nature, the left-to-right shunt may persist even when the pulmonary vascular resistance is markedly increased.

The effects of obligatory shunting on the pulmonary circulation are important in infants with atrioventricular septal defects. All the potential determinants for development of pulmonary vascular disease are present. The persistence of the pulmonary vascular smooth muscle makes the vessels less compliant and therefore more subject to intimal proliferation and luminal narrowing. Whereas this development would tend to reduce pulmonary blood flow and left-to-right shunt in patients with dependent shunts, thus decreasing the shear stress on the endothelium, in patients with obligatory shunting the high flow through the pulmonary vessels would be maintained, hastening the progression of pulmonary vascular intimal disease. In most infants, however, pulmonary vascular resistance falls in the first 6–8 weeks after birth and cardiac failure commonly occurs. Also, the right-to-left ductus arteriosus shunt noted in the neonate disappears (Figure 9.5).

Many aspects of the hemodynamic and clinical features of patients with atrioventricular canal defects are not well understood. Infants with complete atrioventricular septal defects that are not associated with Down syndrome tend to develop severe, rapidly progressive cardiac failure within the first few weeks after birth. The failure is quite difficult to control, and without surgery there is a high mortality within the first 6 months. Infants with Down syndrome and complete atrioventricular septal defects do not usually develop early severe cardiac failure. This could be related to the fact that pulmonary vascular resistance tends to be maintained at relatively higher levels in patients with Down syndrome.

The mechanisms responsible for the increased pulmonary vascular resistance in patients with Down syndrome have not been defined. One possible factor is the frequency of respiratory infections, producing mild hypoxemia, which causes pulmonary vasoconstriction (see Chapter 5). It has also been suggested that the development of the pulmonary arterial tree is somewhat restricted in

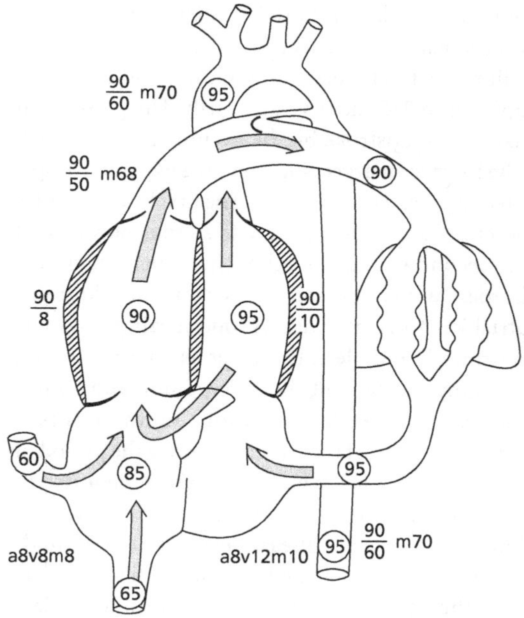

Figure 9.5 Atrioventricular septal defect with obligatory left-to-right shunt in later infancy: course of the circulation, oxygen saturations (circled), and pressures in the heart and great vessels. m, mean pressure.

patients with Down syndrome. Increased flow resulting from left-to-right shunt, through a pulmonary circulation with a decreased cross-sectional area, would stimulate rapid pulmonary vascular changes. Pulmonary vascular disease of severe degree may develop at an early age, and cyanosis often presents by 3–4 years of age. Another possibility that has been raised is that the small pulmonary vessels have an intrinsic abnormality in children with Down syndrome.

Complete atrioventricular septal defect with right ventricular outflow tract stenosis

Right ventricular outflow tract obstruction is occasionally associated with atrioventricular septal defects. The stenosis is usually predominantly infundibular, but the pulmonary valve annulus and pulmonary arteries may also be small; it is thought that this grouping of anomalies represents the association of atrioventricular septal defect with tetralogy of Fallot. It is of interest that it has been observed when the morphology of the atrioventricular septal defect is of the Rastelli type, but not in association with Rastelli type A defects.

The hemodynamic alterations are dependent on the severity of the right ventricular outflow obstruction. If severe, marked right-to-left shunting occurs, resulting in the appearance of cyanosis soon after birth. Most infants with this combination of lesions have moderate to marked degrees of outflow tract stenosis of the right ventricle and therefore do not develop large left-to-right shunts with cardiac failure. This reduces the likelihood for mitral regurgitation to develop.

Clinical features

The clinical manifestations of atrioventricular septal defects are variable and related to the hemodynamic disturbances described above.

Incomplete atrioventricular septal defect

In patients with ostium primum defects, the symptoms and signs are similar to those noted with the fossa ovalis type of atrial septal defect. They are related to the magnitude of the atrial left-to-right shunt. Although the atrial communication may be small, in most individuals it is of moderate to large size and therefore the left-to-right shunt is substantial. However, additional factors are the amount of mitral valve regurgitation and left ventricular to right atrial shunt. As mentioned above, these are not usually prominent components of the lesion during infancy.

Infants

Most infants develop well, but some may be slightly physically retarded. The arterial pulse may have a small volume, but is usually normal. The precordium is hyperactive and there is a prominent impulse along the left sternal border, reflecting volume overload of the right ventricle. Cardiomegaly, if present, is usually mild. The first heart sound is normal or accentuated at the lower left sternal border. The second sound in the pulmonary area is of normal intensity and well split during all phases of respiration. It is usually grade 2–3/6 in intensity. A medium-frequency ejection (crescendo–decrescendo) systolic murmur of grade 2–3/6 intensity is usually heard over the upper left sternal border, often radiating to both lung fields. A short low-frequency diastolic murmur may be heard at the lower left sternal border in the early part of the cycle, starting at about the time of the normal third heart sound. It is thought to be related to relative tricuspid stenosis associated with high flow across the valve. If mitral incompetence develops, the features change to those described for children.

Children

During childhood and adolescence, most patients still show only atrial shunting and the mitral valve is competent. These individuals do not have many symptoms. They may be somewhat underdeveloped and tire easily. The clinical findings are similar to those in infancy and are indistinguishable from those in patients with fossa ovalis defects. As mentioned above, mitral valve function may deteriorate with growth and mitral insufficiency and obligatory shunting may develop. When this occurs there is increasing dyspnea on exertion, and cardiac failure may develop by 4 or 5 years but may be delayed to adolescence or early adulthood. In addition to the clinical findings mentioned above there is also cardiomegaly and the left ventricular impulse becomes hyperactive. There is also a decrescendo systolic murmur heard at the apex or at the lower left sternal border. This varies from grade 2 to grade 4 in intensity, and it may be heard to radiate to the right side of the lower sternum.

Pulmonary vascular disease rarely develops before late adolescence, and the course is similar to that of atrial septal defect of the fossa ovalis type. When it occurs there is cyanosis on exertion, limitation of exercise and, later, cyanosis at rest and right-sided heart failure. The pulmonary component of the second heart sound becomes accentuated and the splitting of the sound is decreased.

Complete atrioventricular septal defect

The clinical manifestations of the complete form of atrioventricular septal defect vary as determined by the diverse morphology and hemodynamic disturbances. The following clinical presentations may be encountered.

Patients who have only a small ventricular septal defect, a large atrial septal defect, and good atrioventricular valve function behave like those with ostium primum defects (see Chapter 9).

If there is a large ventricular septal defect with competent atrioventricular valves, the manifestations are similar to those in patients with isolated ventricular septal defect (see Chapter 7). Cardiac failure, first left-sided and then right-sided, develops within 2–3 months after birth. The pulse often has a brisk upstroke but blood pressure is normal. The heart is enlarged and there is a hyperactive apical and parasternal impulse. The first heart sound is accentuated at the lower left sternal border and the second sound is loud at the upper left sternal border; it may be split if there is an additional atrial left-to-right shunt. A loud harsh pansystolic murmur is audible at the lower left sternal border, radiating throughout the precordium, and a mid-diastolic low-frequency diastolic murmur is present at the apex. If the patient survives the period of failure, there may be gradual improvement due to the development of pulmonary vascular disease. Pulmonary vascular disease develops in early childhood and is associated with cyanosis, first on exertion, then at rest, and finally cardiac failure in late adolescence or even adulthood.

Atrioventricular valve dysfunction, when significant, causes symptoms early in infancy. It is usually associated with Rastelli type C or type B morphology, and a large ventricular septal defect is usually present. The baby shows tachypnea and dyspnea, tires readily, particularly during feeding, perspires excessively, and has poor weight gain, all evidence of persistent cardiac failure. The symptoms progress rapidly, and in most instances death occurs within 1–3 months if the baby is not treated. The infant is usually pale, has poor pulses, tachycardia and hepatomegaly, and often has rales at the lung bases. The sternum and anterior chest may bulge due to cardiomegaly. The heart is markedly enlarged and there is a very hyperactive impulse at both the apex and the lower left sternal border.

The second sound may be palpable at the upper left sternal border. The first heart sound is usually markedly accentuated at the lower left sternal border. This is a striking finding, particularly in view of the fact that the PR interval is often prolonged; it probably represents abnormal atrioventricular valve motion. The second sound almost always is well split and the second component is loud. There is a grade 3–5/6 pansystolic murmur, usually heard best at the lower left sternal border, but it is also prominent over the whole precordium and is invariably very well transmitted to the right parasternal region. A grade 2–3 low-frequency mid-diastolic murmur is usually present at the apex and may also be heard parasternally.

If the ductus arteriosus is patent, the pulse pressure may be widened; however, the typical continuous murmur may not be heard, but rather a prominent systolic murmur may be present at the upper left sternal border. This is related to the increase in pulmonary arterial pressure with reduced diastolic pressure gradient between the aorta and pulmonary artery. If aortic isthmus narrowing is present, the femoral pulses may be weak, and blood pressure will be decreased in the lower compared with the upper extremities.

The response to therapy with diuretics, as well as afterload reducers, is usually poor in these infants; although digoxin was used routinely in the past, currently its use is controversial. Patients show initial improvement, but mild-to-moderate degrees of failure persist, weight gain is slow, the baby is irritable and scrawny, and respiratory distress persists and pulmonary infections may markedly aggravate the cardiac failure. If babies do survive beyond infancy, they have persistent cardiac failure and pulmonary vascular disease tends to develop early. The increase in pulmonary vascular resistance may not result in dramatic improvement in symptoms of cardiac failure if the valvar regurgitation persists. However, as mentioned above, reduction in the magnitude of the left-to-right shunt may reduce ventricular size and improve atrioventricular valve function by decreasing annular diameter.

Investigations

Electrocardiography

Characteristic changes are noted in patients with endocardial cushion defects. Classically, there is left axis deviation in the range 0° to −150°. The axis is more likely to be markedly shifted to the left (−90° to −150°) with complete atrioventricular septal defects and to be in the 0° to −90° range with incomplete defects, but may be at either end of the spectrum with either complete or incomplete defects. The QRS vector shows a superiorly oriented loop with a counterclockwise inscription in the frontal plane. It is not yet clear why the axis is deviated to the left. It is not related to the size or pressures of the ventricles, and it persists even after surgical repair. It has been suggested that it is due to an abnormality in development of conduction tissue. Frequently, atrioventricular conduction is prolonged, and in infants with complete atrioventricular septal defects the PR interval is invariably prolonged. There are variable degrees of ventricular hypertrophy. In patients with ostium primum defects, moderate right ventricular hypertrophy with an rsR′ pattern in the right precordial leads is present. The left precordial leads show either a qRs or a qRS pattern, reflecting a variable degree of right ventricular hypertrophy. With complete atrioventricular septal defects the pattern of hypertrophy varies. Some patients have increased right and left forces; pure left ventricular hypertrophy is uncommon. However, pure right ventricular hypertrophy may be present. The QRS complex is frequently wide and occasionally complete right bundle-branch block may be noted.

Radiography

Ostium primum defect is associated with varying degrees of cardiac enlargement. Usually the right ventricle is enlarged, the pulmonary artery segment is large, and pulmonary vasculature is increased. If an obligatory shunt develops, the heart is larger and left ventricular enlargement also occurs. In complete atrioventricular septal defects, the heart is usually enlarged, with both ventricles contributing, the main pulmonary artery is large, and pulmonary arterial markings are prominent. Right atrial enlargement is also common. The vascular markings may be hazy due to pulmonary edema and hilar shadows are increased. Areas of atelectasis or hyperinflation due to bronchial compression by enlarged pulmonary arteries are frequently evident. There is nothing characteristic about the radiographs in these patients to distinguish them from infants with large ventricular septal defects or many other congenital cardiac anomalies.

Echocardiography

Echocardiography has to a large extent superseded cardiac catheterization and angiocardiography in confirming the diagnosis and definition of the precise morphology of atrioventricular septal defect. The important feature that can be defined by two-dimensional studies is that the atrioventricular valves are on the same plane. As mentioned above, normally the tricuspid valve is displaced toward the apex relative to the mitral valve, so that a short segment of septum separates the left ventricle from the right atrium. In patients with atrioventricular septal defects, the mitral and tricuspid components of the common valve are at the same level. The orientation of the mitral orifice is thus changed, so that the orifice tends to point toward the ventricular septum or right ventricle. Normally the axis of the mitral orifice points toward the free wall of the left ventricle distally. The advantages of ultrasound compared with cardiac catheterization are that it is superior in defining the atrioventricular valve morphology, attachments and motion, as well as in examining the sites and direction of shunting.

Two-dimensional echocardiography should be used to provide information about whether the atrioventricular septal defect is incomplete or complete. In incomplete defects, the mitral and tricuspid valve leaflets attach to the upper margins of the ventricular septum; two separate atrioventricular orifices and no ventricular communication are evident. In complete defects, the atrioventricular valve components bridge the ventricular septum and a ventricular septal defect of varying size is present; the anterior and posterior bridging leaflets do not have fibrous continuity across the atrioventricular junction. Other important features that should be defined by ultrasound are the size of the atrial and ventricular communications, the magnitude and patterns of left-to-right shunt, the morphology and function of the atrioventricular valves, an estimate of right ventricular pressure, and the presence of other cardiovascular anomalies.

The atrial septal defect is seen to extend to the atrioventricular valves with no intervening rim of septum. In complete defects it continues across the annulus into the ventricular component of the defect. The defect varies in size, but often extends to the crista dividens; occasionally a separate fossa ovalis defect is noted. When the defect is small, it is best visualized during ventricular diastole, when the atrioventricular valves open and move away from the atrial septum.

The ventricular septal defect also varies in size from a very small defect to almost complete absence of the septum; the latter is most likely to be encountered in patients with isomerism. The ventricular component of the defect is in the posterior portion of the septum. When the defect is small, it is best visualized during ventricular systole, as the atrioventricular valves move away from the ventricles when they close.

The pattern of flow across the insufficient atrioventricular valve can be defined by color flow Doppler study. Usually the flow from the left ventricle across the valve is directed to the right atrium across the atrial component of the defect, but it may be directed to the body of the left atrium. Although it may be difficult to detect when there is a large left ventricular to right atrial shunt, the presence of regurgitation from the right ventricle to the right atrium should be defined.

The magnitude of the atrial and ventricular shunts can be estimated from Doppler studies and estimation of pulmonary and aortic blood flows. Right ventricular pressure can be estimated by calculating the left-to-right ventricular pressure gradient from measurement of the velocity of the jet across the ventricular septal defect. Caution should be exercised in making this calculation: the jet from the left ventricle to the right atrium is not analyzed, because this would provide a large calculated gradient, and the right ventricular pressure could be underestimated.

It is important to describe the atrioventricular valve morphology and attachments. With incomplete defects, the mitral and tricuspid valves both have three leaflets; the septal portion of the mitral leaflet is split by the cleft into two separate leaflets. In complete defects, as mentioned above, the posterior bridging leaflet is usually rather poorly developed and the anterior leaflet to a large extent determines the atrioventricular valve function and the likelihood of a successful surgical result. The anterior leaflet may be divided into fairly distinct mitral and tricuspid components, each of which is attached by chordae to the crest or upper margin of the ventricular septum; this defines the Rastelli type A arrangement. This is by far the commonest form of complete atrioventricular septal defect. The anterior bridging leaflet may be partly separated but attaches by chordae to a papillary muscle on the right side of the ventricular septum (Rastelli type B). It may not be divided and have no attachment to the ventricular septum, but may have chordal attachment to a papillary muscle on the lateral wall of the right ventricle. The thickness and mobility of the atrioventricular valves should also be assessed because this has important surgical implications. Another important feature to examine is the commitment of the common atrioventricular valve to either ventricle. Usually, the valve is evenly divided between the two ventricles, but on occasion it is committed to a greater extent to the left or right ventricle, and the opposite ventricular chamber is hypoplastic. Greater commitment to, and dominance of, the right ventricle is a more common occurrence; the left ventricle is hypoplastic and aortic coarctation may be associated. The presence of a hypoplastic left or right ventricle has critical surgical implications.

The presence of associated anomalies should also be explored by ultrasound. If significant narrowing of the left ventricular outflow tract is observed, the degree of obstruction to left ventricular outflow should be estimated by Doppler technique. The possibility of aortic isthmus narrowing or coarctation of the aorta should be assessed and, if present, its severity estimated. The presence of an additional left-to-right shunt through a patent ductus arteriosus should be excluded by color flow Doppler examination. Because outflow tract stenosis of the right ventricle is not uncommonly associated with atrioventricular septal defect, this should be assessed by ultrasound.

In view of the association of atrioventricular septal defect with heterotaxia, the presence of left or right atrial isomerism and the anomalies encountered in these syndromes should be assessed. It is particularly important to define pulmonary venous drainage.

Cardiac catheterization and angiocardiography

Since the introduction of echocardiography, cardiac catheterization is currently not usually indicated in the assessment of patients with atrioventricular septal defects. It is occasionally necessary to perform the procedure to determine the level of pulmonary vascular resistance and the response of the pulmonary circulation to vasoactive agents, prior to recommending surgery to correct the defects.

Approach and catheter manipulation

From the groin approach, the catheter commonly tends to pass into the left atrium and ventricle through the defect. The course of the catheter as it passes across the atrial component of the defect may be helpful in defining the position of the defect (Figure 9.6). Since the atrial septal defect is related to the atrioventricular valve annulus, the catheter usually crosses low in the septum, and frequently then passes through the cleft in the anterior leaflet of the mitral valve in ostium primum defects or through the common atrioventricular valve to enter the left ventricle. This contrasts with the position of the catheter when it passes through a fossa ovalis defect, which is more superior in the atrial septum. The catheter is preferentially directed toward the left atrial appendage and must then be curved inferiorly to enter the left ventricle. With atrioventricular septal defects, in the anteroposterior view, it is not possible to distinguish whether the catheter tip is in the left or right ventricle, because its course appears similar (Figure 9.6). Although the course of the catheter is usually fairly characteristic, it is not reliable in differentiating between fossa ovalis defects and ostium primum defects or between partial and complete atrioventricular septal defects. When a large fossa ovalis defect extends to the region of the atrioventricular valve, the course of the catheter may be similar to that in an endocardial cushion defect. Also, on occasion, the foramen ovale is patent, or there may be an additional fossa ovalis defect, in patients with atrioventricular septal defects. It may be difficult to maneuver a stiff catheter into the right ventricle

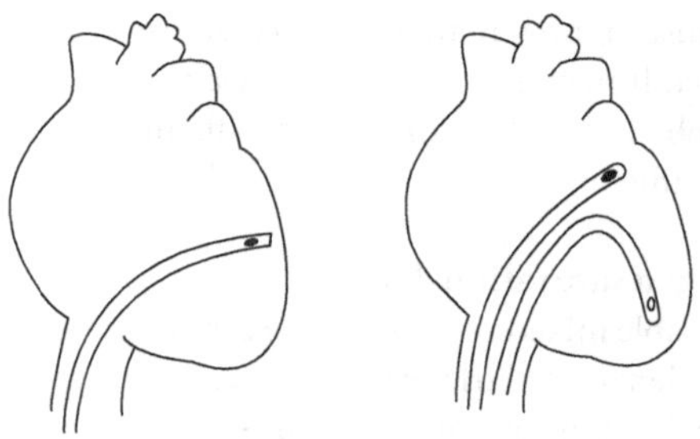

Figure 9.6 Course of the catheter in entering the left ventricle is different in atrioventricular septal defects compared with fossa ovalis defects. In endocardial cushion defects (left) it crosses the low portion of the atrial septum and enters the left ventricle with the tip often under the mitral valve. In fossa ovalis defects (right), the catheter passes across the septum in a more cranial position and usually passes to the left atrial appendage. The catheter takes a more acute bend to enter the left ventricle.

because it preferentially passes across the septal defect. It may be necessary to use a tip deflector or to substitute a balloon-tipped catheter to accomplish this.

Oxygen saturation data

A reliable mixed venous sample cannot be obtained in patients with atrioventricular septal defects. Left-to-right shunting increases the oxygen saturation in the right atrium; right atrial blood refluxes to a greater or lesser extent into the lower SVC, and into the IVC, often beyond the hepatic veins. This further contributes to the unreliability of an IVC sample as a reflection of mixed venous blood oxygen saturation A blood sample from high in the SVC therefore usually represents the best mixed venous oxygen saturation. This saturation is usually normal, but it may be decreased to 45–50% when systemic blood flow is reduced because cardiac failure has ensued, particularly in infants. Depending on the magnitude of the shunt, there is a greater or lesser increase in oxygen saturation in right atrial blood; with large shunts, it may reach 85–90%. There is usually a further increase in oxygen saturation in the right ventricle; in fact, in many instances, the increase in oxygen saturation is larger in right ventricular blood, even in incomplete atrioventricular septal defects. It is due to streaming of shunted blood directly through the tricuspid valve, which is closely related to the defect, and cannot be interpreted as being due to additional shunting at the ventricular level. The amount of increase in oxygen saturation at different levels is therefore completely unreliable in differentiating between partial and complete defects. Usually no further increase in oxygen saturation is noted beyond the body of the right ventricle, but if a patent ductus arteriosus is present, an additional increase may occur at the pulmonary arterial level. However, if there is a very large oxygen saturation increase at the atrial and ventricular level to 88–90%, a large patent ductus arteriosus left-to-right shunt may produce an insignificant increase in pulmonary arterial oxygen saturation of 2–3%. The possibility of a patent ductus should never be excluded under these circumstances; because of this and the relative frequency of an associated patent ductus arteriosus in infants with severe cardiac failure, it should be excluded by other means.

Pulmonary venous oxygen saturation is frequently reduced to 93–95% in older individuals with very large left-to-right shunts through ostium primum defects, presumably related to the high velocity through the pulmonary circulation. In infants with severe cardiac failure, oxygen saturation in pulmonary venous blood is often reduced to 90–92%, due to pulmonary edema or to alveolar hypoventilation or areas of atelectasis due to bronchial compression. The oxygen saturation may also vary in different pulmonary veins. Po_2 is also reduced to a variable degree; with significant atelectasis, it may be as low as 45–50 mmHg and pH may be reduced to 7.25–7.30. These changes are also noted in left atrial blood. Left atrial and left ventricular oxygen saturation is often decreased to as low as 86–88%, especially in patients with complete atrioventricular septal defects, because some degree of right-to-left shunt may occur at the atrial or ventricular level. In patients with elevated pulmonary vascular resistance there may be even greater reductions in oxygen saturation. Oxygen saturation in the systemic arteries is usually similar to that in the left ventricle. If there is a patent ductus arteriosus and pulmonary arterial hypertension, there may be right-to-left shunting, with a lower oxygen saturation in descending as compared with ascending aortic blood. As mentioned above, right-to-left shunting can occur through the ductus even though there is a large left-to-right shunt of the obligatory type.

Pressures

The vascular pressure changes are quite variable and depend on the type and severity of the atrioventricular septal defect. In ostium primum defects, pressures are usually similar to those described for fossa ovalis defects (see Chapter 8). However, if there is considerable atrioventricular valve insufficiency, a prominent *v* wave may be noted in the atrial pressure recordings. Right and left atrial mean pressures may be increased to as high as 15–18 mmHg as cardiac failure develops. With complete atrioventricular canal defects, right ventricular systolic pressure is increased, but the level depends on the size of the ventricular septal component of the defect. The larger the ventricular septal defect, the more likely will right ventricular systolic pressure equal systemic systolic pressure. In infants beyond 3 months of age and in children, equal right and left ventricular pressures almost always signify the presence of a large ventricular communication as part of the defect. In younger infants, even in those with incomplete defects, right ventricular and pulmonary arterial systolic pressures may be increased because pulmonary vascular resistance has not fallen normally postnatally. End-diastolic pressures may be normal in ostium primum defects, but when there are large ventricular shunts or atrioventricular valve insufficiency, both left and right ventricular end-diastolic pressures are increased, and they increase further with onset of cardiac failure.

Pulmonary arterial pressure is variable and depends on the magnitude of the shunt, the size of the ventricular septal defect, and the pulmonary vascular resistance. Often it is normal in ostium primum defects. As in fossa ovalis defects, there may be a flow gradient across the pulmonary valve of 10–15 mmHg. Pulmonary arterial diastolic pressure is usually low when pulmonary blood flow is markedly increased and pulmonary vascular resistance is normal or only slightly increased. If a large patent ductus arteriosus is present, the pulmonary and systemic arterial pressures are equal.

Systemic arterial pressure is usually normal; it may be somewhat reduced in the presence of cardiac failure. A systolic pressure difference across the outflow tract of the left ventricle may be present due to stenosis, resulting from abnormal attachment of the anterior leaflet of the mitral valve to the ventricular septum or a papillary muscle in the right ventricle. When there is moderate to marked aortic isthmus narrowing, descending aortic pressure may be reduced. However, even with severe aortic isthmus obstruction, the descending and ascending aortic pressures may be equal if the ductus arteriosus is widely patent.

Blood flows and shunts

Systemic blood flow is usually normal but may be reduced when failure occurs. Calculation of systemic flow by the Fick method is most unreliable, because it is not possible to obtain a true mixed venous sample and the use of a high SVC sample may introduce considerable error. Furthermore, in these patients, calculation of systemic flow by indicator dilution methods, as has been used in the fossa ovalis type of atrial septal defect, cannot be applied if there is any shunting of left ventricular blood or mitral valve regurgitation.

Calculation of pulmonary blood flow is also subject to serious errors. With large left-to-right shunts, the arteriovenous oxygen difference across the pulmonary circulation will be small and thus small errors in measurement of oxygen content in the pulmonary artery or veins could produce major differences in estimated blood flow. Furthermore, oxygen content of blood in different pulmonary veins may vary considerably, thus making it impossible to determine a reliable value for mixed pulmonary venous oxygen content. Pulmonary blood flow is usually high, but as pulmonary vascular resistance increases, flow falls unless the shunt is mainly of the obligatory type. In view of the potential errors in calculation of both systemic and pulmonary blood flows, values for the pulmonary to systemic flow ratio are equally unreliable.

Vascular resistances

Systemic vascular resistance is usually normal but may be increased in the presence of cardiac failure. Pulmonary vascular resistance varies greatly, depending on the lesion and the type of shunting, as outlined above. In view of the difficulties in measuring pulmonary blood flow, the estimation of pulmonary vascular resistance is also not reliable. If pulmonary vascular resistance is increased, the ability of the pulmonary vessels to dilate should be examined by determining whether pulmonary vascular resistance can be reduced by 100% oxygen inhalation or use of pulmonary vasodilator agents (see Chapter 5). The level of pulmonary vascular resistance is discussed further below in regard to decisions regarding surgical correction of the defects.

Angiocardiography

Prior to the use of ultrasound, angiocardiography was used to define several important issues. These included the site and size of the atrial and ventricular communications, the degree of mitral and tricuspid valve insufficiency, and the presence of associated lesions such as left ventricular outflow obstruction, patent ductus arteriosus, aortic arch obstructions, and anomalous pulmonary venous connections. These features can now be clearly

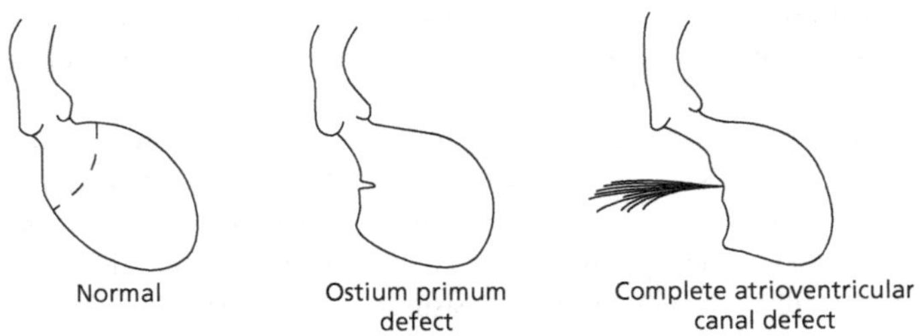

Figure 9.7 Angiographic appearance of the left ventricle in the frontal projection in the normal individual, in the presence of an ostium primum defect with no mitral insufficiency, and in an atrioventricular septal defect with an obligatory shunt. The "gooseneck" deformity is related to the abnormal mitral valve leaflet attachment and aortic displacement.

delineated by two-dimensional echocardiography with color flow Doppler studies.

The left ventricular angiogram shows features characteristic of atrioventricular septal defects. Some features are best revealed in the hepatoclavicular orientation, to provide the so-called four-chamber view, whereas others are seen more clearly in the long axial view. The left ventricular outflow tract is elongated and appears narrow (Figure 9.7), although true obstruction is not common, Normally, the contour of the left ventricle in the subaortic region is convex, bulging toward the right ventricle. In atrioventricular septal defect there is a concavity of the medial border that extends along the outflow region to the aorta. This is due to the abnormal attachment of the anterior leaflet of the mitral valve; if it attaches to the ventricular septum or right papillary muscle, left ventricular outflow obstruction may be evident. The appearance of the left ventricle, its outflow, and the ascending aorta has been designated the gooseneck deformity.

The left ventricular angiogram provides the best evidence of the type of shunting present. Even though the gooseneck deformity and the mitral valve cleft may be seen, there is frequently no evidence of valvar regurgitation. In ostium primum defects, no shunt from the left to the right ventricle is evident. If mitral valve insufficiency is present, the jet from the left ventricle is usually seen to pass directly through the left atrium across the atrial septal defect into the right atrium. Sometimes contrast medium may reach the SVC and IVC. Often only a small amount of contrast medium is seen to enter the body of the left atrium. With complete atrioventricular canal defects, the left ventricular angiogram demonstrates left-to-right shunting through the ventricular septal defect.

In infants, if it has not been possible to definitively exclude the presence of an associated patent ductus arteriosus, an injection should be made into the ascending aorta through a catheter inserted retrogradely from the femoral artery. Not infrequently, it is possible to manipulate the venous catheter through the atrioventricular septal defect into the ascending aorta to perform the angiogram in this site. The aortogram will also define the presence and degree of narrowing of the aortic isthmus, as well as the association of aortic coarctation.

An injection into the right ventricle may be made to try to assess the presence of tricuspid insufficiency. Unfortunately, this is not always satisfactory, as the catheter may recoil into the atrium if the tip is not well positioned in the apex of the ventricle. Also, the presence of a stiff catheter through the valve could possibly deflect a leaflet and induce insufficiency.

It is important to appreciate that endocardial cushion defects are frequently associated with other congenital cardiac anomalies. One should not be satisfied only with confirming the diagnosis; an intensive study to exclude other lesions should be carried out. In asplenia and polysplenia syndromes, it is necessary to consider the position of the great vessels, presence of obstruction, and drainage of pulmonary veins.

Differential diagnosis

Atrioventricular septal defects must be considered in all infants with cardiac failure and evidence of large left-to-right shunt. Lesions such as ventricular septal defect, aortopulmonary transposition with ventricular septal defect, truncus arteriosus communis, tricuspid atresia with ventricular septal defect, double-outlet right ventricle, total anomalous pulmonary venous drainage, single ventricle and others may present features similar to those of endocardial cushion defect. Clinical examination and radiography are not especially helpful in differentiating between these lesions. The electrocardiogram is quite helpful because the left axis deviation or indeterminate axis in the frontal plane is found in only a few of the lesions mentioned. The more important lesions to be considered are double-outlet right ventricle and tricuspid atresia with ventricular septal defect. Echocardiography and, if necessary, cardiac catheterization and angiocardiography usually clarify the diagnosis.

In older infants and children, ostium primum defects must be differentiated from fossa ovalis and other atrial septal defects. The presence of left axis deviation on the electrocardiogram is almost always diagnostic but rarely the axis may be normal. In fossa ovalis defects, the axis is usually deviated to the right, but it may be normal. The differentiation can almost invariably be made by ultrasound studies.

Severe pulmonary stenosis associated with atrioventricular septal defect results in right-to-left shunt and cyanosis. This complex must be differentiated from tetralogy of Fallot because surgical repair may be considerably more complicated. The presence of left axis deviation in the electrocardiogram in patients with atrioventricular septal defect is again usually diagnostic. Ultrasound studies will usually differentiate between the two conditions.

Principles of management

Most atrioventricular septal defects can now be managed surgically. The defects in the atrial and ventricular septa are closed by either a single or double patch, and the atrioventricular valve is repaired as best as possible. Several important issues need to be considered with regard to the timing and type of procedure.

Atrioventricular valve function

As mentioned above, there is a tendency for the severity of mitral valve regurgitation to progress with advancing age. This could be related either to the effects of the left-to-right shunt with enlargement of the left ventricle and atrioventricular valve annulus, or to increase in heart size with advancing age, or both. Mitral insufficiency is not commonly a significant feature in children with partial defects; it usually does not develop until the age of 20–30 years. In patients with complete atrioventricular septal defects, evidence is accumulating that valvar regurgitation is unusual in early infancy, but within 6–12 months it begins to become evident. It is of interest that in Rastelli type C morphology, despite the more primitive development, significant degrees of left-sided atrioventricular valve regurgitation are unusual before the age of about 12 months, whereas in Rastelli type A morphology regurgitation tends to occur earlier. It is also becoming apparent that more effective repair of the atrioventricular valve, with less risk of residual insufficiency, can be achieved if surgery is done before regurgitation has become evident by ultrasound.

Pulmonary vascular obstruction

The risk of early onset of pulmonary vascular disease is a major concern in patients with complete atrioventricular septal defects. Many of the factors contributing to the development of pulmonary vascular obstruction are present in these patients. Right ventricular and pulmonary arterial systolic pressures are frequently elevated to systemic arterial levels. Atrioventricular valve regurgitation may increase left atrial and pulmonary venous pressures, and if an obligatory left-to-right shunt is present, a high pulmonary blood flow is maintained even though some increase in pulmonary vascular resistance occurs. Unlike in infants with ventricular septal defects, which often tend to get smaller with increasing age, the size of atrioventricular septal defects does not change. Surgery is therefore indicated at an early age. Patients with complete atrioventricular septal defect and Down syndrome appear to be prone to the development of early pulmonary vascular obstructive changes [5,9].

In those individuals who have already developed an increase in pulmonary vascular resistance, the decisions regarding surgery will be based on the level of resistance and its responsiveness to pulmonary vasodilator agents (see Chapter 5).

Unbalanced atrioventricular septal defects

The presence of left or right ventricular dominance complicates the decision about whether the ventricular septal defect can be closed, because of concerns that the hypoplastic ventricle will not provide adequate output. No reliable criteria have as yet been developed to decide whether the size of the left or right ventricle will be adequate if they are separated. In infants with dominant right ventricle, the size of the left ventricle may be underestimated if septal deviation is not taken into consideration. By estimating a potential left ventricular volume by taking ventricular septal bowing into consideration, van Son *et al.* [10] determined that a preoperative potential left ventricular volume of 15 mL/m^2 was compatible with adequate left ventricular output after surgery. As mentioned above, left ventricular outflow tract obstruction may complicate the problem of the unbalanced atrioventricular valve commitment. The combination of subaortic obstruction, hypoplastic left ventricle, and atrioventricular valve insufficiency denotes a poor prognosis.

In those children in whom one or other ventricle is considered to be too small to proceed with intracardiac repair, consideration should be given to performing palliative banding of the pulmonary artery if a large left-to-right shunt with cardiac failure is present (see below). This would reduce the left-to-right shunt and pulmonary arterial pressure and thus reduce the risk of pulmonary vascular disease. If the left ventricle is dominant and the right ventricle is thought to be too small to sustain adequate pulmonary blood flow after separating the ventricles, a cavopulmonary anastomosis (bidirectional Glenn procedure) can be performed. This would require that pulmonary vascular resistance is low. Subsequently completing a modified Fontan procedure can be considered.

Banding of the pulmonary artery

Considerable controversy has arisen over the past 25 years regarding the efficacy of banding of the pulmonary artery in infants and children with complete atrioventricular septal defects. In early attempts to perform the procedure, there was a high perioperative mortality of 30–40%. I had proposed that banding of the pulmonary artery was contraindicated in the presence of significant atrioventricular valve regurgitation with obligatory left-to-right shunting, because it would not reduce the volume load but would add a pressure load on the right ventricle. As mentioned above, atrioventricular valve insufficiency is not a prominent feature in the first 6–12 months after birth, so pulmonary arterial banding would not usually be contraindicated. Subsequently, with improvements in surgical technique and perioperative management, the risks declined dramatically, with a mortality of about 5%. However, as with many other lesions, pulmonary arterial banding is now performed infrequently in infants with atrioventricular septal defect because the surgical risks of intracardiac repair are not significantly greater than the palliative procedure. Banding is reserved for those few patients in whom intracardiac repair is likely to be associated with a high risk, because the defect is accompanied by a single papillary muscle, severe left ventricular outflow obstruction, or unbalanced commitment of the atrioventricular valve to the ventricles.

Recommendations

Cardiac failure, if it develops, should be treated in similar manner to that outlined in Chapter 7. Early surgical attempts to correct both partial and complete atrioventricular septal defects were accompanied by high perioperative mortality, particularly during infancy. If the child survived, mitral and/or tricuspid regurgitation frequently developed, resulting in cardiac failure. However, more recently, survival and success with surgery has improved daramatically.

Ostium primum atrial septal defects

Although the atrial septal defect can be readily closed, attempts to repair the cleft in the mitral valve often created or increased mitral insufficiency. Some surgeons recommended that repair of the mitral valve should not be attempted. Recently, with improved understanding of the mitral valve mechanism, the valve can be repaired, with no evidence of regurgitation on postoperative ultrasound study. The mortality associated with surgical repair of partial defects, even during the first 3–6 months after birth, is currently negligible in many centers. However, as information on natural history of ostium primum defects has become available, it is evident that clinical problems do not usually arise before 20–30 years of age. There is therefore no pressing reason to subject them to repair in early infancy. In previous years, there was controversy as to whether the mitral valve cleft should be closed, because a number of patients developed mitral insufficiency. Recently, however, with appreciation of mitral valve anatomy, this is not a significant problem. My recommendation is that surgery be performed by about 6 months of age because there is little mortality associated with repair in infancy. The risk of progressive enlargement of the mitral orifice with increasing insufficiency can thus be avoided.

Complete atrioventricular septal defects

Early surgical attempts at intracardiac repair were associated with a high mortality, particularly during infancy. The repair of the atrioventricular valve is complicated by the fact that a bridging leaflet often provides for both mitral and tricuspid valve function. This valve has to be fashioned into two separate components for the mitral and tricuspid valves respectively. Early attempts to repair the valve were associated with a high incidence of severe mitral or tricuspid valve insufficiency. Therefore this procedure was not recommended in infants because it was difficult to perform these delicate procedures in small hearts. With improved understanding of the attachments of the mitral and tricuspid valves, it has become possible to perform the procedure with far less risk of postoperative valvar insufficiency, even within the first 6 months after birth.

Surgical repair of complete atrioventricular septal defects should be performed within 4–6 months after birth because there is a risk of early pulmonary vascular disease, particularly in patients with Down syndrome (see above). In younger infants, if cardiac failure that cannot be readily controlled is present, surgery is recommended at any age.

In fact, there is now increasing evidence indicating that if surgery is performed before atrioventricular valve regurgitation is evident, there is less likelihood for postoperative regurgitation than if it had already developed. These infants should receive optimal treatment for cardiac failure; if they respond and are thriving reasonably well, surgery should be performed by the age of 4–6 months. However, if cardiac failure is not controlled and the infant fails to thrive, surgery may be necessary earlier, sometimes by 2–4 months of age.

Although the immediate results of surgery for complete atrioventricular septal defects in infancy are quite promising, a major concern is the effectiveness of repair of the atrioventricular valves. In some patients, it is not possible to accomplish adequate repair because of concerns for inducing stenosis. About 5% of patients have moderate to severe residual left atrioventricular valve insufficiency and may require further surgery to attempt to improve valve function. Between 20 and 25% have mild residual left atrioventricular valve insufficiency within the first few years after surgery. Little information is available regarding the long-term outlook for the valve; possibly, with growth and increase in heart size, regurgitation will develop or progress in the repaired valve. Also, the incidence or severity of tricuspid regurgitation should be evaluated.

These patients should be carefully followed to define the long-term outlook after surgery. An additional consideration is the need for antibiotic prophylaxis therapy for infective endocarditis following surgery. Prophylaxis was previously advised because the atrioventricular valve is still abnormal. However, recent guidelines of the American Heart Association do not recommend the use of prophylaxis for this group of patients [11].

Unbalanced commitment of the atrioventricular valve complicates the approach to surgical repair. Dominance of the right ventricle is associated with reduction in the size of the left ventricle. As mentioned above, it is often difficult to predict whether the size of the left ventricle will be sufficient to sustain adequate output after separation of the ventricles to provide a two-ventricle repair. Outflow obstruction of the left ventricle may be severe in these infants and require intracardiac relief. Furthermore, repair of the atrioventricular valve is often associated with residual insufficiency of the mitral or tricuspid valve. The surgery is complicated and associated with a high immediate mortality; if the infant survives, there is frequently serious morbidity during the succeeding months. This has prompted some to recommend cardiac transplant for this syndrome.

References

1 Huggon IC, Cook AC, Smeeton NC, Magee AG, Sharland GK. Atrioventricular septal defects diagnosed in fetal life: associated cardiac and extra-cardiac abnormalities and outcome. J Am Coll Cardiol 2000;36:593–601.

2 Allan LD. Atrioventricular septal defect in the fetus. Am J Obstet Gynecol 1999;181:1250–1253.

3 Fesslova V, Villa L, Nava S, Boschetto C, Redaelli C, Mannarino S. Spectrum and outcome of atrioventricular septal defect in fetal life. Cardiol Young 2002;12:18–26.

4 Al-Hay AA, MacNeill SJ, Yacoub M, Shore DF, Shinebourne EA. Complete atrioventricular septal defect, Down syndrome, and surgical outcome: risk factors. Ann Thorac Surg 2003;75:412–421.

5 Kobayashi M, Takahashi Y, Ando M. Ideal timing of surgical repair of isolated complete atrioventricular septal defect. Interact Cardiovasc Thorac Surg 2007;6:24–26.

6 Rastelli GC, Kirklin JW, Titus JL. Anatomic observations on complete form of persistent common atrioventricular septal defects: its implications concerning conduction tissue disposition. Mayo Clin Proc 1966;41:296–308.

7 Macartney FJ, Zuberbuhler JR, Anderson RH. Morphologic considerations pertaining to recognition of atrial isomerism. Consequences for sequential chamber localisation. Br Heart J 1991;44:657–667.

8 Karl TR. Atrioventricular septal defect with Tetralogy of Fallot or double-outlet right ventricle: surgical considerations. Semin Thorac Cardiovasc Surg 1997;9:26–34.

9 Lange R, Guenther T, Busch R, Hess J, Schreiber C. The presence of Down syndrome is not a risk factor in complete atrioventricular septal defect repair. J Thorac Cardiovasc Surg 2007;134:304–310.

10 van Son JA, Phoon CK, Silverman NH, Haas GS. Predicting feasibility of biventricular repair of right-dominant unbalanced atrioventricular canal. Ann Thorac Surg 1997;63:1657–1663.

11 Wilson W, Taubert KA, Gewitz M *et al.* Prevention of infective endocarditis: guidelines from the American Heart Association: a guideline from the American Heart Association Rheumatic Fever, Endocarditis, and Kawasaki Disease Committee, Council on Cardiovascular Disease in the Young, and the Council on Clinical Cardiology, Council on Cardiovascular Surgery and Anesthesia, and the Quality of Care and Outcomes Research Interdisciplinary Working Group. Circulation 2007;116:1736–1754.

10

CHAPTER 10

Bicuspid aortic valve and aortic stenosis

The normal aortic valve has three cusps. A relatively large proportion of individuals have an abnormality of the aortic valve, characterized by the presence of only two cusps. This anomaly, bicuspid aortic valve, is reported to occur in at least 1% of the population, and some consider the incidence to be as high as 2%. It is of interest that despite the recognition of this high incidence of bicuspid aortic valve for at least half a century, unless it was associated with aortic stenosis, it has not been included as one of the congenital cardiovascular malformations. The incidence of congenital cardiac lesions is usually quoted as 8 per 1000; this includes those individuals who have bicuspid aortic valve, only if associated with stenosis. The incidence of bicuspid aortic valve is as high as, and perhaps higher, than that of all other congenital cardiovascular lesions combined. The reason that it was not included in the classification of congenital cardiac lesions probably relates to the fact that although it was recognized in autopsy studies, it was not detected clinically. It was only diagnosed during life following the introduction of echocardiography during the past 15–20 years. The importance of bicuspid aortic valve is being appreciated with the recent understanding that it represents one aspect of a vascular abnormality that affects the aorta and perhaps other vessels. Furthermore, it is becoming increasingly apparent that related hereditary factors are involved in bicuspid aortic valve, coarctation of the aorta, ascending aortic aneurysm, and aortic dissection and hypoplastic left heart syndrome. Recently, mutations in the *NOTCH1* gene have been implicated in the manifestations of bicuspid aortic valve syndrome (see Chapter 10).

The term *aortic stenosis* is used to indicate an obstruction to left ventricular outflow in the region of the aortic valve. Generally, three main groups of lesions are recognized: valvar stenosis, subvalvar stenosis, and supravalvar stenosis. Valvar stenosis is much more common in males, with a male to female ratio of 4:1, whereas subvalvar and supravalvar stenosis are only somewhat more common in males. Aortic stenosis is one of the more common forms of congenital cardiac disease, comprising about 6–7% of infants born with congenital heart disease. Congenital aortic stenosis probably occurs more frequently than has been recognized previously, because in many adult patients who have aortic stenosis it had been assumed that the lesion was acquired. However, many individuals who develop aortic stenosis as adults have a bicuspid aortic valve, indicating that they have a congenital anomaly of the valve. We now suspect that a significant number of individuals who have bicuspid valves and either insignificant or mild congenital aortic stenosis during childhood may develop progressive obstruction associated with calcification of the valve during adult life. As many as 1–2% of all individuals have been reported to be born with bicuspid aortic valve, so the incidence of "congenital" aortic stenosis is considerably higher than has been previously recognized.

Several congenital lesions may be associated with obstruction to blood flow into the aorta not related to anomalies of the aortic valve or the immediate subvalvar area. Thus in patients with tricuspid atresia and aortopulmonary transposition and a ventricular septal defect, blood flows from the left ventricle through the ventricular septal defect into the right ventricle and aorta. A small ventricular septal defect

Congenital Diseases of the Heart, 3rd edition. By A. Rudolph

would create an obstruction to left ventricular outflow and function as an aortic stenosis. Similarly, patients with single ventricle with a small chamber from which the aorta arises may develop functional aortic stenosis if the bulboventricular foramen connecting the main ventricular chamber to the rudimentary chamber becomes narrowed. The condition of idiopathic hypertrophic subaortic stenosis (IHSS) produces a varying degree of obstruction to outflow of the left ventricle. It is the result of hypertrophy of the left ventricular myocardium, often in an asymmetric manner, involving predominantly the septum. This condition is not discussed in this chapter; it is primarily a disorder of myocardial growth.

Although the term *hypoplastic left heart syndrome* has been used to describe a complex in which the left ventricle and ascending aorta are poorly developed, the majority of patients included in this syndrome have aortic atresia. Aortic atresia possibly represents the extreme end of the spectrum of aortic stenosis; this is supported by observations in human fetuses of progression of aortic stenosis to aortic atresia and hypoplastic left ventricle during gestational development. However, because of the possibility that hypoplastic left ventricle may arise from factors other than aortic stenosis and because the management of patients with aortic atresia and aortic stenosis are so different, I have elected to discuss aortic atresia in Chapter 11. I have decided to discuss hypoplastic left ventricle associated with aortic stenosis in this chapter because the size of the left ventricle in the infant with aortic stenosis is not infrequently an important consideration in deciding whether the ventricle will be able to sustain an adequate systemic blood flow if the stenosis is relieved.

Morphological considerations

Bicuspid aortic valve

Bicuspid aortic valve is much more frequent in males (male to female ratio 2:1) [1]. The two leaflets are sometimes of equal size, but more frequently are of different sizes. The larger of the two leaflets may have been formed by fusion of two of the cusps, because a median raphe is often present. The large cusp is most likely the result of fusion of the right coronary and left coronary leaflets; this is present in most of the patients with aortic coarctation and is less likely to be associated with significant aortic stenosis or insufficiency [2]. Fusion of the right coronary to the noncoronary leaflet is less common, but is more likely to be associated with moderate to severe stenosis and may be associated with insufficiency. The commissures are adherent for varying lengths and this to a great extent determines the degree of stenosis.

The importance of bicuspid aortic valve in patients with aortic stenosis has been documented by Roberts and Ko [3]. They examined the aortic valves in over 900 adults undergoing valve replacement for severe stenosis. Those considered to be caused by rheumatic fever and those on which previous surgery had been performed were excluded. Of the 7% in which surgery was performed below 50 years of age, about two-thirds had bicuspid valves and one-third unicuspid valves. In those 50–70 years of age at the time of surgery, about two-thirds had bicuspid valves and one-third tricuspid valves. In those over 70 years of age, only 40% had bicuspid valves and 60% had tricuspid valves. Thus it is evident that, below the age of 50 years, nonrheumatic valvar aortic stenosis is usually, if not always, associated with a developmental abnormality of the valve, with two cusps, or only one leaflet. In older individuals, aortic valve stenosis is associated with calcification of bicuspid valves or of normally developed tricuspid valves.

Bicuspid aortic valve is frequently noted in patients with coarctation of the aorta. The incidence varies from 25 to 80%. In a recent report, about 70% of patients who had coarctation repair were documented to have bicuspid aortic valves [4]. In a study of infants and children with coarctation of the aorta, bicuspid aortic valve was present in 63% [2].

Dilation of the ascending aorta may be noted in patients with bicuspid aortic valve, even in the absence of significant aortic stenosis. [5]. Enlargement of the ascending aorta had been noted in patients with congenital aortic stenosis and had been ascribed to the effects of turbulence on the aortic wall, so-called poststenotic dilatation. This was supported by the fact that the dilation is frequently related to the portion of the aortic wall subjected to the jet of blood ejected through the stenotic aortic valve. However, sometimes the dilation is diffuse, involving the whole circumference of the ascending aorta. Dilation of the ascending aorta has been observed in fetuses with valvar aortic stenosis. It seems unlikely that this can be accounted for by turbulence because, in the fetus, if there is obstruction to left ventricular outflow, the volume of blood ejected into the aorta will be reduced and thus significant turbulence is unlikely. There is now increasing evidence that there is a structural defect in the aortic wall, which may also be responsible for the abnormal aortic valve. Fedak *et al.* [6] propose that the integrity of the aortic wall is disrupted by deficiency of the microfibrillar proteins fibrillin-1 and fibulin. The authors maintain that these proteins regulate formation of both the aortic valves and the aortic wall. In patients with bicuspid valve the ascending aorta shows structural changes including deficient elastic fibers and smooth muscle cell disorientation as well as varying degrees of cystic fibrosis of the media. This also explains the relatively high incidence of dissection of the ascending aorta in adult life, an incidence five to ten times that of individuals with tricuspid aortic valves. It therefore seems likely that the poststenotic dilation is the result of the inherent abnormality in aortic wall structure and that the turbulence is a contributing factor in the dilation of the aorta.

The reason for the high incidence of bicuspid aortic valve in males is unexplained, but it is of interest that women with Turner syndrome, in whom only one X chromosome is present, have a relatively high incidence of bicuspid aortic valve of about 10%; coarctation of the aorta is also common in these patients. Genetic aspects of bicuspid aortic valve are discussed below.

Valvar aortic stenosis

This is the type encountered most frequently, accounting for about three-quarters of all patients. Based on the study of Roberts and Ko [3], the valve is bicuspid in about two-thirds of individuals with valvar aortic stenosis. The majority of the remaining patients with valvar stenosis has a unicuspid valve, with no clear distinction of separate leaflets. The orifice is usually small and shaped like a teardrop, with the wide portion in the center of the valve. It is not clear whether this valve represents fusion of the three cusps or lack of formation of two of the cusps. It is thus apparent that presence of a tricuspid valve is most unusual with valvar aortic stenosis. This suggests that the concept that aortic stenosis could develop as a result of prenatal infection is unlikely. The valve cusps are often thickened and immobile, but may have the normal mem branous appearance. Calcification of the valve is not usually prominent in individuals below the age of 25–30 years, but becomes increasingly frequent and severe with advancing age. Calcification makes the valve cusps more immobile and thus may aggravate the stenosis or, in individuals with non-stenotic bicuspid valves, may induce stenosis. Following surgery on the valve, calcification tends to occur much sooner and has been observed in adolescents and young adults. It may contribute to recurrence of stenosis after surgical relief or after balloon dilation of the valve.

The morphology of the aortic valve is distinctly different in infants with severe valvar stenosis. Frequently, the valve annulus is narrow and the cusps are thickened, often described as myxomatous, or fleshy. They are also often irregular and have a "knobbly" appearance. These features of the cusps do not persist and within a few months after birth they become thinner and more membranous in appearance, although the leaflets may still be thick and relatively immobile. Occasionally, newborn infants with a hypoplastic left ventricle have a narrow aortic annulus, but the aortic valve may have three relatively normal, thin cusps. These infants are often thought to have aortic stenosis by clinical examination, but the valve is normally developed, although small.

The ascending aorta is often dilated, particularly in its anterior portion, and this has been considered to be due to the turbulence associated with ejection through the stenotic valve. However, as discussed above, it is probably the result of structural abnormality of the aortic wall; the turbulence could be a contributing factor. The ascending aorta frequently has an area of intimal thickening a short distance above the valve related to the jet from the stenotic valve. This is not usually the site for the development of infective endocarditis. The infection most frequently involves the upper surface of the valve cusps or the adjacent aortic sinus; this is the area of least turbulence, proximal and lateral to the narrow stenotic jet flow (vena contracta).

Other cardiac anomalies are frequently associated with aortic valvar stenosis. As above, coarctation of the aorta and aortic stenosis are commonly associated, particularly if the valve is bicuspid. Patent ductus arteriosus is also commonly noted in infants with aortic stenosis; it may be important in providing systemic blood flow in infants with critical stenosis (see Chapter 10). Also during infancy, the foramen ovale may be widely patent because it is stretched by dilatation of the left atrium. Occasionally, ventricular septal defects of various size and location may occur in association with valvar aortic stenosis.

Subvalvar aortic stenosis

This form of stenosis is present in about 20% of patients with left ventricular outflow obstruction. When it occurs as an isolated lesion it presents in two forms. A discrete fibromuscular ring just beneath the aortic valve is the most common type of subvalvar stenosis. A fibrous membrane may extend from the ring into the lumen, adding to the obstruction of left ventricular outflow. Although previously a thin membranous type of obstruction had been described, it appears that most if not all so-called membranous obstructions are components of the fibromuscular ring. The fibromuscular ring may involve one of the valve cusps and this may interfere with valve function, creating mild degrees of insufficiency. The aortic valve may be normal, but often the cusps are thickened. It has been proposed that this results from the turbulence of the jet created by the subvalvar stenosis. The second type of subvalvar stenosis is a more extensive narrowing that is elongated and has been described as tunnel-like. It is most commonly associated with other anomalies such as the Shone complex (supravalvar stenosing ring of the mitral valve, parachute mitral valve, coarctation of the aorta, and subvalvar aortic stenosis). Frequently, subaortic stenosis occurs in association with other intracardiac lesions, including ventricular septal defect and septal malalignment with displacement into the left ventricular outflow tract, double-outlet right ventricle of the Taussig–Bing type, and atrioventricular septal defect with abnormal mitral valve attachment. The aortic valve is bicuspid in about 20% of patients with subvalvar stenosis, particularly those with associated lesions.

Discrete fibromuscular subvalvar stenosis is rarely evident in early infancy and is recognized in later childhood or in adults. The stenosis is invariably progressive, but the rate of increase in stenosis is variable. It may be quite rapid during childhood, but is usually fairly slow in adult life [7]. Also, progression is usually quite slow in the milder forms, but may be rapid if stenosis is more severe. Recurrence after surgery is quite common [8]. Furthermore, aortic valve regurgitation, which may not be evident or is only mild before surgery, is apparent in 50–70% of patients after surgery. It is of variable severity, but may require aortic valve replacement.

Supravalvar aortic stenosis

This type of stenosis is infrequent. Although it may occur as an isolated lesion, it is commonly associated with other anomalies. One-third to half of these individuals have Williams syndrome, characterized by growth delay, developmental delay, stellate iris, elfin facies, dental anomalies, hypoplastic nails and, occasionally, hypercalcemia in early infancy. Stenoses of other arteries, especially the pulmonary arteries, may also occur. The syndrome is thought to be associated with an elastin gene mutation on chromosome 7q11.23. A familial form of supravalvar stenosis has also been described without the associated features of Williams syndrome. The aortic valve is bicuspid in about 20% of patients with Williams syndrome and supravalvar aortic stenosis. [9].

Supravalvar stenosis most commonly presents as a constricting ring located at the superior margins of the sinuses of Valsalva. The media is thickened and collagen in the wall and the intima is increased. The narrowing may extend some distance into the ascending aorta. Although a membranous obstruction has been described, it probably represents a narrow hourglass constriction. Because the stenosis often involves the margins of the cusps, the coronary ostia may be partly covered and the arteries may be small. The intramyocardial arteries usually have thick walls involving both the medial and intimal layers.

Other features in aortic stenosis

Left ventricular size varies in older children and adults with aortic stenosis, depending on the severity of stenosis. With mild stenosis, ventricular myocardial thickness and cavity size may be normal.

With severe stenosis, the left ventricle is hypertrophied but the chamber is not enlarged. However, if aortic insufficiency is associated, the ventricle is enlarged. Myocardial fibrosis is noted in children who have had severe stenosis from infancy, but with milder stenosis may not be evident until adult age.

Infants born with severe stenosis frequently show marked endocardial fibroelastosis. The ventricular wall is markedly thickened, but cavity size varies greatly. Infants who develop cardiac failure several weeks after birth usually have marked chamber enlargement. However, those presenting with early postnatal symptoms may have a small or large ventricle. When the chamber is small, there is often marked endocardial fibroelastosis. Also, papillary muscle abnormalities may occur, involving the posterior papillary muscle more commonly. Infarction with fibrosis and shortening may result in mitral insufficiency. Abnormalities of the small coronary arteries have been described in infants with severe stenosis, especially with small ventricles. The size and function of the left ventricle is an important consideration in making decisions about the surgical approach to be adopted. This is discussed in detail on p. 235.

Occasionally, the left ventricle is small and the aortic annulus narrow. However, the valve may appear to be a normal, but small, tricuspid valve. The left atrium is often small and subendocardial fibroelastosis may occur in the region of the mitral valve or more extensively. The foramen ovale may be of normal size, but frequently is small or closed when the left ventricle is hypoplastic.

Embryological and genetic considerations

There is considerable controversy about the causes of aortic stenosis. Two main hypotheses have been proposed for the occurrence of valvar stenosis: the aortic valve may be deformed by an abnormality during embryological development of the endocardial tubercles from which the cusps form; the other proposal is that an intrauterine insult, such as an infection or metabolic disturbance, causes damage to the valve that results in stenosis. It has been suggested that the frequent finding of a bicuspid valve supports the concept that stenosis is a primary developmental defect. However, as mentioned above, the morphology of the bicuspid valve varies. In most individuals with valvar stenosis, the size of the leaflets is unequal, and the larger leaflet has a median raphe. It is possible that this could be the result of endocarditis with fusion of two of the three cusps. Infants with severe aortic stenosis frequently have associated left ventricular endocardial fibroelastosis and it has been proposed that this may be the result of endocarditis, supporting the concept that an intrauterine infection has involved both the valve and the endocardium. However, subendocardial fibroelastosis could be the result of aortic stenosis. If left ventricular pressure is elevated, there may be interference with coronary flow, which primarily affects the subendocardial region of the myocardium and may cause ischemia resulting in fibrosis. It is thus not yet resolved whether valvar aortic stenosis is a genetic or an acquired developmental anomaly.

The frequent observation of bicuspid aortic valves by echocardiography of relatives of patients with valvar aortic stenosis, coarctation of the aorta, or hypoplastic left heart syndrome suggests that hereditary factors could be important in their etiology. Recently, detailed analysis of families of children with these lesions has confirmed the heritability of these lesions and the association with bicuspid aortic valve [10], and it has been proposed that bicuspid aortic valve and its associated anomalies are linked to the chromosomal regions 18q, 5q, and 13q [11].

A recent study of five generations of one family identified 11 members with aortic stenosis. Eight had bicuspid valves with or without calcification and three had calcified tricuspid valves. A mutation of the *NOTCH1* gene was identified in the affected individuals and it was proposed that this was responsible for the abnormal development of the valve, as well as for the calcification [12].

The mechanisms responsible for subvalvar aortic stenosis are also not known. Postnatal development of fibrous subvalvar obstruction has been observed in the Newfoundland breed of dog. Genetic transmission of the lesion lends support to a developmental cause of some instances of subvalvar stenosis. However, this type of stenosis is unusual, accounting for only 10–15% of patients with subvalvar obstruction. Most have a membranous obstruction, and it is not known what may cause this type of obstruction. As mentioned above, subvalvar obstruction may be associated with other intracardiac lesions; it is usually the result of malalignment of the ventricular septum with displacement into the left ventricular outflow tract. The obstruction is not usually manifest in the fetus and develops postnatally.

Supravalvar aortic stenosis is frequently associated with Williams syndrome, which may be associated with idiopathic infantile hypercalcemia [13]. The suggestion that there may be some relationship between vitamin D and this lesion comes from experimental studies in which administration of large doses of vitamin D to pregnant rabbits may produce supravalvar aortic stenosis and dental anomalies in the offspring. However, little is known about the mechanisms that account for supravalvar stenosis.

Hemodynamic considerations

Fetal circulation

The effects of valvar, isolated subvalvar, and supravalvar stenosis on the course of the circulation in the fetus are probably similar. The effects of aortic stenosis in the fetus will be determined by the time during gestation when the obstruction develops and its severity. Initially, aortic stenosis will decrease left ventricular stroke volume, because the fetal heart is incapable of maintaining stroke volume when afterload is increased (see Chapter 1). Diastolic volume will increase, but inflow into the ventricle will be reduced. Left atrial pressure will tend to rise and flow through the foramen ovale into the left atrium will be reduced. The total volume entering and leaving the ventricle is limited and it might be expected that over time the left ventricle would not develop normally. Several ultrasound studies in human fetuses with aortic stenosis have shown a relative decrease in left ventricular size with advancing gestation. This suggests either that aortic stenosis may become more severe with advancing gestation or that a moderately stenotic valve may not grow and therefore will become more obstructive. In 1995 in serial studies in human fetuses with various types of left ventricular outflow obstruction, Hornberger *et al.* [14] observed that the left ventricle developed normally with advancing gestation in some fetuses, but in others left ventricular volume did not increase proportionately with advancing gestation and thus the left ventricle was hypoplastic at birth. Because the fetuses in this study had diverse diagnoses, including aortic coarctation, it was difficult to define the specific effect of aortic stenosis.

In a study by Axt-Fliedner *et al.* [15], aortic stenosis was suspected in a fetus at about 11 weeks' gestation; by about 16 weeks the left ventricle was hyperechogenic and dysfunctional, suggesting the presence of subendocardial fibroelastosis, and subsequently became hypoplastic. The most comprehensive observations have been made at the Children's Hospital in Boston. In a series of fetuses with aortic stenosis and normal left ventricular dimensions at less than 30 weeks' gestation, 17 of 23 had developed hypoplastic left heart syndrome by the time of delivery. Factors strongly associated with progression to hypoplastic left heart syndrome were retrograde flow in the transverse aortic arch, left-to-right flow across the foramen ovale in contrast to the normal right-to-left flow, monophasic mitral valve filling suggesting abnormal diastolic filling of the left ventricle, and left ventricular dysfunction [16]. The observations of poor left ventricular development in these reports has formed the basis for therapy to relieve aortic stenosis in the fetus in an attempt to prevent the development of hypoplastic left heart syndrome (see Chapter 11).

Evidence supporting the effect of stenosis on ventricular development has been derived from studies in fetal lambs. We produced left ventricular outflow obstruction of moderate severity by placing a band around the ascending aorta in lambs at 0.6–0.7 gestation [17]. Within a few days to 3 weeks, the left ventricular wall was markedly thickened, but cavity size was considerably reduced. The increase in muscle mass was accomplished by increase in the number of myocytes (i.e., hyperplasia), with no evidence of hypertrophy or increase in cell size. These changes are similar to those observed in the right ventricle in fetal lambs in which we banded the pulmonary artery. The development of the coronary circulation in the left ventricular myocardium was not examined in the lambs with aortic banding. If the response was the same as in the right ventricular myocardium of lambs with pulmonary stenosis, the number of capillaries did not match the increase in cell numbers. This resulted in an increase in the intercapillary distance (see Chapter 15).

Based on these observations of left ventricular growth, it can be hypothesized that, at the time of birth, the left ventricle will be small if aortic stenosis develops early in gestation. However, the later aortic stenosis develops, the more opportunity the ventricle would have had to grow normally and the larger it would be at birth. The severity of stenosis would also influence ventricular growth; severe stenosis, although appearing fairly late in pregnancy, could almost completely prevent further growth. However, mild stenosis may permit some further growth. As mentioned above, stenosis that is relatively mild in early gestation could progress to severe obstruction if the valve orifice remains the same.

In another study on fetal lambs, a nonconstricting band was placed around the ascending aorta at 0.3–0.4 gestation [18]. Aortic stenosis developed as the fetus grew *in utero*. Some of the fetuses had marked left ventricular hypertrophy at term and although the ventricles appeared to have small cavities at autopsy, ultrasound studies *in utero* did not demonstrate small left ventricular chambers. It was suggested that the small cavities noted at autopsy were the result of contraction. Other fetuses developed enlarged left ventricles with mitral regurgitation and a number died *in utero* with severe fetal hydrops. Despite a very high left ventricular end-diastolic pressure, none of the fetuses showed any evidence of subendocardial fibroelastosis, unlike human fetuses with aortic stenosis.

It is possible that the site of stenosis in this model could account for the different manifestations. In the experimental model in fetal lambs, the obstruction is beyond the origin of the coronary arteries; thus, with the high pressure in the aorta proximal to the obstruction, coronary blood flow could be well maintained and the reduction in coronary blood flow to the subendocardial region that has been incriminated as the cause of subendocardial fibroelastosis may not occur. In the human fetus with valvar aortic stenosis, coronary blood flow may be impaired and this would contribute to the development of subendocardial ischemia in the presence of high end-diastolic pressure in the ventricle.

Although some human fetuses with severe aortic stenosis or hypoplastic left heart may succumb *in utero* with hydrops, infants born with aortic stenosis, even of severe degree, appear normally developed at birth and do not show any evidence of having suffered from intrauterine hypoxemia or lack of nutrient supply. Therefore, it can be assumed that the fetus with aortic stenosis probably has a normal combined ventricular output (CVO) and normal umbilical–placental blood flow.

There is as yet no published information available in human fetuses regarding right and left ventricular output and umbilical blood flow to confirm this. Because left ventricular output is reduced in the presence of aortic stenosis, right ventricular output would have to increase to maintain a normal CVO. In studies in late-gestation fetal lambs, we found that graded constriction of the aortic isthmus decreased left ventricular output. With mild to moderate degrees of constriction, right ventricular output increased to maintain CVO, but it could not compensate adequately when constriction was severe and CVO fell. The question to be considered is whether the right ventricle can adapt over a longer period to increase output sufficiently to maintain a normal CVO. We examined cardiovascular dynamics a few days and up to 3 weeks after acute banding of the ascending aorta in fetal lambs [17]. Left ventricular systolic pressure achieved levels as high as 110 mmHg, compared with a normal of about 70 mmHg. Left ventricular output decreased markedly; it is interesting, though, that in this relatively acute preparation, right ventricular output did not increase adequately to maintain a normal CVO. Umbilical–placental blood flow fell modestly but flows to fetal body organs were reasonably well maintained. The apparently normal CVO in human fetuses with aortic stenosis could be accounted for by the ability of the right ventricle to fully compensate for the reduction in left ventricular output if the stenosis is induced slowly. Decreased flow through the foramen ovale diverts venous return to the tricuspid valve, increasing right ventricular volume load. This will increase right ventricular volume and induce right ventricular myocardial hyperplasia and possibly hypertrophy. The increased muscle mass will be able to increase right ventricular stroke volume to provide a normal CVO.

The course of the circulation in a fetus with aortic stenosis in which right ventricular output has adjusted is shown in Figure 10.1. Superior vena

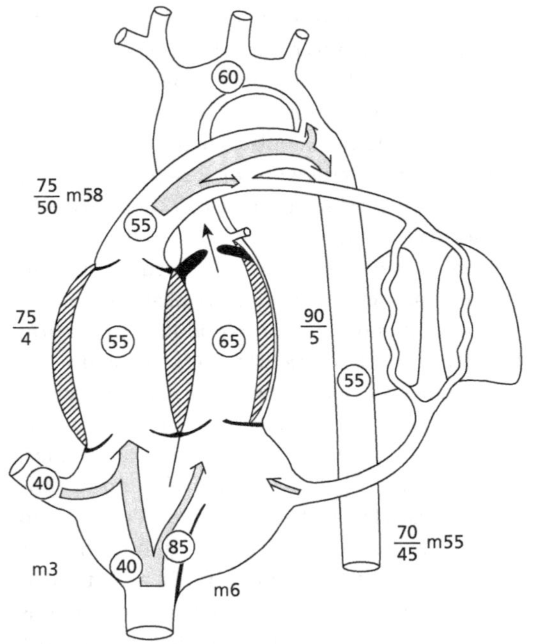

Figure 10.1 Severe valvar aortic stenosis in a fetus: course of the circulation, oxygen saturations (circled), and pressures. It has been assumed that the right ventricle has compensated by increasing its output to provide a normal combined ventricular output. m, mean pressure.

cava blood passes across the tricuspid valve as it does normally. Because left ventricular outflow is obstructed and compliance of the ventricle is decreased, the inflow of inferior vena cava (IVC) blood into the left atrium and the left ventricle is impeded. Thus, a greater proportion of IVC blood passes into the right ventricle and the volume of blood flowing through the foramen ovale is reduced. The right ventricle contributes a greater percentage to CVO, and left ventricular output is reduced to a variable degree, depending on the severity of the stenosis. The ductus arteriosus carries a greater flow than it does normally. Typically, in the lamb fetus, 55–60% of CVO passes through the ductus, but if right ventricular output is increased and lung flow does not increase greatly, flow across the ductus will increase because the contribution to descending aortic flow from the ductus arteriosus increases. Flow across the aortic isthmus is reduced because the contribution to descending aortic flow from the ductus arteriosus increases. The reduction in IVC return to the left atrium results in a larger contribution of blood with higher oxygen saturation to the right ventricle and pulmonary artery. This may result in some degree of pulmonary arteriolar vasodilatation and lack of development of pulmonary vascular smooth muscle (see Chapter 5). The greater IVC contribution to right ventricular output will also result in a decrease in the difference between oxygen saturations in the ascending and descending aortae. Left ventricular systolic pressure will be increased to a modest degree; even though left ventricular muscle mass increases, very high pressures are not generated, because inflow into the ventricle is reduced and end-diastolic pressure is not significantly increased.

The pattern of blood flow in the aortic arch and ascending aorta is a useful indicator of the severity of stenosis and the ability of the ventricle to provide blood flow to the systemic circulation. If aortic stenosis is severe, little or no blood will be ejected into the ascending aorta. Flow to the large arteries arising from the arch will be provided by blood passing through the ductus arteriosus and then coursing in a retrograde direction across the aortic isthmus to the arch. If there is minimal flow through the aortic valve, blood may also flow retrogradely in the ascending aorta to provide coronary blood flow. The pattern of flow in the arch and ascending aorta has been examined by Doppler flow study *in utero* in human fetuses with aortic stenosis. These observations have confirmed the fact that retrograde flow in the arch and ascending aorta is a useful predictor of the severity of stenosis. A similar pattern has been noted with aortic atresia and also in fetuses with a small aortic annulus and hypoplastic left ventricle but without severe valvar stenosis.

If the fetus has mild left ventricular outflow obstruction, left ventricular pressure will increase and myocardial hyperplasia will occur. The increase in muscle mass may allow the ventricle to maintain a normal stroke volume without a significant increase in left ventricular end-diastolic pressure. Left ventricular filling and output will be maintained and therefore left ventricular development will be normal. The contribution of right ventricular blood through the ductus arteriosus to the descending aorta may be somewhat greater than normal, so that the difference between ascending and descending aortic oxygen saturations may be slightly reduced (Figure 10.2).

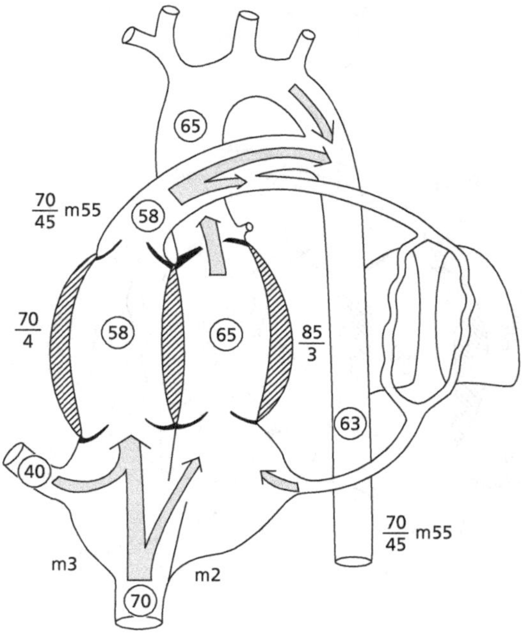

Figure 10.2 Mild valvar aortic stenosis in a fetus: course of the circulation, oxygen saturations (circled), and pressures are only minimally affected, since left ventricular output is only slightly reduced. m, mean pressure.

The pattern of the circulation during fetal life with other types of aortic stenosis is probably similar to that described for the fetus with valvar aortic stenosis. However, if subaortic narrowing is associated with other intracardiac lesions (see Chapter 10), the patterns of blood flow may be modified.

Circulatory changes after birth

The postnatal adaptations of infants with aortic stenosis are dependent on the severity of the obstruction. It is convenient to discuss the hemodynamic changes in four groups of patients: the newborn infant with severe valvar aortic stenosis; the infant with moderately severe discrete valvar, subvalvar or supravalvar stenosis; the child with moderate aortic stenosis and the individual with mild aortic stenosis. The normal aortic valve area is about 2.0 cm^2/m^2 body surface area; stenosis is considered to be severe when the valve area is less than about 0.6 cm^2/m^2, and to be moderately severe when the valve area is below about 1.0 cm^2/m^2. Valve areas above this level are considered to be moderate to mild. Similar criteria can probably be applied to membranous subvalvar stenosis and to localized supravalvar stenosis, but may not be valid for diffuse subvalvar fibromuscular stenosis or a long supravalvar stenosis.

Severe aortic stenosis in the neonate

The systemic circulation in the fetus is largely provided by flow from the pulmonary artery through the ductus arteriosus. After birth, elimination of the low-resistance placental circulation may increase afterload on the left and right ventricles. This may further reduce the ejection of any small volume of blood that the left ventricle was capable of ejecting in the fetus. All or most of the systemic blood flow would have to be provided by flow from the pulmonary artery through the ductus arteriosus. Arterial Po_2 would therefore be reduced in the descending aorta. The Po_2 in the left subclavian and carotid arteries and in the innominate artery will depend on the volume ejected by the left ventricle. With minimal output, retrograde flow in the aortic arch would result in similar reduced Po_2 in all the head and neck vessels. If the left ventricle can provide a modest output, the Po_2 in the innominate artery may be normal but that in the left subclavian artery may be reduced. Except with very severe stenosis, the left ventricle will eject a volume adequate to provide coronary blood flow.

Although left ventricular muscle mass increases during fetal life, the ventricle does not maintain its output, and left ventricular pressure is only modestly increased. After birth the ventricular pressure is increased, but the systolic pressure is usually in the range 100–120 mmHg, and it rarely exceeds these levels in the neonate. Frequently, only a small pressure gradient of 10–15 mmHg can be recorded, because flow through the valve is restricted. The systolic pressure gradient is not usually greater than about 30 mmHg.

Role of the ductus arteriosus

The ductus arteriosus plays an important role in postnatal circulatory adjustments, particularly in those infants in whom left ventricular output is markedly limited (Figure 10.3). In the immediate postnatal period, if left ventricular output is low, aortic pressure tends to fall. However, right-to-left flow of blood from the pulmonary artery through the ductus arteriosus may maintain adequate

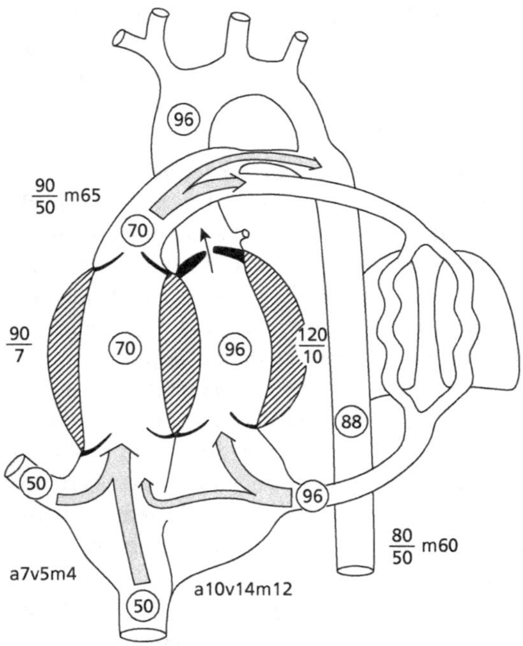

Figure 10.3 Severe valvar aortic stenosis in a newborn infant in whom the ductus arteriosus still is patent: course of the circulation, oxygen saturations (circled), and pressures demonstrate the important role of the ductus in maintaining systemic blood flow. m, mean pressure.

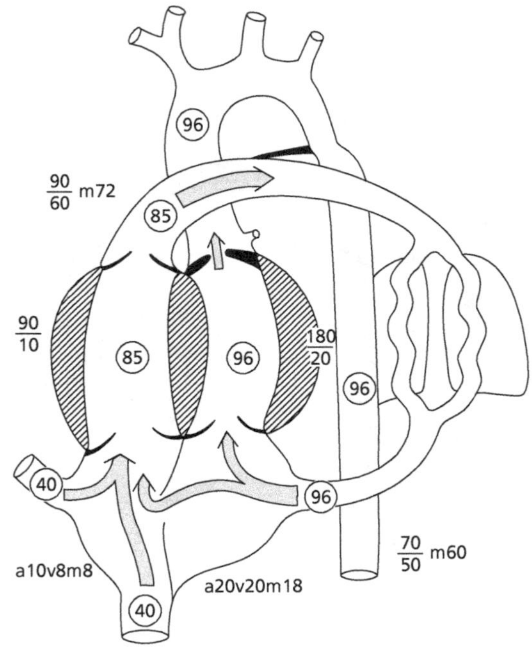

Figure 10.4 Severe valvar aortic stenosis in a newborn infant in whom the ductus arteriosus has constricted: course of the circulation, oxygen saturations (circled), and pressures show the marked deterioration due to interference with blood supply to the systemic circulation. m, mean pressure.

systemic blood flow and systemic arterial pressure. Shunting of pulmonary arterial blood away from the lungs will tend to lessen the severity of pulmonary edema by delaying the development of very high left atrial pressures (see Chapter 10). The infant may thus have little evidence of pulmonary edema and have adequate systemic circulation but cyanosis, particularly in the lower body, may be noted. Blood oxygen saturation and Po_2 in the descending aorta will be reduced compared with the ascending aorta. Depending on the volume of blood entering the ascending aorta, the right subclavian arterial oxygen saturation may also be reduced.

As the ductus arteriosus closes, total systemic blood flow will have to be maintained by left ventricular ejection (Figure 10.4). Left ventricular systolic and end-diastolic pressures will increase, and this may permit the ventricle to maintain an adequate cardiac output and systemic arterial pressure. However, if it is not able to do so, systemic arterial pressure and cardiac output will fall. Peripheral perfusion will be decreased, with the development of metabolic acidemia. Associated with the closure of the ductus arteriosus, pulmonary arterial pressure and blood flow into the lungs will increase. Left atrial and pulmonary venous pressures will tend to rise and pulmonary edema may develop.

Role of the foramen ovale

The level of left atrial pressure is an important determinant of left ventricular output. However, if left atrial pressure increases markedly, pulmonary venous and pulmonary capillary pressures will rise and pulmonary edema will ensue. At birth, elimination of the umbilical venous contribution to IVC return reduces flow through the foramen ovale. This, associated with the increased pulmonary venous return to the left atrium, will tend to close the valve of the foramen ovale. The resulting rise in left atrial pressure enhances filling of the left ventricle, but compliance of the ventricular wall will also determine the degree of filling. As mentioned above, many infants with severe aortic stenosis have subendocardial fibroelastosis, which probably decreases ventricular compliance, thus restricting end-diastolic volume and stroke volume. A more compliant ventricle will permit greater filling and a high atrial pressure may be effective in maintaining adequate left ventricular output (see Figure 10.3). However, if the left ventricle is not able to eject adequate volume across the obstructed valve, left atrial pressure will rise to very high levels and pulmonary edema will develop. The degree to which left atrial pressure rises is also influenced by the behavior of the foramen ovale. If the valve of the foramen is competent, left atrial pressure can rise to high levels, with mean pressures up to 25–30 mmHg. However, elevation of left atrial pressure may stretch the atrial septum and the foramen may become incompetent. This will permit left-to-right atrial shunting that limits the increase in left atrial pressure. The lowered filling pressure reduces the ability of the left ventricle to maintain an adequate output, but there is less likelihood for severe pulmonary edema to develop. If the ductus arteriosus closes, rapid deterioration will occur.

Coronary circulation

Normally, the left ventricle increases stroke volume and stroke work after birth, so that there is increased energy utilization and oxygen requirement. The increased Po_2 of ascending aortic and coronary arterial blood after birth will help to supply additional oxygen. With severe aortic stenosis, aortic pressure may fall when the ductus arteriosus constricts and coronary perfusion may be reduced. Left ventricular systolic and diastolic pressures are elevated so that myocardial blood flow, particularly to the inner layers of the ventricle, will be restricted. This could further interfere with its ability to maintain systemic output across the stenotic valve and aggravate the failure

Effect of oxygen administration

Administration of high-oxygen gas mixtures may potentially have adverse effects in infants with severe aortic stenosis. If systemic blood flow is being maintained by flow from the pulmonary artery through the ductus arteriosus, an increase in systemic arterial Po_2 may constrict the ductus and thus decrease flow into the systemic circulation. Oxygen may also decrease pulmonary vascular resistance and lower pulmonary arterial pressure; this will tend to decrease the flow from the pulmonary artery through the ductus arteriosus, further reducing systemic blood flow.

Effect of prostaglandin E_1

If the left ventricle is unable to provide adequate systemic output after birth, it is mandatory that the ductus arteriosus remain open so that blood can flow from the pulmonary artery to the aorta. The time after birth that the ductus closes varies, but administration of prostaglandin (PG)E_1 dilates the ductus or maintains its patency. Potential adverse effects may be associated with PGE_1 infusion. The vasodilator effect on the systemic circulation may result in a fall in aortic pressure, and interfere with coronary blood flow to both the left and right ventricular myocardium. It is therefore important to monitor arterial pressure; if it falls significantly with PGE_1, intravenous fluids should be infused and catecholamines, such as dopamine or dobutamine, administered. The reduction in pulmonary vascular resistance resulting from PGE_1 may allow pulmonary arterial blood to pass preferentially to the lungs rather than through the ductus into the aorta. This is not a significant concern if right ventricular output is adequate. It is therefore important to provide intravenous fluids and, if necessary, catecholamines. The vasodilator effect of PGE_1 on the pulmonary circulation may increase pulmonary blood flow and possibly induce pulmonary edema by increasing left atrial pressure. This also does not appear to be a major problem.

Adequacy of left ventricle to maintain systemic blood flow

Newborn infants with severe aortic stenosis frequently have small left ventricles; there is often serious question as to whether the ventricle is capable of maintaining an adequate systemic output even if the stenosis is relieved. Cardiac output is the product of heart rate and stroke volume. Stroke volume can be expressed as the proportion of left ventricular diastolic volume that is ejected. Diastolic volume is determined by ventricular cavity size and compliance, as well as by filling pressure. The ejection fraction is related to myocardial contractility. Until recently, it was immaterial whether the left ventricle was capable of providing an adequate output, because no alternative was available other than attempting to relieve the stenosis. Now, with the possibility that the Norwood procedure can be used as in aortic atresia, the decision has to be made whether the left ventricle can become an adequate systemic ventricle. Numerous measurements have been proposed for determining whether the cardiac output is likely to be adequate if the stenosis is relieved.

The diameter of the aortic valve annulus has been proposed as an indicator of likelihood for survival after surgery. The size below which survival is unlikely has varied in different reports. Generally, if annulus diameter is greater than 10 mm most infants will survive, whereas if it is below 7.5 mm survival is unlikely. However, others report survival with annulus diameters of 5 or 6 mm; thus this measurement is not reliable in decision-making. Measurement of ventricular size at end diastole by ultrasound technique has also been used to assess the potential for adequate cardiac output. In one report, left ventricular diameter was 18.4 mm in survivors and 11.3 mm in nonsurvivors. Ventricular volume (V) has also been estimated by two-dimensional ultrasound from the following equation:

$$V = 6.83b^3$$

where b is the minor or short-axis dimension. Normal left ventricular end-diastolic volume is about 40 mL/m^2. Survival is unlikely after surgery if the volume is less than 20 mL/m^2. With volumes of 20–30 mL/m^2, survival after valvotomy is 70%; with volumes greater than 30 mL/m^2, survival is about 90%. Estimating ventricular volume using the above formula presents a serious problem. Minor variations in measurement of the minor axis introduce large differences in calculated volume, because the value is cubed. Thus a minor-axis measurement of 18 mm produces an estimated volume of 40 mL; however, a minor-axis measurement of only 2 mm less (16 mm) produces an estimated volume of 28 mL. To overcome this concern, various other measurements to predict the likelihood for survival after aortic valvotomy have been proposed. The criteria proposed by Rhodes *et al.* [19] based on echocardiographic study are favored because, based on the experience with 46 neonates with aortic stenosis, the outcome for two-ventricle repair could be predicted with 95% accuracy. The equation used is as follows:

$$\text{Score} = 14.0\,(\text{BSA}) + 0.943\,(\text{AoR/m}^2) + 4.78\,(\text{LAR}) + 0.157\,(\text{MVA/m}^2) - 12.03$$

where BSA indicates body surface area, AoR aortic root diameter (cm) indexed to body surface area, LAR ratio of the long-axis dimension of the left ventricle to the long-axis dimension of the heart, and MVA mitral valve area (cm^2) indexed to body surface area. A score less than −0.35 was considered not compatible with survival after two-ventricle repair. However, with more experience, it was found that this formula was predictive in somewhat less than 80% of the patients, so it has now been modified to the following:

$$\text{Score} = 10.98\,(\text{body surface area}) + 0.56\,(\text{aortic annulus } z\text{-score}) + 5.89\,(\text{left ventricular to heart long-axis ratio}) - 0.79\,(\text{grade 2 or 3 endocardial fibroelastosis}) - 6.78$$

Using a cutoff of less than −0.65, outcome could be predicted in 90% of the patients [20].

The calculation of this score involves several measurements in small hearts and is therefore also subject to potential error. Furthermore, all these estimates of morphology do not take into consideration functional aspects of the left ventricle. Thus infants with ventricles with volumes that are only modestly reduced may not be able to maintain an adequate output after relief of stenosis if there is significant endocardial fibroelastosis. Also, the presence of mitral insufficiency may limit the ability of the ventricle to sustain systemic blood flow. One of the most reliable predictors of the inability of the ventricle to provide an adequate cardiac output after relief of aortic stenosis is the pattern of blood flow in the aorta, assessed by Doppler ultrasound study. The observation of retrograde systolic blood flow in the arch and ascending aorta indicates that there is no significant flow across the aortic valve; even in the presence of severe valvar stenosis, this still predicts unlikelihood of survival with attempted two-ventricle repair. The issues relating to surgical choices are discussed on p. 250. Despite the various criteria that have been suggested to assess the likelihood that the left ventricle will be capable of providing an adequate systemic flow, none are reliable indicators. As techniques have improved, many infants in whom previous attempts to provide two functioning ventricles have not been successful may now survive.

Hypoplastic left ventricle

As mentioned above, occasionally the aortic valve has three thin leaflets and no obvious stenosis is evident, but flow into the aorta is severely restricted because the left ventricle is small. The aortic annulus and ascending aorta are also small, as is the mitral valve annulus. Endocardial fibroelastosis is present, involving the papillary muscles and mitral valve and it may be more extensive. This complex may be truly described as hypoplastic left ventricle. If the ventricular size is estimated to be too small to sustain adequate output, or if flow in the aortic arch is retrograde, it is unlikely that a two-ventricle repair is feasible.

Moderately severe aortic stenosis in infants and children

Associated with ventilation at birth, pulmonary venous return increases and the left ventricle is required to increase stroke volume. In the infant with moderately severe stenosis and with a well-developed ventricular cavity, the ventricle is able to provide adequate output across the obstructed valve in the immediate postnatal period. The subsequent hemodynamic events are variable, depending on the severity of stenosis. With moderate stenosis, left ventricular systolic pressure increases to maintain stroke volume, but because the high afterload induced by the stenosis lowers ejection fraction, end-diastolic volume and pressure increase. Initially, to maintain adequate ventricular filling, the height of the left atrial *a* wave is increased, but with more severe obstruction or greater flow demands, mean left atrial pressure increases. The requirements for cardiac output increase over the first 6–8 weeks postnatally in association with the physiological fall in hemoglobin concentration (see Chapter 2). During this period the left ventricle undergoes hypertrophy and may be able to provide an increase in stroke volume with only a modest increase in end-diastolic pressure. However, evidence of increased sympathoadrenal stimulation often become manifest (see Chapter 7). If left atrial pressure is markedly increased, pulmonary edema with tachypnea and increased respiratory effort will develop. The drop in hemoglobin concentration reduces arterial oxygen content and this may interfere with oxygen supply to the myocardium. The increased workload on the ventricle associated with the rise in systolic pressure demands a higher oxygen consumption. In addition the higher mass of the left ventricular muscle demands an increase in total oxygen supply. If coronary flow cannot be increased adequately to meet the increased oxygen demands, myocardial ischemia may result, and this will be evidenced by electrocardiographic changes. Frequently, the infant tolerates the postnatal circulatory changes with only mild symptoms, but may develop acute cardiac failure as a result of infection, which increases the requirements for cardiac output and therefore myocardial oxygen supply. Cardiac failure most frequently develops within about 8 weeks after birth in infants with moderately severe stenosis as a result of the increased demands for cardiac output, as mentioned above. Occasionally, failure develops later, within 6–8 months, particularly as a result of infection.

Usually left ventricular pressure is not higher than about 120 mmHg in newborn infants, even with severe aortic stenosis. Postnatally, cardiac output requirements increase with growth (see Chapter 2). If the aortic valve orifice does not enlarge in proportion with the increased blood flow, the pressure gradient required to provide the flow will increase and left ventricular pressure will rise. In order to generate the higher pressure and stroke volume, myocardial mass subsequently increases, mainly by hypertrophy of myocytes but possibly with some hyperplasia. Left ventricular systolic pressure thus increases, sometimes achieving levels as high as 180–200 mmHg within the first few months after birth. Systemic arterial blood pressure may be normal, but often pulse pressure is somewhat reduced. The increase in myocardial muscle mass usually parallels the increase in pressure gradient and left ventricular pressure required to provide increased output requirements, so that cardiac failure is most unusual with valvar or discrete subvalvar stenosis beyond infancy.

The pressure gradient required for maintaining flow across the stenotic valve depends on the magnitude of flow during systole. The relationship between valve area, pressure and flow has been described by Gorlin and Gorlin [21] in the following equation:

$$\text{Aortic valve area (cm}^2\text{)} = \frac{\text{Stroke volume (mL)/Systolic ejection time (s)}}{44.5\sqrt{\text{Mean systolic pressure gradient}}}$$

It is apparent that if aortic valve area does not change, the volume of blood flowing through the valve in systole is related to the square root of the mean pressure gradient. The mean pressure gradient is therefore related to (stroke volume during systole)^2. A doubling of flow will be associated with a fourfold increase in mean pressure gradient. Not only will an increase in stroke volume elevate the pressure gradient, but it also increases the duration of ejection. The decrease in systolic duration occurring with the increased heart rate associated with sympathetic stimulation, exercise or anxiety contributes to the rise in pressure gradient, in addition to the rise in stroke volume. Infusion of catecholamines such as isoproterenol, dobutamine, or low doses of dopamine increases cardiac output by raising heart rate as well as stroke volume. These agents increase the pressure gradient across the valve and they have been used to simulate the effects of exercise in individuals with aortic stenosis. The relationship between pressure gradient and stroke volume is similar to that in patients with pulmonary stenosis; this is shown in Figure 15.7 (p. 399).

As with severe aortic stenosis in the neonate, the foramen ovale may influence the hemodynamic and clinical features in older infants with moderate or severe aortic stenosis. The increased left atrial pressure that develops when left ventricular failure occurs distends the left atrium and the atrial septum and may open the foramen ovale. A left-to-right shunt develops, and because left-sided pressures are elevated it may be substantial, even though the atrial septal opening is not very large. Pulmonary to systemic flow ratios as great as 3:1 have been encountered. Pulmonary arterial pressure is elevated, partly as a result of increased left atrial pressure but also because of increased pulmonary blood flow. The left-to-right shunt prevents the left atrial pressure from rising to high levels and thus will reduce the likelihood for pulmonary edema to develop. However, the filling pressure of the left ventricle is not able to increase and left ventricular

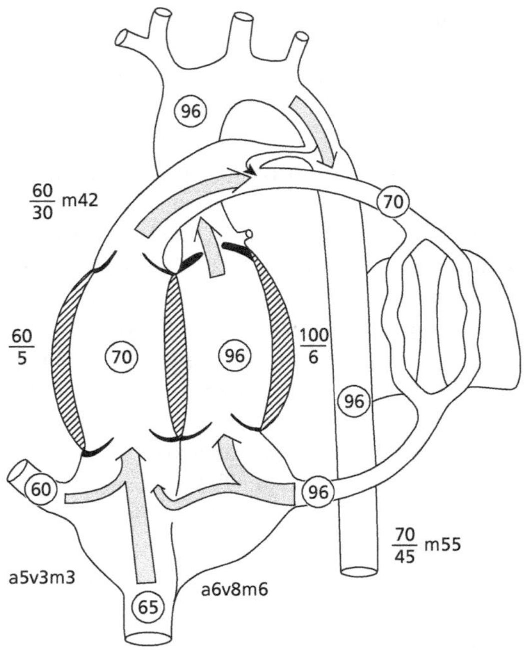

Figure 10.5 Moderate valvar aortic stenosis in a newborn infant: course of the circulation, oxygen saturations (circled), and pressures. m, mean pressure.

output may be somewhat compromised. The large volume load on the right ventricle, associated with modest right-sided hypertension, may result in right-sided failure.

Less severe degrees of aortic stenosis induce moderate increases in left ventricular pressure after birth (Figure 10.5). The ventricle is able to maintain adequate cardiac output without significant increases in end-diastolic pressure and no symptoms are evident during infancy. We do not know what determines the natural history of the anatomical lesions in children with aortic stenosis. If the valvar or subvalvar orifice enlarges with growth of the patient, no significant changes in pressure gradient may occur. However, there is considerable evidence suggesting that the orifice is usually relatively fixed, so that stenosis progressively becomes more severe relative to body size and cardiac output requirements. Serial observation during infancy has demonstrated that in most infants, growth of the stenotic orifice has not matched growth in body size and the stenosis becomes relatively more severe. The heart rate decreases as the child grows (see

Chapter 2). In order to maintain adequate cardiac output, stroke volume has to increase. This requires an elevation of left ventricular systolic pressure. Associated with the lower heart rate, the duration of systole is longer, because the stroke volume is ejected over a longer period. This increase in the period of systolic ejection may not be adequate to significantly modify the increase in pressure gradient required for the greater flow across the obstructed outlet.

Individuals with aortic stenosis do not develop cardiac failure during childhood or adolescence; the most common disturbances are syncope, infective endocarditis, or sudden death. Syncopal episodes usually occur above the age of 6 years and are probably related to inability of the left ventricle to maintain an adequate stroke volume, and cerebral blood flow falls. Syncope is often associated with or immediately follows exertion, but other physiological mechanisms may be involved. Syncope usually occurs in patients with aortic stenosis when they are forced to stand erect and still for long periods, particularly in a warm environment. The peripheral venous dilatation and pooling decreases venous return to the heart, and results in a fall in systemic blood flow. Infective endocarditis may occur at any age but is unusual before the age of 2–3 years. Following recovery from an episode of infective endocarditis, aortic insufficiency may develop.

The cause of sudden death in children or young adults with aortic stenosis is not known, but it is probably due to the sudden increased demand on the left ventricle for greater cardiac output. Sudden death occurs most frequently during or immediately after exertion. Normally, vasodilatation occurs during exercise, but arterial pressure is usually elevated because cardiac output increases. In individuals with aortic stenosis, if the increase in left ventricular stroke volume is restricted, systemic blood pressure will not be maintained. This interferes with coronary perfusion of the left ventricular myocardium, and because the demand on the left ventricle is increased during exercise, oxygen supply is inadequate and acute myocardial ischemia will result. The most likely cause of sudden death is ventricular fibrillation resulting from myocardial hypoxia. The risk of sudden death is greatest in those individuals who have electrocardiographic evidence of marked left ventricular hypertrophy, and especially in those with ST- and T-wave changes in the left precordial leads. Although sudden death is most likely to be encountered in children with more severe degrees of stenosis, it has been known to occur with only moderately severe stenosis. The degree of stenosis and the severity of the stress determine when syncopal episodes or sudden death occur. Generally, it is considered unlikely that children who have a resting systolic pressure difference of less than 50 mmHg between the left ventricle and the aorta will die suddenly. In most of these children in whom there is valvar stenosis, the calculated orifice area is above 0.6–0.7 cm^2/m^2.

Maintenance of coronary blood flow is important in individuals with aortic stenosis because the increased left ventricular muscle mass necessitates greater oxygen consumption. Although blood flow per gram of myocardium is probably the same as in the normal heart, the total coronary flow must be increased in the hypertrophied ventricle. Because coronary flow is largely determined by aortic diastolic pressure, a fall in pressure could decrease flow and thus oxygen supply to the ventricle. A fall in aortic pressure, which may result from peripheral vasodilatation, may therefore compromise left ventricular output. Vasodilator drugs or anesthesia could be dangerous in patients with aortic stenosis and it is mandatory to monitor arterial pressure and to provide vasoconstrictor agents if arterial pressure falls significantly.

The physiological effects of discrete subvalvar and supravalvar stenosis are similar to those of valvar aortic stenosis in children. However, with supravalvar stenosis, the coronary arteries, arising from the sinuses of Valsalva, are placed between the aortic valve and the stenosis and are therefore subjected to the same elevated left ventricular systolic pressure. Systolic flow in the arteries is increased early after experimental supravalvar aortic constriction, but diastolic blood flow is reduced because the diastolic pressure in the aorta proximal to the stenosis is lower than normal. This is comparable to the very low diastolic pressure observed in the main pulmonary artery proximal to a band. The low diastolic pressure results in reduced flow to the subendocardial layers of the myocardium. The coronary arteries become markedly dilated and tortuous and the small coronary arteries develop marked medial thickening and intimal proliferation and occlusion, which may interfere with coronary perfusion.

Left ventricular outflow obstruction associated with other lesions

As mentioned above, obstruction proximal to the aortic valve may be associated with other intracardiac defects. The hemodynamic disturbances are influenced by the specific lesions as well as by the subvalvar stenosis. The subvalvar aortic stenosis is not usually very severe and is frequently not appreciated, because other features dominate. During the neonatal period, blood supply to the aorta is derived partly through the ductus arteriosus and either a small or zero pressure gradient is noted between the ventricle and the aorta. After the ductus arteriosus closes, systemic arterial flow must be provided by flow into the aorta from the left ventricle. The disturbances associated with different lesions are discussed briefly.

In infants with double-outlet right ventricle of the Taussig–Bing type, there is a malalignment ventricular septal defect and the pulmonary artery overrides the left ventricle. The postnatal fall in pulmonary vascular resistance results in preferential flow from the left ventricle into the pulmonary circulation and the resulting high pulmonary blood flow may induce cardiac failure. Flow into the aorta is limited and arterial pressure may be reduced, but because flow is restricted, a large pressure gradient between the ventricle and the aorta is not evident. The stenosis may become manifest after a surgical procedure. Banding the pulmonary artery will reduce pulmonary blood flow, but left ventricular pressure rises, blood flow into the aorta increases, and a pressure gradient becomes evident. A similar phenomenon may occur in the infant with a posteriorly malaligned ventricular septum with a ventricular septal defect. Also, with this lesion, the stenosis may become evident after the ventricular septal defect is closed. If careful attention is not directed to the aortic outflow during repair, subvalvar stenosis may become evident after surgery.

A different mechanism is responsible for the development of outflow obstruction in infants with tricuspid atresia, ventricular septal defect, and aortopulmonary transposition. Postnatally, after the ductus arteriosus has closed, aortic blood flow is derived from the left ventricle through the ventricular septal defect and right ventricular infundibulum. The postnatal fall in pulmonary vascular resistance results in preferential flow into the pulmonary artery. If the ventricular septal defect is large, no gradient will be noted between the left and right ventricles, but flow into the aorta would be somewhat limited, because blood flows preferentially into the low-resistance pulmonary vascular bed. If the ventricular septal defect were restrictive, a gradient between the left and right ventricle would be evident but, because flow into the aorta would be restricted, it would not be a large gradient. Banding of the pulmonary artery will limit flow into the pulmonary circulation and increase left ventricular pressure. A greater flow across the restrictive ventricular septal defect will occur and a larger pressure gradient across the ventricular septal defect will develop. Because the ventricular septal defect usually becomes smaller with growth, the functional subvalvar aortic stenosis increases in severity and the pressure gradient between the ventricles increases.

Mild aortic stenosis and bicuspid aortic valve

Because it is a common lesion and has not previously appeared to be associated with serious hemodynamic or clinical disturbance, bicuspid aortic valve has been considered a relatively benign lesion. Mild aortic stenosis is encountered most frequently when there is a bicuspid valve with some adhesion at the margins of the raphe and slight limitation of valve opening. The systolic pressure gradient across the aortic valve may be as low as 5–10 mmHg, and the presence of a definite aortic valve lesion may be confirmed only after an ultrasound study has demonstrated the bicuspid valve with thickening and limitation of motion of the leaflets. A resting systolic pressure gradient of up to about 30 mmHg does not appear to influence normal development or exercise tolerance during childhood (Figure 10.6). Usually, left ventricular systolic pressure is not raised to more than 140–150 mmHg and cardiac output can be maintained during exertion. The main concern with these individuals is that there may be progression of the stenosis in adult life. Calcification of the valve is rare in childhood and adolescence, but it is thought that many instances of severe aortic stenosis occurring in the third to fifth decade are due to fibrosis and calcification of congenital bicuspid valves associated with mild

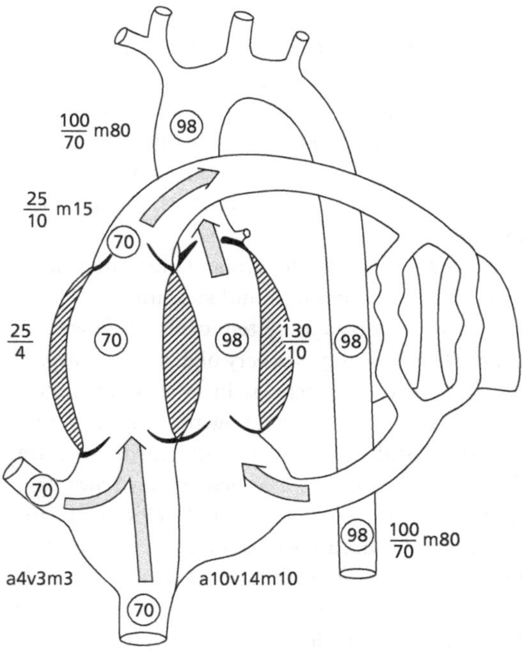

Figure 10.6 Mild valvar aortic stenosis in a child: course of the circulation, oxygen saturations (circled), and pressures indicate that apart from left ventricular hypertension there is little interference with the circulation. m, mean pressure.

stenosis in childhood. Bicuspid aortic valve also raises other concerns: in children and adolescents, bicuspid aortic valve is the lesion, second only to ventricular septal defect, with which infective endocarditis is most commonly associated.

It has also been proposed that thinning of the ascending aortic wall may occur in association with bicuspid aortic valve. As discussed above, bicuspid aortic valve, defective aortic wall, and aortic coarctation are probably associated with a common developmental abnormality (p. 229). Almost 30% of individuals below the age of 40 years who develop dissection of the aorta have associated bicuspid aortic valves. Also dissection of the aorta is five to ten times more common in individuals with bicuspid, compared with tricuspid, aortic valves. In addition to these concerns is the occurrence of aortic insufficiency in adults with bicuspid aortic valves.

Clinical features

The clinical features of aortic stenosis are discussed in relation to the same groups outlined above, namely severe aortic stenosis in the newborn infant, moderately severe stenosis in older infants and children, and mild aortic stenosis.

Severe aortic stenosis in the newborn infant

The infant may appear normal at birth, but mild to moderate cyanosis is evident, due to shunting of pulmonary arterial blood through the ductus arteriosus. If the aortic valve provides adequate flow to supply the ascending aorta and branches arising from the arch, the Po_2 of blood in the lower body will be reduced compared with blood distributed to the upper body and differential cyanosis may be appreciated. Descending aortic Po_2 may be reduced to 35–40 mmHg and pH may fall to below 7.0 due to severe metabolic acidemia. If the ascending aortic blood flow is derived across the aortic valve, right arm arterial Po_2 may be normal at 90–100 mmHg. A reduced Po_2 in right radial arterial blood similar to that in descending aortic blood indicates that ascending aortic flow is derived retrogradely across the arch from the ductus arteriosus. It indicates that the aortic stenosis is very severe or that the left ventricle is markedly hypoplastic. Pco_2 may be normal but is often slightly increased due to pulmonary edema; it rarely exceeds 45 mmHg. Administration of 100% oxygen usually increases Po_2 considerably, and if systemic blood flow is reduced, Po_2 may reach levels above 250 mmHg. There is a potential risk with oxygen administration because it could constrict the ductus arteriosus and restrict systemic arterial blood flow. This effect of oxygen is largely prevented by infusion of PGE_1.

In the early postnatal period, mild tachypnea may be noted, but severe respiratory distress does not usually occur. The pulse volume is usually normal or slightly reduced and heart rate is increased to 160–180/min. The cardiac impulse is also normal in this period. The first heart sound may be soft; the second sound is either single or narrowly split, because the aortic second sound is not heard or is soft, because flow through the valve is greatly reduced. A systolic ejection murmur of grade 2–3/6 intensity is often heard along the mid-left parasternal border. Occasionally the murmur is transmitted to the upper right sternal border. However, in many infants with severe aortic stenosis, a murmur may not be audible, because flow across the valve is negligible. As the ductus arteriosus constricts, cyanosis may improve, but the infant shows evidence of hypoperfusion, with pallor and weak pulses. Respiratory rate and effort increase and hepatomegaly may develop. If an atrial left-to-right shunt occurs through the foramen ovale, the precordial activity over the lower sternum becomes prominent. The infant may show some improvement with diuretic therapy and other supportive measures such as inotropic support (see Chapter 10), but the response may be minimal and the infant's condition usually deteriorates progressively, with pulmonary edema, inadequate perfusion, and increasing metabolic acidemia. Infusion of PGE_1 usually results in improvement of peripheral perfusion by opening the ductus arteriosus.

Moderately severe aortic stenosis in older infants and children

When aortic stenosis is not critical in the newborn period but is moderately severe, significant symptoms may not arise until 8–10 weeks after birth. The infant is often anxious and irritable and has increased perspiration, tires during feeding, and respiratory rate increases. Frequently a murmur has been detected even prior to the onset of symptoms. The symptoms progress to severe cardiac failure with pallor, tachypnea to 60–80/min, and marked respiratory distress. The heart rate is increased to 160–180/min and the pulses are poorly felt. Blood pressure is reduced to 50–60 mmHg systolic and pulse pressure is narrow.

The liver is usually enlarged and, if right-sided failure has resulted from a large atrial left-to-right shunt, it may extend 4–5 cm below the costal margin. Rales are sometimes heard at the lung bases posteriorly. The heart is enlarged and the impulse may be prominent at the apex. If an atrial left-to-right shunt is present, the precordial impulse may be increased beneath the lower sternum. The first sound may be soft or of normal intensity and the second sound is normal and split. Paradoxical splitting of the second sound, which is occasionally heard in older individuals with severe aortic valvar stenosis, is unusual in infants. A systolic ejection click may be heard in some infants along the left sternal border, but is not, as is usual in older children, always heard with valvar stenosis in infants. A harsh crescendo–decrescendo systolic murmur of grade 4–5/6 extending throughout most of systole is heard at the mid-left sternal border and radiates to the upper right sternal border; it is particularly loud in the suprasternal notch. The clinical features of the cardiac examination do not differ significantly in relation to the site of stenosis. The presence of an ejection click suggests valvar stenosis, but it is occasionally heard with a subvalvar membrane.

Infants who develop cardiac failure may show progressive deterioration and succumb to cardiac failure or inadequate systemic blood flow with shock. The mortality was very high in early surgical attempts to relieve stenosis in infants. Treatment with digoxin and diuretic agents was occasionally successful in relieving acute cardiac failure. The infants usually continued to have sweating, respiratory distress, and poor development, and subsequently succumbed to infection or persistent failure before the end of their first year.

Infants with moderate or less severe stenosis frequently do not develop any symptoms during infancy. The clinical presentation is that of an incidental finding of a systolic murmur. As mentioned above, even if the valve orifice does not increase in proportion with body size during growth, hypertrophy of the left ventricle compensates for the increase in cardiac output requirements so that ventricular failure does not develop. These individuals are commonly encountered as older children or adults with moderate degrees of aortic stenosis. These children usually have no symptoms and often have normal exercise tolerance, but occasionally fatigue is experienced with relatively limited exertion. The severity of the stenosis may not change greatly, but progressive increase in severity over time has been recorded in some children. The clinical examination in these children varies, depending on the severity of the stenosis.

The arterial pulse may be normal, but with more severe stenosis the upstroke may be delayed and the pulse volume may be weak. The left ventricular impulse is increased at the apex and is thrusting in character.

The first heart sound is normal and commonly a systolic ejection click is heard at the cardiac apex and along the left sternal border. The click is usually indicative of valvar stenosis, but occasionally an ejection click may be heard with discrete subvalvar stenosis. Due to the prolongation of left ventricular ejection, the second heart sound tends to be narrow and the aortic component soft. The normal increased splitting of the second sound during inspiration may not occur and, in severe valvar stenosis, widening of the sound on expiration and narrowing on inspiration (paradoxical splitting) may be evident. A prominent third sound is heard quite frequently at the apex and, in severe stenosis, an atrial or fourth sound may also be present. A loud systolic murmur of grade 3–5/6 intensity is characteristic of aortic stenosis; the murmur usually starts with the first sound, reaching a crescendo early in systole with milder stenosis and in mid-systole with more severe stenosis. It may also occupy only the first two-thirds of systole when stenosis is less severe but extends throughout systole with severe stenosis. In older children the murmur is most prominent at the upper right sternal border in patients with valvar or supravalvar stenosis and radiates well to the right side of the neck. With subvalvar stenosis the murmur is often heard best at the mid-left sternal border. Diastolic murmurs are not heard often, but a short grade 2–3/6 decrescendo blowing murmur following the second sound may be present along the mid-left or at the upper right sternal border. This murmur does not differentiate between valvar and subvalvar stenosis and is more frequently heard with membranous subvalvar stenosis. The cause of the aortic regurgitant murmur in these patients is not known, but it may be due to interference with normal valve closure by the subvalvar membrane or fibrous ring. The aortic insufficiency is rarely severe enough to produce a significant hemodynamic effect unless there has been complicating infective endocarditis. This may damage the valve and produce marked regurgitation, with enlargement and hyperactivity of the ventricle, an increase in the systolic murmur, a loud prolonged diastolic murmur, and a widening of pulse pressure.

Supravalvar stenosis is frequently associated with other anomalies and, as mentioned above, the features of Williams syndrome are commonly associated. These include mental retardation, abnormal facies consisting of a prominent forehead, a small mandible, up-turned nose with poorly formed nasal bridge, well-developed epicanthal folds, and usually poorly developed and widely spaced teeth. Individuals also often have outgoing personalities. In children with supravalvar stenosis, blood pressure in the right arm may be as much as 15–20 mmHg higher than in the left arm. This is thought to be due to the fact that the jet created by the stenosis is directed into the innominate artery and thus kinetic energy is transferred into this vessel. This phenomenon is known as the Coanda effect. Apart from the specific features mentioned, these patients are otherwise normal in appearance.

Mild aortic stenosis

Individuals with bicuspid aortic valve may have no symptoms and no abnormal physical findings. Females with findings consistent with bicuspid aortic valve should be carefully evaluated for physical features of Turner syndrome. Occasionally, a systolic ejection click is heard at the mid-left sternal border, with no accompanying murmurs.

The patient with mild stenosis has no symptoms during childhood. The lesion is diagnosed by the presence of a systolic murmur at the upper right sternal border radiating to the right side of the neck. In contrast to patients with severe stenosis, the second heart sound is normal, the pulse and blood pressure are normal, and there is no increased left ventricular impulse. A systolic ejection click is usually present at the mid-left sternal border. The systolic murmur is usually of grade 2–3/6 intensity, rarely occupies more than the first two-thirds of the systolic cycle, is less harsh, and peaks early in systole. In late adolescence or adulthood, progressive stenosis may occur due to calcification of the valve. Some individuals develop aortic insufficiency in adult life. As mentioned above, the incidence of aortic dissection is increased in individuals with bicuspid aortic valve. In addition these individuals are subject to the risk of infective endocarditis.

The chest radiograph shows a normal-sized heart, possibly with some left ventricular prominence and the ascending aorta may be mildly enlarged. The electrocardiogram is usually normal.

Investigations

Electrocardiography

Severe aortic stenosis in the newborn infant

The usual pattern is that of right axis deviation and right ventricular hypertrophy within the normal limits for age. However, in some infants, significant right ventricular hypertrophy is noted, evidenced by tall right precordial R waves and upright T waves in the right precordial leads. The left ventricular forces may be of normal amplitude in the left precordial leads, but infants with hypoplastic left ventricle may show R waves of low amplitude in left precordial leads. Increased left ventricular forces are infrequently present in the newborn period but may be seen in older infants with moderately severe stenosis (see below). The P waves are usually normal, but occasionally a bifid P wave is observed in leads I and II, reflecting left atrial enlargement. The T waves may be inverted or flattened in leads I, aVL, V5, and V6.

Moderately severe aortic stenosis in older infants and children

Electrocardiography usually provides a reasonable indication of the severity of stenosis, but there are enough examples in which there is a discrepancy between the electrocardiogram and the degree of stenosis that the relationship cannot be relied on. In infants, there is often right axis deviation up to 3–4 months postnatally and right ventricular precordial voltages may be increased in addition to increased left ventricular forces. In older children, left ventricular voltages are usually increased in moderate to severe stenosis. The absence of ST depression and/or T-wave flattening or inversion does not exclude severe aortic stenosis, but the presence of these changes almost invariably confirms that the stenosis is severe. They should also raise concern that the coronary arterial ostia may be narrowed by growth of fibrous tissue in the region of the supravalvar ridge in patients with supravalvar stenosis.

Chest radiography

Severe aortic stenosis in the newborn infant

Chest radiography usually shows modest cardiomegaly during the fist day or two postnatally, but heart size increases progressively and pulmonary edema becomes evident. Cardiomegaly is generalized and usually it is not possible to specify which ventricle is predominantly enlarged. The left atrium is often prominent.

Moderately severe aortic stenosis in older infants and children

Chest radiography in the infant with cardiac failure shows cardiomegaly involving particularly the left ventricle and the left atrium, with prominent pulmonary venous markings and pulmonary edema. In older individuals who do not have any symptoms, the transverse cardiac diameter is not increased but there may be left ventricular enlargement, evidenced by downward displacement and rounding of the apex. In infants in whom foramen ovale dilation has occurred, resulting in a large atrial left-to-right shunt, the right ventricle may be enlarged and the pulmonary vascular markings are prominent.

There is usually prominence of the ascending aorta in patients with valvar stenosis; this may be due to poststenotic dilatation, but is most likely related to abnormal structure of the aortic wall associated with the occurrence of bicuspid aortic valve (see Chapter 10). In patients with supravalvar stenosis, the ascending aorta is not usually prominent but may be mildly enlarged in some individuals. With subvalvar stenosis the ascending aorta is not enlarged. It has been mentioned that a discrete subvalvar membranous obstruction may be associated with poststenotic dilation, but I have never encountered this. In patients with more severe degrees of stenosis, left atrial enlargement may be noted.

Echocardiography

Ultrasound examination is capable of confirming the presence of aortic stenosis and assessing its severity. The presence of bicuspid aortic valve, which may not have any clinical manifestations, is also detectable by ultrasound technique. The need for cardiac catheterization for diagnosis or evaluation of the severity of stenosis has largely been eliminated. Recently, however, catheterization is being performed more frequently for treatment by balloon valvoplasty. Important information that should be obtained by ultrasound examination includes the following:

- location and nature of the obstruction;
- morphology of the aortic valve;
- assessment of the severity of obstruction;
- estimation of the diameter of the aortic annulus;
- assessment of the size of the left ventricle;
- evaluation of left ventricular wall thickness;
- assessment of left ventricular function;
- presence of endocardial fibroelastosis;
- patency of the ductus arteriosus and flow through it;

• atrial left-to-right shunting through the foramen ovale;
• presence of associated cardiac lesions.

The severity of obstruction is assessed by measuring peak instantaneous and mean pressure drops. Also, if possible, aortic valve area should be estimated from the continuity equation:

$$A_1V_1 = A_2V_2$$

where A_1 denotes flow area of the left ventricular outflow tract, V_1 mean flow velocity in the left ventricular outflow tract, A_2 effective valve orifice area, and V_2 mean velocity in the vena contracta. The equation should be solved for A_2.

Two-dimensional ultrasound studies demonstrate the site of obstruction at the valve or in the subvalvar or supravalvar region. The aortic valve is frequently dysplastic and markedly thickened in newborn infants with valvar stenosis. The valve may show little motion and frequently the annulus is narrow. In older infants and children, the valve is membranous, but often the leaflets are thick. Commonly the valve is bicuspid; the two cusps may be of equal size, but often one cusp is considerably larger and in diastole a median raphe is evident, giving the appearance that the valve is bicuspid. However, in systole, the typical fish-mouth appearance of the orifice confirms the bicuspid nature of the valve. The stenotic valve domes upward during systole. Subvalvar stenosis may be related to a fibrous membrane immediately beneath or a few millimeters proximal to the valve cusps. It may also dome during systole and the membrane may restrict motion of the valve cusps during diastole. Also, in some patients a discrete subvalvar membrane may develop into a fibromuscular obstruction with a more diffuse obstruction some distance proximal to the valve.

The severity of the stenosis has been evaluated by various techniques. One method used M-mode measurements of the thickness of the posterior wall of the left ventricle and the dimension of the cavity during systole to assess left ventricular systolic pressure. This is of no particular value in newborn or young infants and the technique has now been largely replaced by use of Doppler flow techniques. Continuous-wave Doppler allows measurement of peak velocity in the jet beyond the stenosis. The direction of the jet may vary, depending on the orientation of the orifice, so it is important to attempt to use color Doppler to align the transducer accurately in order to measure the maximal velocity. Based on the Bernoulli principle, with flow across a thin membrane, the instantaneous pressure gradient (P) can be calculated from the equation $P = 4V^2$, where V is peak velocity. Peak instantaneous pressure gradients recorded by this method have yielded results that correlate fairly well with peak-to-peak systolic pressure gradients measured by cardiac catheterization. However, the gradients measured by Doppler technique are generally higher than those measured by catheterization. The pressure gradient measured by catheters reflects the difference in peak systolic pressures recorded in the left ventricle and the aorta. These peaks may not be reached simultaneously. The gradient calculated from peak Doppler flow velocity represents the difference in pressures at the instant peak velocity is reached. This could explain the difference in the gradients measured by the two methods. Recently, the discrepancies between gradients measured by the two methods has been explained on the basis of the phenomenon of pressure recovery, i.e., an increase in pressure distal to a stenosis resulting from conversion of kinetic into potential energy. By making adjustments in the Doppler gradients to correct for pressure recovery, the correlation between pressure gradients measured by Doppler and catheter techniques is greatly improved.

Although the estimation of systolic pressure gradient by means of continuous-flow Doppler examination is very useful, it must be recognized that the overestimation compared with the gradient measured on pressure recordings varies greatly. The differences reported have varied from 5 to about 80 mmHg. Until such time as a reliable method for predicting the gradient recorded by pressure measurements using Doppler equipment is developed, decisions about treatment should not be based on the Doppler gradient alone (see Principles of management, p. 250). The pressure gradients measured by Doppler technique are probably reasonably reliable when stenosis is due to a subvalvar membrane or to a localized supravalvar stenosis. However, the gradients may be unreliable with subvalvar tunnel-like stenosis or a long supravalvar constriction.

In infants, increased echodensity in the region of the papillary muscles is often noted and the whole endothelial surface of the ventricle may show the increased echodensity, which probably represents endocardial fibroelastosis. The importance of this finding has not been resolved, because severe fibroelastosis has been observed in fetal hearts that did not demonstrate increased echodensity when examined prior to death. Also, infants with marked echocardiographic changes often have apparently normal left ventricular function.

Assessment of ventricular size is extremely important in newborn infants, because detection of a hypoplastic ventricle requires a decision about whether it is capable of maintaining an adequate systemic blood flow if the stenosis is relieved. This will influence the surgical procedure that will be attempted. This assessment is now generally made from ultrasound studies; these have been discussed on p. 236. In addition, the ejection fraction of the ventricle can be calculated to try to assess ventricular function. However, this is not at all reliable in the presence of stenosis, because the high afterload will markedly reduce ejection from the ventricle. This assessment is of greater value after the stenosis has been relieved, when a low ejection fraction is a more useful indicator of poor function. The use of color flow Doppler techniques to assess direction of flow in the aortic arch and ascending aorta is also helpful in making theses decisions. The presence of retrograde flow indicates that flow is being derived through the ductus arteriosus and that flow through the aortic valve is severely restricted. It is unlikely that the left ventricle will provide adequate flow, even if aortic stenosis is relieved.

The ultrasound examination should determine whether other lesions, such as aortic coarctation or mitral valve anomalies, are present. If subvalvar stenosis is present, the lesions frequently associated should be excluded.

Cardiac catheterization and angiocardiography

As mentioned above, ultrasound examination has largely replaced cardiac catheterization for diagnosis and assessment of severity of aortic stenosis. In many centers, patients with aortic stenosis, including newborn infants, are referred for surgery with information obtained by ultrasound study alone. However, in recent years, cardiac catheterization is again being performed in a number of individuals with aortic stenosis for the purpose of relieving the obstruction by balloon valvoplasty (see Chapter 10).

Approach and catheter manipulation

Prior to proceeding with the procedure in a newborn infant, measures should be instituted to improve the hemodynamic and metabolic status by correcting acidemia, hypoglycemia, and hypocalcemia, administering diuretic therapy if the infant has cardiac failure and oxygen if hypoxemia is present. Intravenous PGE_1 should be administered to open the ductus arteriosus if it has constricted or to maintain its patency, so as to provide systemic blood flow if the aortic stenosis is critical. Usually a right heart catheterization is performed to confirm the findings of ultrasound examination and also to measure mixed venous oxygen saturation in order to calculate blood flows by the Fick method. The venous catheter is inserted first from the femoral approach; after routine catheterization of the right heart, attempts are made to pass the catheter across the foramen ovale into the left ventricle. If this can be accomplished, the pressure difference across the aortic outflow may be measured by advancing a catheter inserted into the umbilical artery to the central aorta. It may not be possible to pass a catheter into the left atrium and ventricle because the foramen ovale may have been sealed by elevation of left atrial pressure. In this event a long trans-septal sheath can be used to pass a catheter into the left ventricle. From here it may be possible to manipulate a catheter across the outflow tract into the aorta. If it is not possible to enter the left ventricle across the atrial septum, an arterial catheter is inserted into either an umbilical or femoral artery and passed retrogradely across the aortic valve into the left ventricle. This may be a difficult procedure in a newborn infant. Slow withdrawal of the catheter either from the aorta into the left ventricle or from the ventricle into the aorta may make it possible to establish whether the stenosis is subvalvar, valvar, or supravalvar. This may be difficult in an infant because the catheter may flip so that the pressure transition is not well visualized.

In children, after performing the right heart study, a trans-septal approach is used to manipulate a catheter into the left ventricle and then into the aorta. Slow withdrawal across the outflow tract will demonstrate the site of stenosis. However, it may be difficult to distinguish between a valvar stenosis and stenosis due to a membrane immediately beneath the valve. The distance between the valve and the membrane may be so short that, on withdrawal of the catheter, no transitional pressure can be recorded between the aorta and the main left ventricle.

Oxygen saturation and blood gases

In infants with cardiac failure, mixed venous oxygen saturation is low because cardiac output is reduced. Frequently right atrial, right ventricular, and pulmonary arterial oxygen saturations are increased by an atrial left-to-right shunt. Oxygen saturations may be increased to as high as 85–88%. Oxygen saturation in the descending aorta may be lower than that in the ascending aorta due to right-to-left shunting through the ductus arteriosus. However, when there is a large left-to-right shunt at the atrial level, the pulmonary arterial blood shunted into the descending aorta may have a relatively high saturation and this will to some extent mask the difference in upper and lower body saturation. If flow through the aortic valve is severely restricted, oxygen saturation in the ascending aorta may be reduced to levels similar to that in the descending aorta because ductus arteriosus-derived blood will flow retrogradely across the arch.

When systemic blood flow is markedly reduced, systemic arterial pH may fall to below 7.0. Pco_2 may be slightly increased up to 45 mmHg if pulmonary edema is present. Po_2 in descending aortic blood may be reduced to 35–40 mmHg. Oxygen administration usually increases Po_2 levels; occasionally, 100% oxygen will raise ascending aortic Po_2 above 250 mmHg because of the high pulmonary blood flow and low systemic flow.

In children with aortic stenosis at any site, oxygen saturations and blood gases on the right and left sides of the heart are normal unless there are complicating lesions.

Pressures

In infants with cardiac failure, right atrial pressure is increased and mean levels of 8–10 mmHg are common. Right ventricular and pulmonary arterial pressures vary greatly; in the newborn period, they may exceed aortic systolic pressure, and mean pulmonary arterial pressure may be higher than mean aortic pressure. In later infancy, right ventricular and pulmonary arterial pressures may be normal, but are often moderately elevated, with systolic pressure in the range 40–60 mmHg. The pulmonary arterial wedge and left atrial pressures are increased, sometimes to mean levels of 20–25 mmHg. Left atrial pressure shows equal *a* and *v* waves or a dominant *a* wave; left ventricular end-diastolic pressure may reach 25–35 mmHg. Left ventricular systolic pressure is rarely greater than about 120 mmHg in the newborn infant, but in the older infant it may be raised to 180–200 mmHg. Aortic systolic pressure in the presence of cardiac failure is usually below 70 mmHg. The pressure gradient across the outflow may be relatively low in infants with severe stenosis when systemic blood flow is very low. It is not usually greater than about 50 mmHg and even smaller gradients of 10–20 mmHg may be recorded with severe stenosis. Also, when the left ventricle is hypoplastic, left ventricular output may be severely restricted and a minimal gradient may be recorded even though stenosis is severe.

In children with aortic stenosis, the right atrial, right ventricular, and pulmonary arterial pressures are usually normal. The left atrial *a* wave and left ventricular end-diastolic pressure may be increased to 25–30 mmHg in children with severe stenosis. Left ventricular systolic pressure may be increased to 280–300 mmHg, but with mild stenosis it may be in the normal range.

The systolic pressure difference across the obstruction may be as high as 200 mmHg, but with mild stenosis the gradient may be only 10–15 mmHg. In individuals with bicuspid valve, no systolic pressure gradient may be recorded, even though valve motion is seen to be restricted on ultrasound examination. Proximal to the obstruction, with severe stenosis, the left ventricular pressure contour shows a slower than normal upstroke and downstroke. The site of stenosis can usually be determined by careful withdrawal of the catheter from the ventricle into the aorta. With supravalvar stenosis, the systolic pressure is higher in the aorta just beneath the obstruction. The diastolic pressure in the chamber between the stenosis and the aortic valve is often lower than that in the aorta beyond the stenosis. A sudden change in systolic pressure as the catheter is moved across the valve indicates the presence of valvar stenosis. When subvalvar stenosis is some distance proximal to the valve, the left ventricular chamber between the stenosis and the valve shows a lower systolic pressure but similar diastolic pressure as the left ventricle. With discrete subaortic stenosis, it may be difficult to record a decrease in systolic pressure below the aortic valve, because the stenosis is just proximal to the valve and the catheter may flip across the membrane and valve, giving the appearance that the stenosis is valvar. No systolic pressure difference is recorded across the valve. In assessing the presence or severity of stenosis, it is important to appreciate that the peripheral arterial pressure, when recorded with a needle or a cannula in the femoral, brachial or radial artery, may show a considerably higher systolic pressure than that in the ascending aorta, due to reflected waves. Thus, if left ventricular pressure is recorded by a catheter passed into the ventricle across the atrial septum, it is possible that a mild degree of aortic stenosis may be overlooked.

Blood flow and shunts

In infants in cardiac failure, cardiac output is decreased. Systemic blood flow may be reduced to 1.5–2.0 L/min per m^2. Pulmonary blood flow may be reduced, but is often normal or increased due to an atrial left-to-right shunt. The pulmonary to systemic flow ratio may be increased to as much as 3.0–3.5:1. This reflects a decrease in systemic blood flow as well as maintenance or an increase in pulmonary blood flow. Some right-to-left shunt may occur through the ductus arteriosus, but it may be difficult to detect from oxygen saturation measurements when right ventricular oxygen saturation is increased, because of the left-to-right shunt at the atrial level.

In older children, cardiac output is usually normal at rest. During exercise, the cardiac output does not increase normally in patients with severe stenosis, but heart rate increases and stroke volume may fall. The response to exercise is normal in children with mild stenosis.

Vascular resistances and valve area

Pulmonary vascular resistance is usually increased in infants in cardiac failure, but is otherwise normal. Systemic vascular resistance is increased when failure is present or in severe stenosis with reduced cardiac output. The valve area calculation is probably not reliable except with valvar and possibly discrete subvalvar membranous stenosis. The valve area reflects the pressure–flow relationship across the valve and should be viewed in this way, rather than as a reliable anatomical measurement of the size of the orifice. The area of the aortic valve is similar to that of the pulmonary valve, and the normal changes in valve area are similar to those of the pulmonary valve. Aortic valve area is normally about 2 cm^2/m^2 body surface area. Usually a valve area less than about 0.6 cm^2/m^2 is considered to represent severe stenosis and is associated with a systolic pressure difference of at least 70 mmHg across the valve in older infants and children. Smaller valve areas are associated with much larger gradients. Because cardiac output and heart rate may vary considerably during a cardiac catheterization study, the stroke volume and thus pressure difference across the valve may vary. The calculation of aortic valve area has been used in considering recommendations for surgery, as it takes into account the pressure variations associated with changes in flow.

Response to catecholamines

Cardiac output increases during exercise and this is associated with an increase in systolic gradient across the stenosis. It is technically difficult to measure the response of the gradient to exercise during cardiac catheterization. To simulate the response to exercise, catecholamines have been used to increase heart rate and cardiac output. Isoproterenol or dobutamine have been infused while left ventricular and aortic pressures are being recorded. Isoproterenol produces a marked increase in heart rate that, together with the increased cardiac activity, may produce considerable artifact in pressure recording due to catheter movement. It is preferred to place a pigtail catheter in the ventricle for this procedure, but it does not eliminate the problem of pressure interpretation completely. Dobutamine has been used recently and has the advantage that it does not produce marked tachycardia. The changes in pressure gradient can thus be assessed more reliably. Although the change in pressure gradient has been used for decisions about treatment, there are, as yet, no guidelines for making this determination. It is therefore difficult to justify the use of catecholamines for assessing severity of stenosis.

Angiocardiography

Angiograms are usually performed in both the left ventricle and the ascending aorta in patients with aortic stenosis. Prior to the introduction of ultrasound techniques, angiograms were important in defining whether the stenosis was valvar or immediately subvalvar in position, because pressure recordings are not always reliable. They also provide details about the anatomy of the outflow, the size of the annulus and, usually, the number of leaflets and sinuses. An injection into the aorta just above the valve, or in supravalvar stenosis just above the obstruction, is often more useful in showing the location of the obstruction and function of the valve than is a left ventricular injection. The angiograms are best performed with biplane equipment and projections are designed to demonstrate the left ventricular outflow tract and to clearly visualize the valve and supravalvar and subvalvar areas. The vertical tube is usually positioned to obtain about 45° in left anterior oblique and about 20° of craniocaudal angulation. The lateral tube is placed to provide about 30° right anterior oblique and 20° craniocaudal angulation.

In newborn infants with severe stenosis, the left ventricle may be small and empty slowly. The aortic valve annulus is often narrow, the sinuses are poorly developed, and the valve is thickened and moves poorly. The ascending aortic diameter is variable in newborn infants with severe stenosis; it may be relatively small, but is occasionally somewhat dilated. A central or eccentric jet during systole is evident. An injection into the aorta may show slow clearing of contrast medium if only a small amount of blood enters the aorta from the left ventricle.

In older infants, the left ventricular cavity is usually enlarged and the residual volume is increased. The valve is not as thick and is seen to dome during systole and a jet is seen centrally or sometimes directed posteriorly. In infants with markedly reduced systemic blood flow there is a risk of myocardial depression and renal complications from contrast material. It is therefore advisable to limit the amount of contrast medium and to use nonionic agents.

In older children with discrete stenosis, left ventricular cavity size is usually normal; the thickened wall is usually evident when stenosis is severe. When valvar stenosis is present, usually only two leaflets are noted and the leaflets are thickened, move poorly, and dome upward in systole. With mild stenosis no jet is noted, but in moderate or severe cases a systolic jet is seen, often eccentric in position and most commonly directed to the posterior right wall of the ascending aorta. The width of the jet through the valve orifice may reflect the severity of the stenosis. With mild valvar stenosis there is almost always a bicuspid valve with some thickening and restricted motion. Subvalvar stenosis presents as a diffuse narrowing in the outflow just below the valve, often more severe in the septal region. When a membrane is present, it may be seen to move up and down during the cardiac cycle. With supravalvar stenosis there is dilatation of the supravalvar portion of the aorta and marked dilatation and tortuosity of the main coronary arteries. The aorta is usually narrowed just above the valve, but frequently the wall of the aorta at the level of the attachments of the valve cusps is involved in the stenosis. Mild degrees of aortic regurgitation may be seen with the ascending aortogram in both valvar and discrete subvalvar stenosis.

Cardiac catheterization and angiocardiography are associated with high risk in patients with marked supravalvar aortic stenosis. Hypotension and decreased cardiac output may occur at any time during the procedure. It has been proposed that an acute decrease in diastolic pressure may induce coronary insufficiency with rapid deterioration.

Differential diagnosis

The diagnosis of aortic stenosis is most likely to be missed or not considered in the newborn period. Because the systolic murmur may be soft or absent, the diagnosis of aortic atresia, coarctation of the aorta, cardiomyopathy, or acute myocarditis may be considered. Aortic atresia presents many similar features, namely weak pulses, minimal cyanosis, increased right ventricular activity, similar radiological appearance, and an electrocardiogram with dominant right forces. In infants with aortic coarctation, the finding of prominent pulses in the upper extremities and absent or weak femoral pulses is usually diagnostic. The possibility should be considered that the right subclavian artery may have an anomalous origin below the coarctation and that the left subclavian artery may be involved in the coarcted segment. For this reason it should be routine practice to palpate carotid pulses if the arm pulses are diminished. Both arm pulses would be weak in these circumstances. Myocardial disease, particularly acute myocarditis, may present with poor peripheral circulation, weak pulses, and a large heart with poor sounds and no murmurs. The heart is usually markedly enlarged on radiography, but this is of no help in differentiation. The electrocardiogram usually shows low voltages with ST segment and T-wave changes in the left precordial leads. In cardiomyopathies, voltages may be increased. Murmurs are not usually noted, but a systolic apical murmur due to left ventricular enlargement and mitral incompetence may be heard. Arrhythmias, particularly multiple ventricular ectopic beats, are more frequent in infants with myocarditis. The diagnosis may be difficult to make from clinical examination alone, but ultrasound examination will differentiate between the various lesions.

In older infants, on clinical examination, the differentiation between aortic stenosis and ventricular septal defect may be difficult. The murmur of aortic stenosis is often maximal at the mid-left sternal border in this age group. Usually, however, the murmur radiates to the upper right sternal border and neck with aortic stenosis and to the xiphoid with ventricular septal defect. Increased pulmonary vascular markings would support the diagnosis of ventricular septal defect, but if there is an atrial left-to-right shunt with aortic stenosis, pulmonary vessels may also be prominent. Marked left ventricular hypertrophy on the electrocardiogram would support the diagnosis of aortic stenosis. Ultrasound study clearly differentiates the lesions.

In children, a ventricular septal defect may be confused with aortic stenosis, and the differentiation is similar to that in infants. Occasionally, it may be difficult to distinguish between aortic and pulmonary stenosis because the systolic murmur is heard on both sides of the upper sternum and radiates to both sides of the neck. Other clinical features, electrocardiography, and radiography usually help to differentiate. An ultrasound study will demonstrate the lesions.

Principles of management

The management of patients with aortic stenosis depends on age and on the severity and location of the obstruction.

Aortic stenosis in the fetus

Aortic stenosis does not appear to cause serious symptoms in the fetus. Although hydrops fetalis is not common in fetuses with aortic stenosis, it has occasionally been observed. Whether this is due to the presence of associated lesions has not been resolved. In one report, two fetuses with aortic stenosis and hydrops were treated by maternal digoxin administration. The edema resolved and balloon valvoplasty was performed after birth. It would thus appear that, if hydrops is detected, maternal digoxin therapy should be attempted.

The progression or development of left ventricular hypoplasia in fetuses with aortic stenosis examined serially by ultrasound has raised the question of whether relief of the stenosis will allow normal development of the ventricle. This is discussed in detail in Chapter 11.

Severe aortic stenosis in newborn infants

These infants frequently require urgent management because they develop poor perfusion when the ductus arteriosus constricts and metabolic changes follow. In addition to tracheal intubation it is important to gain intravascular access rapidly, either through an umbilical vessel if this is possible or through a peripheral vein. The infant should be maintained at optimal environmental temperature. Hypoglycemia and hypocalcemia should be treated. It is advisable to infuse PGE_1 to attempt to open the ductus arteriosus if it is constricted, or to maintain its patency. It is important to monitor respiration carefully when infusing PGE_1 because it may induce apnea and assisted ventilation may be required. Arterial pressure should be observed because PGE_1 may cause a considerable fall in arterial pressure and this could seriously affect coronary blood flow to the myocardium. Intravascular fluids and possibly catecholamine infusion (e.g., dopamine or epinephrine) should be administered to attempt to maintain arterial pressure. Recently, the value of these agents in treatment is being questioned. Infants with aortic stenosis who present with circulatory shock or cardiac failure in the neonatal period do not usually survive more than several days. It is therefore mandatory that an additional procedure be attempted.

Various surgical approaches have been used to relieve aortic valvar stenosis in infants, but cardiopulmonary bypass with open valvotomy became the standard procedure. Mortality was extremely high; in the early experience, only about 20% of infants survived. More recently, optimal results have been about 70% survival with surgery. However, it was difficult to assess whether the infants died as a result of the procedure or whether the left ventricle was unable to maintain an adequate cardiac output. With the introduction of the Norwood procedure for treatment of aortic atresia, we have two options: (i) relieving the stenosis and hoping that the left ventricle will be able to sustain an adequate systemic circulation; or (ii) avoiding any attempt to allow the left ventricle to provide systemic blood flow. This currently poses a serious dilemma, because, if possible, it would always be preferable to perform a two-ventricle repair. The decision is based largely on an assessment of left ventricular size. This issue is discussed in detail above (Adequacy of the left ventricle to maintain systemic blood flow). As mentioned, factors other than ventricular cavity size, such as ventricular contractility and presence of mitral valve disease, will affect the ability of the ventricle to provide an adequate output if the stenosis is relieved. A useful indication of the probability that output is *not* likely to be adequate is the finding of retrograde flow in the aortic arch and especially in the ascending aorta, because it indicates that there is minimal flow from the left ventricle into the aorta. However, as mentioned above, a number of infants who had small ventricles and who would previously not have been considered likely to maintain adequate systemic output have done well with aortic valvotomy or valvoplasty.

If it is decided that the ventricle will be incapable of providing adequate output, a Norwood procedure can be performed (see Chapter 11). If the decision is made to relieve the stenosis, two approaches are now possible: surgical valvotomy and balloon valvoplasty. The early experiences with balloon valvoplasty were not very favorable, because of complications and mortality. However, the results of the procedure have improved over the past 15 years and results are comparable with, if not perhaps better than, those of surgery. The procedure is performed via either a prograde or retrograde approach. In the prograde approach, the catheter is passed across the atrial septum to the left atrium and ventricle and then into the aorta. It may then be possible to pass a wire and the balloon catheter across the aortic valve and perform the valvoplasty. One disadvantage of this approach is that damage to the mitral valve may occur occasionally. If this is not technically feasible a retrograde approach from an umbilical or femoral artery is used and the wire and balloon catheter passed through the aortic valve. This may require considerable manipulation and there is some risk of damage to the valve, with perforation and valvar insufficiency. There is also a risk of perforation of the left ventricle. If the femoral approach is used, 50% or more of the infants develop obstruction of the artery, which may not respond to thrombolytic therapy. The possibility that this will interfere with limb growth has to be considered. Balloon valvoplasty has been quite successful in producing sufficient relief of stenosis that cardiac failure is relieved and adequate systemic blood flow maintained. The mortality of the procedure is 10–15% in infants as a group but may be somewhat higher in newborns. Survival varies in different series, but at about 6–8 years 75–80% of those in whom the procedure was performed in infancy are alive. Many require repeat valvoplasty, and aortic regurgitation is common, being moderate to marked in about 20% of patients. Residual stenosis is common and many patients continue to have pressure gradients as high as 50 mmHg or more. The indications for repeat valvoplasty vary in different centers, but many recommend it if the gradient is greater than 50 mmHg.

Some reports of both surgical aortic commissurotomy and balloon dilation of the valve are rather disappointing, with a higher mortality, especially in those with associated coarctation or depressed ventricular performance Agnoletti *et al.* [22] reported a 19% mortality with surgery and a 56% mortality after balloon dilation. Although many survivors required additional surgery including valve replacement, they have done well and have good left ventricular function.

There is a relatively high incidence of subendocardial fibroelastosis in infants with severe aortic stenosis. Despite the appearance of marked echodensity of the inner surface of the left ventricle, in some infants it does not appear to have a significant effect on left ventricular filling or performance. In others, there is serious impairment of ventricular performance. Some attempts have been made in several centers to improve left ventricular function in some of these infants by surgical relief of the stenosis and stripping the fibroelastic layer from the septal surface and free wall of the left ventricle. Some infants have survived the procedure and shown improvement in left ventricular performance, but the long-term outlook of these patients is yet to be assessed.

The subsequent management of those infants who have had balloon dilation or surgery of the aortic valve is discussed below in the section on stenosis in older infants and children. With these improvements in the results of balloon valvoplasty, the approach to infants with aortic stenosis and hypoplastic left ventricle can be reassessed. If the ventricle cannot sustain an adequate cardiac output after surgical valvotomy, a second major operation to perform a Norwood procedure would entail a high mortality. However, if there is uncertainty about the potential ability of the ventricle to provide adequate output, the response to balloon valvoplasty can be tested. If not successful, the single-ventricle Norwood approach can be used.

Older infants and children with moderate to severe stenosis

In older infants with moderate to severe aortic stenosis and cardiac failure, surgery or balloon valvoplasty is recommended. Current practice is tending toward balloon valvoplasty in patients with valvar stenosis, whereas surgery is preferred in those with subvalvar and supravalvar stenosis. When the subvalvar stenosis is due to a tunnel-like obstruction of the left ventricular outflow, it is often necessary to do an extensive resection of tissue and complex techniques have been developed to relieve the stenosis. The Konno procedure has been performed in these individuals; this operation is also indicated if the aortic annulus is small. The procedure involves incising the root of the aorta and the right ventricular outflow tract. The ventricular septum is then incised to open the aortic annulus. Previously, a prosthetic valve was inserted into the widened annulus. A patch was then used to close the aorta and the ventricular septum. If necessary a patch was placed over the right ventricular infundibulum. More recently, the favored approach is to use a pulmonary valve and artery autograft instead of a prosthetic valve (see Chapter 10). The pulmonary autograft placement in the aortic position was developed by Ross. The combined surgical technique is now known as the Ross–Konno procedure.

Supravalvar stenosis is currently treated surgically. The aorta is incised across the constriction and a patch is used to relieve the stenosis. Care must be exercised to avoid damaging the coronary arteries and the aortic valve mechanism during the procedure. A long segment of stenosis is more difficult to relieve and may require more extensive grafting in the ascending aorta. Although it is feasible to relieve supravalvar stenosis by balloon angioplasty, the concern is that there is a similar risk for hemorrhage and aneurysm as occurs with aortic coarctation.

Discrete subvalvar aortic stenosis

The risks of syncope or sudden death are not significantly different in patients with subvalvar stenosis compared with those with valvar stenosis. Many centers recommend surgical treatment for this lesion when left ventricular outflow pressure gradients are considerably lower than those used as indications for treating aortic valvar stenosis. This approach is based on two concerns: first, that the aortic valve may become progressively damaged by the impact of the jet arising from the subvalvar stenosis; and second, that the stenosis may progress to produce a more diffuse stenosis, which would require more extensive surgery at a later time.

Subvalvar stenosis associated with intracardiac lesions

When subvalvar stenosis is the result of ventricular septal malalignment, as with double-outlet right ventricle of Taussig–Bing type or single ventricle with rudimentary outlet chamber leading to the aorta, a procedure has been used to bypass the obstruction. The Damus–Kaye–Stansel operation involves anastomosing the proximal cut end of the transected pulmonary artery to the side of the ascending aorta. This allows blood from the left or dominant ventricle to flow through the pulmonary artery directly into the aorta, thus bypassing the obstructed area. The distal end of the pulmonary artery is sutured and pulmonary flow is provided first by a modified Blalock–Taussig systemic-to-pulmonary arterial shunt in young infants or, in older infants and children, by a bidirectional superior cavopulmonary anastomosis and later by a Fontan or modified Fontan procedure (see Chapter 16).

Valvar aortic stenosis in children

This group of children includes those treated by surgery or balloon valvoplasty in infancy, and the much larger number of individuals who did not have clinical concerns during infancy or early childhood. Most of these patients do not have symptoms, although they are at risk of developing infective endocarditis.

The indications for treating these individuals are still not clearly defined. We do know that the tendency is for the stenosis to become more severe with growth. However, there is no reliable information regarding the natural history of the disease in individuals with different levels of gradient across the valve. The recommendations for management are based on subjective views rather than on any firm documentation of the course and risks of the lesion. Certain clinical features are generally regarded as definite indications, namely electrocardiographic evidence of strain as shown by ST- and T-wave changes, cardiomegaly, repeated syncopal attacks, and angina. In the majority of individuals, these criteria are not present. The recommendations for either initial or repeat valvoplasty or surgery are based on the magnitude of the pressure gradient across the valve. However, these recommendations are arbitrary.

It is important to appreciate that all current recommendations for intervention based on the magnitude of the pressure gradient refer to the systolic gradient recorded across the valve by pressure measurement. The recommendations do *not* apply to gradients estimated from Doppler velocity recordings. Furthermore, the recommendations refer to gradients measured at rest and *not* to gradients during exercise or during infusion of catecholamines. Because the gradients estimated from Doppler velocity are likely to be overestimates, it is crucial that if relief of stenosis is being considered solely on the basis of the pressure gradient, then this should be evaluated by cardiac catheterization prior to the valvoplasty or valvotomy.

At present, the recommendation of most pediatric cardiologists is that if the systolic pressure difference across the aortic obstruction is greater than 70–75 mmHg, surgery is definitely indicated. This usually corresponds to a valve area of less than 0.5–0.6 cm^2/m^2. This recommendation is based on the fact that ST- and T-wave abnormalities are most likely to be associated with pressures above this level, and that individuals who have died suddenly have usually demonstrated ST- and T-wave changes. When the pressure difference across the obstruction is less than 25–30 mmHg, surgery is not recommended. No restrictions are placed on their activities, but these patients are observed for possible increase in severity of stenosis with growth. During early childhood, they are examined at about 6-monthly intervals and subsequently at 1-year and later 2-year intervals if no significant change has occurred in the electrocardiogram or the ultrasound examination. If the stenosis has progressed, they are managed as discussed below. Patients with valvar stenosis with gradients of 30–55 mmHg are also followed carefully. When the child is cooperative an exercise study is performed to assess electrocardiographic responses. Although no restrictions are usually recommended for normal activities, many advise that participation in competitive activities be discouraged. These children are usually evaluated annually beyond infancy clinically and by electrocardiography and ultrasound study.

There is considerable diversity regarding management of individuals with valvar stenosis and systolic pressure gradients of 55–70 mmHg. When surgery was the only method of relieving the stenosis, a pressure gradient of about 70 mmHg was considered the level at which the operation should be performed, unless other symptoms or signs were evident (see above). However, with the introduction of the interventional procedure of balloon valvoplasty, several centers are now recommending that the procedure be performed if the gradient is greater than 55 mmHg. There is no known rationale for this recommendation. It has been suggested that it is likely that, over time, these individuals are at risk of developing myocardial hypertrophy and fibrosis and that relief of the obstruction will inhibit or slow this process. If valvotomy or valvoplasty is not performed in this group of patients, they should be observed closely. Active sports and especially competitive activities should be avoided. Exercise and ultrasound studies should be done every 6–12 months. If there is evidence of electrocardiographic abnormalities or increase in the gradient, valvoplasty or valvotomy should be considered.

Although the results of surgical valvotomy are excellent in older infants and children with valvar stenosis, it is generally agreed that the surgery is not ideal. Rarely there is a tricuspid aortic valve with adherent raphe that can be separated readily to provide an effective valve with no regurgitation. Usually, however, the valve is bicuspid and the surgeon must compromise between partial relief from the stenosis and complete relief, with a high risk of producing aortic insufficiency. When there is a unicuspid valve, the results of surgery are even less predictable and the risks of insufficiency are even greater. The majority of patients do experience excellent relief from stenosis and the mortality is well below 5%. Balloon valvoplasty also has a very low mortality beyond infancy and achieves excellent relief of stenosis. Currently, there does not appear to be any justification for surgical valvotomy as the initial procedure for valvar aortic stenosis in children. As with valvotomy, valvoplasty may result in aortic insufficiency of variable degree. With both valvotomy and balloon valvoplasty, recurrence of stenosis usually develops after a variable period. It is therefore important to follow these patients carefully, and if stenosis again becomes severe, repeat valvoplasty may be indicated. Subsequent procedures are likely to be less successful in relieving stenosis and aortic regurgitation may be considerably greater. After either valvotomy or valvoplasty, the valve is still abnormal. Prior to the middle of 2007, it was strongly recommended that these individuals be provided with antibiotic prophylaxis for infective endocarditis, but with the change in recommendations for prophylaxis it is no longer indicated, as long as a prosthetic valve is not used for valve replacement [23]. Prophylaxis is still recommended for those individuals in whom there is a high risk of infection and in whom infection may have serious consequences. The guidelines of the American Heart Association state that "IE prophylaxis for dental procedures may be reasonable, even though we acknowledge that its effectiveness is unknown." Some pediatric cardiologists consider the risk of infective endocarditis to be so high in patients who have had previous palliative surgery on the aortic valve that prophylaxis should be recommended in these individuals.

If, after the initial or subsequent procedures, it is considered that the stenosis cannot be adequately relieved, or that aortic insufficiency is likely to be severe, the possibility of valve replacement has to be considered. There used to be reluctance to use prosthetic valves in children for several reasons. A major consideration is that the prosthesis provides a valve of fixed orifice and with growth it would have to be replaced. A second concern is that anticoagulants are necessary to prevent thrombosis on the prosthetic valve; it is inconvenient and sometimes difficult to regulate therapy and active children are prone to injury with risk of hemorrhage. Recently, the Ross procedure has been performed in infants and children in several centers. The aortic valve and annulus are replaced by the individual's own pulmonary annulus and valve – a pulmonary autograft. The pulmonary artery is then replaced by a valved conduit from the right ventricle to the pulmonary artery, such as an aortic homograft.

The results of this approach have been gratifying. Preliminary results suggest that the autograft grows in proportion to the child's growth. Initially there was concern that the postvalvar pulmonary artery became dilated and that aneurysmal dilatation may occur. However, it appears that after the first few months no further expansion occurs. A significant advantage is that anticoagulation is not necessary. The survival of the pulmonary valve in the aortic position is of some concern. In a large series of Ross's adult patients there was no evidence of deterioration of valve function over two decades; it remains to be seen how the valve will perform over decades in children. If the Ross procedure is performed during infancy, it is very likely that the pulmonary conduit will have to be replaced at intervals. This, and the possibility of associated pulmonary valve abnormalities, has begun to raise some questions about the desirability of performing Ross procedures in infants.

It is also being recognized that the pulmonary valve is sometimes abnormal in patients who have bicuspid aortic valves. In one study, about 15% of patients with bicuspid aortic valve had bicuspid pulmonary valves or pulmonary valve fenestrations and valve insufficiency. This precluded the application of the Ross procedure [24]. Because the majority of children with aortic stenosis have bicuspid aortic valves, it is important to exclude the possible association of pulmonary valve abnormalities in those in whom a Ross procedure is being contemplated.

Bicuspid aortic valve without stenosis

In the past, little attention was directed toward individuals in whom a bicuspid aortic valve had been detected. Generally, in the era when antibiotic prophylaxis for infective endocarditis was still being recommended, it was not usually recommended unless the valve was stenotic. This is surprising, because it is known that those with a bicuspid valve alone are prone to develop endocarditis. With the change in guidelines for prophylaxis in 2007, this is no longer an issue. However, the valve may develop stenosis with advancing age and insufficiency may occur. Also, with the recognition that patients with bicuspid aortic valve have associated abnormalities of the aortic wall and are prone to development of ascending aortic dilation, as well as aortic dissection, these individuals should be monitored by ultrasound examination to assess aortic valve morphology and function and the size of the ascending aorta. This examination does not need to be performed frequently during childhood, but becomes increasingly important with advancing age.

References

1 Fernandes SM, Sanders SP, Khairy P *et al.* Morphology of bicuspid aortic valve in children and adolescents. J Am Coll Cardiol 2004;44:1648–1651.

2 Ciotti GR, Vlahos AP, Silverman NH. Morphology and function of the bicuspid aortic valve with and without coarctation of the aorta in the young. Am J Cardiol 2006;98:1096–1102.

3 Roberts WC, Ko JM. Frequency of unicuspid, bicuspid and tricuspid aortic valves by decade in adults having aortic valve replacement for isolated aortic stenosis. Circulation 2005;111:920–925.

4 Roos-Hesselink JW, Schölzel BE, Heijdra RJ *et al.* Aortic valve and aortic arch pathology after coarctation repair. Heart 2003;89:1074–1077.

5 Lewin MB, Otto CM. The bicuspid aortic valve. Adverse outcomes from infancy to old age. Circulation 2005; 111:832–834.

6 Fedak PW, Verma S, David TE, Leask RL, Weisel RD, Butany J. Clinical and pathophysiological implications of a bicuspid aortic valve. Circulation 2002;106:900–904.

7 Oliver JM, Gonzalez A, Gallego P, Sanchez-Recalde A, Benito F, Mesa JM. Discrete subaortic stenosis in adults: increased prevalence and slow rate of progression of the obstruction and aortic regurgitation. J Am Coll Cardiol 2001;38:835–842.

8 Gersony WM. Natural history of discrete subvalvar aortic stenosis: management implications. J Am Coll Cardiol 2001;38:843–884.

9 Hallidie-Smith KA, Karas S. Cardiac anomalies in Williams–Beuren syndrome. Arch Dis Child 1988;63: 809–813.

10 McBride KL, Pignatelli R, Lewin M *et al.* Inheritance analysis of congenital left ventricular outflow tract obstruction malformations: segregation, multiplex relative risk, and heritability. Am J Med Genet A 2005; 134:180–186.

11 Martin LJ, Ramachandran V, Cripe LH *et al.* Evidence in favor of linkage to human chromosomal regions 18q, 5q and 13q for bicuspid aortic valve and associated cardiovascular malformations. Hum Genet 2007;121:275–284.

12 Garg V, Muth AN, Ransom JF *et al.* Mutations in NOTCH1 cause aortic valve disease. Nature 2005;437: 270–274.

13 Garcia RE, Friedman WF, Kaback MM, Rowe RD. Idiopathic hypercalcemia and supravalvular aortic stenosis. Documentation of a new syndrome. N Engl J Med 1964;271:117–120.

14 Hornberger LK, Sanders SP, Rein AJ, Spevak PJ, Parness IA, Colan SD. Left heart obstructive lesions and left ventricular growth in midtrimester fetus. A longitudinal study. Circulation 1995;92:1531–1538.

15 Axt-Fliedner R, Kreiselmaier P, Schwarze A, Krapp M, Gembruch U. Development of hypoplastic left heart syndrome after diagnosis of aortic stenosis in the first trimester by early echocardiography. Ultrasound Obstet Gynecol 2006;28:106–109.

16 Makikallio K, McElhinney DB, Levine JC *et al.* Fetal aortic valve stenosis and the evolution of hypoplastic left heart syndrome: patient selection for fetal intervention. Circulation 2006;113:1401–1405.

17 Fishman NH, Hof RB, Rudolph AM. Models of congenital heart disease in fetal lambs. Circulation 1978; 58:354–364.

18 Eghtesady P, Michelfelder E, Altaye M, Ballard E, Hirsh R, Beekman RH III. Revisiting animal models of aortic stenosis in the early gestation fetus. Ann Thorac Surg 2007;83:631–639.

19 Rhodes LA, Colan SD, Perry SB, Jonas RA, Sanders SP. Predictors of survival in neonates with critical aortic stenosis. Circulation 1991;84:2325–2335. Erratum Circulation 1995;92:2005.

20 Colan SD, McElhinney DB, Crawford EC, Keane JF, Lock JE. Validation and re-evaluation of a discriminant model predicting anatomic suitability for biventricular repair in neonates with aortic stenosis. J Am Coll Cardiol 2006;47:1858–1865.

21 Gorlin R, Gorlin SG. Hydraulic formula for calculation of the area of the stenotic mitral valve, other cardiac valves,

and central circulatory shunts. Am Heart J 1951;41:1–29.

22 Agnoletti G, Raisky O, Boudjemline Y *et al.* Neonatal surgical aortic commissurotomy: predictors of outcome and long-term results. Ann Thorac Surg 2006;82:1592–1593.

23 Wilson W, Taubert KA, Gewitz M *et al.* Prevention of infective endocarditis: guidelines from the American Heart Association: a guideline from the American Heart Association Rheumatic Fever, Endocarditis, and Kawasaki Disease Committee, Council on Cardiovascular Disease in the Young, and the Council on Clinical Cardiology, Council on Cardiovascular Surgery and Anesthesia, and the Quality of Care and Outcomes Research Interdisciplinary Working Group. Circulation 2007;116: 1736–1754.

24 Favaloro R, Stutzbach P, Gomez C, Machain A, Casabe H. Feasibility of the Ross procedure: its relationship with the bicuspid aortic valve. J Heart Valve Dis 2002; 11:375–382.

CHAPTER 11

Aortic atresia, mitral atresia, and hypoplastic left ventricle

In 1952, Lev [1] introduced the term "hypoplasia of the aortic tract complex" to describe a group of congenital cardiac lesions in which severe aortic stenosis or atresia, severe stenosis or atresia of the mitral valve, hypoplastic ascending aorta, and a small left ventricle were associated. Noonan and Nadas [2] recognized that the clinical presentation with severe cardiac failure and inadequate systemic perfusion, which is common in these infants, is also observed in infants with aortic isthmus atresia or interruption and aortic coarctation of the so-called preductal type. They suggested the term *hypoplastic left heart syndrome* to describe all these infants. This term and clinical concept have now been widely accepted. This is unfortunate, because these lesions may differ considerably in their hemodynamic effects and the type of surgical procedure recommended may be greatly influenced by the precise anatomical and physiological disturbance. It has become apparent that the hypoplastic left ventricle associated with aortic arch obstructions is usually adequate to maintain systemic cardiac output when the obstruction is relieved. However, the hypoplastic left ventricle associated with critical aortic stenosis may not be capable of providing adequate systemic blood flow even if the stenosis is relieved (see Chapter 10). The etiological factors resulting in the development of these lesions are not known. As discussed in Chapter 11, there is a strong hereditary association between some of the lesions, whereas others such as aortic arch interruption could be associated with a distinct genetic anomaly (see Chapter 12). The precise classification of these lesions is therefore not merely semantic, as has been suggested by some, but most important with regard to embryological, hemodynamic, and therapeutic implications. Furthermore, the left ventricle may be hypoplastic in association with other congenital cardiac lesions. Occasionally an atrioventricular septal defect is committed predominantly to the right ventricle, resulting in hypoplasia of the left ventricle; also, the left ventricle may rarely be hypoplastic in individuals with double-outlet right ventricle. The grouping of all lesions associated with a small left ventricle creates considerable confusion in the literature, because it is difficult to assess results of surgery in specific lesions causing hypoplasia of the left ventricle. I have elected to discuss the hypoplastic left ventricle associated with aortic stenosis in Chapter 10 and the hypoplastic ventricle associated with aortic arch obstructions in Chapter 12. This chapter presents a discussion on aortic atresia and mitral atresia. In various reviews, 65–80% of hypoplastic left ventricles are related to aortic atresia, whereas the remainder are associated with aortic stenosis or aortic arch obstructions and other lesions. The variability in reported incidences may be accounted for by differences in the criteria used for the assessment of left ventricular size in the latter groups.

Morphological observations

Mitral and aortic atresia with intact ventricular septum

Aortic atresia is associated with an intact ventricular septum in 95% of patients and with mitral atresia in about 40% [3,4]. If mitral atresia is present, there may be no evidence of a valve, or a blind dimple may be noted at the atrioventricular junction; occasionally, atretic mitral valve tissue may be noted. In these instances, the left ventricular cavity

Congenital Diseases of the Heart, 3rd edition. By A. Rudolph
© 2009 Blackwell Publishing, ISBN: 9781405162456

may not be distinguishable or it may be diminutive and represented by a small slit. The cavity of the ventricle is separated from the atretic aortic valve by fibromuscular tissue. The free wall of the ventricle is fairly thin and, in the presence of both mitral and aortic atresia, fibrosis of the left ventricular myocardium and the presence of endocardial fibroelastosis are considerably less evident compared with hearts with aortic atresia and a patent mitral valve [5]. The ascending aorta is very narrow; in the neonate the diameter is 3 mm or less along its length to the origin of the innominate artery. It then becomes somewhat wider at the origins of the left carotid and subclavian arteries but the whole aortic arch is narrow and even the arteries arising from the arch may be narrowed. The ascending aorta ends blindly proximal to the origin of the coronary arteries; it is often somewhat wider in the region of the sinuses of Valsalva and the coronary arteries usually originate normally. Coarctation of the aorta is almost always present; the degree of constriction varies, but it is marked in 70–80% of all patients. The coarctation is at the junction of the isthmus with the ductus arteriosus and thus could restrict flow from the ductus and descending aorta into the aortic arch and its branches, as well as the coronary circulation. The main pulmonary artery and ductus arteriosus are large.

The left atrium is usually small; the superior attachment of the septum primum is often displaced toward the left, making the left atrium very small. The atrial septum is small as a result of the small size of the chamber. There is frequently endocardial fibrosis involving both the wall of the atrium and the septum, and the muscular tissue of the septum is replaced by fibrous or elastic tissue. This is important with regard to possible attempts to perform balloon atrial septostomy (see Chapter 11). The size of the foramen ovale is variable but is usually small. In a small proportion of patients, the foramen ovale is tiny, with an orifice as small as 1 mm. In these individuals, the walls of the pulmonary veins are often thickened and the endothelium is also thick and white. In addition, the small intrapulmonary vessels have increased medial smooth muscle development. Rarely, mitral valve atresia is associated with a sealed foramen ovale and the exit of blood from the left atrium is through a levoatriocardinal vein.

Aortic atresia with patent mitral orifice and intact ventricular septum

Although the mitral orifice is patent in about 60% of patients with aortic atresia, the valve is usually abnormal. Valve cusps are usually thickened, and the chordae are thickened and usually short and attached to short papillary muscles. The mitral valve orifice is stenotic to varying degrees. Compared with patients with mitral atresia, the left ventricular cavity is larger and the myocardial wall is thickened. Myocardial fibrosis is common and endocardial fibroelastosis is also usually a prominent feature in these individuals. Abnormalities of the coronary arteries occur in 30–50% of patients with aortic atresia and open mitral valve. The coronary arterial walls may be thickened and ventricular to coronary arterial communications have been described [6]. The other features of the heart and great vessels are similar to those described above in the hearts with both mitral and aortic atresia.

Aortic atresia, mitral atresia, and ventricular septal defect

In the presence of a large ventricular septal defect associated with mitral or aortic atresia, the left ventricular cavity may be of normal size and the ventricular wall may be of normal thickness. Aortic atresia with ventricular septal defect and a normal left ventricle is observed in only 5% of patients with aortic atresia [7]. With aortic atresia and ventricular septal defect, flow into the aorta is still derived through the ductus arteriosus, so the ascending aorta and arch are small.

With mitral atresia and ventricular septal defect, the left ventricle may be of normal size, because blood can enter the ventricle through the defect. In the absence of aortic atresia, flow into the ascending aorta could be derived from the left ventricle and the ascending aorta and aortic arch may be of normal size.

Proposed causes of hypoplastic left heart syndrome

The causes of aortic and mitral atresia with hypoplastic left ventricle are not known, but several hypotheses have been suggested.

Genetic factors

In a study of the heritability of bicuspid aortic valve, it was observed that, in addition to occurrence of bicuspid valve and aortic coarctation in first-degree relatives, hypoplastic left heart syndrome was also noted [8]. Subsequently, the heritability of this malformation as well as other cardiovascular anomalies was examined in 38 probands with hypoplastic left heart; 55% of families had more than one affected individual and there was a high incidence of abnormalities of other cardiac valves, leading to the conclusion that "hypoplastic left heart syndrome is determined largely by genetic factors" [9]. Specific genes that may be involved have not been identified, but it has been suggested that possibly a mutation of the *HAND* genes could explain failure of left ventricular development. Knockout mice lacking *HAND2* do not form a right ventricle and those lacking *HAND1* and *HAND2* do not form either ventricle [10].

Interference in blood flow

The concept has been proposed that reduction in the volume of blood entering the left ventricle could interfere with its normal development during growth of the heart prenatally. Experimentally, occlusion of the mitral valve in the chick embryo results in a hypoplastic ventricle [11]. It has been suggested that premature closure of the foramen ovale in the fetus could result in left ventricular hypoplasia [12]. The cause of the foramen ovale narrowing has not been defined. If the foramen ovale is narrowed early in fetal development, filling of the left atrium from the inferior vena cava (IVC) stream will be reduced. Because pulmonary flow in the fetus is low, the total volume of blood entering the left atrium and ventricle will be less than normal and this could interfere with development of the left side of the heart. It has also been suggested that the effect of prenatal constriction of the foramen ovale on cardiac development may be related to the period during gestation when it occurs. If the foramen ovale narrows in early gestation, the left ventricle would be almost absent, with complete atresia of mitral and aortic valves. If it constricts at a later stage of gestation, the left ventricle would have the opportunity to develop, with normal mitral valve and aortic valve leaflets, but this development would subsequently be arrested or limited. Closure of the foramen ovale in late fetal life would not interfere with development of the left ventricle but may cause a delayed postnatal decrease in pulmonary vascular resistance, because a large flow into the right ventricle and pulmonary artery may create fetal pulmonary arterial hypertension. However, it is just as likely that the initial insult is obstruction at the mitral, ventricular, or aortic valve level. The resulting increase in left atrial pressure would tend to close the foramen ovale and reduce flow from the right to the left side of the atrial septum. Ultrasound study of the foramen ovale in fetuses with hypoplastic left heart usually demonstrates the small foramen ovale and often shows an exclusive flow of blood from the left to the right atrium.

The volume of blood entering the left ventricle could also be reduced by obstruction to left ventricular output. Thus aortic stenosis in the fetus would tend to reduce stroke volume and increase end-systolic volume. This could limit the volume of blood entering the left ventricle by increasing left atrial pressure, thus restricting foramen ovale right-to-left flow. In experimental studies in fetal lambs, we showed that when the ascending aorta is constricted by a band in fetal lambs at 0.6–0.7 gestation [13], the left ventricle first showed marked thickening of the muscle but the cavity progressively decreased in size; left ventricular output was markedly reduced. Nevertheless, we thought it possible that if aortic obstruction occurs in the embryo or in early fetal development, the left ventricle may not develop further. However, in a recent report of ascending aortic banding in fetal lambs at 0.3–0.4 gestation, the left ventricle was hypertrophied but cavity size was not reduced [14]. It is difficult to explain this difference in response. Several reports have described progressive reduction in the size of the left ventricle in human fetuses in association with aortic stenosis [15,16]. These observations have suggested that the presence of aortic stenosis in the fetus interferes with flow out of and into the left ventricle, resulting in progressive reduction in volume during fetal development and culminating in hypoplasia of the ventricle. The progressive decrease in left ventricular dimensions in human fetuses has been noted in numerous studies and it has been proposed that relief of aortic stenosis *in utero* could prevent the progression to hypoplastic left heart syndrome and allow normal growth of the ventricle. This has led to the application of balloon dilation to attempt to relieve the obstruction at the aortic valve. The procedure, guided by ultrasound imaging, consists of passage of a needle through the maternal abdominal wall and uterus into the fetal left ventricle, manipulating a wire into the aorta and then passing a balloon dilation catheter over the wire [17,18].

The concept that hypoplastic left heart is commonly the result of increasing severity of aortic valvar stenosis during fetal growth is now widely accepted. However, in most reports, the left ventricle has been abnormal at the initial examination of the fetus by ultrasound; usually there is echodensity suggesting the presence of endocardial fibroelastosis, ventricular dysfunction, and sometimes enlargement. Subsequent studies show lack of left ventricular growth, with progressive reduction in size relative to fetal growth. There are only scattered reports of fetuses in whom, on initial study, aortic valvar stenosis with an apparently normal left ventricle was observed, with subsequent progression to fibroelastosis and ventricular dysfunction and then left ventricular hypoplasia. In one report, a fetus first observed at about 11 weeks' gestation showed increased ascending aortic flow velocity with an otherwise normal heart. About 5 weeks later the left ventricle showed increased echodensity and was dysfunctional, suggesting the development of hypoplastic left heart syndrome; at birth the infant had typical hypoplastic left heart syndrome [19].

Primary left ventricular dysfunction

Left ventricular dysfunction and echocardiographic evidence of endocardial fibroelastosis are not always associated with aortic stenosis. Sharland *et al.* [20], in a study of 30 fetuses with echocardiographic features of left ventricular dysfunction, noted that the aortic valve was bicuspid but not obstructive in six. One of these had hypoplasia of the left ventricle and the others had endocardial fibroelastosis. Also, three newborn infants with left ventricular hypoplasia were noted at autopsy to have myocardial hypertrophy and endocardial fibroelastosis; however, even though the left ventricular outflow tract and aortic valves were small, no stenosis was present [21].

These observations have raised the question as to whether hypoplastic left heart could be the result of myocardial damage resulting from intrauterine infection or exposure to toxins. It is of interest that, in the fetus, the course of the circulation may favor involvement of the left rather than the right ventricle. As discussed in Chapter 1, about half of umbilical venous return passes through the ductus venosus and flows preferentially across the foramen ovale into the left atrium and ventricle. Thus any infectious agent or toxin traversing the placenta from the mother would be preferentially directed to the left ventricle.

Viral infection, particularly coxsackievirus B, may cause myocarditis and result in ventricular dysfunction. It is also possible that endocarditis of the aortic and mitral valve could occur and result in damage to the valve leaflets, with development of stenosis. Another possible mechanism that could affect the valve is reduced output of the left ventricle resulting from disturbed myocardial function. If the output is reduced, the aortic valve may not open adequately and potentially stenosis or even atresia could result.

Although the role of toxin exposure as a cause of hypoplasia of the left heart has not been entertained seriously, one study supports the possible role of environmental toxins as a factor in its occurrence. Over an 18-year period, all infants born with hypoplastic left heart syndrome in Maryland and the District of Columbia were analyzed. A region of Baltimore was identified in which the incidence was twice as high as in other areas. In this region industrial release of dioxin, polychlorinated biphenyls, and solvents into the atmosphere were documented, suggesting that environmental toxins could have a role in the occurrence of hypoplastic left heart syndrome [22].

It is possible that there is not a single etiology for the development of hypoplastic left ventricle and that any of the mechanisms mentioned above, or a combination, may be involved. It is also possible that the period during fetal development when the insult is introduced could influence the type of abnormality, as well as the severity of the cardiovascular malformation. Thus if aortic stenosis is the initial lesion, not only will the severity of the stenosis be important in interfering with left ventricular development, but also the gestational age at which it becomes manifest. Stenotic lesions of the aortic and pulmonary valve tend to increase with advancing age in many infants postnatally. The likelihood for progressive stenosis of the aortic valvar stenosis would be greater, as well as more rapid, *in utero* because of the relatively much more rapid rate of growth. The earlier in gestation that significant aortic stenosis becomes manifest, the more likely would left ventricular as well as mitral valve development be affected.

The presence of endocardial fibroelastosis predominantly in those fetuses that have a patent mitral valve in association with aortic stenosis or atresia is of considerable interest. The hypothesis currently favored regarding the development of fibroelastosis postulates that it is the result of high end-diastolic pressure in the left ventricle interfering with coronary blood flow into the subendocardial layers of the myocardium. Thus if aortic stenosis were the primary lesion, reduced output from the left ventricle could result in an increase in diastolic volume and pressure. Poor growth of the ventricle could interfere with mitral valve growth and perhaps also result in mitral insufficiency, which could further increase diastolic pressure.

In the 40% of the patients with mitral atresia as well as aortic atresia, it is difficult to explain the absence of subendocardial fibroelastosis. Based on current concepts, if aortic stenosis was the primary lesion and if it was severe enough to cause left ventricular and mitral valve hypoplasia with resultant atresia, it is most unlikely that an increase in ventricular diastolic pressure would not have occurred. Thus, the lack of fibroelastosis suggests that aortic stenosis is unlikely to be the primary lesion. One would have to postulate that the mitral valve anomaly is primary and that the left ventricular and aortic valve manifestations are secondary to interference with flow through the mitral valve. Possibly foramen ovale obstruction could be the primary anomaly.

These hypotheses assume that the main factors determining coronary blood flow are the degree of aortic stenosis and the magnitude of increase in left ventricular diastolic pressure. However, aortic stenosis or atresia is associated with a small ascending aorta and aortic arch and the majority of these individuals also have coarctation of the aorta between the ductus arteriosus and the aortic arch. If flow into the ascending aorta from the left ventricle is markedly restricted, blood supply to the coronary circulation would have to be derived from retrograde flow into the aortic arch from the ductus arteriosus. If the aortic coactation is severe, coronary blood flow could be severely restricted. It would be interesting to determine the severity of the coarctation in those individuals in whom there is mitral and aortic atresia, as compared with those with a patent mitral valve.

Hemodynamic considerations

Fetal circulation

Congenital cardiovascular malformations result in alterations in blood flow patterns and it has long been postulated that these changes may result in additional abnormalities of the circulation during prenatal development. The interrelationships between blood flow and morphological changes associated with hypoplastic left heart syndrome in the developing circulation have been well documented in human fetuses by serial echocardiographic studies (see Chapter 11). It is also apparent that the period of gestation when the malformation manifests its effects is important in determining the type of anomaly as well as its severity. For these reasons, the hemodynamic features of the circulation may vary considerably. In this section I propose to first discuss features of specific malformations and then to consider the following possible concerns in the fetus:

- development of cardiac failure;
- adequacy of coronary blood flow;
- adequacy of cerebral blood flow;
- foramen ovale restriction;
- development of the pulmonary circulation;
- distribution of oxygen to the tissues.

Specific malformations

Mitral and aortic atresia with intact ventricular septum

With complete obstruction to output from the left ventricle, the right ventricle has to maintain the total cardiac output. The course of the circulation in the fetus is shown in Figure 11.1.

If mitral as well as aortic atresia is present, the normal flow of blood from the IVC across the foramen would be abolished and most of the IVC blood

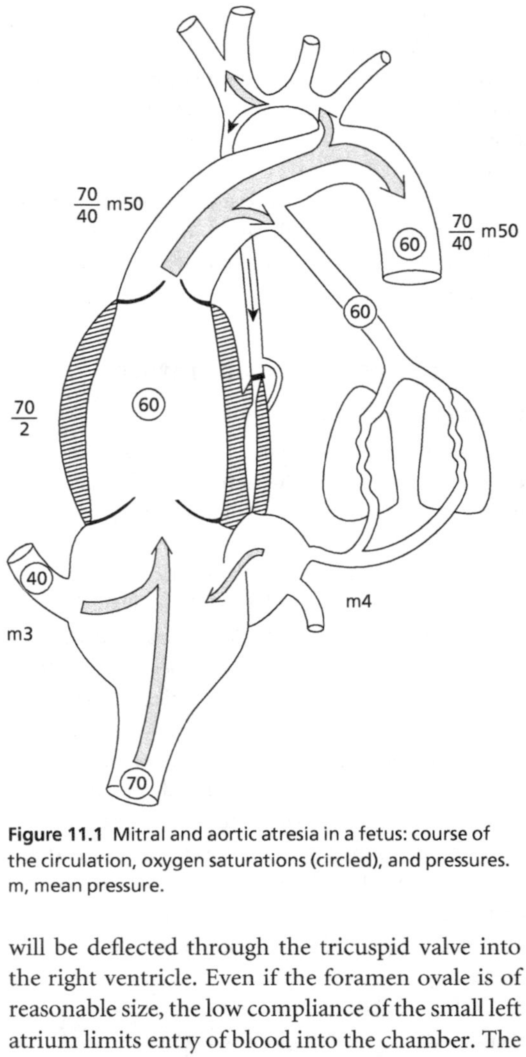

Figure 11.1 Mitral and aortic atresia in a fetus: course of the circulation, oxygen saturations (circled), and pressures. m, mean pressure.

will be deflected through the tricuspid valve into the right ventricle. Even if the foramen ovale is of reasonable size, the low compliance of the small left atrium limits entry of blood into the chamber. The right ventricle also receives all the superior vena cava (SVC) return. The pulmonary venous blood enters the left atrium; if the mitral valve is open but hypoplastic, a small amount of blood may enter the left ventricle. However, with no egress from the ventricle, all pulmonary venous blood must pass through the foramen ovale to the right atrium. If the foramen ovale is restrictive, left atrial and pulmonary venous pressures will be markedly elevated. Observations of pulmonary venous flow patterns by Doppler technique in fetuses with hypoplastic left heart have shown decreased systolic velocity and exaggerated flow reversal [23]. The pattern of pulmonary venous flow was found to be predictive of the degree of obstruction at the foramen between the left and right atrium. Continuous forward flow with minor reversal during atrial systole was associated with a mean foramen ovale size of 4.5 mm. With continuous but reduced forward flow and a prominent *a*-wave reversal, the mean foramen ovale size was 1.6 mm. When flow was briefly forward and reverse, there was no atrial septal communication [24]. The pattern of flow in the pulmonary veins is helpful in determining whether attempts should be made to enlarge the foramen ovale in the fetus or immediately after birth (see Chapter 11).

The blood ejected from the right ventricle enters the main pulmonary artery. The proportion that enters the pulmonary circulation will depend on pulmonary vascular resistance, as well as the degree of obstruction at the foramen ovale, but the remainder, which consists of almost the total cardiac output, flows through the ductus arteriosus into the descending aorta. The head, brain, and upper extremities, as well as the coronary circulation, receive their blood from the ductus by retrograde flow across the isthmus. The lower body and the placenta receive blood supply from the descending aorta in the usual manner. It is not known whether total cardiac output in the fetus is restricted in hypoplastic left ventricle, because it is all ejected by the right ventricle. In the normal fetal lamb, acute complete occlusion of the ascending aorta results in an increase in right ventricular output, but total output falls by 10–15%. However, in the lamb, the left ventricle ejects only about 33% of combined ventricular output (CVO), so the right ventricle has to increase its output by only 50% of its usual output to maintain normal CVO. In the human fetus, left ventricular output is about 45% of CVO, so the right ventricle would have to almost double its output to maintain a cardiac output similar to that in the normal fetus. It has generally been assumed that cardiac output is close to normal levels because infants born with hypoplastic left heart syndrome do not usually show evidence of intrauterine growth retardation. The normal fetal development and normal hemoglobin levels usually found in neonates suggest that placental blood flow and systemic blood flow to the lower body are adequate to provide sufficient nutritional and oxygen requirements to the fetus.

However, it is very likely that pulmonary blood flow is less than normal because, as discussed on p. 265, pulmonary vascular changes may result in elevation of pulmonary vascular resistance and restriction of the foramen ovale could further interfere with flow into the lungs. Furthermore, flow into the ascending aorta and its branches will be restricted to a variable degree, depending on the severity of the preductal coarctation of the aortic isthmus that is usually present. Thus the total cardiac output may be lower than in the normal fetus and the demand on the right ventricle to maintain the total output may be increased only modestly.

In the normal human fetus it is estimated that about 75% of descending aortic blood flow is provided through the ductus arteriosus and 25% from the ascending aorta across the arch and isthmus (see Table 1.3). In the fetus with aortic atresia, the total descending aortic flow as well as blood passing retrogradely into the arch and its branches traverses the ductus arteriosus. This represents a substantial increase in ductus blood flow and this, combined with the fact that there is no forward flow in the aortic isthmus, may account for the development of the coarctation just above the junction of the aorta with the ductus, as proposed by Hutchins [25]. However, it is possible that the aortic arch malformation may be a component of abnormal development of the left side of the heart.

Normally, because the ductus venosus stream in the IVC passes preferentially through the foramen ovale, the oxygen content of ascending aortic blood is higher than that in the descending aorta. However, with aortic atresia, little if any blood from the IVC crosses the foramen ovale. Pulmonary venous blood, which enters the right atrium across the foramen ovale, and IVC and SVC blood mix in the right atrium. The completely mixed venous blood enters the right ventricle and pulmonary artery. The oxygen contents of pulmonary arterial, ascending aortic, and descending aortic blood are identical. The $P\text{O}_2$ of blood to the upper body is therefore slightly lower than normal, whereas $P\text{O}_2$ of blood to the lungs and lower body will be slightly higher than normal. The small decrease in $P\text{O}_2$ in blood supplied to the head could possibly have some effect on oxygen availability to the brain, particularly if blood flow is also restricted. The fetal blood oxygen dissociation curve is steep, and a difference of 2–3 mmHg in $P\text{O}_2$ could produce a change in oxygen content of as much as 1.0–1.5 mL/dL. However, cerebrovascular resistance may adjust to these changes, permitting an increase in flow and normal oxygen and substrate supply.

With the complete mixing of venous return, pulmonary arterial blood will also have a higher $P\text{O}_2$ than normal; this difference could be as much as 3–5 mmHg. The fetal pulmonary circulation is very sensitive to even small changes in $P\text{O}_2$ (see Chapter 5) and the higher level could produce relaxation and possibly reduce the degree of medial smooth muscle development. However, other factors could also affect pulmonary vascular development. Infants suspected of having had premature closure of the foramen ovale *in utero* have been found to have increased pulmonary arteriolar smooth muscle development. This is thought to be related to the higher flow into the right ventricle and pulmonary artery, creating pulmonary arterial hypertension in the fetus. Constriction of the ductus arteriosus *in utero* also results in pulmonary hypertension and increased thickness of the pulmonary arteriolar smooth muscle layer (p. 96). Both these factors could be operative in fetuses with aortic atresia. The total systemic and umbilical blood flow traverses the ductus arteriosus and if the ductus does not distend to accommodate the large flow, pulmonary arterial hypertension could result. If the foramen ovale is small in association with aortic atresia, even the small amount of pulmonary venous blood returning to the right atrium could result in left atrial and pulmonary venous hypertension and this could induce increased pulmonary arteriolar smooth muscle formation.

The amount of smooth muscle in the pulmonary arterioles at birth could vary, depending on the factors influencing the fetus. If the foramen ovale is small or the ductus arteriosus does not dilate to accommodate the increased flow, pulmonary vascular smooth muscle development will be increased. Newborn infants with aortic atresia and a small foramen ovale have been noted to have pulmonary venous changes and increased pulmonary arteriolar smooth muscle. If the foramen ovale is large enough to readily accommodate pulmonary venous flow and the ductus is wide enough to accommodate systemic and umbilical blood flow with no elevation in pulmonary arterial pressure, the higher $P\text{O}_2$ of pulmonary arterial blood may limit pulmonary arteriolar smooth muscle development. There is some evidence supporting this possibility. In a report of two infants with aortic atresia, the walls of the pulmonary arterioles were noted to be unusually thin.

In the presence of aortic atresia, coronary circulation must be maintained by retrograde flow through the hypoplastic ascending aorta. It appears that this channel is usually adequate to provide myocardial oxygen and nutritional requirements during fetal growth. In association with fetal hypoxemia, coronary blood flow increases markedly. It is possible, however, that the long narrow ascending aorta may not be able to accommodate the increased demands for flow and myocardial hypoxia could occur.

Mitral and aortic atresia with ventricular septal defect
Mitral atresia with ventricular septal defect may occur with or without aortic atresia. Complete mixture of all venous return to the fetal heart occurs in the right atrium. If aortic atresia is also present, blood ejected by the right ventricle may pass through the ductus arteriosus and be distributed in the same manner described above. Blood may pass through the ventricular septal defect into the left ventricle, but then would be ejected back into the right ventricle. The ventricular septal defect would have no influence on the course of the circulation, but by providing flow into the left ventricle it could permit its normal development. If the aortic orifice is patent, blood entering the left ventricle through the ventricular septal defect can be ejected into the ascending aorta and provide blood flow to the coronary circulation and the upper body. The left ventricle may not be normally developed and the ascending aorta may be smaller than normal. Although the ascending aorta is supplied by blood from the left ventricle, the oxygen saturation and Po_2 of blood in the ascending and descending aortae and the pulmonary circulation will be similar because there is complete admixture in the right atrium. Usually the aortic isthmus is narrow, suggesting that although the left ventricle may provide the blood supply to the coronary circulation, upper extremities and head, very little blood crosses the isthmus in the fetus. Probably most blood supplied to the descending aorta is derived by flow from the pulmonary artery across the ductus arteriosus.

Development of cardiac failure

The occurrence of hydrops fetalis resulting from cardiac failure in the fetus with hypoplastic left heart syndrome has been recognized for many years [26]. With the introduction of ultrasound examination, hydrops fetalis due to cardiac failure can be detected *in utero* in fetuses with hypoplastic left heart syndrome [27]. It has also been observed in fetuses with critical aortic stenosis [28].

Hydrops fetalis is the manifestation of cardiac failure in the fetus, associated with high venous pressure (see Chapter 1). Although the right ventricle is required to eject a larger volume of blood than normal in the fetus with hypoplastic left heart, as discussed above, the output is probably not equal to CVO in the normal fetus and it is unlikely that the increased output alone causes venous pressure to increase. Several factors may contribute to raising venous pressure. If the left ventricle is dysfunctional and enlarged, the septum may be deviated to project into the right ventricle, thus limiting diastolic flow into the chamber and increasing venous pressure. If pulmonary vascular resistance is increased because of either pulmonary vascular changes or an increase in left atrial pressure due to a restricted foramen ovale, the right ventricle will be required to eject a larger volume against a higher afterload and this may result in elevation of diastolic and thus venous pressure. If the aortic coarctation is severe, retrograde flow into the ascending aorta may be inadequate to provide coronary blood flow to meet the oxygen and energy requirements of the right ventricle, with resultant failure and elevated venous pressure.

Adequacy of coronary blood flow

In the presence of aortic atresia or severe aortic stenosis, coronary blood flow is provided by retrograde flow from the ductus arteriosus into the aortic arch and ascending aorta. The severity of preductal coarctation is probably the most important factor in determining coronary flow. However, blood flows retrogradely in the aortic arch and ascending aorta and if the ascending aorta is very small, flow to the coronary circulation could be more compromised than flow to the upper extremities, head, and brain. Inadequate coronary blood flow could contribute to the severity of endocardial fibroelastosis and, as mentioned above, to induction of cardiac failure.

Adequacy of cerebral blood flow

Studies of patients with hypoplastic left heart syndrome have shown disturbances in cognitive development in a number of these individuals [29]. The initial hypotheses were that this was the result of the complex procedures associated with palliative surgery. However, studies of patients who had transplantation indicated that they also showed neurodevelopmental delay [30].

The possibility was then considered that cerebral development could be impaired during fetal life as a consequence of inadequate cerebral blood flow resulting from the small aortic arch and particularly the presence of preductal aortic coarctation. This concept received support from several observations of a considerable incidence of decreased head circumference in newborn infants with hypoplastic left heart syndrome [31–33]. Attempts have been made to evaluate cerebral blood flow in fetuses with hypoplastic left heart syndrome by measuring the pulsatility index in Doppler flow recordings from cerebral arteries. In two reports, the presence of a low pulsatility index was interpreted as indicating that cerebral vascular resistance was low and that this reflected a "brain-sparing effect" in an attempt to maintain cerebral oxygen supply [34,35]. Although cerebral vascular resistance may be reduced in these fetuses, it is inappropriate to derive this conclusion from the low pulsatility index. The majority of fetuses with hypoplastic left heart have preductal aortic coarctation and this is most likely the main factor responsible for the reduced pulsatility index. Oxygen supply to the brain is probably reduced in fetuses with aortic atresia; whereas normally blood provided to the brain is derived from the ascending aorta and has a relatively high oxygen saturation, in fetuses with aortic atresia the blood distributed to the whole body is mixed and thus oxygen saturation of blood to the brain would be lower than normal (see Chapter 11). However, a reduced volume of flow is probably more important than the modestly reduced oxygen saturation, because this will interfere not only with oxygen supply but with delivery of energy substrates.

The severity of coarctation that will affect cerebral perfusion in the human fetus is not known. In fetal lambs autoregulation of cerebral blood flow has been shown to function over a relatively small range of pressures. Also, the mean perfusion pressure can be decreased by only a small amount without reducing cerebral blood flow [36]. If these relationships are present in the human, it is likely that even a relatively mild degree of obstruction by aortic coarctation could significantly compromise cerebral flow.

A recent report by Hinton *et al.* [37] indicates there is a high incidence of reduced head circumference in fetuses with aortic atresia and in many, white matter injury in the brain was demonstrated. Of interest is the fact that the reduced head size developed during the second or third trimester. I propose that the findings could be explained by the development of aortic coarctation, resulting in cerebral ischemia. It would be interesting to examine the relationship between the presence and severity of aortic coarctation and head size in fetuses with aortic atresia.

Foramen ovale restriction

The foramen ovale is usually small in fetuses with aortic atresia. In the normal fetus about 25% of CVO passes through the foramen ovale into the left atrium and about 20% of CVO returns from the lungs to the left atrium. With aortic or mitral atresia, there is no egress from the left ventricle. Blood returning from the lungs can return to the general circulation only by passing through the foramen ovale to the right atrium. Left atrial pressure is increased and this tends to close the foramen ovale and limit flow from the IVC into the left atrium. The smaller the foramen ovale, the higher the left atrial pressure. This elevation of left atrial pressure may result in the development of pulmonary lymphangiectasis. As mentioned on p. 262, restriction of the foramen ovale can be recognized by a change in the pattern of pulmonary venous blood flow. The high left atrial pressure is reflected in high pulmonary venous pressure and the pulmonary veins become thickened. The high venous pressure may also affect pulmonary vascular development and pulmonary vascular resistance may be increased (see below). Infants with a restricted foramen ovale often have serious cardiopulmonary distress at the time of birth and prognosis is very poor. The serious implications of a restricted foramen ovale have prompted some centers to attempt to dilate the opening *in utero* (see Chapter 11).

Development of the pulmonary circulation

In the normal human fetus about 20% of CVO is distributed to the lungs from the pulmonary trunk. It returns to the left atrium and ventricle and is ejected into the aorta. In the fetus with aortic atresia and intact ventricular septum, pulmonary venous blood has to exit the left side of the heart through the foramen ovale. If the foramen ovale is restricted, left atrial and pulmonary venous pressures are elevated and, as mentioned above, pulmonary lymphangiectasis and thickening of pulmonary veins may be noted.

In adults with increased left atrial pressure, obstructive lesions of small pulmonary vessels are frequently noted. There is increasing evidence indicating that fetuses with high left atrial pressure may have abnormalities in development of small pulmonary arteries. Not only is there increased thickening of the walls, but the number of small arterioles is reported to be decreased. It is proposed that the smaller pulmonary vascular bed may be responsible for the critical condition of newborn infants who have hypoplastic left heart syndrome with restricted foramen ovale [38,39].

Distribution of oxygen to tissues

In the normal fetus oxygen content of ascending aortic blood is higher than that in the descending aorta. This is the result of preferential streaming of well-oxygenated umbilical venous blood through the ductus venosus and foramen ovale into the left atrium and ventricle and of systemic venous blood into the right ventricle and pulmonary artery and then through the ductus arteriosus to the descending aorta. In the fetal lamb, oxygen saturation in the ascending aorta is about 65% and in the descending aorta about 52%.

In the fetus with aortic atresia, blood does not flow from the right to the left atrium across the foramen ovale and thus all umbilical and systemic venous blood enters the right atrium. Pulmonary venious blood passes through the foramen ovale from the left to the right atrium and mixes with the other venous blood. The mixed venous blood enters the right ventricle and pulmonary artery. The oxygen saturations of pulmonary arterial, ascending aortic, and descending aortic blood are identical. The oxygen saturation of blood distributed to the upper body, brain, and heart is therefore somewhat lower than normal, whereas oxygen saturation of blood distributed to the lungs and lower body is slightly higher than normal. An estimate of the magnitude of change in these saturations can be derived, using assumed values for umbilical and systemic venous blood flows and oxygen saturations.

In the sheep, umbilical blood flow is about 200 mL/min per kg and systemic venous return about 250 mL/min per kg. In the human the assumption is made that umbilical blood flow is about 150 mL/min per kg and systemic venous return about 300 mL/min per kg. Oxygen saturations in umbilical venous blood in both lamb and human are about 80% and in systemic venous blood about 40%. With complete admixture, mixed oxygen saturation would be about 58% in the sheep and about 53% in the human.

The decrease in oxygen in blood supplied to the head is considerable and, combined with a probable reduction in blood flow resulting from the aortic obstruction, could substantially limit oxygen availability to the brain. Similarly, the oxygen saturation as well as the volume of blood flow to the coronary circulation may be compromised and thus reduce oxygen availability to the myocardium.

With the complete mixing of venous return, pulmonary arterial blood will have an oxygen saturation higher than normal. The fetal pulmonary circulation is very sensitive to even small changes in Po_2 (see Chapter 5) and the higher level could produce relaxation and possibly reduce the amount of medial smooth muscle development. However, other factors could also affect pulmonary vascular development. As mentioned above, restriction of the foramen ovale *in utero* has been found to be associated with a reduction in the number of small arteries in the lung and an increase in pulmonary vascular smooth muscle development. Thus the increase in left atrial pressure appears to have a more important effect than oxygen saturation change on pulmonary vascular development.

Changes in the circulation after birth

The elimination of the placental circulation results in a marked increase in systemic vascular resistance, and it is necessary for an increased pulmonary circulation to be established to provide adequate postnatal oxygenation. If there is a diminutive or absent left ventricle, all pulmonary venous blood must cross the atrial septum to enter the right atrium, except in the rare instance when a levoatriocardinal vein is present.

Aortic and mitral atresia with diminutive left ventricle

Survival of the infant postnatally depends on the presence of an adequate atrial communication to

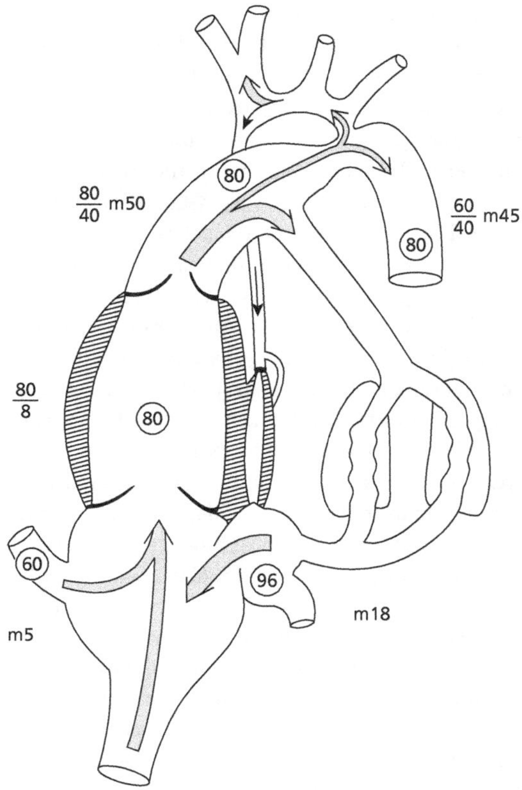

Figure 11.2 Mitral and aortic atresia in a newborn infant: course of the circulation, oxygen saturations (circled), and pressures. The systemic blood flow is derived through the ductus arteriosus. m, mean pressure.

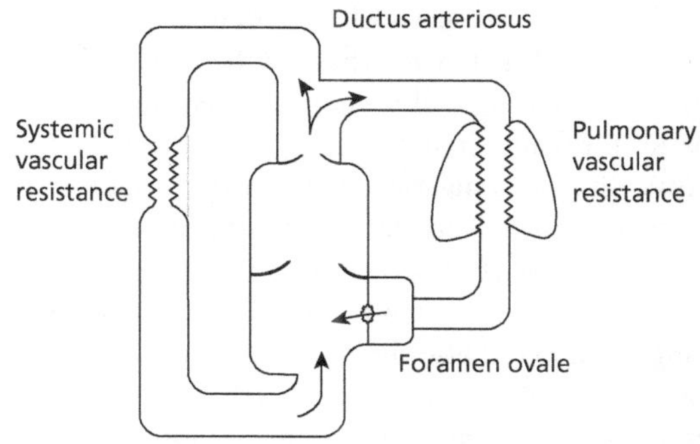

Figure 11.3 The circulation in a newborn infant with aortic and mitral atresia demonstrating the various vascular resistances that determine the circulatory distribution. Detailed description is given in the text.

permit pulmonary venous drainage to enter the systemic circulation and an adequate ductus arteriosus to maintain systemic blood flow. The hemodynamic and clinical features vary greatly, as determined by the relative resistances imposed by the foramen ovale, ductus arteriosus, and systemic and pulmonary vascular resistances (Figure 11.2). Also, the severity of coarctation of the aorta proximal to the ductus arteriosus has an important role in determining systemic blood flow distribution.

The course of the circulation postnatally is similar to that in the fetus. All the SVC and IVC blood passes into the right atrium and right ventricle (Figure 11.3). The pulmonary venous blood also passes into the right atrium across the foramen ovale. Complete mixing of all pulmonary and systemic venous bloods occurs in the right atrium or, if there is streaming of the various venous flows, in the right ventricle. This mixed systemic and pulmonary venous blood is ejected into the main pulmonary artery, and blood of similar oxygen saturation is distributed to the lungs through the pulmonary arteries and to the systemic circulation across the ductus arteriosus. Flow to the vessels arising from the aortic arch is provided in a retrograde manner across the aortic isthmus from the ductus arteriosus; coronary circulation is derived from flow down the hypoplastic ascending aorta to the aortic root.

The hemodynamic features and clinical manifestations of hypoplastic left ventricle are influenced by a number of factors, and these are discussed separately. It should be appreciated, however, that various combinations of these features can modify the circulatory dynamics and clinical presentation. It is also not unusual that the clinical manifestations may change as the factors are modified at different periods after birth.

Foramen ovale

The foramen ovale has a crucial role in the circulatory dynamics and clinical manifestations of aortic atresia both before and after birth. It may be restricted *in utero* and this may result in increased fluid transudation into the lungs and some fetuses develop pulmonary lymphangiectasis. Postnatal adaptation will be difficult, because the large amount of interstitial fluid may interfere with lung expansion and gas exchange. In a series of fetuses with hypoplastic left heart and a foramen ovale orifice of less than 2 mm, postnatal survival was severely compromised. In seven fetuses with very severe restriction delivered by planned cesarean section, only two survived [40]. Restriction of the foramen ovale in the fetus has now been recognized by the abnormal pulmonary venous blood flow pattern. Because it adversely affects postnatal survival, it has been suggested that the foramen should be enlarged by balloon inflation in the fetus.

The adverse effect of a restricted foramen ovale may be the result of not only the effect on the lung *in utero* but also the postnatal changes in the circulation. With transfer of the function of gas exchange to the lungs after birth, pulmonary blood flow has to increase to provide adequate oxygen uptake. With aortic atresia all pulmonary venous blood must pass through the foramen ovale. Even if the foramen is of moderate size, the large increase in flow through it may create a relative obstruction and further increase left atrial and pulmonary venous pressures, with the likelihood that pulmonary edema will develop. The high venous pressure in the lungs will tend to limit pulmonary blood flow; this reduction in flow would help to reduce pulmonary venous pressure, but would result in a reduction of oxygen uptake in the lungs. If the foramen ovale is restricted, even a small increase in pulmonary blood flow will raise left atrial and pulmonary venous pressures.

Pulmonary blood flow and pulmonary venous pressure are determined to some extent by the behavior of the ductus arteriosus. If the ductus arteriosus is widely patent, pulmonary arterial pressure will not exceed systemic arterial pressure. The limitation in pulmonary arterial pressure will restrict the volume of blood flow into the lungs; this will interfere with oxygen uptake and the infant may therefore be quite cyanotic. However, because the volume of blood returning to the left atrium is relatively low, pulmonary venous and left atrial pressures will not increase markedly and the tendency for pulmonary edema to occur would be reduced. If the ductus arteriosus constricts, pulmonary arterial pressure can exceed aortic pressure and result in an increase in pulmonary blood flow; however, particularly if the foramen ovale is small, left atrial and pulmonary venous pressures would be increased and pulmonary edema will tend to develop.

Ductus arteriosus

In infants with hypoplastic left ventricle, systemic blood flow is dependent on the size of the ductus arteriosus and the ratio of pulmonary to systemic vascular resistance. After birth there is a dramatic decrease in blood flow through the ductus arteriosus. In the fetus, the ductus arteriosus conducts both total systemic and umbilical blood flow (see Chapter 1). In the fetal lamb, this represents a flow of about 400 mL/min per kg fetal body weight. Since about 40% of CVO, or 200 mL/min per kg, is directed to the placenta, this will be eliminated after the umbilical cord is clamped. If systemic blood flow is in the usual postnatal range of about 300 mL/min per kg, only this amount will flow through the ductus arteriosus from the pulmonary artery to the aorta. The flow across the ductus arteriosus will therefore drop by about 25% from the prenatal level. However, although measurements in the human fetus vary considerably, in the fetus with aortic atresia with no significant aortic coarctation it can be estimated that about 340 mL/min per kg would flow through the ductus arteriosus during fetal life, of which about 110 mL/min per kg would be directed to the umbilical circulation. Eliminating the placental circulation after birth will result in a fall of 33% from prenatal levels.

If the ductus arteriosus remains widely patent, there will be no interference with flow to the systemic circulation after birth. In fact, since flow across the ductus postnatally is considerably smaller than that prenatally, some constriction could occur without producing obstruction to flow. Using the Poiseuille equation, I have estimated that the diameter of the ductus arteriosus could be reduced by 20–25% after birth without any change in the pressure gradient required to produce a flow that is half the prenatal level.

If the ductus arteriosus constricts to a greater degree, the pressure in the systemic circulation will fall unless pulmonary arterial pressure is increased sufficiently to maintain the same flow across the ductus. Usually, at the time of cardiac catheterization there is a pressure difference between the pulmonary artery and the aorta, and aortic pressure is often lower than normal. These findings suggest that by the time symptoms develop, the ductus arteriosus has constricted and systemic blood flow has dropped.

The increased oxygenation of arterial blood after birth contributes to the constriction of the ductus arteriosus. If systemic and pulmonary arterial Po_2

levels are increased by administering high-oxygen gas mixtures to the infant, greater constriction of the ductus arteriosus may be induced, resulting in a further decline in systemic blood flow. The role of other mechanisms, such as sympathoadrenal stimulation and other hormonal influences (see Chapter 6), in producing constriction of the ductus arteriosus in aortic atresia has not been explored. It is conceivable that decreased peripheral perfusion could aggravate ductus arteriosus constriction by release of catecholamines or other vasoactive hormones. Dilation of the ductus arteriosus by infusion of prostaglandin (PG)E_1 has been effective in maintaining systemic blood flow (see Chapter 11).

The pattern of flow in the ductus arteriosus after birth will be determined by the resistances in the systemic and pulmonary circulations and is phasic in some infants with hypoplastic left heart syndrome [41]. During systole blood will flow from the pulmonary artery to the aorta but if pulmonary vascular resistance is low, there may be a small amount of backflow from the aorta to the pulmonary artery during diastole. If systemic vascular resistance represented by the combined resistance of the systemic circulation and the preductal coarctation is high, the left-to-right ductus flow in diastole will be relatively large. If pulmonary vascular resistance is high as a result of foramen ovale restriction, this flow will be a relatively small proportion of the right-to-left flow in systole.

Pulmonary and systemic vascular resistances

Both the pulmonary and systemic circulations are perfused by blood ejected by the right ventricle; in the absence of constriction of the ductus arteriosus, perfusion pressures are the same. The relative proportions of blood distributed to the pulmonary and systemic circulations are determined by the ratio of total pulmonary vascular resistance to total resistance to systemic perfusion. Total pulmonary resistance is related to pulmonary vascular resistance and the resistance to flow of pulmonary venous blood across the foramen ovale into the right atrium. Total systemic resistance is determined by the resistance imposed by the ductus arteriosus and the systemic vascular bed (see Figure 11.3). The roles of the foramen and of the ductus arteriosus have been discussed above. If total pulmonary resistance is lower than total systemic vascular resistance, blood flows preferentially to the lungs and is diverted away from the systemic circulation, thus interfering with systemic perfusion. A very important consideration in infants with aortic atresia is the possibility that flow into the upper body, heart and brain may be affected to a much greater extent than flow to the lower body, because a preductal aortic coarctation imposes a resistance to upper body flow distal to the ductus arteriosus. Furthermore, with the decrease in systemic blood flow resulting from constriction of the ductus arteriosus, flow to the upper body will be compromised to a greater extent than that to the lower body. The effect of pulmonary and systemic vascular resistance on patterns of flow in the ductus arteriosus is discussed above.

Systemic blood flow and systemic arterial pressure

The decrease in systemic blood flow associated with ductus constriction will tend to result in a drop in systemic arterial pressure. Upper and lower extremity blood pressures may be similar. However, I know of no information regarding pressure in the aortic arch and ascending aorta distal to the obstruction to flow imposed by the coarctation. The status of baroreceptor function is also not known. It is possible that it may have adapted to a reduced pressure in the ascending aorta and its branches during fetal life and may be relatively insensitive. However, if baroreceptor function is normal, the marked reduction in aortic and carotid arterial pressure that would result with ductus arteriosus constriction could produce reflex vasoconstriction in the peripheral circulation, as well as catecholamine release. Thus baroreceptor response would tend to raise pressure in the aorta by causing vasoconstriction. Because the peripheral and gastrointestinal circulations would be affected to a greater extent than the coronary and cerebral circulations, there may be some protective effect on cerebral and coronary blood flow.

The low blood flow to the peripheral tissues results in a reduction in total oxygen delivery and a fall in tissue oxygen availability. Anaerobic glycolysis results and lactic acid production is increased, resulting in lactic acidemia and a reduction in blood pH. As a result of the anaerobic glycolysis, there is greater metabolic turnover of glucose by the tissues. The increased catecholamine production stimulates gluconeogenesis from the liver, but the infant is prone to develop hypoglycemia when liver glycogen content has been depleted.

Coronary blood flow

In aortic atresia, coronary blood flow must be provided by retrograde flow from the ductus arteriosus through the narrow hypoplastic ascending aorta. Rare instances of coronary sinusoids in the left ventricle, similar to those seen in the right ventricle in infants with pulmonary atresia, have been described (see Chapter 11). If the left ventricle is functional, it is possible that some coronary flow may be provided by retrograde flow through these sinusoids. Usually, however, the magnitude of coronary blood flow will depend on the severity of the preductal aortic coarctation and the size of the ascending aorta and pressure in the aortic arch.

The ascending aorta usually appears to be adequate to transmit coronary blood flow in the fetus. Normally, associated with the increase in Po_2 after birth, coronary blood flow falls. With aortic atresia, unless pulmonary blood flow is reduced by foramen ovale restriction, arterial Po_2 will increase in blood entering the aortic arch and ascending aorta so that, unless the coarctation is severe, there may be adequate oxygen delivery to the myocardium. However, the level of systemic arterial pressure is very important in determining blood flow to the right ventricle. The fall in systemic arterial pressure resulting from ductus arteriosus constriction could seriously affect coronary perfusion. Furthermore, constriction of the ductus arteriosus will result in an increase in pulmonary arterial pressure; the increased workload placed on the right ventricle increases myocardial oxygen consumption and there is a greater demand for increased coronary blood flow. At the lower aortic perfusion pressure, the limits of compensatory coronary vasodilatation may not permit adequate coronary blood flow to provide the increased oxygen and metabolic requirements. Right ventricular performance may become impaired and output may be reduced. This further compromises systemic blood flow, resulting in a decrease in aortic pressure. A vicious circle thus develops, which results in rapidly progressive right ventricular and peripheral circulatory failure.

A major concern relating to adequacy of coronary blood flow is the pattern of flow in the ductus arteriosus. As mentioned above, if pulmonary vascular resistance is low, flow in the ductus arteriosus is in the left-to-right direction during diastole and there is retrograde flow in the descending aorta as well as the arch. Because the major proportion of coronary blood flow occurs in diastole, coronary perfusion could be seriously affected.

Cerebral blood flow

Microcephaly is a relatively common finding in infants with hypoplastic left heart syndrome and, as discussed on p. 265, the possibility that brain blood flow is compromised by the aortic arch obstruction has been considered. In a recent report it was observed that the ascending aorta, but not the transverse arch, was small in infants with microcephaly associated with hypoplastic left heart syndrome [42]. However, the severity of the coarctation was not considered as a possible factor contributing to the development of microcephaly. Cerebral blood flow after birth is normally reduced because, with the increase in arterial oxygen saturation, less flow is required to provide oxygen delivery.

Right ventricular performance

The right ventricle provides both pulmonary and systemic blood flows in infants with aortic atresia. In order to provide adequate systemic perfusion, right ventricular systolic pressure must be maintained. The greater the degree of ductus arteriosus constriction, the greater must be the elevation in right ventricular pressure. A decrease in pulmonary vascular resistance would result in an increase in pulmonary venous return and a larger volume load on the right ventricle. This increase in volume ejected at high pressure places a large workload on the ventricle; right ventricular pressure will increase and clinical evidences of right heart failure, predominantly presenting as hepatomegaly, will occur.

If there is interference with pulmonary venous return to the right atrium because the foramen ovale is small, left atrial and pulmonary venous pressures will increase, causing further elevation in pulmonary arterial pressure and thus placing a greater workload on the right ventricle. However, a rise in pulmonary venous pressure may decrease pulmonary blood flow and thus lower the right ventricular load.

Systemic arterial oxygenation

In mitral and aortic atresia there is complete admixture of pulmonary and systemic venous returns in the right atrium; thus, the oxygen saturation and Po_2 of pulmonary and systemic arterial blood are the same. The level of saturation is determined by the ratio of pulmonary to systemic blood flow and by the levels of oxygen saturation of mixed venous and pulmonary venous blood (see Chapter 4). Obstruction of the foramen ovale is associated with low pulmonary blood flow and oxygen saturation of the mixed blood will be reduced. However, in the absence of foramen ovale restriction, arterial blood oxygen saturation is usually high because pulmonary blood flow is increased and systemic blood flow is reduced. Constriction of the ductus arteriosus will further reduce systemic blood flow, thereby increasing the pulmonary to systemic blood flow ratio and thus arterial oxygen saturation and Po_2 will increase. Reduction of systemic blood flow will result in greater oxygen extraction by the tissues and oxygen saturation of mixed venous blood is low. Pulmonary venous oxygen saturation may be normal or only slightly reduced. However, if pulmonary edema is present as a result of foramen ovale restriction, it will be reduced. The effects of the flow relationships on oxygen saturation are illustrated in the following example.

> If pulmonary blood flow is twice normal (6 L/min per m^2), systemic blood flow 50% normal (1.5 L/min per m^2), pulmonary venous oxygen saturation 95%, and systemic mixed venous saturation 45%, the final mixed saturation would be:
>
> $$\frac{(6 \times 95) + (1.5 \times 45)}{7.5} = 85\%$$
>
> This level of oxygen desaturation may not be detected in an infant, particularly if there is peripheral vasoconstriction that results in pallor of the skin.

The effects of oxygen administration on arterial oxygen saturation and Po_2 are of considerable importance. In the absence of significant pulmonary edema, administration of 100% oxygen will raise oxygen saturation in pulmonary venous blood to 100% and Po_2 will increase to levels above 400 mmHg. Because pulmonary blood flow may be considerably greater than systemic blood flow, the final mixed oxygen saturation may be close to 100%. The effects of oxygen on the pulmonary circulation and the ductus arteriosus may further enhance the effects of oxygen. A fall in pulmonary vascular resistance and an increase in ductus arteriosus constriction may further increase pulmonary blood flow and decrease systemic blood flow, thus increasing the pulmonary to systemic flow ratio. These effects may combine to produce a marked increase in arterial Po_2; I have noted levels of 250–280 mmHg in infants with aortic atresia during 100% oxygen administration.

The roles of the ductus arteriosus, pulmonary vascular resistance, and size of the foramen ovale are similar to those outlined above.

Mitral atresia with ventricular septal defect

The pattern of circulatory changes after birth differs considerably from that in infants with aortic and mitral atresia with intact ventricular septum. Several features are quite similar. The total pulmonary venous return must pass through the foramen ovale from the left atrium to the right atrium, and thus there is complete admixture of pulmonary and systemic venous returns. The blood distributed to both the pulmonary and systemic circulation has the same blood oxygen saturation and Po_2; these levels are determined by the pulmonary to systemic flow ratios, as described above. If foramen ovale obstruction is present, pulmonary blood flow will not increase sufficiently after birth and severe cyanosis will be evident. With an adequate foramen ovale, and with aortic but not mitral atresia, the circulatory pattern will be similar to that described above. It is still necessary that systemic blood flow be provided through the ductus arteriosus. However, if the aortic outflow is patent, blood can pass from the right to the left ventricle through the ventricular septal defect and provide either all or part of the systemic blood flow. A large pulmonary blood flow is established after birth as pulmonary vascular resistance falls. The infant may develop cardiac failure but survival is much more likely than with aortic atresia. With growth after birth the foramen ovale may become restrictive and pulmonary edema may develop.

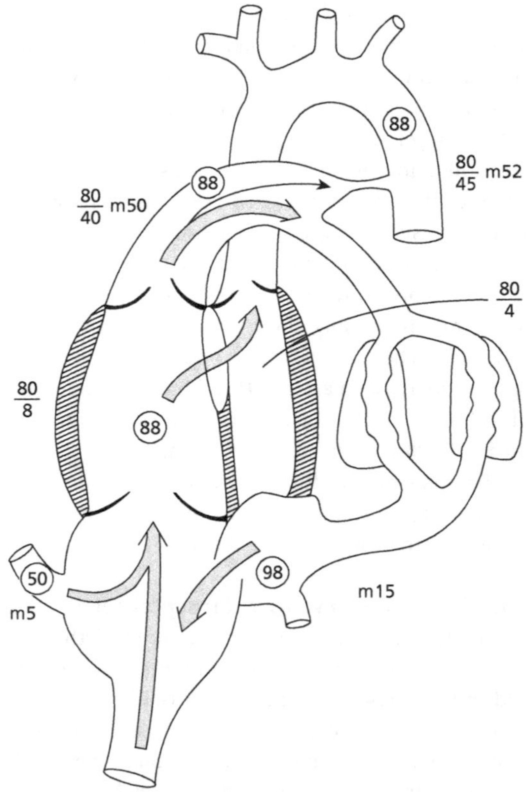

Figure 11.4 Mitral atresia with large ventricular septal defect in a newborn infant: course of the circulation, oxygen saturations (circled), and pressures. Systemic blood flow is maintained through the ventricular septal defect. m, mean pressure.

The pattern of flow into the aorta depends on the degree of development of the isthmus and on the behavior of the ductus arteriosus. If the isthmus is well developed, the right ventricle can supply the total systemic blood flow through the ventricular septal defect after the ductus arteriosus constricts (Figure 11.4). If the aortic isthmus is narrow, blood to the descending aorta may be supplied partly through the ductus arteriosus from the pulmonary arteries. If the ductus arteriosus constricts, pressure in the descending aorta will fall whereas pressures in the ascending aorta may be well maintained. Since pulmonary arterial pressure is at systemic arterial levels, there is a serious risk of the development of early pulmonary vascular obstruction. This will result in a decrease in pulmonary flow, with increasing cyanosis.

Clinical features

Despite the high heritability of hypoplastic left heart syndrome, associated congenital cardiac anomalies are not common. Some infants show mild growth retardation at birth and about 20% have a decreased head circumference. A small percentage of patients have Turner syndrome. Symptoms may appear within an hour or two after birth but are usually noted after 24–48 hours; there may be a delay of several days and rarely of weeks.

Infants who have had severe foramen ovale restriction *in utero* may have pulmonary lymphangiectasis and edema and are likely to suffer immediate distress after birth because adequate respiration cannot be established. The clinical features are variable and depend on the combination of circulatory disturbances described above.

Aortic and mitral atresia

The clinical features in the early neonatal period are influenced by the severity of obstruction at the foramen ovale during fetal life.

Severe foramen ovale restriction

Infants born with severe obstruction of the foramen ovale usually have severe early symptoms, sometimes within a few minutes after birth, but usually within a few hours. The most prominent manifestation is respiratory distress and severe cyanosis, related to inability to establish adequate alveolar ventilation, and low pulmonary blood flow. Systemic arterial $P\text{O}_2$ is often 30 mmHg or less and metabolic acidemia soon develops, with pH falling to below 7.2 and sometimes to 7.0. $P\text{CO}_2$ is increased to 50–55 mmHg or even higher, due to disturbed ventilation, as well as low pulmonary blood flow. No difference in oxygen saturation between the upper and lower extremities is noted. Assisted ventilation may be difficult to establish because of pulmonary edema, and even with high inspiratory pressures adequate ventilation may not be possible. The severe hypoxemia and acidemia induce sympathoadrenal stimulation, which results in peripheral vasoconstriction and poor skin perfusion with a grayish pallor due to associated cyanosis; the extremities also become cold. The peripheral pulses may be normal initially, but soon become weak. The liver may be slightly enlarged to

2–3 cm below the costal margin. The cardiac impulse is prominent at the lower left sternal border, as in normal infants, and is not hyperactive. The first heart sound is normal and the second sound is loud, but single, at the upper left sternal border. No murmurs may be audible, but a grade 2–3/6 medium-frequency systolic murmur may be heard at the lower left sternal border due to tricuspid insufficiency. Associated with the severe hypoxemia and metabolic acidemia, hypoglycemia and hypocalcemia may develop. These infants deteriorate rapidly and require urgent treatment (see below); even though treatment, including dilation of the foramen ovale, is instituted immediately after birth, there is a high mortality. The rapid onset and progression of respiratory distress and cyanosis within a few hours after birth is unlikely with other congenital cardiac lesions except total pulmonary venous return with severe obstruction to pulmonary venous drainage (see Chapter 11).

Foramen ovale unobstructed

Ductus arteriosus patent

If the size of the foramen ovale is adequate to accommodate pulmonary venous return and the ductus arteriosus is patent, the infant may manifest no symptoms for several days. Mild to moderate cyanosis is often present in the early neonatal period, but as pulmonary blood flow increases cyanosis lessens and may not be appreciated clinically because arterial oxygen saturation may be as high as 88–92%. Arterial blood Po_2 is usually in the range 40–55 mmHg, while Pco_2 is either normal or may be reduced to 35 mmHg; pH is normal or slightly reduced. Tachypnea and dyspnea are first noted and feeding becomes difficult. Heart rate is increased to 160–180/min and pulses are palpable but often weak and peripheral perfusion may be reduced. No difference in pulses in the upper and lower extremities is evident. Systolic blood pressure is often reduced to 40–50 mmHg and pulse pressure is reduced. Liver enlargement to 3–5 cm below the costal margin is often noted. The cardiac impulse is hyperactive and prominent beneath the lower sternum due to the high right ventricular volume load. The first heart sound is normal, but the second sound is single and loud at the upper left sternal border. No murmurs may be heard, but often a medium-frequency grade 2–3/6 systolic murmur is audible over the lower sternum due to tricuspid insufficiency resulting from ventricular enlargement. Occasionally a soft crescendo–decrescendo systolic murmur is heard over the upper left sternal border, radiating to the left chest, related to the high flow through the pulmonary valve and pulmonary arteries. As right ventricular failure progresses, its output falls and this seriously affects systemic blood flow with resulting fall in arterial pressure with systolic levels below 40 mmHg and narrow pulse pressure. Pulses are weak and pallor, mottling, and cold extremities develop. The child succumbs to right heart failure and inadequate output.

Ductus arteriosus constricted

Although the ductus arteriosus normally closes within a few hours after birth, in infants with aortic atresia it often remains patent for several days and occasionally for several weeks. The early manifestations are those of the increased pulmonary blood flow and right ventricular output described above. Ductus constriction may develop gradually over several days, but not infrequently it occurs rapidly over a few hours, creating the need for urgent treatment. The predominant features are those related to the reduction in systemic blood flow. The pulses are very weak, if not impalpable, and peripheral perfusion is poor, with generalized pallor, mottling of the skin, and coldness of the extremities. Systolic arterial pressure is reduced to 30–40 mmHg and pulse pressure is low. Due to reduced tissue perfusion, with anaerobic metabolism, metabolic acidemia rapidly develops. Arterial blood oxygen saturation is only slightly reduced, usually to about 88–92% and Po_2 is about 50–60 mmHg; pH is usually about 7.2 at presentation but may fall to 7.0, and Pco_2 is normal or reduced to 30–35 mmHg. The other physical findings are similar to those described above. The poor perfusion of the kidneys results in oliguria, progressing to anuria and elevation of serum nonprotein nitrogen and creatinine levels.

Hypoglycemia and hypocalcemia are also frequently noted. The infant's condition sometimes fluctuates over several hours or even days, due to variability in the degree of constriction of the ductus arteriosus. The weak pulses and poor perfusion may spontaneously improve and the infant's general condition, including blood gas status, also improves for several hours, after which the condition deteriorates again.

Moderate restriction of foramen ovale

The foramen ovale may be large enough to accommodate the increase in pulmonary blood flow that occurs immediately after birth, but the size may not be adequate as pulmonary blood flow progressively increases as pulmonary vascular resistance falls further. The onset of manifestations will depend on the degree of restriction. The initial clinical manifestations are similar to those in infants with no restriction to flow, but as the obstruction becomes significant, evidence of pulmonary edema becomes manifest. Respiratory distress becomes more severe and cyanosis may become more marked. Rales may be heard at the lung bases. The increase in left atrial and pulmonary venous pressures results in some diminution of pulmonary blood flow, so that the degree of precordial hyperactivity may become less prominent. If the ductus arteriosus constricts, in addition to the evidence of reduced systemic blood flow, the increase in pulmonary arterial pressure will tend to increase pulmonary blood flow and aggravate the pulmonary edema.

Mitral atresia with ventricular septal defect and open aortic valve

The infant with this combination of lesions may be moderately cyanotic at birth, but as soon as pulmonary vascular resistance falls there will be a decrease in the degree of cyanosis. The symptoms and signs will be related to the hemodynamic disturbances that predominate. If the ductus arteriosus constricts early, the pulses in the lower extremities will become weak and perfusion to the lower body will be poor, with mottling and pallor, but pulses in the arms will be well felt. As pulmonary blood flow increases, the heart will become hyperactive, with the maximal impulse at the lower left sternal border. The first heart sound is accentuated at the lower left sternal border and the second sound is accentuated at the upper left sternal border; the second sound may be split but is usually narrow. A systolic ejection click is present occasionally and a third sound is heard frequently. No murmurs may be heard, but a grade 2–3/6 systolic murmur may be present at the mid-left sternal border. Cardiac failure occurs early, with pulmonary rales, hepatomegaly, and respiratory distress. If the foramen ovale is small, pulmonary edema may be severe and evidence of right-sided failure not so prominent; cyanosis will also be more marked because pulmonary venous return will be limited.

The ductus arteriosus remains widely patent in some infants, and the main clinical features are those of cardiac failure. If the failure can be controlled, the infant may progress favorably. One of two possible courses may then develop. With growth, the foramen ovale may become relatively small, resulting in a high left atrial pressure with, first, intermittent and, later, persistent severe pulmonary edema. Some patients who survive the period of infancy do well for many years and then develop increasing cyanosis and cardiac failure when pulmonary vascular obstruction develops.

Investigations

Electrocardiography

In infants with aortic atresia and a small left ventricle, the electrocardiogram shows right axis deviation and right ventricular hypertrophy. One finding that may be helpful is the absence of a Q wave and absent R waves in the left precordial leads, suggesting the left ventricle is small or absent. ST- and T-wave changes, with inversion of T waves in all the precordial leads, have been observed in some infants and could be associated with endocardial fibroelastosis but could be related to inadequate coronary perfusion in the presence of increased workload on the right ventricle. If the left ventricle is hypoplastic, the presence of left axis deviation should suggest the diagnosis of atrioventricular septal defect, with malalignment and major commitment to the right ventricle. The P wave is often tall and peaked in standard leads II and III and right precordial leads.

Chest radiography

In the early postnatal period the heart is not usually enlarged. If the foramen ovale is severely obstructed, the lungs are poorly aerated due to the presence of pulmonary lymphangiectasis and pulmonary edema. With less severe restriction, increased hilar vascular markings due to pulmonary venous engorgement may be evident. When the foramen ovale is adequate, heart size enlarges as pulmonary blood flow increases, and the pulmonary arterial markings become prominent. Constriction of the ductus arteriosus does not result in further major changes, but pulmonary arterial markings may become more prominent. The heart is often globular in shape, with absence of the left ventricle, so that the apex is tilted upward.

Echocardiography

Fetal studies

With advances in technology and diagnostic skills, the presence of aortic valve obstruction is being recognized at a younger fetal age than previously possible. As mentioned above, aortic stenosis was suspected in an 11-week fetus that showed an increase in ascending aortic blood flow velocity. With subsequent observation it was observed that left ventricular function was disturbed and it became progressively hypoplastic [19]. Numerous serial studies have confirmed the development of atresia in fetuses that showed aortic stenosis on initial examination. Many infants are born with aortic stenosis and do not develop hypoplastic ventricles. It is therefore important to be able to predict whether a particular fetus with aortic stenosis is likely to develop hypoplasia of the left ventricle. Ultrasound examination has also been useful in assessing the degree of restriction imposed by the foramen ovale. Because foramen ovale restriction *in utero* is associated with a very high mortality after birth, its recognition in the fetus, with the possibility of treatment in the fetus or immediately after birth, has become an important part of fetal studies. These issues are discussed in the section on therapy below.

Postnatal studies

The introduction of ultrasound examination has largely eliminated the need for cardiac catheterization in the infant with aortic or mitral atresia prior to surgery. A detailed evaluation should include assessment of:

- aortic and mitral valve morphology;
- sizes of the left and right ventricles;
- right ventricular function and presence and severity of tricuspid regurgitation;
- bowing of the atrial septum, size of the foramen ovale, and displacement of the septum primum;
- size of the ascending aorta and aortic arch, presence of preductal coarctation, and pattern of flow in the arch and ascending aorta;
- degree of constriction and pattern of flow in the ductus arteriosus;
- presence of a ventricular septal defect;
- connections of the pulmonary veins;
- presence of associated lesions.

The right ventricle is large and usually contracts well. Tricuspid regurgitation is very common and has been observed in about half of all patients, but is usually mild. However, it is important to note the presence of marked regurgitation, because this has surgical implications. The left ventricle may not be identifiable, but if aortic atresia with a ventricular septal defect without mitral atresia is present, the size of the left ventricle should be evaluated to decide if it might support an adequate systemic blood flow. A reasonably well developed left ventricular cavity in the presence of mitral or aortic atresia indicates the presence of a ventricular septal defect; its location and size should be assessed.

The direction of bowing of the atrial septum should be examined. With aortic and mitral atresia, it bulges into the right atrium, whereas in infants with total anomalous pulmonary venous drainage it may bulge into the left atrium. The size of the foramen ovale should be assessed from two-dimensional ultrasound as well as Doppler flow analysis. The connections of all pulmonary veins should be determined to ensure they are draining to the left atrium. The pattern of flow in the pulmonary veins should be examined carefully. An increase in the reverse flow during atrial systole and a reduction in forward flow is indicative of the presence of foramen ovale restriction (see Chapter 11).

With aortic atresia, the diameter of the ascending aorta is usually less than 5–6 mm and flow is retrograde toward the coronary arteries. The aortic arch and the isthmus are narrow; in 70–80% of infants, aortic coarctation is present in the isthmus just above the junction with the ductus arteriosus. The ductus arteriosus is usually widely patent in early infancy but constriction may be observed later. Bidirectional flow is commonly evident on Doppler flow study; during systole blood flows from the pulmonary artery into the descending aorta and the isthmus and arch, but when pulmonary vascular resistance falls, diastolic flow from the descending aorta through the ductus to the pulmonary artery may be seen. The absence of aortic to pulmonary artery diastolic flow suggests that pulmonary vascular resistance is high, or that the foramen ovale is severely obstructed.

Infants with aortic and mitral atresia with severe obstruction at the foramen ovale are usually very cyanosed and distressed soon after birth. Urgent management is necessary. Therefore the most important information to obtain is confirmation of the diagnosis and demonstration of foramen ovale obstruction. Once these are documented, it is inappropriate to extend the examination to assess other features prior to treatment.

Cardiac catheterization and angiocardiography

General considerations

Prior to the advent of ultrasound techniques, cardiac catheterization was performed in the infant suspected of having hypoplastic left ventricle to confirm the diagnosis. The specific indications were to clarify:

- whether both the mitral and aortic valves were atretic;
- size of the left atrium and foramen ovale and the degree of obstruction of the foramen ovale;
- presence of a ventricular septal defect;
- size of the ascending aorta and the aortic isthmus;
- size and functional capacity of the left ventricle;
- degree of constriction of the ductus arteriosus.

As mentioned above, these issues can now almost always be resolved by ultrasound examination, so there is little indication to perform cardiac catheterization in these often very sick infants. Currently, the main indications for the procedure are (i) to relieve obstruction to pulmonary venous flow into the right atrium imposed by the atrial septum in the critically ill neonate with severe cyanosis; and (ii) to determine the feasibility of proceeding with additional surgery after the first stage of palliation (Norwood procedure) (see section on therapy below).

Infants with aortic and mitral atresia are often extremely ill. Oxygen should be administered if severe cyanosis is present, with arterial Po_2 below 30–35 mmHg. Hypoglycemia and hypocalcemia should be corrected and temperature controlled and maintained (see Chapter 3). Prostaglandin should be administered to maintain ductus arteriosus patency. Although the cardiac catheterization procedure is now rarely done for diagnosis, the findings are presented because they form the basis for our understanding of the hemodynamic disturbances.

Aortic and mitral atresia

Oxygen saturation data

The oxygen saturations of SVC and IVC blood are variable and depend on the magnitude of systemic blood flow. Initially saturation may be near normal at 60–65%. As systemic blood flow falls there is increasing oxygen extraction and vena cava saturation falls to as low as 25–30%. Oxygen saturation increases at the right atrial level; with foramen ovale obstruction, it may increase to only 50–60%, but if there is no obstruction right atrial oxygen saturation may be about 85–90% or even higher. Frequently, there is a further small increase in right ventricular oxygen saturation due to streaming of the blood shunted across the atrial septum directly into the tricuspid valve orifice. Pulmonary and systemic arterial oxygen saturations are identical. The level of oxygen is determined by the pulmonary to systemic blood flow ratio (see Chapter 4). Pulmonary venous and left atrial saturations are normal or slightly decreased to about 95%. If pulmonary blood flow is markedly reduced, pulmonary venous oxygen saturation may be normal with room air, and with 100% oxygen Po_2 above 400 mmHg may be achieved. In infants who have severe respiratory distress associated with pulmonary edema, pulmonary venous and left atrial saturations may be reduced to 85–90%. Arterial blood gases show variable levels of Po_2 depending on the magnitude of pulmonary blood flow; it is markedly reduced to 30 mmHg or less with severe foramen ovale obstruction, but may be as high as 65–70 mmHg if pulmonary blood flow is large. Arterial Pco_2 is usually normal or reduced to about 35 mmHg, but it may be raised to about 45 mmHg if pulmonary edema is present. Arterial pH also varies; it may be normal but with severe hypoxemia it is often 7.20 or less. Ductus arteriosus constriction with reduced systemic blood flow results in a fall in pH to 7.2–7.0 associated with a Po_2 above 50–60 mmHg and an oxygen saturation of 85–92% in systemic arterial blood.

Pressures

Pulmonary venous and left atrial pressures are usually elevated; mean pressure is usually greater than 15 mmHg, and with foramen ovale obstruction may be as high as 25–30 mmHg. The *a* and *v* waves are prominent and usually equal in magnitude. A pressure difference is recorded as the catheter is withdrawn across the foramen ovale into the right atrium. Usually right atrial mean pressure is increased to 10–12 mmHg, but higher levels may be recorded when severe right ventricular failure is present. The right atrial pressure pulse shows a dominant *a* wave that may reach 15–20 mmHg.

The left ventricular pressure cannot be recorded. Right ventricular systolic pressure is usually 70–100 mmHg, and end-diastolic pressures are increased to levels similar to the right atrial *a* wave.

Systolic pressure in the pulmonary artery is similar to that in the right ventricle. Diastolic pressure is variable but is usually maintained above 35 mmHg, despite the relatively low pulmonary vascular resistance. If foramen ovale obstruction is present, pulmonary arterial systolic and diastolic pressure are elevated and may reach 110/70 mmHg or even higher, depending also on the degree of constriction of the ductus arteriosus. Without prostaglandin infusion there is usually a pressure difference across the ductus arteriosus when the catheter is withdrawn from the descending aorta to the pulmonary artery. This may be small, with a systolic and mean pressure difference of only 8–10 mmHg and no significant diastolic pressure gradient; however, with ductus arteriosus constriction, a mean pressure difference of as much as 20–25 mmHg may be recorded. The gradient has been observed to increase during administration of 100% oxygen, but it is considerably lower during prostaglandin infusion. Ductus constriction may reduce systemic pressure markedly, with systolic pressures of 35 mmHg or less.

I know of no reports of pressure measurement in the aortic arch but presumably if the coarctation is severe, pressures in the ascending aorta and the arch and its branches would be low.

Blood flows

Calculation of flows is difficult in infants with aortic and mitral atresia; there are large potential errors in calculation of both systemic and pulmonary blood flows because the measurement of arteriovenous differences may be unreliable. Pulmonary and systemic flows can be calculated from the usual Fick equations (see Chapter 4). A reliable mixed venous sample cannot be obtained because there is a large shunt across the atrial septum. SVC and IVC oxygen saturations may differ greatly and mixed venous oxygen saturation must be estimated between the two values. Although saturations from different pulmonary veins may vary slightly, left atrial oxygen saturation is a reasonable representation of mixed pulmonary venous blood. However, when pulmonary blood flow is high, the actual level of flow may be difficult to calculate accurately, because the pulmonary arteriovenous oxygen difference is very small (see Chapter 4). This problem is compounded if oxygen is being administered to the infant. Oxygen saturation in both pulmonary venous and pulmonary arterial blood may be 100%. It is then necessary to calculate dissolved oxygen from Po_2 measurements. The calculation of flow is therefore subject to considerable error.

Systemic blood flows may be near normal levels, but when the ductus arteriosus is constricted may fall to 2.0 L/min per m^2 or less. Pulmonary blood flow may be increased to levels estimated as high as 8–15 L/min per m^2, but these values may be high because of potential errors in the calculation. If the foramen ovale is obstructed, pulmonary blood flow is reduced.

Shunts

As in many other congenital heart lesions, there is a difference between the volumes of blood actually shunted left to right and right to left and the volumes that recirculate in the pulmonary and systemic circulations. The concept of anatomical and physiological shunting may be applied to differentiate between these (see Chapter 4).

1 The anatomical left-to-right shunt in infants with aortic and mitral atresia is the volume of blood that crosses the foramen ovale from the left atrium to the right atrium and represents total pulmonary blood flow. In addition, a small amount of blood may flow from the aorta through the ductus arteriosus into the pulmonary artery during diastole.

2 The anatomical right-to-left shunt is the volume of blood passing from the pulmonary artery to the aorta through the ductus arteriosus and represents total systemic blood flow.

3 The physiological left-to-right shunt reflects the volume of pulmonary venous blood that recirculates through the lungs and is calculated from the equation:

$$\text{Left-to-right shunt} = \dot{Q}p - \dot{Q}ep$$

where $\dot{Q}p$ denotes pulmonary flow and $\dot{Q}ep$ effective pulmonary flow.

4 The physiological right-to-left shunt represents the portion of systemic venous blood that returns to the systemic arteries without passing through the lungs and is calculated from the equation:

$$\text{Right-to-left shunt} = \dot{Q}s - \dot{Q}ep$$

where $\dot{Q}s$ denotes systemic flow.

Angiocardiography

A contrast injection into the left atrium shows the size of the chamber, whether there is any mitral valve opening and, if contrast medium enters the left ventricle, the size of the chamber. It also delineates the foramen ovale and provides an estimate of its size. An injection into the descending aorta just beyond the ductus arteriosus demonstrates the anatomy of the aortic isthmus, the great vessel origins from the arch, and usually clearly shows the size of the ascending aorta, because flow occurs retrograde to the coronary arteries. The aortic injection also demonstrates whether a preductal coarctation is present.

An injection should be made into the right ventricle to demonstrate a ventricular septal defect and define the size of the defect and of the left ventricle. The right ventricular injection will also show the pulmonary arteries, ductus arteriosus, and aorta; the ascending aorta may not be seen clearly because the contrast medium is diluted by the large pulmonary blood flow. For this reason, the pulmonary veins and left atrium are not visualized clearly, as the right atrium and ventricle fill rapidly and no specific chambers can be seen well.

Mitral atresia with ventricular septal defect

In many respects the cardiac catheterization findings are similar to those of aortic and mitral atresia. Since there is complete admixture of pulmonary and systemic venous blood, the oxygen saturation data are similar. The atrial pressure data are also similar. The diagnosis may be established if the catheter is passed from the right ventricle through the ventricular septal defect into the left ventricle and the ascending aorta. A left atrial angiogram will show that there is no filling of the left ventricle, and all the contrast medium enters the right atrium. A right ventricular angiogram will demonstrate passage of contrast medium across the ventricular septal defect, to fill the ascending aorta as well as the pulmonary artery.

Differential diagnosis

Most infants with aortic or mitral atresia or hypoplastic left heart develop symptoms within a few days after birth. It is most important to make the diagnosis rapidly in the infant who has severe obstruction of the foramen ovale, because progressive hypoxemia may result in early demise. Although many congenital cardiac lesions with marked cyanosis should be considered, the most important condition that can simulate the findings of severe cyanosis with respiratory distress is total anomalous pulmonary venous drainage with obstruction to pulmonary venous return.

Total anomalous pulmonary venous return

The clinical features of moderate to severe cyanosis, respiratory difficulty, weak pulses, and pallor are similar in both lesions. Clinical examination of the heart reveals an accentuated second sound, with no significant murmurs, in both. The electrocardiogram usually shows absent left ventricular forces in both lesions. Chest radiography shows an increase in pulmonary vascular markings, with variable degrees of pulmonary edema, and the heart may be variably enlarged in either lesion.

In general, symptoms and signs tend to be delayed for several days in infants with total anomalous pulmonary venous return, and to appear earlier in those with aortic atresia and foramen ovale obstruction, but this is not reliable in the differentiation. Most of the other lesions associated with severe cyanosis present after a few days, because the ductus arteriosus provides a reasonable pulmonary blood flow and deterioration occurs when the ductus constricts. However, aortopulmonary transposition with a very small or closed foramen ovale may present early. Ultrasound examination readily makes the differentiation.

Idiopathic respiratory distress syndrome

During the first day after birth, the possibility of respiratory distress syndrome should be considered. The differentiation from aortic atresia is not usually difficult. Infants with respiratory distress syndrome with marked cyanosis demonstrate much greater respiratory difficulty, with sternal retraction and grunting. Examination of the chest or heart is not especially contributory. However, the presence of a markedly enlarged liver would tend to lead one away from the diagnosis of respiratory distress syndrome. The chest radiograph may be helpful; infants with aortic atresia with obstructed foramen ovale show increased hilar pulmonary venous plethora, but those with respiratory distress syndrome usually have diffuse pulmonary changes. The electrocardiogram is not of much help, as it usually shows dominant right forces, but if R waves are seen in the left precordial leads, the diagnosis of hypoplastic left ventricle is unlikely. Measurement of arterial blood gases may be helpful; in respiratory distress syndrome the $P\text{CO}_2$ is usually markedly elevated, often to 50–60 mmHg, whereas with aortic atresia it is either normal or only slightly increased.

In infants with mild obstruction of the foramen ovale, the occurrence within a few days after birth of the characteristic picture of pallor, mild cyanosis, often with mottling, respiratory distress and weak pulses should lead one to suspect the lesion. There are, however, several disease entities that should be considered.

Severe aortic stenosis

Infants with severe aortic stenosis but with well-developed left ventricles may present a clinical picture similar to that seen in aortic atresia, because they may have markedly decreased cardiac output with poor peripheral perfusion. In infants with aortic stenosis a harsh systolic ejection murmur is usually heard at the mid to lower left sternal border, but if cardiac output is severely reduced the murmur may be soft. Chest radiography usually shows marked cardiomegaly in the infant with aortic stenosis, but this is not a reliable differentiating feature. The pulmonary arterial markings are usually very prominent with aortic atresia, but not with aortic stenosis. However, some infants with aortic stenosis have left-to-right shunts through the foramen ovale, which results in prominent pulmonary vasculature. The newborn infant with severe aortic stenosis often has dominant right-sided forces with right axis deviation on the electrocardiogram but, unlike in aortic atresia, R waves (indicating left ventricular forces) are usually present in the left precordial leads.

The diagnosis can be made readily by ultrasound study, demonstrating the markedly hypoplastic ascending aorta with retrograde flow toward the coronary arteries in aortic atresia. In patients with hypoplastic left ventricle with aortic and mitral stenosis, the clinical picture may be very similar to that in aortic and mitral atresia. The differentiation is made by ultrasound examination, including Doppler flow studies. The presence of a small ventricle with flow through both the mitral and aortic valves differentiates the condition from aortic atresia.

Acute myocarditis

Newborn infants with acute viral myocarditis may present with acute cardiovascular collapse, pallor, very weak pulses, and respiratory difficulty. The clinical features may be indistinguishable from those of aortic and mitral atresia. The heart is usually quiet to palpation as compared with aortic atresia and murmurs are not usually heard. Chest radiography is not helpful, as it shows a large heart with pulmonary edema. The electrocardiogram may show low voltage of the QRS complex in all leads, but in early infancy right-sided forces may be dominant. In the absence of an epidemic or evidence of viral infection in the mother or other infants, the differentiation clinically may be difficult. Ultrasound study readily provides the correct diagnosis.

Principles of management

Fetal diagnosis and management

The introduction of ultrasound examination of the fetus has led to the ability to recognize hypoplastic left heart syndrome by mid-gestation and often even earlier. Currently, the main interest in fetal diagnosis is related to the hypothesis that hypoplastic left heart frequently develops in fetuses with a primary lesion of valvar aortic stenosis during gestational growth (see Chapter 11).

It is hoped that by relieving the aortic stenosis by balloon dilation of the valve *in utero*, the left ventricle would be able to develop a size and function that would permit it to sustain an adequate systemic output postnatally. If this concept that the left ventricle becomes progressively hypoplastic with advancing gestation is correct, the earlier the dilation of the valve is performed, the more likely optimal ventricular development is achieved. It would therefore be important to make the diagnosis of aortic stenosis as early as possible *in utero*. This requires identification of at-risk populations, recognizing the earliest evidence of the lesion and skillful interpretation of ultrasound studies.

Hypoplastic left heart syndrome has high heritability, as discussed above. Therefore, if there is a history in the parents' families of hypoplastic left heart syndrome, aortic stenosis, coarctation of the aorta, or bicuspid aortic valve, the fetus should be carefully studied, probably by 11 or 12 weeks of gestation for possible presence of aortic stenosis. Sequential studies should be conducted every 4–5 weeks. The presence of increased nuchal fold thickness in the fetus during ultrasound screening in the first trimester has been found to be associated with chromosomal anomalies or congenital cardiovascular malformations; hypoplastic left heart is one of the malformations noted in the fetus with increased nuchal fold thickness.

With current approaches, most fetuses are recognized to have aortic obstruction because they have left ventricular enlargement and usually dysfunction and often manifest endocardial fibroelastosis. However, several observers have suspected the presence of stenosis when left ventricular size and function are normal. In one report [19], aortic stenosis was suspected in a fetus at about 11 weeks' gestation, based on the observation of increased flow velocity in the ascending aorta by Doppler examination; by about 16 weeks the fetus had developed a dysfunctional left ventricle and then progressed to typical hypoplastic left heart syndrome. With current techniques, it is probably unlikely that a stenotic aortic valve could be identified from imaging of the valve itself. Thus the finding of turbulence and increased flow velocity in the ascending aorta may be the best evidence available to suspect the diagnosis. It will be necessary to develop data for normal aortic flow velocity in fetuses during early gestation and criteria for what represents an abnormal velocity.

A major concern in the USA is the fact that currently most ultrasound technicians performing studies of cardiac structure in fetuses have not had adequate training in the identification of cardiovascular abnormalities. There is a relatively high incidence of failure to recognize lesions subsequently shown to be present. Certainly there is a general lack of ability to interpret more sophisticated aspects of Doppler examination of flow patterns in the heart and great vessels. This concern will have to be addressed if earlier diagnoses are to be made.

Several centers around the world are now capable of performing balloon dilation of the aortic valve in the fetus by transabdominal and transuterine insertion of a needle into the fetal left ventricular apex and then passage of a wire and balloon dilation catheter across the aortic valve, but the largest experience has been reported from the Children's Hospital in Boston [18]. Many infants are born with mild, moderate or severe aortic stenosis with left ventricles that may show hypertrophy but which have normal function and no endocardial fibroelastosis. It is not known what factors determine whether a fetus with aortic stenosis will progress to hypoplastic left heart. This is crucial in making the decision whether to attempt balloon dilation of the valve *in utero*. In an attempt to resolve this question, Makikallio *et al.* [16] assessed what circulatory disturbances *in utero* were associated with development of hypoplastic left heart syndrome and found that hypoplasia developed in a high proportion of those with retrograde flow in the transverse aortic arch, left-to-right flow across the foramen ovale, monophasic mitral inflow, and significant left ventricular dysfunction. However, by the time these changes are observed, the majority of fetuses have markedly impaired left venticular function as well as considerable endocardial fibroelastosis. My concern is that if one waits for these advanced changes to occur, the degree of damage sustained by the left ventricle may limit its ability to provide an adequate systemic blood flow after birth. Better criteria need to be developed to decide when therapeutic intervention should be considered.

Another therapeutic procedure that has been considered in the fetus is the relief of a restricted foramen ovale. Restriction of the foramen ovale in the fetus is associated with the development of pulmonary lymphangiectasis and severe pulmonary edema and a high early mortality after birth. The possibility that relief of the obstruction during fetal life could prevent the high mortality after birth has been entertained. However, it is necessary to be able to detect the presence of foramen ovale restriction *in utero*. As discussed above, the pattern of blood flow in pulmonary veins has been shown to be predictive of foramen ovale restriction (p. 262). With restriction, reverse flow during atrial systole is exaggerated and forward flow is progressively reduced. Using techniques similar to those developed for balloon dilation of the aortic valve, a balloon catheter is passed across the foramen ovale and it is dilated to relieve the obstruction. This procedure has been performed successfully in a number of fetuses by the group at the Children's Hospital, Boston. Its effectiveness is yet to be assessed.

When the diagnosis of hypoplastic left heart syndrome is confirmed in a fetus, there are several options that should be presented to the parents, including:

- termination of pregnancy;
- term delivery, but no intervention apart from supportive care;
- plan to proceed with palliative procedure;
- plan for cardiac transplantation.

It is important to inform the parents about such issues as limited availability of hearts for transplantation, the several surgical procedures required for the palliative surgery, and the stress endured by the parents, patient, and siblings. Also, the potential complications and long-term outlook should be discussed. The ensuing discussion is presented on the assumption that the decision has been made to proceed with active intervention.

General considerations

Prior to the early 1980s, although sporadic attempts to palliate infants with aortic atresia were made, it was generally accepted that no effective treatment was available. Norwood *et al.* [43] developed palliative reconstructive surgery consisting of a two-stage approach. In the first procedure, with cardiopulmonary bypass, the main pulmonary artery was transected and anastomosed to the undersurface of the aortic arch. The distal stump of the pulmonary artery was sutured and pulmonary blood flow was provided by a subclavian-to-pulmonary artery anastomosis. The right ventricle thus ejected through the pulmonary artery into the aorta to provide systemic blood flow and it also maintained pulmonary blood flow through the shunt. In the second procedure, performed 2–4 years later, the right atrium was connected to the pulmonary arteries (Fontan procedure) to relieve some of the volume load on the single right ventricle. Although initial results were not very encouraging, modifications in technique and experience have considerably improved the results. Soon after this approach was developed, successful cardiac transplantation was performed in newborn infants with aortic atresia.

Currently, survival after surgery under optimal conditions is comparable. With palliative reconstruction the survival is 65–80% at 1 year and 60–70% at 5 years at various institutions. For infants treated by cardiac transplantation, survival is 75–80% at 1 year and 70–75% at 5 years. Both of these approaches have advantages and disadvantages. Palliative reconstruction is done with the use of native tissues and therefore the use of immunosuppressive therapy with its attendant risks is not necessary. The right ventricle provides systemic blood flow and may not be able to tolerate this load through adult life, so that right ventricular failure may develop. This is particularly prone to develop if tricuspid regurgitation is present. Following the atriopulmonary connection, there is a high incidence of atrial arrhythmias, which may be disabling or life-threatening. Although modifications of the procedure have reduced the incidence of arrhythmias, they are still potentially serious sequelae. The complications of palliative reconstruction are discussed in more detail below. The real advantage of cardiac transplantation is that it provides a heart with two functioning ventricles. The disadvantages of cardiac transplantation are that only few hearts of appropriate size are available for infants and many with aortic atresia have succumbed while awaiting transplantation. In addition, immunosuppressive therapy is required throughout life and this imposes risks such as infection. Also, despite appropriate immunosuppressive therapy, risks of rejection as well as early coronary artery disease must be considered.

The clinical presentation of infants with aortic and mitral atresia is influenced by the presence of severe foramen ovale obstruction and this also determines initial management.

Aortic and mitral atresia with foramen ovale obstruction

The infant with severe cyanosis requires urgent therapy. Concern has been expressed about administration of oxygen because of the perceived risk of causing constriction of the ductus arteriosus. However, when pulmonary blood flow is very low, 100% oxygen will have only a small effect on total oxygen uptake in the lung and arterial blood Po_2 will increase only slightly. This may provide a small increase in oxygen delivery to the tissues (see Chapter 3) but will not have a significant effect on the ductus arteriosus (see Chapter 6). Therefore, if the arterial Po_2 is below about 35 mmHg, oxygen should be administered. Tracheal intubation should be performed and ventilation assisted, particularly if pulmonary edema is present. Hypoglycemia and hypocalcemia should be treated. PGE_1 should be infused intravenously to dilate the ductus arteriosus if it is constricted or to maintain its patency. After having initiated these measures, the most immediate concern is to relieve the foramen ovale obstruction. Two approaches are possible.

1 If palliative surgery is planned and it is possible to perform the procedure without significant delay, immediate surgery could be performed. However, there is an increasing reluctance to subject the infant to extensive surgery before attempting to stabilize the clinical status first; creating an opening in the atrial septum is thus recommended.

2 If surgery has to be delayed for some days or if it is decided to await availability of a heart for transplant, an attempt should be made to create an atrial septal opening as soon as possible. The difficulty in creating an atrial septal opening by balloon or blade septostomy, as well as the possibility of perforating the septum, followed by serial dilatation of the septum are discussed below.

Atrial septostomy

Enlargement of the foramen ovale or creation of an atrial septal opening is indicated if the foramen ovale is restrictive. As mentioned above, this procedure may be required urgently in the immediate newborn period in the infant with severe cyanosis. The technique of balloon atrial septostomy first developed by Rashkind has been very successful in enlarging the foramen ovale in several congenital cardiac lesions, particularly aortopulmonary transposition. Rapid withdrawal of a balloon dilated in the atrium across the atrial septum creates a tear in the inferior margin of the foramen and enlarges the lumen. However, this procedure is often not successful in aortic and mitral atresia for several reasons: the left atrium is often small, so the balloon cannot be inflated adequately; the atrial septum is thick and fibrous, making it difficult or impossible to withdraw the balloon across it; and the septum is tough and will not tear. Blade septostomy, as developed by Park *et al.* [44], has been used to incise the septum prior to attempting to dilate the opening with the balloon, but this has risks because of the small size of the left atrium as well as the thickness of the septum. The technique that has been most successful is the creation of an atrial septal opening by passage of a Brockenbrough needle through a catheter to puncture the septum. More recently, trans-septal puncture of the thick atrial septum has been accomplished by use of radiofrequency perforation of the septum. The opening is then enlarged by serial balloon inflation; because an adequate opening often cannot be maintained, it is becoming common practice to place a trans-septal stent.

Aortic and mitral atresia with adequate foramen ovale

In these infants, the clinical manifestations are a combination of right ventricular failure due to the high volume load, poor systemic circulation resulting from ductus arteriosus constriction, and possibly some degree of pulmonary edema if the foramen ovale is mildly restrictive. Attention should be directed to correction of hypoglycemia and hypocalcemia and consideration should be given to the following measures.

Oxygen administration

It has become an almost routine part of management of an infant in severe respiratory distress to administer high concentrations of oxygen. In the infant with aortic atresia, administration of oxygen could have a possible beneficial effect, but it could also be deleterious. The beneficial effect would be derived from increasing Po_2 in arterial blood, thus providing a greater amount of oxygen for delivery to the tissues, thereby tending to relieve local hypoxia due to decreased blood flow. This potential beneficial effect is limited, because arterial oxygen saturation is already high with the infant breathing room air. A limited increase in arterial oxygen content will be achieved by raising Po_2 from 50–60 mmHg to 100–150 mmHg. Dissolved oxygen would increase by only about 0.4–0.6 mL/dL of blood. This small increase in arterial oxygen content will have only a minor effect on availability of oxygen to the tissues if systemic blood flow is inadequate. The rise in arterial Po_2 associated with oxygen administration could have an adverse effect by constricting the ductus arteriosus, thus further reducing systemic blood flow and oxygen availability even though arterial Po_2 is increased. In addition the fall in systemic arterial pressure could interfere with coronary blood flow to the right ventricle. The high inspired oxygen concentration could also have an adverse effect by reducing pulmonary vascular resistance, thus permitting a further increase in pulmonary blood flow, with accentuation of right ventricular failure. In addition, pulmonary arterial pressure may fall and flow across the ductus arteriosus could be reduced.

Maintaining patency of the ductus arteriosus

Administration of PGE_1

If there is evidence of constriction of the ductus arteriosus, PGE_1 is indicated to dilate the ductus and also to maintain its patency. Arterial pressure should be carefully monitored at the start of the PGE_1 infusion. If necessary, additional fluids may be required to prevent significant hypotension. Although PGE_1 usually increases systemic blood flow and perfusion, it could have deleterious effects. PGE_1 is a peripheral vasodilator and this effect will be particularly prominent if the systemic vascular resistance is high. Even though flow across the ductus may increase, systemic arterial pressure may fall and possibly compromise coronary blood flow. It is therefore important to attempt to limit large decreases in arterial pressure by use of inotropic agents such as dopamine. Potentially, PGE_1 may have an adverse effect by reducing pulmonary vascular resistance, thus diverting blood away from the systemic circulation.

Stenting of the ductus arteriosus

Although PGE_1 has been effective in maintaining ductus patency, the disadvantage is that it is necessary to administer it continuously by intravenous infusion until either palliation or transplant is performed. Several attempts have therefore been made to maintain ductus patency by inserting a stent by peripheral vascular approaches as a palliative procedure while awaiting transplant [45]. Maintaining patency of the dictus arteriosus alone is not adequate to promote survival because, with the decline in pulmonary vascular resistance after birth, blood would flow preferentially into the pulmonary circulation and thus systemic flow and perfusion is not well maintained; in addition, the large volume load from the high pulmonary blood flow may result in right ventricular failure. For this reason, bilateral banding of the pulmonary arteries has been performed surgically to restrict pulmonary blood flow. It is quite difficult to judge the degree of constriction of the pulmonary arteries that should be achieved. If it is too severe, pulmonary flow would be inadequate and cyanosis will develop. If it is inadequate, cardiac failure and poor systemic perfusion will persist. For this reason, attempts have been made to apply adjustable cuffs on the left and right pulmonary arteries at the time of surgery. The degree of constriction can be controlled by inflating or deflating the cuffs by subcutaneous injection or withdrawal of fluid into chambers connected to the cuffs [46]. Although stents have been successfully introduced, the long-term survival has been variable, from a few months to as long as a year [47].

Treatment of cardiac failure

Diuretics should be given after systemic blood flow has been improved by PGE_1, in order to improve pulmonary edema. Digitalis has been used but is not generally recommended because it has not been observed to have a significant effect. Attempts have been made to improve right ventricular function by infusing catecholamines, particularly dobutamine and dopamine. They have been administered as inotropic agents to improve right ventricular function and thus increase systemic blood flow. It is important that these agents be used in relatively low doses, below about 5 μg/kg per min, because larger doses of dopamine may also cause an increase in systemic vascular resistance and thus have a deleterious effect on systemic blood flow and tissue perfusion. Recently, their effectiveness has been questioned.

Increasing pulmonary vascular resistance

It has been suggested that pulmonary vascular resistance be increased either by lowering the concentration of oxygen in inspired gas, or by increasing arterial $P\text{CO}_2$ by hypoventilation or by increasing the CO_2 concentration in inspired gas. The potential benefits of this approach are to reduce pulmonary blood flow and improve right ventricular failure by decreasing the volume load on the right ventricle. Lowering pulmonary blood flow could potentially also improve pulmonary edema if the foramen ovale is somewhat restrictive. In addition, by diverting blood away from the lungs, the flow across the ductus arteriosus could increase, and provide greater systemic blood flow. The suggested concentration of oxygen in inspired air is 15–17%. Arterial blood gases should be monitored repeatedly to ensure that $P\text{O}_2$ is not falling to very low levels and that arterial pH is not decreasing. Hypoventilation is accomplished by mechanical ventilation of the intubated infant. Muscle relaxants are also usually necessary to regulate ventilation to achieve an arterial $P\text{CO}_2$ of about 45–50 mmHg. These measures would be appropriate only in an attempt to stabilize the infant while awaiting surgery for palliation or cardiac transplant. Little information is available regarding their effectiveness, nor how long they can be maintained.

Decreasing systemic vascular resistance

Because blood flow to the systemic and pulmonary circulations depends on the relative resistances, an approach to increasing systemic blood flow has been to reduce systemic vascular resistance by administering systemic vasodilators. The α-adrenoceptor blocker phenoxybenzamine has been used, particularly in the postoperative period after a Norwood procedure [48].

Palliative surgery (Norwood procedure)

As mentioned above, Norwood originally designed a two-stage procedure. The first consisted of connecting the pulmonary artery to the aorta, with provision of pulmonary blood flow through a systemic arterial–pulmonary arterial shunt. In the second stage, the right atrium was connected to the pulmonary artery (Fontan procedure). The second stage was delayed for 2–4 years after the first stage, because it was not well tolerated if done earlier. There were several disadvantages associated with this relatively long delay. If the aortopulmonary shunt did not adapt with growth, marked cyanosis developed. If the shunt was too large, the high pulmonary flow and increased pulmonary arterial pressure imposed the risk of pulmonary vascular disease. An additional concern was that the right ventricle was responsible for providing both pulmonary and systemic blood flow and the risk of failure was considerable. In addition, there is the concern that the excessive load on the ventricle could result in myocardial fibrosis with permanent damage. The approach has now been modified and a three-stage procedure is currently recommended by many centers. This palliative procedure is not recommended if marked tricuspid insufficiency is detected, because when the right ventricle assumes the role of the systemic ventricle, it is subject to a high afterload and this may accentuate the insufficiency, with rapid onset of failure. Some surgeons have attempted to perform tricuspid valvuloplasty at the time of the initial palliation, with variable success. The alternative approach is to schedule a transplantation procedure.

First stage

The main pulmonary artery is divided and the proximal portion is anastomosed to a long segment of the aorta, extending from the ascending aorta along the undersurface of the arch to the descending aorta beyond any coarcted segment. Coarctation, which is frequently present, is also relieved. The distal pulmonary artery segment is sutured. Pulmonary blood flow is provided by a tube graft placed between the aorta and the distal pulmonary artery segment. In this stage the atrial septum is excised to create as large a septal opening as possible. A concern following this procedure is that systemic perfusion during the early postoperative period is often poor. It was postulated that this could be the result of a high diastolic flow from the aorta through the aortopulmonary shunt into the low-resistance pulmonary circulation. A modification was developed by Sano *et al.* [49] to attempt to prevent this runoff, by introducing a conduit from the right ventricle to the pulmonary arteries. It was thought this would provide better systemic perfusion, but although systemic arterial diastolic pressure was higher in the infants who had this procedure, there was no consistent benefit to systemic perfusion or oxygenation [50].

In view of the not infrequent occurrence of cognitive delay in patients with hypoplastic left heart syndrome who have had a Norwood procedure, one hypothesis proposed that the introduction of an aortopulmonary shunt resulted in a decrease in diastolic pressure with compromise of cerebral blood flow. It was thought that a right ventricular to pulmonary arterial conduit may help to avoid the steal of blood flow to the brain. However, infants who had the right ventricular to pulmonary artery conduit procedure have somewhat higher systemic arterial diastolic pressure, but there was no difference in cerebral blood flow or oxygenation [51]. It is perhaps most important to completely relieve obstruction due to coarctation of the aorta in order to provide maximal cerebral flow.

Many infants who have had a Norwood procedure have problems with maintaining systemic blood flow and oxygen delivery in the perioperative period. The tendency was to infuse catecholamines in large amounts in an attempt to increase cardiac output. Recently, however, the concept that systemic perfusion could be improved by reducing systemic vascular resistance has led to the administration of the α-adrenoceptor blocker phenoxybenzamine during surgery and in the early postoperative period. This has considerably improved systemic oxygen delivery [48].

Second stage: bidirectional cavopulmonary anastomosis

The SVC is divided and anastomosed to the distal pulmonary artery segment. This is performed at about 4–6 months of age, but if the aortopulmonary shunt is inadequate and the infant has severe cyanosis, it can be done at 2–3 months. The aortopulmonary shunt or ventricular–pulmonary arterial conduit is obliterated. Various modifications of the procedure have been developed to attempt to facilitate the accomplishment of the third stage.

Third stage: total cavopulmonary connection (modified Fontan procedure)

The IVC is diverted into the pulmonary artery by creating a tunnel with woven material sutured to the atrium, using the right atrial wall as one side of the tube. This is then connected to the pulmonary artery. A 3–4 mm perforation is made in the lateral tunnel to allow decompression of the IVC should pressure increase as a result of relatively high pulmonary vascular resistance. This procedure is now performed at about 18–24 months of age. An alternative approach is to introduce an external conduit, which does not involve the right atrial wall. More recently, the IVC return has been directed so that all or part of hepatic venous blood continues to drain directly into the right atrium. Cavopulmonary anastomoses are discussed in detail in Chapter 15.

Survival and long-term prognosis

Survival after the first stage varies in different centers, but as many as 75–90% of infants may be alive at 1 month. During the early postoperative period, the infant will require assisted ventilation and treatment for cardiac failure with diuretics, digitalis and possibly afterload reducers. The main postoperative concerns are (i) development of severe cyanosis because the aortopulmonary shunt is thrombosed or obstructed at the suture site; (ii) manifestations of aortic coarctation, because the affected segment was not adequately removed; and (iii) onset of severe cardiac failure due to tricuspid regurgitation. Ultrasound studies and, if necessary, cardiac catheterization should be performed to evaluate these problems. If the shunt is inadequate, it may be necessary to introduce an additional shunt, or, beyond about a month, possible earlier cavopulmonary anastomosis could be considered. If residual aortic coarctation is severe, it may be necessary to relieve it surgically in the early postoperative period. If tricuspid regurgitation is severe, annuloplasty can be attempted, but the results have not generally been too successful and mortality is high in these infants.

Prior to proceeding with the second stage, the infant should be evaluated by ultrasound study and cardiac catheterization for the purposes of assessing pulmonary vascular resistance and morphology of the pulmonary arteries to decide if cavopulmonary anastomosis is appropriate and whether pulmonary arteries may require reconstruction because of distortion. Retrograde arterial catheterization with manipulation of the catheter through the shunt provides a measure of pulmonary arterial pressure and, with an estimate of pulmonary blood flow, pulmonary vascular resistance can be calculated. An angiogram in the pulmonary artery or in the aorta proximal to the shunt will demonstrate distortion or stenosis of the pulmonary arteries. In addition, right ventricular performance should be evaluated. A similar evaluation should be performed prior to the third stage of palliation. The pulmonary arteries can be catheterized from an upper extremity vein prior to the third stage. There is growing interest in using ultrasound or magnetic resonance imaging in evaluating infants for the second or third stage, but at present these techniques are not proven to provide reliable information on pulmonary vascular resistance.

The cavopulmonary anastomosis relieves the right ventricle of the need to provide total pulmonary blood flow and thus reduces the volume load on the ventricle. This procedure is usually well tolerated and is attended by a relatively small risk. The practice of staging the diversion of all systemic venous blood into the pulmonary arteries directly has significantly reduced the incidence of postoperative complications as compared with the original Fontan procedure. It has also made it possible to perform the partial diversion by cavopulmonary anastomosis at a considerably younger age with greater success.

The long-term outlook in individuals who have had the staged palliative procedure is yet to be determined. However, several complications have been described within a few years. Atrial arrhythmias are common; although the incidence appears to be less since the traditional Fontan procedure has been modified, sick sinus syndrome and tachyarrhythmias, particularly atrial flutter, are still a significant problem. Systemic venous hypertension may result in protein-losing enteropathy with ascites and peripheral edema 2–5 years after surgery. This is a severely disabling condition that is difficult to treat. If symptoms are severe, it may be necessary to reduce venous pressure by creating an opening between the IVC and right atrium, but this has the disadvantage of causing cyanosis (see Chapter 16 for further discussion).

Another serious concern has been the issue of neurological and intellectual development. Because the child is subjected to complex therapeutic procedures for a prolonged period in early childhood, there is considerable risk of brain damage. The results in reported studies vary considerably. One study showed considerable functional disturbances in neurodevelopmental outcome in school-age children, with learning disability in one-third and developmental retardation in 13%. Other studies in younger children have shown normal intellectual development. It is possible that neurological disturbances were more common in the early experience but that, with improvement in techniques, the outcome has improved.

Following the palliative procedure, the right ventricle continues to function as the systemic ventricle. It is not known whether it will be able to maintain systemic blood flow over a normal lifespan. The frequent association of tricuspid insufficiency places an additional load on the ventricle. There is a significant risk that right ventricular failure will develop, but the time period over which this will occur is not known.

Heart transplantation

Heart transplantation is considered the primary therapy in some centers. Limited availability of donor hearts is a serious problem and 25% or more infants succumb while awaiting transplant. Prostaglandin is administered to maintain patency of the ductus arteriosus until the procedure is performed. An alternative approach, allowing the infant to survive until transplant is feasible, is the so-called hybrid procedure, performed simultaneously by a surgeon and an interventional cardiologist. A stent is placed transthoracically into the ductus arteriosus and banding of the left and right pulmonary arteries is performed. Following surgery, circulatory support with inotropic agents is often required for several days. Immunosuppressive therapy must be administered throughout the life of the patient, and avoidance of infection is a major issue, as is the risk of secondary malignancies. Survival is comparable to that of the palliative procedure, with 1-year survival of about 80% and 5-year survival of 70–75%. The long-term outlook for these patients is yet to be determined. Some information on patients who had transplantation for hypoplastic left heart syndrome 20 years or more ago has indicated the development of coronary artery disease, with the need for repeat transplantation.

References

1 Lev M. Pathologic anatomy and interrelationship of hypoplasia of the aortic tract complex. Lab Invest 1952;1:61–70.

2 Noonan JA, Nadas AS. The hypoplastic left heart syndrome: an analysis of 101 cases. Pediatr Clin North Am 1958;5:1029–1056.

3 Bharati S, Lev M. The surgical anatomy of hypoplasia of aortic tract complex. J Thorac Cardiovasc Surg 1984;88: 97–101.

4 Roberts WC, Perry LW, Chandra RS, Myers GE, Shapiro SR, Scott LP. Aortic valve atresia: a new classification based on necropsy study of 73 cases. Am J Cardiol 1976;37:753–756.

5 Cook AC. The phenotype during fetal develoment. In: Anderson RH, Smith AC, Pizzo M, eds. Hypoplastic Left Heart Syndrome. Singapore: Springer-Verlag, 2005.

6 Sauer U, Gittenberger-de Groot AC, Geishauer M, Babic R, Buhlmeyer K. Coronary arteries in the hypoplastic left heart syndrome. Histopathologic and histometrical studies and implications for surgery. Circulation 1989; 80:I168–I176.

7 Freedom RM, Culham JA, Rowe RD. Aortic atresia with normal left ventricle: distinctive angiocardiographic findings. Cath Cardiovasc Diagn 1977;3:283–295.

8 Cripe L, Andelfinger G, Martin LJ, Shooner K, Benson DW. Bicuspid aortic valve is heritable. J Am Coll Cardiol 2004;44:138–143.

9 Hinton RB Jr, Martin LJ, Tabangin ME, Mazwi ML, Cripe LH, Benson DW. Hypoplastic left heart syndrome is heritable. J Am Coll Cardiol 2007;50:1590–1595.

10 Olson EM. A decade of discoveries in cardiac biology. Nat Med 2004;10:467–474.

11 Harh JY, Paul MH, Gallen WJ, Friedberg DZ, Kaplan S. Experimental production of hypoplastic left heart syndrome in the chick embryo. Am J Cardiol 1973;31:51–56.

12 Schall SA, Dalldorf FG. Premature closure of the foramen ovale and hypoplasia of the left heart. Int J Cardiol 1984;5:103–107.

13 Fishman NH, Hof RB, Rudolph AM. Models of congenital heart disease in fetal lambs. Circulation 1978; 58:354–364.

14 Eghteshady P, Michelfelder E, Altaye M, Ballard E, Hirsh R, Beekman RH III. Revisiting animal models of aortic stenosis in the early gestation fetus. Ann Thorac Surg 2007;83:631–639.

15 Hornberger LK, Sanders SP, Rein AJ, Spevak PJ, Parness IA, Colan SD. Left heart obstructive lesions and left ventricular growth in the midtrimester fetus. A longitudinal study. Circulation 1995;92:1531–1538.

16 Makikallio K, McElhinney DB, Levine JC *et al.* Fetal aortic valve stenosis and the evolution of hypoplastic left heart syndrome: patient selection for fetal intervention. Circulation 2006;113:1401–1405.

17 Maxwell D, Allan L, Tynan MJ. Balloon dilatation of the aortic valve in the fetus: a report of two cases. Br Heart J 1991;65:256–258.

18 Tworetzky W, Wilkins-Haug L, Jennings RW *et al.* Balloon dilation of severe aortic stenosis in the fetus: potential for prevention of hypoplastic left heart syndrome. Candidate selection, technique, and results of successful intervention. Circulation 2004;110:2125–2131.

19 Axt-Fliedner R, Kreiselmaier P, Schwarze A, Krapp M, Gembruch U. Development of hypoplastic left heart syndrome after diagnosis of aortic stenosis in the first trimester by early echocardiography. Ultrasound Obstet Gynecol 2006;28:106–109.

20 Sharland GK, Chita SK, Fagg NL *et al.* Left ventricular dysfunction in the fetus: relation to aortic valve anomalies and endocardial fibroelastosis. Br Heart J 1991; 66:419–424.

21 Ursell PC, Neill CA, Anderson RH, Ho SY, Becker AE, Gerlis LM. Endocardial fibroelastosis and hypoplasia of the left ventricle in neonates without significant aortic stenosis. Br Heart J 1984;51:492–497.

22 Kuehl KS, Loffredo CA. A cluster of hypoplastic left heart malformation in Baltimore, Maryland. Pediatr Cardiol 2006;27:25–31.

23 Better DJ, Apfel HD, Zidere V, Allan LD. Pattern of pulmonary venous blood flow in the hypoplastic left heart syndrome in the fetus. Heart 1999;81:646–649.

24 Taketazu M, Barrea C, Smallhorn JF, Wilson GJ, Hornberger LK. Intrauterine pulmonary venous flow and restrictive foramen ovale in fetal hypoplastic left heart syndrome. J Am Coll Cardiol 2004;43:1902–1907.

25 Hutchins GM. Coarctation of the aorta explained as a branch-point of the ductus arteriosus. Am J Pathol 1971;63:203–214.

26 Leake RD, Strimling B, Emmanouilides GC. Intrauterine cardiac failure with hydrops fetalis. Case report in a twin

with the hypoplastic left heart syndrome and review of the literature. Clin Pediatr 1973;12:649–651.

27 Sahn DJ, Shenker L, Reed KL, Sobonya R, Anderson R. Prenatal ultrasound diagnosis of hypoplastic left heart syndrome in utero associated wth hydrops fetalis. Am Heart J 1982;104:1368–1372.

28 Schmider A, Henrich W, Dähnert I, Dudenhausen JW. Prenatal therapy of non-immunologic hydrops fetalis caused by severe aortic stenosis. Ultrasound Obstet Gynecol 2000;16:275–278.

29 Mahle WT, Clancy RR, Moss EM, Gerdes M, Jobes DR, Wernovsky G. Neurodevelopmental outcome and lifestyle assessment in school-aged and adolescent children with hypoplastic left heart syndrome. Pediatrics 2000;105: 1082–1089.

30 Ikle L, Hale K, Fashaw L, Boucek M, Rosenberg AA. Developmental outcome of patients with hypoplastic left heart syndrome treated with heart transplantation. J Pediatr 2003;142:20–25.

31 Yang SS, Chen YC, Brough AJ, Bernstein J. Correlation of head circumference and crown-rump length in newborn infants. A potential indicator of congenital maldevelopment. Biol Neonate 1975;27:308–317.

32 Rosenthal GL. Patterns of prenatal growth among infants with cardiovascular malformations: possible fetal hemodynamic effects. Am J Epidemiol 1996;143:505–513.

33 Manzar S, Nair A, Pai MG, Al-Khusaiby SM. Head size at birth in neonates with transposition of great arteries and hypoplastic left heart syndrome. Saudi Med J 2005; 26:453–456.

34 Donofrio MT, Bremer YA, Schieken RM *et al.* Autoregulation of cerebral blood flow in fetuses with congenital heart disease: the brain sparing effect. Pediatr Cardiol 2003;24:436–443.

35 Kaltman JR, Di H, Tian Z, Rychik J. Impact of congenital heart disease on cerebrovascular blood flow dynamics in the fetus. Ultrasound Obstet Gynecol 2005;25:32–36.

36 Papile L, Rudolph AM, Heymann MA. Autoregulation of cerebral blood flow in the preterm fetal lamb. Pediatr Res 1985;19:159–161.

37 Hinton RB, Andelfinger G, Sekar P, Hinton AC, Gendron RL, Michelfelder EC, Robitaille Y, Benson DW. Prenatal head growth and white matter injury in hypoplastic left heart syndrome. Pediatr Res 2008;64:364–369.

38 Rychik J, Rome JJ, Collins MH, DeCampli WM, Spray TL. The hypoplastic left heart syndrome with intact atrial septum: atrial morphology, pulmonary vascular histopathology and outcome. J Am Coll Cardiol 1999;34: 554–560.

39 Maeda K, Yamaki S, Kado H, Asou T, Murakami A, Takamoto S. Hypoplasia of the small pulmonary arteries in hypoplastic left heart syndrome with restrictive atrial septal defect. Circulation 2004;110(suppl 1):139–146.

40 Glatz JA, Tabbutt S, Gaynor JM *et al.* Hypoplastic left heart syndrome with atrial level restriction in the era of prenatal diagnosis. Ann Thorac Surg 2007;84:1633–1638.

41 Rychik J, Gullquist SD, Jacobs ML, Norwood WI. Doppler echocardiographic analysis of flow in the ductus arteriosus of infants with hypoplastic left heart syndrome: relationship of flow patterns to systemic oxygenation and size of interatrial communication. J Am Soc Echocardiogr 1996;9:166–173.

42 Shillingford AJ, Ittenbach RF, Marino BS *et al.* Aortic morphometry and microcephaly in hypoplastic left heart syndrome. Cardiol Young 2007;17:189–195.

43 Norwood WI, Lang P, Casteneda AR, Campbell DN. Experience with operations for hypoplastic left heart syndrome. J Thorac Cardiovasc Surg 1981;82:511–519.

44 Park SC, Zuberbuhler JR, Neches WH, Lenox CC, Zoltun RA. A new atrial septostomy technique. Cathet Cardiovasc Diagn 1975;1:195–201.

45 Ruiz CE, Gamra H, Zhang HP, García EJ, Boucek MM. Brief report: stenting of the ductus arteriosus as a bridge to cardiac transplantation in infants with the hypoplastic left-heart syndrome. N Engl J Med 1993;328:1605–1608.

46 Assad RS, Zamith MM, Silva MF *et al.* A novel adjustable pulmonary artery banding system for hypoplastic left heart syndrome. Ann Thorac Surg 2007;84:2081–2084.

47 Michel-Behnke I, Akintuerk H, Marquardt I *et al.* Stenting of the ductus arteriosus and banding of the pulmonary arteries: basis for various surgical strategies in newborns with multiple left heart obstructive lesions. Heart 2003;89:645–650.

48 Hoffman GM, Tweddell JS, Ghanayem NS *et al.* Alteration of the critical arteriovenous oxygen saturation relationship by sustained afterload reduction after the Norwood procedure. J Thorac Cardiovasc Surg 2004; 127:738–745.

49 Sano S, Ishino K, Kawada M *et al.* Right ventricle–pulmonary artery shunt in first-stage palliation of hypoplastic left heart syndrome. J Thorac Cardiovasc Surg 2003;126:504–509.

50 Ghanayem NS, Jaquiss RD, Cava JR *et al.* Right ventricle-to-pulmonary artery conduit versus Blalock–Taussig shunt: a hemodynamic comparison. Ann Thorac Surg 2006;82:1603–1609.

51 Kussman BD, Gauvreau K, DiNardo JA *et al.* Cerebral perfusion and oxygenation after the Norwood procedure: comparison of right ventricle-pulmonary artery conduit with modified Blalock–Taussig shunt. J Thorac Cardiovasc Surg 2007;133:648–655.

12

CHAPTER 12
Aortic arch obstruction

Lesions of the aortic arch or proximal portion of the descendyng aorta are common and account for about 5–8% of congenital disorders of the heart and great vessels. The term *coarctation of the aorta* indicates that the aortic lumen is narrowed, whereas *interruption of the aortic arch* implies a complete occlusion or absence of a segment of the aortic arch. Although these two conditions are discussed in this chapter, there is increasing evidence that the mechanisms responsible for these anomalies may differ.

In some of the earlier descriptions of coarctation of the aorta, the lesions were classified as the infantile type of coarctation, which it was thought usually produced severe symptoms in infancy, and the adult type, which usually produced symptoms in older children or adults. The infantile type of coarctation, also known as tubular hypoplasia of the aorta, or preductal coarctation was characterized by diffuse narrowing of the aorta proximal to the ductus arteriosus. Because the ductus arteriosus is patent during infancy and blood may flow from the right ventricle and pulmonary artery to the descending aorta, the term "coarctation of the aorta with systemic right ventricle" was used to describe this anomaly. The adult type of coarctation was defined as a localized narrowing of the aorta at the junction of the ductus arteriosus or ligamentum arteriosum with the aorta. In older individuals there is usually a circumferential narrowing that often produces a greater degree of obstruction of the lumen than is suggested by the external appearance.

The classification of coarctation of the aorta into infantile and adult types is no longer acceptable, because infants with localized aortic narrowing in the region of the ductus arteriosus may develop severe cardiac failure in the newborn period.

Congenital Diseases of the Heart, 3rd edition. By A. Rudolph

Morphological considerations

The ascending aorta arches to the right and the transverse aorta gives rise to the innominate, left carotid and left subclavian arteries and is then directed caudally. In the adult, the diameter of the aorta beyond the origin of the innominate artery decreases only slightly and the cross-sectional area of the upper portion of the descending aorta is about 0.95 of that between the left subclavian artery and the site of attachment of the ligamentum arteriosus. However, in the newborn infant and term fetus, the diameter of the descending aorta is reported to be about 1.5 that of the aorta between the left subclavian artery and the ductus arteriosus [1]. In a study of aortic dimensions by both echocardiography and measurement in aborted fetuses, the ratio of the diameter of the aortic isthmus to that of the ascending aorta was 0.6–0.7 [2]. Based on these reports, the cross-sectional area of this portion of the aorta, termed the aortic isthmus, is only about 0.5 that of the descending aorta. This marked narrowing of the isthmus in the normal fetus and neonate has been explained on the basis of the patterns of blood flow in the fetus. A more recent echocardiographic study found that the ratio of the isthmus to ascending aortic diameter in human fetuses at 16–38 weeks' gestation was 0.81 [3], so that the cross-sectional area of the isthmus was about two-thirds that of the ascending aorta. In five fetuses in whom coarctation of the aorta was confirmed postnatally, the isthmus diameter was below the third percentile for gestational age.

In the normal fetal lamb in late gestation, the right ventricle ejects about 66% of combined ventricular output (CVO); 8–10% of CVO perfuses the lungs and 56–58% passes through the ductus arteriosus to the descending aorta. The left ventricle ejects only 33% of CVO. About 3–5% goes to the coronary circulation, the remaining 28–30% passing into the ascending aorta. About 20% of CVO is distributed to the head, neck and upper extremities, so that only about 10% crosses the aortic isthmus to the descending aorta (see Figure 1.6), which carries about 66% of CVO. The diameters of the vessels reflect the magnitude of the flows through them. The pulmonary trunk and the descending aorta are very large, the ductus arteriosus slightly less so, and the ascending aorta is smaller than the descending aorta, but the isthmus is narrow, with a cross-sectional area only about half that of the descending aorta. The amounts of blood flowing through the large arteries in the human fetus have not been measured precisely. Blood flow into the ascending aorta is considerably larger in the human compared with the sheep fetus and pulmonary blood flow is also greater (see Table 1.3). However, it is recognized that the volume flowing across the aortic isthmus is also quite low, and probably only about 8% of CVO. The diffuse narrowing of arch and isthmus of the aorta has been referred to as "fetal coarctation" and "tubular hypoplasia of the aorta." However, it is important to appreciate that this portion of the aorta is normally narrowed in the fetus and neonate.

The influence of blood flow on development is apparent from examination of the aortic arch and the ductus arteriosus in several congenital cardiac anomalies, in which blood flow patterns can be assumed. In the fetus with a lesion where the right ventricle ejects little or no blood, the left ventricle ejects the total CVO into the ascending aorta. Lesions that produce this type of flow pattern include pulmonary atresia (see Figure 15.1) and tricuspid atresia with normal origin of the aorta and pulmonary artery (see Figure 16.1). In these lesions, of the 100% of CVO that enters the ascending aorta, a small percentage is distributed to the coronary circulation and, in the human fetus, probably about 30–35% supplies the upper body including the brain. The remaining 65–70%, which includes blood to be distributed through the ductus arteriosus to the lungs, passes across the aortic isthmus. In infants with these anomalies, the ascending aorta is larger than normal, the isthmus at least as wide as the descending aorta, and the ductus arteriosus seems to be quite narrow.

Narrowing of the arch of the aorta and of the aortic isthmus is frequently associated with several congenital cardiac anomalies. A feature common to all these lesions is the likelihood that, in the fetus, blood flow into the ascending aorta is reduced by the abnormal intracardiac morphology. The ascending aorta may or may not be narrowed. The diameter of the arch just beyond the origin of the innominate artery is progressively narrowed to the isthmus at the junction with the ductus arteriosus. This represents a degree of narrowing greater than that in the normal fetal aorta. The lesions with which tubular hypoplasia is associated include:

- ventricular septal defect with deviation of the outlet septum causing narrowing of the left ventricular outflow tract;
- atrioventricular septal defect with narrowing of the left ventricular outflow tract;
- tricuspid atresia with aortopulmonary transposition with the aorta arising from a small right ventricle;
- double-outlet right ventricle of the Taussig–Bing type, with narrowing of the subaortic region;
- aortopulmonary transposition with ventricular septal defect and septal deviation to the right, causing narrowing of the subaortic region.

Unfortunately, no reliable information is currently available regarding the degree of narrowing that is hemodynamically significant. In many of these individuals, although the aorta is narrower than normal, after correction of the intracardiac defect there is no evidence of aortic obstruction and the aorta develops normally. In others, clinical manifestations of aortic arch obstruction do develop. The length as well as the degree of narrowing is probably important in determining the severity of obstruction. Coarctation of the aorta or interruption of the aortic arch may also be associated with any of the lesions mentioned.

This lesion is characterized morphologically by a localized intraluminal projection of a shelf from the lateral, posterior, and sometimes anterior wall of the aorta in the region of the ductus arteriosus. The aortic wall may be indented at the site of the shelf projection, but the luminal narrowing is more severe than is apparent from the indentation viewed from the exterior surface. The shelf has been

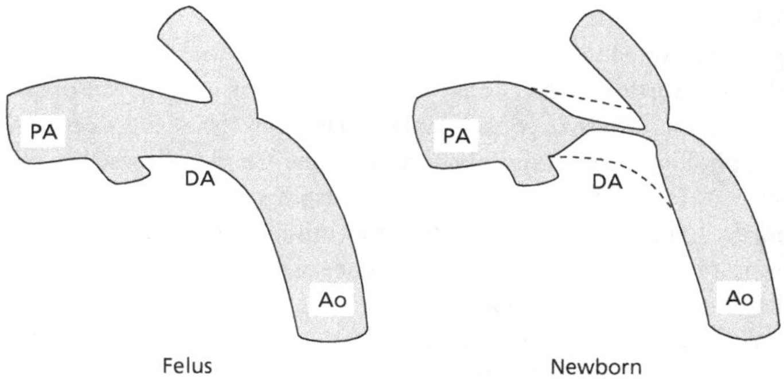

Figure 12.1 Diagram showing the absence of significant aortic obstruction in the presence of a posterior shelf while the ductus arteriosus (DA) is widely patent. Constriction of the ductus results in aortic obstruction becoming manifest. Ao, aorta; PA, pulmonary artery.

observed in the human fetus, but no significant obstruction of the aorta is evident, because the lumen of the patent ductus arteriosus allows flow around the shelf. In the newborn infant, the aortic isthmus is often also narrow; it appears as if the aortic isthmus is attached to the side of the large artery comprised of the ductus arteriosus continuing into the descending aorta (Figure 12.1). The shelf thus appears to be located toward the superior end of the lumen of the ductus arteriosus. This has been referred to, erroneously I believe, as a preductal coarctation. When the ductus arteriosus closes, the shelf is positioned opposite the attachment of the ligamentum arteriosum; after the isthmus has enlarged, the constriction moves somewhat more distally. The location of the shelf is best described as being opposite the ductus arteriosus and the term "juxtaductal coarctation" describes this localized narrowing of the aorta. Normally the aortic wall largely comprises many layers of elastic lamellae, whereas the wall of the ductus arteriosus has a well-developed smooth muscle layer. Ductus tissue extends a short distance onto the wall of the aorta at the site of connection. In the newborn infant with coarctation, the shelf comprises an infolding of the aortic wall in some, but in others there is swelling between the elastic fibers. Ductus arteriosus tissue is usually observed in the shelf and, in addition, there is extension of ductus tissue into the aortic wall to involve about half to almost the total circumference of the aorta. In older individuals, there is also thickening of the intima, which exaggerates the obstruction.

With advancing postnatal age, the aortic constriction appears to be more circumferential and the aortic isthmus tends to dilate. Frequently the aorta beyond the coarctation is dilated due to poststenotic dilatation. Collateral circulation between carotid and subclavian arteries and the descending aorta develops postnatally. The vertebral, transcervical, scapular, internal mammary, and intercostal arteries are all enlarged. The collateral circulation is not developed at the time of birth, because the aorta is not obstructed *in utero*. Within a few months after birth, collateral vessels begin to become evident and their subsequent enlargement depends on the severity of the coarctation.

Coarctation of the aorta is frequently associated with other cardiac lesions. The lesions mentioned above in which tubular hypoplasia occurs may also be associated with coarctation; tubular hypoplasia and coarctation may occur in the same individual. About 75–80% of infants with aortic atresia have associated coarctation; the coarctation is at the junction of the aortic isthmus and the ductus arteriosus and creates an obstruction to flow into the aortic arch and its branches and into the ascending aorta (see Chapter 11). Many patients with aortic coarctation have various degrees of mitral valve involvement, ranging from minor anomalies to moderate stenosis. Severe narrowing of the mitral orifice due to a supravalvar stenosing ring, papillary muscle abnormalities, parachute mitral valve, and subvalvar aortic stenosis may be associated with coarctation of the aorta as the Shone complex. Ventricular septal defects are not infrequently associated with coarctation of the aorta. They are most commonly trabecular or muscular, or perimembranous in location. A bicuspid aortic valve is frequently associated with coarctation of the aorta, but the reported incidence varies widely, from about 30 to 80%. It is generally thought that about

50% of individuals with coarctation have bicuspid aortic valves. However, of all individuals who have bicuspid aortic valves, only about 5–8% have aortic coarctation. There is considerable variation in the morphology of bicuspid aortic valves (see Chapter 10). In most individuals with bicuspid valve, aortic stenosis is either insignificant or mild. However, moderate or severe aortic stenosis may be associated with coarctation.

Although juxtaductal coarctation is usually distal to the origin of the left subclavian artery, occasionally the orifice of the subclavian artery is involved in the coarctation and is partially obstructed. An anomalous origin of the right subclavian artery from the descending aorta below the coarcted segment is also occasionally encountered. These abnormal subclavian arteries are important in clinical diagnosis (see Chapter 12). Juxtaductal coarctation of the aorta is commonly associated with Turner syndrome, being present in about 15% of these individuals. Aneurysms of the circle of Willis, so-called berry aneurysms, are thought to occur in about 10% of individuals with coarctation of the aorta, but their true incidence is not known reliably. They are rarely noted in infants and young children and appear to occur in adult life and to be associated with longstanding hypertension. It is proposed that there is an underlying degenerative change in the media (see below).

Interruption of the aortic arch

Complete interruption of the lumen of the aorta occurs at three sites in the arch. Celoria and Patton [4] have suggested the following classification.

- Type A: interruption between the left subclavian artery and the ductus arteriosus, i.e., interruption of the isthmus.
- Type B: interruption between the left subclavian and left common carotid arteries.
- Type C: interruption between the left common carotid and the innominate arteries.

The incidence of type C is low, constituting less than 5% of all patients. The occurrence of types B and A varies in different series: type B is most common, with an incidence of about 60–80% of all individuals with interruption; type A is found in about 20–35%.

Almost all individuals with aortic arch interruption have associated lesions; a patent ductus arteriosus is almost always present and most have a ventricular septal defect. Rarely the interruption may be observed in an older child or adult in whom the ductus arteriosus is closed; perfusion of the lower body has been achieved by development of an extensive collateral arterial circulation. In individuals with type B interruption, 85–90% have an associated ventricular septal defect and most of these defects are characterized by maldevelopment of the outflow region with malalignment of the infundibular septum that creates narrowing of the left ventricular outflow. Other lesions that may be associated with arch interruption are those associated with tubular hypoplasia, namely Taussig–Bing anomaly, tricuspid atresia with aortopulmonary transposition and ventricular septal defect, and atrioventricular septal defect with subaortic narrowing. Interruption in this group of lesions is usually type B. Interrupted arch is also encountered in patients with truncus arteriosus and with aortopulmonary septal defect. Aortopulmonary septal defect is usually associated with type A interruption. Berry syndrome is a rare combination of interrupted arch, aortopulmonary septal defect, intact ventricular septum, and origin of the right pulmonary artery from the ascending aorta.

Embryological considerations

The causes of coarctation and interruption of the aorta are not known but two mechanisms have been considered: (i) the lesion is primarily due to a disturbance in embryological development; and (ii) the abnormality is secondary to a disturbance in blood flow patterns.

Coarctation of the aorta

Two hypotheses have been proposed relating to possible abnormalities in embryological development. The first, proposed by Craigie and later Skoda, postulates that there is abnormal extension of the ductus arteriosus into the aortic wall and that the factors responsible for closure of the ductus arteriosus after birth constrict the ductus tissue in the aorta and result in coarctation. This is supported by the histological demonstration of extension of ductus arteriosus tissue into about half the circumference of the aortic wall, and sometimes the whole circumference. Ductus tissue is also usually observed in the shelf projecting into the aortic lumen. Furthermore, the aortic obstruction is not usually evident *in utero* by ultrasound examination, but develops after birth when the ductus arteriosus closes. One problem with this hypothesis is that the posterolateral shelf has been demonstrated to be present in fetuses in whom the ductus arteriosus is widely patent, with no evidence of constriction. It is also difficult to explain why the initial obstruction in the aorta is opposite the ductus arteriosus. In those individuals in whom ductus tissue extends into less than the full circumference of the aorta, it would be expected that the constriction of ductus tissue would cause an indentation where the ductus connects with the aorta, rather than on the opposite wall. It is also not necessary to invoke contraction of ductus tissue in the aortic wall to explain the development of coarctation after birth when the ductus closes. We showed that this phenomenon could be related to a simple physical effect of ductus constriction on the aortic lumen when a shelf is present. We simulated a posterolateral aortic shelf opposite the ductus arteriosus by surgically indenting the aorta in late-gestation fetal lambs. In the fetus and during the immediate postnatal period, no pressure difference was detected between the ascending and descending aorta. However, when the ductus arteriosus was constricted by administration of 100% oxygen or by infusing acetylcholine, a pressure gradient developed, indicating the induction of aortic narrowing. The coarctation was demonstrated by injecting silicone rubber into the aorta at autopsy; the cast showed that constriction of the ductus had narrowed the aorta at the site of indentation [5]. The effect of ductus constriction is shown diagrammatically in Figure 12.1. However, these studies do not exclude the possibility that extension of ductus tissue into the aortic wall may play some role in the production of localized aortic coarctation.

The second developmental anomaly that has been proposed as a possible cause of coarctation is related to migration of the left seventh intersegmental artery that forms the left subclavian artery. Normally, in early embryogenesis, this artery arises from the descending aorta distal to the junction with the ductus arteriosus. Over the course of development the subclavian artery migrates cranially so that its origin is proximal to the ductus attachment and the portion of aorta between the subclavian artery and the ductus arteriosus forms the isthmus. The left subclavian artery is abnormal in more than half of individuals with juxtaductal coarctation. As mentioned above, it may be involved in the coarctation and be partly obstructed, or it may arise immediately proximal to the ductus. It has been proposed that this suggests that the disturbances of subclavian artery migration may cause aortic coarctation. There is no evidence to support this hypothesis. It is equally possible that some other factor is responsible for causing the coarctation as well as the disturbance in migration. Also presence of coarctation with a shelf projecting from the wall of the aorta could be the primary lesion and it could interfere with migration of the artery.

A focal obstruction has been described in the zebrafish that is thought to resemble aortic coarctation. It is located where the two anterior dorsal aortae join to form a single midline aorta [6]. The recessive mutant in which this anomaly occurs has been called the *gridlock* (*grl*) mutant. This lesion differs from coarctation of the aorta in that it arises early in embryological development and is thought to be related to abnormalities in endothelial rearrangement to form tubular blood vessels. It is associated with development of shunts or collateral circulation to bypass the obstruction. However, description of this mutant does raise the possibility that the abnormal shelf in coarctation is related to early embryonic disturbance of vessel formation.

The possible role of alteration of blood flow patterns in causing coarctation of the aorta has been discussed above. The decrease in flow across the arch could possibly explain the development of tubular hypoplasia and even aortic arch interruption, but does not by itself explain the development of the aortic shelf and juxtaductal coarctation. The hypothesis has been proposed by Hutchins [7] that the site at which the aortic isthmus joins the ductus arteriosus acts as a branch-point. Normally, the predominant flow pattern is that of blood passing from the ductus to the descending aorta, so that the ductus and descending aorta behave as a continuous channel and the isthmus appears to be a branch entering the side of this channel (Figure 12.1). If flow through the ductus arteriosus is increased and that through the isthmus decreased, the point at the posterolateral junction of the two arteries will become exaggerated and could thus form the shelf characteristic of coarctation. The development of the shelf at this branch-point would, Hutchins hypothesized, be very prone to develop if there were retrograde flow in the isthmus. This proposal is strongly supported by the very frequent association of juxtaductal coarctation with aortic atresia. In this condition the total CVO is ejected into the pulmonary trunk and, apart from that distributed to the lungs, it all passes through the ductus arteriosus. Blood is supplied to the head and neck vessels by retrograde flow of blood through the isthmus into the arch. The possibility that altered flow patterns could also affect growth of the ductus arteriosus and stimulate extension of ductus tissue into the aortic wall should be entertained, but there is no evidence to support or negate this concept.

Bicuspid aortic valve is observed in about 50% of individuals with coarctation of the aorta. It has been proposed that bicuspid valve may interfere with left ventricular output in the fetus, thereby limiting flow across the aortic isthmus and resulting in coarctation. Although this is an appealing concept, there is no evidence to indicate that a bicuspid valve is obstructive in the fetus and that left ventricular output is restricted. The effects of bicuspid aortic valves on flow patterns should be studied further in fetuses by ultrasound examination.

Coarctation of the aorta is rarely encountered in individuals with severe pulmonary stenosis or atresia. This can be explained by the fact that flow into the pulmonary artery is reduced or absent during fetal life. Blood flow through the ductus arteriosus from the pulmonary artery to the aorta is markedly reduced or flow from the aorta to pulmonary artery may occur. Thus the hemodynamic characteristics that would favor the development of a juxtaductal aortic shelf, namely high flow through the ductus and low flow through the isthmus, do not occur with right ventricular outflow obstruction. Aortic coarctation is rarely associated with right aortic arch. When the right arch is a mirror image of the normal arch in terms of the origin of the great vessels, the common association of obstructive lesions of the right ventricular outflow explains the rarity of coarctation. In individuals who do not have right ventricular outflow obstruction, the ductus arteriosus usually connects with the left innominate artery rather than below the isthmus region. Flow from the pulmonary artery would not produce the same hemodynamic effect as with the normal arrangement and thus coarctation is rare. The mechanism responsible for coarctation in these individuals is not known.

Finally, in studies of the hereditability of hypoplastic left heart syndrome, a close relationship was observed between the occurrence of aortic atresia, bicuspid aortic valve, and aortic coarctation. This suggested a genetic relationship between these conditions. Mutations of the *NOTCH* gene have been implicated as a possible factor common to these lesions (see Chapter 11).

Aortic arch interruption

This anomaly is thought to be due to abnormal development of the branchial arterial system. A brief description of this system is provided as a basis for understanding the morphological types of interruption. In the embryo, this system comprises the aortic sac, six arterial arches that evolve at different times, and the paired dorsal aortae. Intersegmental arteries arise from the dorsal aorta and are distributed to the somites. During development various segments of these structures either regress or form portions of the vascular system. The first and second arches regress, but may remain as portions of arteries in the head and neck, such as mandibular or hyoid arteries. The third arches form the common carotid and portions of the internal carotid arteries. The segments of the dorsal aortae between the third and fourth arches on both left and right sides regress. The fifth arches do not appear to be important contributors to permanent vascular structures in humans. The sixth arches contribute to the main pulmonary artery; the right arch forms the right pulmonary artery and the left arch persists as the left pulmonary artery and the ductus arteriosus. On the left side, the fourth arch persists to form the arch of the aorta. On the right side, the dorsal aorta regresses beyond the origin of the fourth arch. Persistence of the third arch instead of the fourth arch on the left probably explains the cervical aortic arch. Regression of the left dorsal aorta between the third and forth aortic arches could explain the presence of right aortic arch. The first six intersegmental arteries do not appear to make significant permanent contributions but may be important in forming the vertebral arteries. The right seventh intersegmental artery forms the distal portion of the right subclavian artery; the proximal portion is derived from the right fourth arch. On the left, the seventh intersegmental artery persists as the left subclavian artery. The aortic arch may be considered to develop from the following components. The ascending aorta and the segment up to the left common carotid artery is derived from the ventral aortic sac. The left fourth arch contributes the portion between the left common carotid artery and the ductus arteriosus, and the dorsal aorta provides that part between the ductus arteriosus and the left seventh intersegmental or subclavian artery. As mentioned on p. 293, this intersegmental artery migrates cranially so that the final position of the left subclavian artery is between the left common carotid artery and the ductus arteriosus.

The hypothesis that interruption of the aortic arch may result from alterations in blood flow patterns during intrauterine development is based on the fact that many intracardiac anomalies are associated with arch interruption (see Chapter 12). The feature common to many of these lesions is the presence of various degrees of obstruction to outflow into the ascending aorta, which may restrict blood flow into the aorta and result in hypoplasia or, if extreme, interruption. In some anomalies, obstructive lesions may not be demonstrable, but other possible reasons for reduced flow across the arch can be surmised. In the fetus with atrioventricular septal defect, mitral insufficiency with shunting to the right atrium through the atrial septal defect may limit ejection from the left ventricle into the aorta and increase pulmonary blood flow. In fetuses with aortopulmonary defects or truncus arteriosus communis, blood in the ascending aorta may flow preferentially through the ductus arteriosus and flow across the arch would be restricted. These lesions are all associated with aortic arch interruption. The concept that restriction of flow in the ascending aorta and arch may result in interruption has received some support from experimental studies in chick embryos, in which it was shown that constriction of the conotruncus frequently resulted in the development of arch interruption.

However, it is difficult to explain the different types of interruption on the basis of this single concept. Type A interruption would result from failure of formation or atresia of the dorsal aorta between the left carotid artery and the ductus arteriosus. It would have to develop after the migration of the intersegmental artery proximal to the ductus arteriosus, because of the location in the aortic isthmus between the left subclavian artery and the ductus arteriosus. One might conjecture that lack of development or atresia of the dorsal aorta segment is not the likely explanation for type A interruption, because the left subclavian artery could not then have migrated proximal to the ductus. Type A interruption therefore appears to have its origin rather late in embryogenesis and is more compatible with the flow theory than the other types. Another possible explanation for type A interruption is that the aorta is somehow constricted in the migration of the subclavian artery to its final position. This concept is based on the fact that the left subclavian artery is frequently involved in the obstruction and is narrowed at its origin or is hypoplastic.

Type B interruption, between the left common carotid and subclavian arteries, must be the result of failure of formation or regression of the left fourth arch or the dorsal aorta between the fourth and sixth arch, or both. Type C interruption, between the innominate and left common carotid arteries, could be the result of atresia of the connection between the aortic sinus and the left third and fourth arches. It is difficult to explain A and B types of interruption on the basis of reduced flow into the ascending aorta. Even if total ascending aortic flow were reduced, it would be expected that flow to the brain through both carotid arteries would be maintained, so that the arch, at least up to the site beyond the left common carotid origin, should develop.

The frequent association of DiGeorge syndrome with aortic arch interruption has led to the view that genetic factors may play a role. In DiGeorge syndrome, immunological disturbances and parathyroid deficiency suggest that maldevelopment of the third and fourth branchial arches is involved. Cardiac defects such as truncus arteriosus communis are commonly associated with DiGeorge syndrome; about one-third of these individuals have aortic arch interruption. Also about two-thirds of infants with aortic arch interruption have been noted to have DiGeorge syndrome. Shprintzen (velocardiofacial) syndrome is also recognized to be associated with conotruncal abnormalities, as well as aortic arch anomalies. In recent years, it has been recognized that DiGeorge and Shprintzen syndromes are related and both are frequently associated with a chromosomal deletion in 22q11. Studies in patients with aortic arch interruption have shown a high incidence of 22q11 deletions, ranging from 50 to 90%. The majority of these individuals have type B interruption and they frequently also have conotruncal anomalies or ventricular septal defect with infundibular septal deviation causing left ventricular outflow obstruction. The association of type A interruption with 22q11 deletions is much less frequent; there are fewer reports but some report no relationship, whereas others report a low incidence of deletions in type A. The relationship of type C interruption to 22q11 deletions has not, as yet, been reported. The mechanisms by which 22q11 deletions result in the cardiac and arch defects are not known. However, it has been proposed that the deletion affects neural crest cells. These cells migrate to the heart and to the arch and are thought to contribute to the development of the fourth aortic arch and to the conotruncus. This could explain the frequent association between conotruncal lesions and interrupted aortic arch, as well as the concept that type A interruption may be associated with reduced blood flow whereas type B interruption is related to abnormal migration of neural crest tissue.

These observations suggest that there are possible differences in the etiological factors involved in the development of type A and B interruption. Type B appears to be related to a primary developmental defect, whereas type A could be explained by disturbances in flow. However, intracardiac defects are associated with both types of interruption. Although it has generally been proposed that the cardiac defect may alter flow patterns in such a way as to contribute to aortic obstruction, the possibility should be considered that the arch abnormality could be the primary defect and that disturbances in flow may result in the intracardiac anomalies. This concept is supported by experimental observations in chick embryos, where constriction of the left sixth aortic arch resulted in intracardiac abnormalities. As mentioned above, it is possible that genetic disturbances could account for both the intracardiac and aortic arch anomalies.

Aortic arch interruption is rarely encountered in patients with right aortic arch. In all the individuals in which the association has occurred the interruption was type B, and DiGeorge syndrome or 22q11 deletion has also been present. Thus it appears that if interruption of the arch is associated with right aortic arch, it is genetically determined and not related to disturbed flow patterns.

Hemodynamic considerations

Fetal circulation

Coarctation of the aorta

Many of the alterations in fetal hemodynamics are related to the intracardiac defects associated with tubular hypoplasia of the aorta. The features common to all these lesions are reduction in flow into the ascending aorta, increased flow into the pulmonary trunk, and greater proportion of CVO carried across the ductus arteriosus to the descending aorta. The presence of the posterolateral shelf can be recognized, but this does not cause obstruction between the ascending and descending aorta during fetal life (Figure 12.2). In the fetus with aortic atresia, blood from the ductus arteriosus is distributed below the shelf to the descending aorta. The aorta is narrowed where the isthmus joins the ductus arteriosus so that there may be varying degrees of obstruction to flow from the ductus arteriosus and descending aorta into the transverse arch and ascending aorta (see Chapter 11).

The associated intracardiac lesions may result in shunting of blood from the left ventricle into the right ventricle or pulmonary artery and thus the Po_2 of pulmonary arterial blood may be slightly above normal. It is unlikely, however, that the magnitude of shunting will be large enough to produce an increase in oxygen saturation that would significantly affect pulmonary vascular tone or smooth muscle development, although this needs further study. The small increase in pulmonary arterial oxygen saturation will provide blood with a slightly higher oxygen content to the descending aorta through the ductus arteriosus, so that the normal difference between ascending and descending aortic oxygen saturation will be somewhat

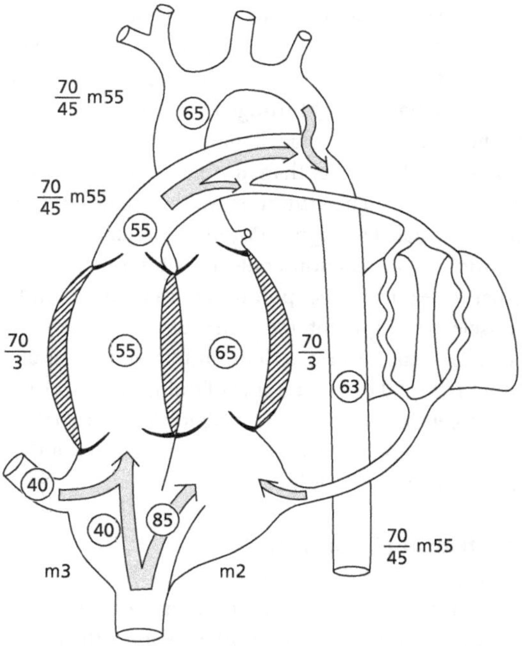

Figure 12.2 Localized aortic coarctation in the fetus: course of the circulation, oxygen saturations (circled), and pressures are all normal, since the widely patent ductus arteriosus permits normal flow around the shelf projecting into the aorta. The relatively small flow of blood across the aortic isthmus is related to the decreased left ventricular output. m, mean pressure.

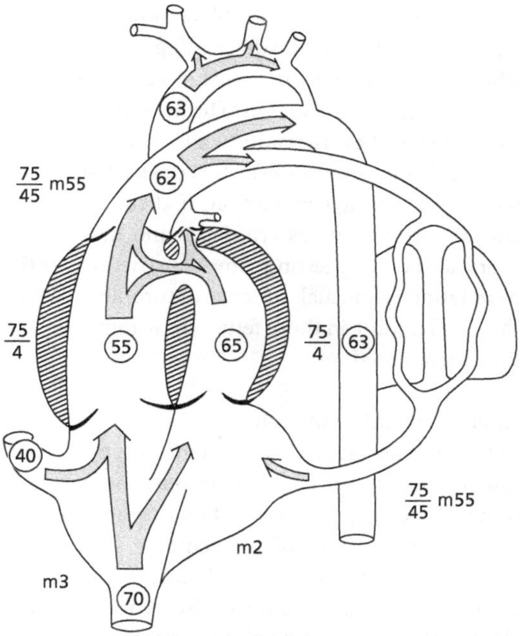

Figure 12.3 Aortic isthmus narrowing, ventricular septal defect, and subvalvar left ventricular outflow obstruction in the fetus: course of the circulation, oxygen saturations (circled), and pressures. The relatively small flow of blood across the aortic isthmus is related to the decreased left ventricular output. m, mean pressure.

reduced. It is unlikely that this will significantly affect perfusion or metabolism in the lower body or placenta. Figure 12.3 depicts the circulation in a fetus with narrowing of the aortic isthmus, a ventricular septal defect, and obstruction of left ventricular outflow into the aorta.

Recently, observations of the size of the cardiac ventricles and of the ascending aorta and pulmonary artery in fetuses with aortic coarctation have raised questions about possible hemodynamic effects in the fetus. Although right ventricular dilation is noted in other conditions, it is not uncommonly observed in fetuses with coarctation [8,9]. In addition, the pulmonary trunk diameter is frequently increased in fetuses with coarcatation and a ratio of pulmonary trunk to ascending aortic diameter greater than 1.6 was considered to be predictive of the presence of coarctation [10]. It is difficult to explain the presence of right ventricular and pulmonary arterial dilation. Possibly it is the result of an increase in output of the right compared with the left ventricle. Narrowing of the aortic arch is often observed in fetuses with coarctation; this may cause modest obstruction to left ventricular ejection and thus decreased left ventricular output. Venous blood returning to the heart may thus be diverted away from the foramen ovale and a greater proportion will be directed through the tricuspid valve, and account for the right ventricular enlargement. An alternative explanation is that although the localized coarctation in the aorta does not interfere with blood flow from the ascending to the descending aorta, it might interfere with blood flow from the ductus arteriosus into the descending aorta, effectively causing mild to modest outflow obstruction to the right ventricle with dilation. I know of no ultrasound studies in which left and right ventricular outputs have been determined in fetuses with coarctation. It would be of great interest to determine ventricular outputs in fetuses with coarctation and also to study blood flow patterns in the ductus arteriosus and descending aorta to assess whether there is abnormal flow or turbulence as a result of partial obstruction. This hypothesis is not supported by the observations of Charles Kleinman (personal communication). He states that in fetuses with right ventricular dilation, if there is turbulent flow in the ductus arteriosus and descending thoracic aorta, suggesting some constriction, aortic coarctation is unusual. Absence of turbulent flow is the usual finding in those fetuses in whom coarctation is diagnosed.

Aortic arch interruption

In the rare instances where arch interruption is not associated with intracardiac lesions, the obstruction will increase the afterload on the left ventricle and thus the output of the ventricle will be decreased. Flow into the ventricle through the foramen ovale and left atrium will also be reduced, but right ventricular output will be increased modestly. The decreased volume loading of the left ventricle could possibly interfere with its development (see Chapter 11). The Po_2 in descending aortic blood, derived through the ductus arteriosus, will be the same as that in the pulmonary artery and lower than in the normal fetus because no blood from the ascending aorta reaches the descending aorta. The difference in oxygen saturation between the ascending and descending aortae will be exaggerated, but the relatively small decrease in oxygen content in descending aortic blood probably has little effect on oxygenation and metabolism of the lower body.

In the majority of fetuses with interruption, the presence of intracardiac lesions will have a major influence on hemodynamics. In those with ventricular septal defect with septal displacement and subaortic obstruction, left ventricular blood will be shunted across the defect into the right ventricle and pulmonary artery, so that it will reach the descending aorta through the ductus arteriosus. Therefore the oxygen saturation difference between ascending and descending aortic blood will probably be similar to normal. In the fetus with tricuspid atresia, ventricular septal defect and aortopulmonary transposition, venous return from all sources mixes in the left atrium. The blood entering the pulmonary artery from the left ventricle has the same oxygen saturation as blood entering the aorta, derived from the right ventricle through the ventricular septal defect. Blood distributed to the lungs as well as that passing through the ductus arteriosus to the descending aorta will have an oxygen saturation somewhat higher than normal, whereas ascending aortic oxygen saturation will be slightly lower than normal. The higher Po_2 of blood entering the pulmonary circulation could possibly reduce vascular tone and restrict pulmonary vascular smooth muscle development (see Chapter 5). In fetuses with truncus arteriosus communis or aortopulmonary septal defect, mixing of pulmonary arterial and ascending aortic blood probably occurs, so that the Po_2 of blood distributed to the lungs and upper and lower body is similar.

Postnatal circulation

Coarctation of the aorta

The circulatory adjustments after birth will be affected by the presence of other lesions, the commonest being ventricular septal defect. A small defect will not have a major effect, but a larger defect will have a significant influence on the hemodynamic changes and clinical manifestations. Coarctation with associated ventricular septal defect is discussed on p. 301.

Coarctation with intact ventricular septum

During the neonatal period, while the ductus arteriosus is still patent, flow from the ascending to the descending aorta may not be impeded by the posterior shelf (Figure 12.4). The circulation does not therefore differ from the normal transitional status. The decreased pulmonary vascular resistance after birth will permit pulmonary blood flow to increase. While the ductus remains patent, a left-to-right shunt will occur because systemic vascular resistance increases with elimination of the umbilical–placental circulation.

The ductus arteriosus usually begins to constrict at its pulmonary arterial end. The narrowing of the ductus allows pulmonary arterial pressure to fall in association with the progressive decrease in pulmonary vascular resistance. The aortic end of the ductus may not constrict for several hours, days or even weeks after the pulmonary arterial portion has constricted. However, when it does constrict, blood flow from the ascending to the descending aorta

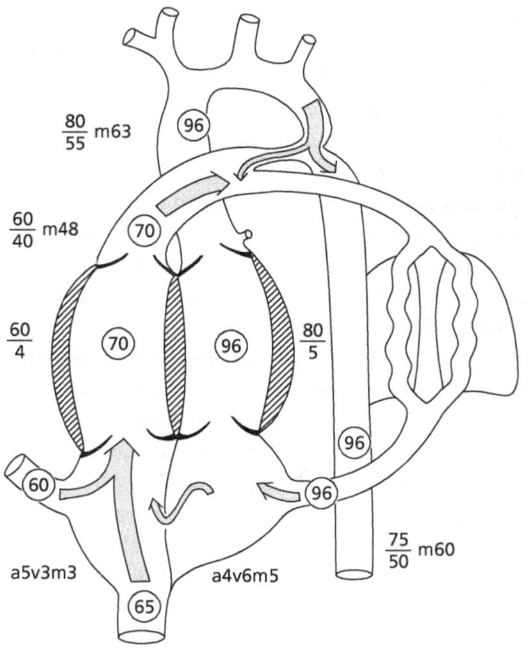

Figure 12.4 Localized juxtaductal coarctation of the aorta in a newborn infant in whom the aortic end of the ductus arteriosus is still patent: course of the circulation, oxygen saturations (circled), and pressures are similar to those observed normally. m, mean pressure.

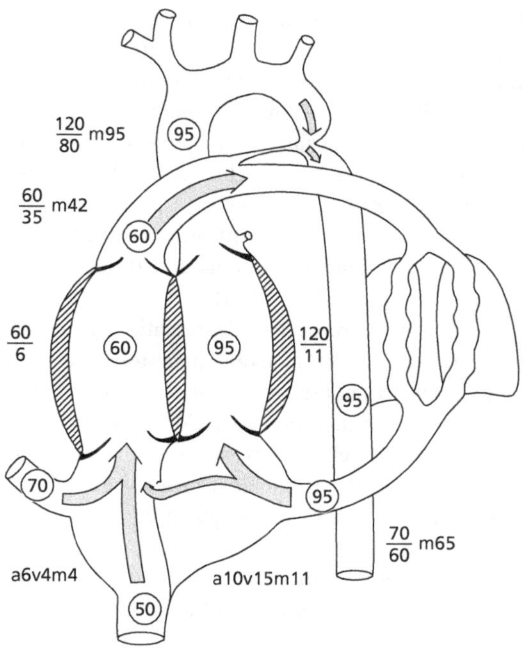

Figure 12.5 Localized juxtaductal coarctation of the aorta in an infant in whom the ductus arteriosus has constricted: course of the circulation, oxygen saturations (circled), and pressures. The constriction of the ductus has resulted in aortic obstruction. m, mean pressure.

will be obstructed by the shelf (Figure 12.5). Questions have been raised about whether the behavior of the ductus arteriosus is normal in infants with aortic coarctation. The ductus normally closes completely within a few days after birth, but in infants with coarctation it often remains patent for several weeks, usually with only a narrow lumen. When the aortic end of the ductus closes, the location of its lumen varies in relation to the shelf in the aorta. It is usually adjacent to the shelf, but may be just below or just above the narrowed eccentric stenotic area in the aorta. A small or modest left-to-right shunt will occur through the ductus and it may contribute to the development of left ventricular failure by adding a volume load to the pressure load created by development of the coarctation. Aortic obstruction may not be demonstrable for several days or weeks after birth. The degree to which the shelf projects, the rapidity of constriction of the aortic end of the ductus, and the time of occurrence after birth will determine the circulatory responses. Because there is no functional obstruction of the aorta during fetal life, no collateral circulation is developed. If the shelf projects well into the aortic lumen and the ductus constricts rapidly, ascending aortic systolic and diastolic pressures will increase. A sudden increase in afterload is presented to the left ventricle; the neonatal myocardium is very sensitive to rapid increases in afterload and left ventricular stroke volume falls. Left ventricular end-diastolic and left atrial pressures increase and if the rise in pressure is large, pulmonary edema will result.

The increase in left atrial pressure results in dilation of the chamber and may result in stretching of the septum with opening of the foramen ovale. An atrial left-to-right shunt develops and this may be large as a result of the large pressure gradient between the left and right atria. The pulmonary arterial pressure may be normal but is often increased to mean levels of 25–30 mmHg and right ventricular systolic pressure is often elevated to

40–60 mmHg. The pulmonary arterial hypertension is the result of the elevated left atrial pressure and the increased pulmonary blood flow. As a result of the combination of the high volume load resulting from the atrial left-to-right shunt and the increased pressure load, right ventricular failure may develop. A patent ductus arteriosus may also result in a left-to-right shunt and shunting may occur through both the ductus and the foramen ovale.

In the absence of collateral circulation, pressure in the descending aorta falls and its systolic pressure may be lower than ascending aortic diastolic pressure. The size of the ductus arteriosus and its relationship to the shelf influences the supply of blood to the lower body and the development of cardiac failure. A large atrial left-to-right shunt will interfere with filling of the left ventricle, thus limiting stroke volume and the pressure that can be developed in the ascending aorta and the gradient for flow across the coarctation to the descending aorta. An additional factor that may aggravate the fall in descending aortic pressure is patency of the ductus arteriosus. If pressure in the aorta is higher than that in the pulmonary artery, blood will shunt left to right and this will divert blood away from the descending aorta. The shunt will be particularly large if the ductus lumen is connected to the aorta above the coarctation, because aortic pressure at this site will be greater. A large left-to-right shunt will develop and cardiac failure will occur as a result of the combined increased pressure and volume load on the left ventricle.

If the aortic shelf is not very prominent, or if the ampulla of the ductus remains open and gradually occludes, the aortic obstruction will develop more slowly over several weeks or even months. Depending on the period over which obstruction develops, a varying hemodynamic and clinical picture will occur. The left ventricle will respond to the increased afterload by progressive hypertrophy and, in the newborn period, possibly hyperplasia. This may allow the ventricle to compensate for the increased pressure load. Thus, cardiac failure may first appear only after 2–3 months, when obstruction becomes severe, or it may be precipitated by an infection; increased cardiac output requirement associated with growth may also be important, because a fixed stenosis will become relatively more severe. An additional factor that may contribute to the development of cardiac failure is the physiological fall in hemoglobin concentration (see Chapter 7 for discussion of factors influencing onset of failure). If the coarctation does not become more severe with growth or if an adequate collateral circulation develops, blood supply to the descending aorta and lower body may not be severely compromised. The main concerns are those relating to ascending aortic hypertension and persistent left ventricular failure over the ensuing months. If the collateral circulation is well developed, the ascending aortic pressure required to maintain flow to the descending aorta will fall; this will decrease left ventricular afterload and cardiac failure may improve (Figure 12.6). Prior to the institution of surgical management of aortic coarctation in early infancy, many infants with persistent cardiac failure would succumb during the first year, often as a result of a complicating infection.

The aortic arch, as mentioned above, is frequently narrow and has been described as hypoplastic. The isthmus and the segment between the

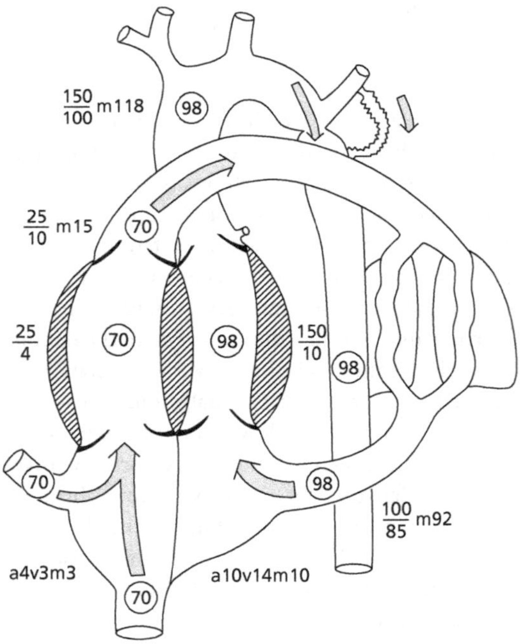

Figure 12.6 Localized juxtaductal coarctation of the aorta in a child in whom a collateral circulation is well developed: course of the circulation, oxygen saturations (circled), and pressures. m, mean pressure.

left carotid and subclavian arteries are usually the segments that are narrowed. There has been considerable concern that the narrow arch may continue to impose obstruction even if the localized juxtaductal coarctation is eliminated. However, this is unusual if the coarctation shelf and the aorta in proximity are effectively removed. An important issue is what size of arch can be expected to be obstructive if the coarctation is eliminated. One suggestion is that if the diameter of the aortic arch is at least as large as that of the carotid artery, it is not likely to be obstructive. Another proposal was that reduction of diameter to below 40% of normal should be considered obstructive. Unfortunately, there is no evidence to support these proposals. Surgeons have, in the past, used subjective impressions to decide whether either extensive resection or arch repair should be attempted. This is probably not necessary in most instances because, with adequate repair of the coarctation, the arch usually develops normally. The recent approach to surgical repair has largely eliminated the need to make the decision (see section on management in Chapter 12).

Effect of prostaglandin E_1

Prostaglandin (PG)E_1 relaxes ductus arteriosus smooth muscle. Because constriction of the ductus arteriosus is important in the development of aortic obstruction in infants with coarctation, PGE_1 has been used effectively in improving left ventricular failure. The exact mechanism of action has not yet been resolved. The effect could be to relax ductus arteriosus tissue extending into the wall of the aorta, constriction of which caused the obstruction. It is possible that opening the lumen of the ductus could allow blood to flow from the ascending to descending aorta around the aortic shelf, thus reducing the obstruction. PGE_1 is usually effective within the first 7–10 days after birth, but there appears to be lesser relaxant effect on the ductus after several weeks.

Effect of oxygen

During the early postnatal period, administration of 100% oxygen could potentially have an adverse effect by causing constriction of the ductus arteriosus and thus induce or worsen the aortic obstruction.

If the degree of obstruction is not very severe and cardiac failure has not occurred within the first 3–6 months after birth, it is unlikely to develop during childhood. There are rarely symptoms until much later in life, and cardiac failure does not usually present until after 30 years of age, when secondary myocardial fibrotic changes may have occurred. The condition may first be recognized when it is appreciated that a child or adolescent has hypertension. The manifestations of coarctation of the aorta beyond early childhood are usually related to infective endocarditis, cerebrovascular accidents, or rupture of the ascending or descending aorta. Neurological symptoms may be due to rupture of an aneurysm of the circle of Willis with subarachnoid hemorrhage or an intracranial hemorrhage related to upper body hypertension. They rarely occur before the age of 8–10 years and are usually noted in adults. Infective endocarditis may occur at any age, usually after the age of 2 years, and the area most commonly involved is the bicuspid aortic valve or the distal aorta just beyond the obstructed segment.

As mentioned above, the degree of hypertension in the ascending aorta and its branches is related to the degree of obstruction and the extent of the collateral circulation. There has been considerable controversy regarding the role of the kidneys in the production of hypertension in coarctation of the aorta. It was suggested that either an actual decrease in pressure or a reduction in pulse pressure may initiate renal production of renin and thus of angiotensin and this contributes to the hypertension. Studies of angiotensin concentrations in the blood of patients with coarctation thus far have presented conflicting results but no convincing evidence that the kidneys are involved in causing the hypertension.

The usual complications of systemic arterial hypertension in adults are also noted in patients with aortic coarctation. Hypertensive encephalopathy is rare but changes in the eyegrounds occur. Left ventricular hypertrophy and fibrosis develops and the aorta may develop early calcification; dissecting aneurysm of the aorta has also been noted.

Coarctation with ventricular septal defect

The presence of a small ventricular septal defect may not have a significant effect in an infant with coarctation. However, the increase in both systolic and diastolic pressures in the left ventricle that develop with obstruction will induce a larger left-to-right shunt. This additional volume load on the left ventricle may contribute to the development of failure. Also in association with the increase in left atrial pressure, the higher pulmonary blood flow may result in modest pulmonary arterial hypertension. In the infant with coarctation and a large ventricular septal defect the increase in afterload on the left ventricle that occurs when the obstruction develops will result in a large left-to-right shunt. If this occurs acutely due to rapid closure of the ductus arteriosus, the left ventricle may not be able to compensate and the volume ejected into the aorta may not be sufficient to provide an adequate cardiac output. Thus circulatory failure develops; although flow to the upper body may be adequate, blood supply to the lower body will be severely compromised and tissue hypoxia will result (see Chapter 3). If the left ventricle does compensate by increasing stroke volume, output into the aorta may be adequate but a large left-to-right shunt will develop. The hemodynamic consequences are similar to those observed with large ventricular septal defects (see Chapter 7). However, two additional factors influence circulation. The increased afterload on the left ventricle will increase left ventricular pressure and thus increases the left-to-right shunt. The high pressure and volume load is likely to produce early and severe cardiac failure. If the ventricular septal defect is unrestrictive, the systolic pressure in the right ventricle and pulmonary artery will be elevated to that in the left ventricle. Elevation of pulmonary arterial pressure to very high levels is likely to result in the development of very early pulmonary vascular disease.

Coarctation of the aorta with reversal of pressures

Aortic coarctation is classically recognized by the presence of higher blood pressure in the ascending aorta and its branches compared with the descending aorta and its branches. Mention has been made of the unusual condition where the pressure in one or both arms may be low, but similar to lower body pressure. However, in rare instances, pressure in the descending aorta may be higher than that in the ascending aorta. Several conditions that may be associated with coarctation could lead to this finding. These are discussed below in the section on aortic arch interruption.

Interruption of the aortic arch

As mentioned above, the vast majority of individuals with arch interruption have an associated large systemic-to-pulmonary communication, most commonly a ventricular septal defect and occasionally a common truncus arteriosus or aortopulmonary septal defect. This communication is very important in determining the hemodynamics and clinical manifestations. When the aortic arch is interrupted, blood flow to the lower body must be provided through a ductus arteriosus or by an adequate collateral arterial circulation, after birth as well as in the fetus. In the immediate postnatal period the removal of the umbilical–placental circulation results in an increase in resistance to flow to the descending aorta. Pulmonary vascular resistance falls as a result of ventilation of the lungs and pulmonary blood flow increases. While the ductus arteriosus is widely patent, flow to the lower body is determined by the ratio of resistances in the pulmonary circulation and the lower body systemic circulation. In the absence of a large systemic-to-pulmonary communication, should pulmonary vascular resistance fall markedly, blood ejected into the pulmonary artery would flow preferentially into the lungs and flow through the ductus to the lower body would be severely restricted. During ventricular systole, the kinetic forces in the pulmonary artery may direct blood through the ductus into the descending aorta, but during diastole flow would occur from the high-resistance systemic circulation into the pulmonary circulation. Blood to the lower body would be provided from the pulmonary artery and thus would have a lower Po_2 than blood distributed to the upper body from the aorta. In addition, because the arch is interrupted, the pressure in the ascending aorta and its branches will be higher than in the descending aorta and its branches.

The presence of a large ventricular septal communication maintains pulmonary arterial systolic pressure at levels in the ascending aorta. Pulmonary arterial diastolic pressure is determined by pulmonary vascular resistance; if it is low, diastolic pressure in the pulmonary artery will be lower than that in the ascending aorta. As mentioned

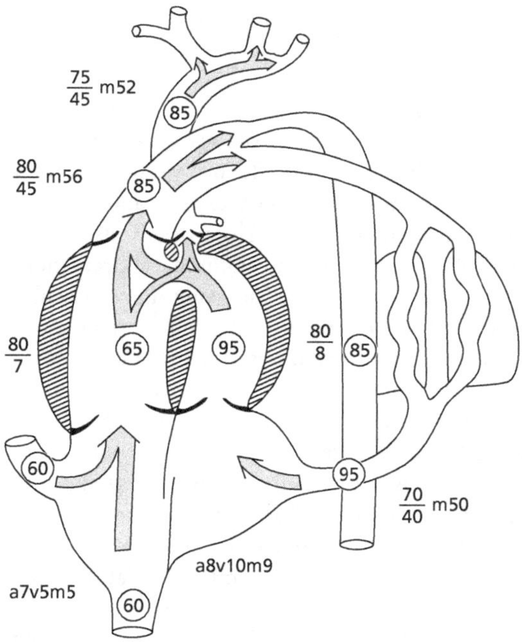

Figure 12.7 Aortic arch interruption, ventricular septal defect, and subvalvar left ventricular outflow obstruction in the newborn period, with the ductus arteriosus widely open: course of the circulation, oxygen saturations (circled), and pressures. Note that the systemic blood flow is maintained by flow through the ductus arteriosus. m, mean pressure.

above, this may interfere with maintenance of an adequate flow to the lower body and facilitate backflow from the descending aorta into the pulmonary circulation in diastole. The course of the circulation in the immediate newborn period is shown in Figure 12.7. An interesting relationship develops between resistances in the systemic circulation in the upper and lower body and in the lungs. With obstruction of the aortic arch, the resistance in the upper body circulation is high; this, with the subvalvar aortic stenosis that is often present, confronts the left ventricle with a very high afterload. The presence of a large systemic-to-pulmonary communication impedes the normal decline of pulmonary vascular resistance (see Chapter 5). Despite the maintenance of a relatively high pulmonary vascular resistance, a left-to-right shunt develops through the systemic-to-pulmonary communication, because the afterload on the left ventricle is markedly increased. This combination of increased volume and pressure load on the left ventricle is likely to result in early development of cardiac failure.

The left-to-right shunt into the ventricle or pulmonary artery increases the Po_2 in pulmonary arterial blood, so that the blood passing through the ductus arteriosus has a higher Po_2 than does systemic venous blood. If the shunt is large, the Po_2 in descending aortic blood may be only slightly lower than that in the ascending aorta. With Taussig–Bing anomaly and arch interruption, the pulmonary artery may receive predominantly left ventricular blood and thus the Po_2 in descending aortic blood is higher than that in the ascending aorta. When systemic and pulmonary venous return is completely or almost completely mixed, as with tricuspid atresia, ventricular septal defect, aortopulmonary transposition and arch interruption, or with truncus arteriosus communis, the Po_2 of blood in the upper and lower body will be the same.

While the ductus arteriosus remains patent, descending aortic pressure and blood flow to the lower body will be maintained and the main concern is the development of left ventricular failure. After a varying period of hours to several days after birth, constriction of the ductus arteriosus may produce rapidly progressive deterioration of the infant's condition. The changes that occur and their effects on circulatory hemodynamics are shown in Figure 12.8. Constriction of the ductus arteriosus interferes with blood flow from the pulmonary artery to the descending aorta. A pressure gradient develops between the pulmonary artery and the descending aorta, and descending aortic pressure falls. The progressive decrease in pulmonary vascular resistance after birth further interferes with the supply of blood to the descending aorta, because blood will flow preferentially through the pulmonary circulation rather than through the ductus. Thus, the left-to-right shunt through the ventricular septal defect becomes very large and results in a progressive increase in pulmonary venous return with marked elevation of left ventricular end-diastolic and left atrial pressures. Left-sided and right-sided cardiac failure with increased respiratory effort and hepatomegaly ensues. Even though the oxygen saturation of blood supplying the lower body may not be greatly reduced, the low blood flow will result in reduced oxygen delivery and result in severe local hypoxia, with progressive

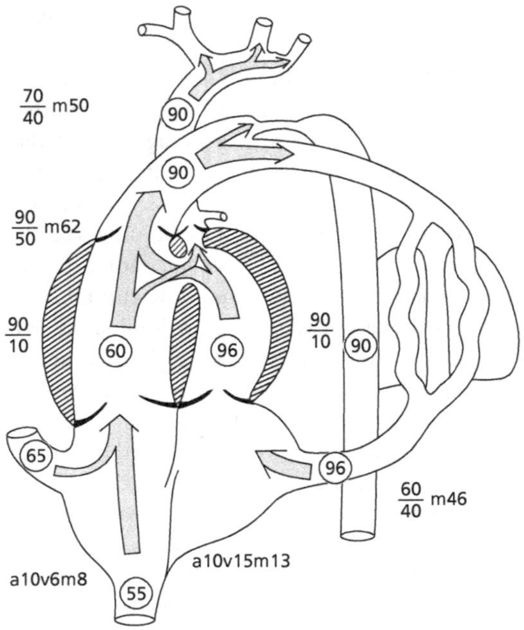

Figure 12.8 Aortic arch interruption, ventricular septal defect, and subvalvar left ventricular outflow obstruction in an infant in whom the ductus arteriosus has constricted: course of the circulation, oxygen saturations (circled), and pressures. Note that the decrease in systemic blood flow causes a fall in aortic pressure. m, mean pressure.

lactic acid accumulation and metabolic acidemia (see Chapter 3). The decreased perfusion pressure in the descending aorta may interfere with renal perfusion, resulting in poor urinary output and, if prolonged, renal tubular damage.

The ductus arteriosus appears to remain patent for a longer period after birth than normal, as in infants with aortic atresia (see Chapter 11), but the factors influencing closure of the ductus in this condition are not well understood.

Effect of oxygen

Administration of 100% oxygen may have adverse effects in these infants. As a result of the left-to-right shunt and increased pulmonary blood flow, oxygen produces a large increase in Po_2 of pulmonary arterial blood; both the ductus arteriosus and the pulmonary circulation will be exposed to the well-oxygenated blood. The higher Po_2 may result in greater constriction of the ductus as well as dilation of the pulmonary circulation; both these changes would further reduce blood flow and pressure in the descending aorta.

Effect of PGE_1

PGE_1 produces relaxation of the ductus arteriosus; when administered soon after birth, it will maintain patency of the ductus and thus flow and pressure in the descending aorta. However, it also has a vasodilator effect on the pulmonary circulation. The resulting decrease in pulmonary vascular resistance will permit a greater left-to-right shunt through the ventricular septal defect or other communication and thus place a larger volume load on the left ventricle. In addition to increasing the likelihood of cardiac failure, the lowered pulmonary vascular resistance may limit flow through the ductus arteriosus because flow will occur preferentially into the pulmonary circulation rather than through the ductus into the systemic circulation. The responsiveness of the ductus arteriosus to PGE_1 appears to be decreased if it is first administered several weeks after birth. However, in the presence of aortic arch interruption, the ductus usually does respond even several weeks after birth.

Interruption of the arch with reversal of pressures

Although pressure in the ascending aorta and the upper limb arteries is usually higher than in the descending aorta and lower extremity arteries, in certain situations lower body arterial pressure is higher. This occurs with several of the lesions associated with arch interruption or aortic coarctation. The common features are that the pulmonary artery is either partly or completely transposed and arises from the left ventricle. If the aorta is transposed and arises from the right ventricle and outflow into the aorta is restricted, pressure in the ascending aorta will be lower than that in the ventricles. Systolic pressure in the pulmonary artery is the same as that in the left ventricle; if the ductus arteriosus is widely patent, pressure in the descending aorta will be similar to that in the pulmonary artery. With tricuspid atresia and aortopulmonary transposition and a ventricular septal defect, if the septal defect is restrictive or if the right ventricular infundibulum is narrow, ascending aortic pressure will be lower than left ventricular pressure. Left ventricular pressure will be transmitted to the pulmonary artery and through the ductus arteriosus to the descending aorta. The reversal of upper and lower extremity pressures with arch interruption or coarctation may also occur with aortopulmonary transposition and ventricular septal defect associated with infundibular stenosis of the right ventricle. Double-outlet right ventricle of the Taussig–Bing variety is characterized by a large ventricular septal defect, origin of the aorta from the right ventricle, and a pulmonary artery that overrides the right and left ventricles. Subaortic stenosis as well as aortic coarctation or arch interruption is often associated. Ventricular pressures exceed aortic pressure and pulmonary arterial and descending aortic pressures are similar to the high ventricular pressure while the ductus arteriosus is widely patent. In all these conditions, when the ductus constricts, pressures in the descending aorta and its branches fall and reach levels lower than those in the ascending aorta. In these lesions, because descending aortic blood is derived through the ductus arteriosus from the transposed pulmonary artery, oxygen saturation in the lower extremities is higher than that in the upper body (see Chapter 3).

Clinical features

Coarctation of the aorta

Coarctation with intact ventricular septum

In the newborn period there may be no evidence of aortic obstruction, and blood pressure and pulses in the legs may be equal to those in the arms. Within a few days to 1–2 weeks, tachypnea with increased respiratory effort and excessive perspiration are noted. Usually the infant is restless and irritable and feeds poorly. Examination reveals tachycardia to 160–180/min; the pulses in the upper extremities are readily palpable and the femoral and dorsalis pedis pulses may be weak but are usually absent. Blood pressure is usually moderately elevated in the arms to 100–110 mmHg systolic and 70–80 mmHg diastolic, but the pressures may be higher. Lower extremity pressure is often not measurable because the pulse pressure is small; if pressure can be measured it is reduced to 50–60 mmHg systolic and 25–40 mmHg diastolic. If the infant is in severe cardiac failure, the upper limb pulses are often also weak and the diagnosis may not be obvious clinically. Occasionally, the pulse in the left arm may be weak or absent and the blood pressure low, because the left subclavian artery is involved in the coarctation. Rarely, the pulse is weak or absent and the blood pressure low in the right arm if the right subclavian artery arises from the descending aorta below the coarctation. If the right and left subclavian arteries are abnormal, the diagnosis of coarctation may not be considered, because it is usually made by recognizing a difference in pulse volume and pressures in the upper and lower extremities. If the pulses in all the extremities are weak, it is important to feel the carotid pulses. If they are full and prominent, the diagnosis of coarctation of the aorta should be considered.

Some infants deteriorate rapidly within a few hours, with progressive respiratory distress, tachycardia, pallor, mottling, and weak pulses in the arms and legs. Pulmonary rales may be heard at the lung bases and hepatomegaly may be noted. The heart is clinically markedly enlarged but is not very active. The second heart sound is usually moderately increased at the upper left sternal border and a third sound may be heard at the apex. A systolic ejection click is often heard at the mid to lower left sternal border due to the presence of a bicuspid aortic valve. Murmurs are not usually present, but a soft decrescendo systolic murmur may be heard at the apex. If the ductus arteriosus is still patent, a continuous murmur may be heard at the upper left sternal border.

Infusion of PGE_1 often results in rapid improvement of symptoms within 15–60 min. The lower extremity pulses become palpable and blood pressure increases, whereas upper limb blood pressure may fall. Respiratory distress becomes less severe and over a few days heart size decreases. If diuretic and digitalis therapy is instituted and PGE_1 stopped, the infant may maintain the improvement. In those who respond, breathing becomes less labored and other signs of cardiac failure improve. The cardiac impulse becomes more evident on palpation, the pulses in the upper extremities become much stronger, and a definite blood pressure difference is noted between the arms and the legs. In the neonatal period, it is unusual for pressure in the upper body to rise above about 120 mmHg systolic and 90 mmHg diastolic, but much higher pressures of up to 200 mmHg systolic and 120 mmHg diastolic may be noted in older infants. If the obstruction has not developed rapidly, the onset of left ventricular failure may be gradual, with several weeks of moderate respiratory distress and excessive perspiration before pulmonary edema occurs. The clinical features in these infants are similar to those described for the infant who has responded to treatment of cardiac failure.

If there has been a good response to treatment, the infant may progress well with no obvious symptoms and develop the clinical features described below in older children. However, some have persistent or repeated episodes of cardiac failure, particularly associated with infection, and may succumb. If the infant survives the first year with no evidence of cardiac failure, it is most unusual for failure to develop before adult life. Associated with the development of collateral supply, the blood pressure in the upper extremities may fall gradually and the difference between arm and leg pressures diminishes.

In children, aortic coarctation rarely produces symptoms unless the complications described above occur. When the obstruction is marked there may be a limited ability to increase blood flow to the legs during exercise and intermittent claudication of the legs has been known to occur. However, this is unusual and is not experienced by most patients. The upper part of the trunk and arms are frequently well developed, whereas the pelvis and the lower extremities are slender. The large collateral arteries may be palpated over the lateral and inferior scapular margins and above the clavicle. The pulses in the arms are strong but the femoral and dorsalis pedis pulses are decreased; the quality of the pulses in the lower limbs depends on the severity of the lesion and the collateral circulation. In severe obstruction, femoral pulses may not be palpable. If obstruction is less severe, or with good collateral circulation, the pulses may be weak but delayed compared with the arm pulses. With mild stenosis, the leg pulses may be readily felt but are weaker and may be delayed compared with those in the arms. Blood pressures in the arm and the leg also vary greatly. Some children have normal blood pressures in the arm and slightly lowered pressures in the leg. Usually, arm pressures are moderately increased to 130–160/90–110 mmHg while leg pressures are 75–100/65–85 mmHg, but higher arm pressures may occur, particularly in adults. If the left subclavian artery is involved in the coarctation, the left arm pulse may be weak and the pressure low. The heart is usually not enlarged clinically but there may be a prominent apical impulse. The first sound is normal; the second sound may be increased at the upper right sternal border when hypertension is marked; a third heart sound is often heard at the apex. A systolic ejection click is frequently heard along the left margin of the sternum, and it usually indicates the presence of a bicuspid aortic valve. Precordial murmurs are not heard often, but occasionally a short mid-diastolic murmur is present at the apex. A soft continuous murmur is sometimes present over the left side of the spine along the scapular margin. This could be due to flow through the coarctation, but could be related to flow through large collateral arteries such as intercostal or scapular vessels. A harsh systolic ejection murmur of grade 2–3/6 intensity may be heard at the upper right sternal border if aortic stenosis is present in association with the coarctation. If the ductus arteriosus is patent, a harsh continuous murmur is usually heard at the upper left sternal border.

Coarctation with ventricular septal defect

If a small ventricular septal defect is associated with aortic coarctation, the clinical features will be similar to those described above, but additional manifestations of ventricular septal defect will be evident. A loud harsh pansystolic murmur will be heard at the lower left sternal margin. If the ventricular left-to-right shunt is large, increased precordial hyperactivity will be noted at the apex and lower sternum, and the second heart sound may be accentuated at the upper left sternal margin. Also, evidence of cardiac failure will tend to occur early and be more marked than with isolated aortic coarctation. If the ventricular septal defect is nonrestrictive, the second sound at the upper left sternal border is markedly accentuated and, in addition to the systolic murmur, a low-frequency mid-diastolic murmur is usually heard at the apex. These infants usually have marked cardiac failure; prior to the current practice of closing the ventricular septal defect when the coarctation is corrected surgically, the failure often persisted if only the coartation was relieved.

Infants with aortic coarctation and a large atrial shunt, either through a stretched foramen ovale or a fossa ovalis defect, also usually manifest more severe cardiac failure. The precordial impulse is hyperactive with prominent right ventricular activity. The second heart sound at the upper left sternal border is usually somewhat accentuated and is well split. When coarctation is associated with lesions that cause reduced ascending aortic blood flow, the clinical manifestations of those lesions will also be evident. These lesions are described in other chapters.

Interruption of the aortic arch

Infants with aortic arch interruption usually develop symptoms soon after birth. Apart from the evidence of the interruption itself, the clinical manifestations are determined by the associated lesions. These are described in other chapters, but early onset of manifestations of cardiac failure almost always present within a few days after birth. In the immediate newborn period there may be no symptoms but mild cyanosis may be present. The presence of arch interruption may be suspected early by the finding of a difference in oxygen saturation or Po_2 in the upper and lower limb. Usually the saturation is lower in the legs, but in infants with aortopulmonary transposition or Taussig–Bing anomaly, the saturation may be lower in the arms. With type A interruption, the saturation in the left arm will be the same as that in the lower extremities, whereas in type B interruption both arms will have higher oxygen saturations. However, if the right subclavian artery has an anomalous origin from the descending aorta, the saturation will be the same as in the legs. While the ductus arteriosus is still widely patent, pulses in the lower extremities are palpable and no blood pressure difference is noted between the arms and legs. As mentioned above, the finding of a lower blood pressure in the arms than the legs may be confusing and the diagnosis of interruption may not be considered. This may be observed in infants with Taussig–Bing anomaly, tricuspid atresia with transposition and ventricular septal defect, and aortopulmonary transposition with ventricular septal defect and subaortic stenosis.

Within hours or a few days, associated with constriction of the ductus arteriosus, femoral arterial pulses become weak and blood pressure in the lower limb is decreased. The subsequent picture is one of acidemia and oliguria or anuria related to inadequate blood flow to the descending aorta and cardiac failure related to the large ventricular septal defect and increased pulmonary blood flow. Heart rate increases to 160–180/min and respiratory rate to 60–80/min. Cardiomegaly occurs, and the precordial impulse is felt over the apex and left sternal border and it becomes hyperactive. The second heart sound is usually accentuated at the upper left sternal border. Although no murmurs may be present postnatally, an increasingly loud pansystolic murmur develops at the mid or lower left sternal border. An apical third heart sound and low-frequency mid-diastolic murmur are heard frequently. Differential cyanosis between the upper and lower parts of the body may be noted, but usually is not striking because of ventricular left-to-right shunting. In patients with aortopulmonary transposition, the upper part of the body may be more cyanotic than the lower; this is not usually observed clinically, but measurement of oxygen saturations may demonstrate a higher saturation in the lower extremities. As right heart failure develops, hepatomegaly is noted. If these infants are not treated surgically, they usually die within a few weeks. In the past, attempts were made to relieve the aortic obstruction surgically, without correcting the associated lesions. Although many infants survived the procedure and showed some improvement in cardiac failure with digitalis and diuretic treatment, they usually had severe persistent cardiac failure and succumbed if additional procedures were not performed.

In addition to the cardiovascular manifestations, patients with aortic arch interruption may have the features associated with 22q11 deletion syndromes. Most of the individuals with type B interruption have the deletion, but it is present in far fewer with type A interruption. In the DiGeorge syndrome, the thymus and parathyroid glands are absent or poorly developed. Thus these infants have a disturbance in cell-mediated immunity with normal serum immunoglobulin concentrations and are susceptible to opportunistic infections with bacteria, viruses, and fungi. They are also prone to develop neonatal tetany and have craniofacial anomalies such as antimongoloid slant to the eyes, hypertelorism, mandibular hypoplasia, low-set ears, and short philtrum of the upper lip.

Investigations

Electrocardiography

With aortic coarctation the electrocardiogram characteristically shows right axis deviation and right ventricular hypertrophy in infants under 3 months of age, and often prominent right forces are present up to 6 or even 9 months. Left ventricular voltages are usually normal after birth but increase within 3–6 months. When severe failure is present, T waves are often flattened or inverted in the left precordial leads and in standard leads I and II. In children, the electrocardiogram is variable; usually it shows a normal pattern or a modest increase in left ventricular forces and right ventricular conduction delay is commonly noted. In older children and particularly in adults, ST depression and T-wave flattening or inversion may be noted in leads I, V5, and V6.

In patients with aortic arch interruption, the electrocardiographic pattern largely depends on the associated lesions. Usually right axis deviation and right ventricular hypertrophy are noted, but in infants with tricuspid atresia with transposition there is left axis deviation and left ventricular dominance. If hypocalcemia is severe, the typical features of prolongation of the QT interval with flattening of T waves may be observed.

Chest radiography

With both aortic coarctation and interrupted arch, in the immediate postnatal period the chest radiograph may be normal. If a left-to-right shunt develops, pulmonary arterial markings become prominent. Generalized cardiomegaly becomes evident as the infant develops cardiac failure; the pulmonary veins may be prominent and the lung fields are hazy due to pulmonary edema. Left atrial enlargement may be evident. Improvement in the failure is associated with a decrease in heart size and pulmonary edema.

In older children with coarctation, the heart size is normal or moderately increased and there is prominence of the left ventricle. The ascending aorta is often dilated and displaces the superior vena cava to the right. This may be associated with a bicuspid aortic valve with mild aortic stenosis and poststenotic dilation of the aorta, but does occur with severe coarctation alone. An indentation may be seen along the left margin of the aortic shadow just beyond the arch; this has been termed the "3 sign." When the esophagus is filled with barium, two indentations may be seen along its left border due to the dilated aortic segment just above the site of coarctation and the poststenotic dilation below it; this has been termed the "E sign." It is important to note if there is a posterior indentation in the barium-filled esophagus to suggest an anomalous origin of the right subclavian artery. Notching of the lower margin of the posterior ends of the fourth to eighth or ninth ribs may be noted due to erosion of the bone by the large intercostal arteries. In adults, calcification of the ascending aorta and the region of the coarctation may be seen. The left ventricle becomes more prominent and generalized cardiomegaly may occur.

The radiological features with aortic arch interruption reflect those characteristic of the associated lesions.

Echocardiography

In the early experience with ultrasound, it was not uncommon that the diagnosis of aortic coarctation or interrupted arch was not recognized, because imaging the aorta, particularly in the region of the ductus arteriosus connection, is often difficult. However, with recent improvement in techniques and in the hands of skilled echocardiographers, the diagnosis can be made with assurance, so that it is usually possible to refer the patient for surgery without additional studies such as catheterization and angiocardiography. The important information that should be obtained by ultrasound includes:

- definition of the presence and site of obstruction;
- presence and severity of aortic arch narrowing;
- site of origin and morphology of the large arteries arising from the aorta;
- estimation of the severity of obstruction;
- patency of the ductus arteriosus;
- definition of associated intracardiac or great vessel anomalies.

The posterolateral shelf of aortic coarctation may be readily demonstrated by two-dimensional ultrasound. It has been observed in the fetus, but it may be readily overlooked because while the ductus arteriosus is patent, no obvious obstruction is apparent. There is also a concern that if the infant is receiving PGE_1 postnatally, aortic coarctation may not be recognized because the ductus is widely patent. The arch of the aorta should be examined to assess its diameter. As mentioned above, the arch is frequently considered to be hypoplastic in infants with coarctation, but there are no reliable indications for determining what degree of narrowing is functionally significant. The site of origin of the left subclavian artery in relation to the coarctation, and the presence of obstruction of the artery if it is involved in the coarcted segment, should be defined. Also the origin of the right subclavian artery should be imaged to determine that it arises normally and not from the descending aorta.

Doppler flow studies are often helpful in defining the site of coarctation. Continuous-wave Doppler flow may demonstrate two flow velocities within a single envelope. A high velocity, representing the flow through the coarctation, presents as the outer envelope, whereas the low velocity, due to flow in the isthmus proximal to the coarctation, is contained within the envelope. The duration of the high-velocity flow does provide some indication of the severity of coarctation; in severe obstruction, it extends through most of the cardiac cycle. The velocity pattern in the descending aorta below the coarctation is also helpful. With severe obstruction the velocity profile shows a slow upstroke and slow descent, resembling a damped pressure tracing. In most infants with cardiac failure related to coarctation, the descending aortic flow profile is essentially flat, with little variation between systole and diastole. With juxtaductal coarctation, it is important to assess whether the ductus arteriosus is still patent and whether there is a left-to-right shunt through it. Also, the atrial septum should be assessed for the presence of bulging into the right atrium and atrial left-to-right shunting. It is important to determine the presence of a ventricular septal defect and its size and to assess the magnitude of left-to-right shunt. The aortic valve should be imaged to determine the presence of a bicuspid aortic valve; valve motion should be examined and Doppler flow velocity analyzed for evidence of aortic stenosis.

An experienced operator can currently make the diagnosis of aortic arch interruption by ultrasound examination with assurance, so that surgery can be recommended without further studies in most patients. However, if there are doubts about arch morphology or origin of great arteries, catheterization with angiocardiography should be used for their definition. The interruption is recognized by the failure to image continuity of the arch from one segment to the next. Thus, in type A interruption, there is lack of continuity of the aorta between the left subclavian artery and the ductus arching to the descending aorta. Also, three large arteries are seen to arise from the aortic arch proximal to the isthmus. With type B interruption, the left carotid artery appears to sweep upward as a continuation of the ascending aorta and the transverse aortic arch cannot be visualized. The left subclavian artery is connected to the ductus arteriosus–descending aorta arch. The ascending aorta is usually considerably smaller than the main pulmonary artery in these individuals. It is important to appreciate that the arch formed by the pulmonary artery extending to the ductus arteriosus and descending aorta may be readily mistaken for the aortic arch, but no vessels directed to the head arise from this arch. This error is particularly likely to occur with truncus arteriosus and interrupted arch. The innominate and carotid arteries arise from a short segment of ascending aorta. The pulmonary artery arising from the truncus connects through a large ductus to the descending aorta and gives the appearance of the aortic arch. Intracardiac morphology should be examined in detail to define the associated anomalies. The lesions likely to be associated with interrupted aortic arch are described above.

Magnetic resonance imaging and computed tomography

These techniques are extremely helpful in delineating the aorta and provide detailed images of the aortic arch and coarctation and are particularly useful for defining abnormalities in the aortic wall following surgery or balloon angioplasty and stent placement.

Cardiac catheterization and angiocardiography

General considerations

Prior to the ability to define the morphology and altered function by ultrasound techniques, a detailed cardiac catheterization study was considered essential in infants in whom aortic arch interruption or coarctation was suspected, so that the severity of the lesion could be assessed and associated lesions diagnosed. However, ultrasound techniques and particularly magnetic resonance imaging (MRI) now provide detailed assessment of the site and severity of obstruction or the presence of interruption in the majority of these patients, so that surgery can be recommended without the need for catheterization. Occasionally, the procedure is indicated in an infant in whom the anatomy cannot be defined accurately, or if a large ventricular septal defect is associated and it is felt necessary to assess pulmonary vascular resistance. Some surgeons considered catheterization and angiography necessary in older individuals thought to have mild coarctation in order to determine whether a collateral circulation had developed, because it is considered to be important during surgery. However, with the introduction of MRI, this is rarely indicated. Recently, cardiac catheterization has been indicated in some patients for therapeutic dilatation of the aorta at the site of coarctation by balloon angioplasty and stent implantation (discussed in the section on therapy on p. 310).

Infants with severe coarctation or with interrupted arch often present with cardiac failure as well as inadequate perfusion of the lower body. Arterial blood gases and pH should be measured and diuretic therapy should be instituted. Although it is common practice to administer alkali to treat acidemia, there is no convincing evidence indicating that it provides any benefit, and it could possibly be harmful [11,12]. PGE_1 infusion should be started prior to proceeding with the catheterization procedure. This will usually help to relieve acidemia by improving perfusion of the lower body. With aortic coarctation it may also improve cardiac failure by decreasing the afterload on the left ventricle. Most centers also recommend administration of inotropic agents such as dobutamine, dopamine or milrinone, but there is no documentation of beneficial effects of these agents. These procedures will all help to reduce the risk attendant with the procedure by improving the infant's condition.

Oxygen saturation and blood gases

In infants with aortic isthmus narrowing or interruption, the oxygen saturation data reflect the associated lesions. Almost always there is atrial or ventricular left-to-right shunting or both. When blood to the descending aorta is supplied either partially or completely by flow through the ductus arteriosus from the pulmonary artery, there is a difference in oxygen saturations in the ascending and the descending aortae (see Chapter 3). However, this difference is often not large, because a large ventricular left-to-right shunt will increase oxygen saturation in the pulmonary artery so that blood shunted into the descending aorta may have an oxygen saturation of 85–88%. In many of the lesions associated with aortic isthmus narrowing, such as double-outlet right ventricle, some venous blood will be directed into the ascending aorta, so that the oxygen saturation is often reduced to 85–90%, a level similar to that in the descending aorta. In infants with aortopulmonary transposition or Taussig–Bing anomaly, pulmonary arterial oxygen saturation is usually higher than aortic oxygen saturation; therefore, saturation in the descending aorta may be higher than that in the ascending aorta. Because oxygen saturations are in the higher ranges, a small difference may not be considered significant. In infants with localized juxtaductal coarctation, an increase in oxygen saturation at the right atrial level is frequent due to shunting through the foramen ovale. Usually the shunt is small, but right atrial saturation may sometimes be increased markedly to 85–88%. If cardiac output is reduced, the venous oxygen saturation is lowered; oxygen saturation in the inferior vena cava is usually considerably lower than that in the superior vena cava and may be as low as 35–40%. With juxtaductal coarctation the presence of a left-to-right shunt through the ductus arteriosus may be appreciated by an increase in oxygen saturation at the pulmonary arterial level as compared with the right ventricle. However, if there is a large increase in oxygen saturation at the right atrial level, a small shunt into the pulmonary artery may not produce enough additional increase in oxygen saturation to make it appear significant (see Chapter 3). The pulmonary venous oxygen saturation and Po_2 are usually normal, but if severe pulmonary edema is present, they may be reduced and this will be reflected in decreases in left atrial and ventricular and systemic arterial levels. In older patients with aortic coarctation, blood oxygen saturations and gases are usually normal. Changes as described above reflecting atrial or ductus arteriosus shunts may be noted.

Blood flows and shunts

In infants with aortic arch interruption the associated lesions determine blood flows and shunts. Calculations are often unreliable because there is bidirectional shunting and because ascending and descending aortic oxygen saturations may be different. Pulmonary blood flow is usually increased and systemic flow is normal or reduced.

In infants with localized coarctation, the cardiac output is reduced if cardiac failure is present. A left-to-right shunt may occur through the foramen ovale or the ductus arteriosus or both; it may vary from a small to a very large shunt with a pulmonary to systemic flow ratio greater than 3:1. In older patients, cardiac output is usually normal and shunts are infrequent.

Pressures

In infants with localized coarctation and an intact ventricular septum, right atrial pressure may be raised, particularly in the presence of cardiac failure. Particularly if atrial left-to-right shunt occurs, right ventricular systolic pressure is usually increased moderately to 40–60 mmHg. Pulmonary arterial pressure is also increased, with mean levels of about 25–30 mmHg. Left atrial pressure is increased, often markedly, with mean levels up to 15–20 mmHg; the *a* and *v* waves are usually equal in height. Left ventricular end-diastolic pressure is raised and may reach 25–30 mmHg. Left ventricular and ascending aortic systolic pressures vary considerably, depending on the severity of cardiac failure and the response to therapy. In infants in severe failure, the pressure may be in the range 80–100 mmHg, but in those no longer in failure, and particularly in older infants, levels may be higher. The descending aortic pressure also varies, but in infants in severe failure it may be reduced to 40–60/25–35 mmHg, with mean levels of 30–40 mmHg. The descending aortic pressure contour shows a slow upstroke and slow descent, often with a very narrow pulse pressure. If the infant has responded well to PGE_1 infusion, no pressure difference may be detected between the ascending and descending aortae. Left ventricular end-diastolic and left atrial pressures will decrease and pulmonary arterial and right ventricular pressures will also fall. If a large ventricular septal defect is associated with localized coarctation, systolic pressure in the right ventricle and pulmonary artery will be the same as that in the left ventricle and ascending aorta.

In children, the pressures on the right side of the heart are usually normal. Left ventricular end-diastolic pressure may be normal but may be increased to 12–20 mmHg if marked hypertension is present. The ascending aortic pressure may be increased to 160–200 mmHg systolic and 90–130 mmHg diastolic, with mean levels of 110–150 mmHg. However, in many children there is only a mild elevation to 120–130 mmHg systolic and 90–100 mmHg diastolic. Although a marked elevation in ascending aortic pressure usually indicates that the stenosis is severe, a mild elevation does not exclude the presence of severe obstruction, because an extensive collateral circulation may be present. The descending aortic pressure is usually in the range 80–100 mmHg systolic and 60–85 mmHg diastolic, with a mean of 70–90 mmHg. Pulse pressure is narrow in the descending aorta in most patients, but in those with mild coarctation it may be almost normal. The pressure contour usually shows a rather damped appearance and there is a slow rise with a late systolic peak and a low descent; usually no dicrotic notch is seen.

In infants with aortic arch interruption, pressure in the descending aorta is lower than that in the pulmonary artery when the ductus arteriosus is constricted. However, if PGE_1 is being administered, no pressure difference may be detected. The associated lesions influence the intracardiac pressures. In most instances, a large ventricular septal defect or aortopulmonary communication is associated with elevation of right ventricular and pulmonary arterial diastolic pressures to systemic levels. Subvalvar aortic obstruction may result in lower systolic pressure in the ascending aorta than in the ventricles. Unusually, pressure in the descending aorta is higher than that in the ascending aorta. In patients with aortic coarctation, exercise or other causes of increased cardiac output may increase the pressure difference across the stenosed area.

Angiocardiography

When descending aortic flow and pressure are reduced, there is a serious risk of renal complications when large amounts of contrast medium are injected in infants. Therefore the number of injections should be limited and one should consider what sites of injection are most important in providing necessary information. The information obtained from ultrasound studies should be used as a basis for deciding what additional material is necessary. The need for other injections should be based on the information obtained from ultrasound studies. If it is considered necessary to define the size and location of a ventricular septal defect, a left ventricular injection can be done.

In infants with juxtaductal coarctation, a left ventricular or ascending aortic injection shows the aorta to be normal in size, but occasionally small. There is a localized posterolateral indentation in the aorta just beyond the arch, which gives the appearance of a shelf projecting into the lumen. The narrowed lumen at this site is eccentric on the medial side of the aorta and is closely related to the ductus arteriosus, which frequently fills with contrast medium from the aorta. The lumen of the ductus is usually narrow. The left subclavian artery may arise from the region of the coarctation and then it is small and fills poorly. The descending aorta is larger and wider than the isthmus in most instances, but sometimes a posterior bulge is noted in the isthmus just above the coarcted segment. The internal thoracic arteries may be enlarged and tortuous but collateral arteries are not usually well developed.

In older infants and children with coarctation, ascending aortic injection frequently shows a bicuspid aortic valve and the aorta may be somewhat dilated. The coarcted segment varies considerably; usually there is a concentric localized narrowing of the aorta just beyond the origin of the left subclavian artery with a dilated arch and poststenotic dilation of the descending aorta. Sometimes there is a longer segment of narrowing of the isthmus and the left subclavian artery may be involved in the narrow area and be quite small. Occasionally, an anomalous right subclavian artery arises from the descending aorta just below the coarcted area. In some children, the stenosis is eccentric, with an appearance similar to that seen in early infancy and a ductus ampulla may still be present. The internal mammary and intercostal arteries and other vessels involved in the collateral circulation are large and tortuous and are usually seen clearly. If collateral vessels are not noted, one should examine the information carefully to assess the severity of the coarctation. Many consider this an important consideration at the time of surgery (see Chapter 12).

With aortic interruption, contrast injection into the ascending aorta shows it is usually narrower than normal and smaller than the main pulmonary artery. In type C interruption, neither the left carotid nor the subclavian artery fills from the ascending aorta. In type B interruption, the innominate and left carotid arteries fill, but the left subclavian artery does not. In type A interruption, all three great vessels arising from the arch will fill with contrast, but none crosses the isthmus to the descending aorta. Contrast injection into the pulmonary artery shows a large vessel with prompt filling of the ductus arteriosus and descending aorta. In type A interruption, the left subclavian artery is well visualized, unless the orifice is constricted. The descending aorta is usually quite large; if the right subclavian artery has not been seen to arise normally from the innominate artery on ultrasound examination, it should be noted whether it has an anomalous origin from the descending aorta.

Contrast injection into other sites will be determined by need, based on the ability of the ultrasound study to define the other lesions present. Thus left or right ventricular injections may be deemed necessary. As mentioned above, a difficult diagnosis to make with assurance by ultrasound examination is that of truncus arteriosus communis with interrupted arch. Similar difficulties arise with angiography; an injection into the truncus shows filling of the ascending aorta and some of its branches. The pulmonary arteries, ductus arteriosus, and descending aorta are also visualized. The sweep of the ductus arteriosus to the descending aorta may easily be interpreted as the aortic arch. If an arch interruption is present, the arteries arising distal to the interruption will fill from the descending aorta by retrograde flow. The exact sequence of filling of the left carotid and subclavian arteries may be difficult to define. An injection of contrast material at the upper end of the descending aorta may help to clarify the filling sequence by showing contrast entering the left subclavian or left carotid artery or both, with a blind end to the aorta proximally.

Differential diagnosis

The diagnosis of aortic arch interruption should be considered if femoral pulses are weak compared with arm or carotid pulses. However, difficulties frequently arise in infants with cardiac failure, in whom all pulses may be weak. Sometimes, the finding of a low pressure with a damped appearance arouses suspicion concerning the diagnosis when an umbilical arterial catheter is passed into the descending aorta. The finding may be discarded as merely representing a problem of catheter position, but if the tip is in the aorta, the possibility that there is aortic obstruction should be considered. As mentioned above, in some infants, although it is unusual, the pressure may be higher in the lower as compared with the upper extremities.

The most frequent problem is that the diagnosis is not considered in a severely ill infant in failure. In all patients with lesions commonly associated with aortic coarctation or interruption, such as double-outlet right ventricle, aortopulmonary transposition with ventricular septal defect and tricuspid atresia or narrowing of the right ventricular outflow, atrioventricular septal defect, or large ventricular septal defect with septal malalignment, the possibility should be considered. I do not propose to discuss the differential diagnosis of the associated lesions in this section, as it is presented in the chapters relating to these defects.

Localized aortic coarctation may also be diagnosed readily in infants by palpation of arm and leg pulses and measurement of pressures. When severe cardiac failure is present, the diagnosis of aortic atresia, severe aortic stenosis, or myocarditis may be considered because all the pulses are weak. The clinical examination is not particularly helpful in differentiation, nor is the chest radiograph; the electrocardiogram is similar in aortic stenosis and coarctation of the aorta, but may show low voltage with severe ST- and T-wave changes with myocarditis. In infants with aortic atresia, right axis deviation and marked right ventricular hypertrophy are accompanied by paucity of left ventricular forces. The diagnosis is usually made by ultrasound examination. As mentioned above, imaging of the isthmus region of the aorta and the site of the ductus arteriosus connection may be challenging in infants and often requires a skilled echocardiographer to diagnose or exclude aortic coarctation. The use of Doppler flow techniques to examine velocities at the site of coarctation and in the descending aorta has been helpful.

In older children, there is usually no difficulty in making the diagnosis by palpating pulses in arms and legs and measuring blood pressures. A lesion in which blood pressure in the arms may be higher than that in the legs and which must be distinguished from coarctation at the usual juxtaductal site is abdominal aortic coarctation. This lesion may cause a continuous murmur in the abdomen. If the ultrasound study does not demonstrate the coarctation in the usual site in a patient with pressure difference between the upper and lower extremities, the abdominal aorta should be imaged carefully for the presence of obstruction. Segmental obstruction of the distal descending thoracic or abdominal aorta may occur with Takayasu arteritis, neurofibromatosis, and Williams syndrome. The term "middle aortic syndrome" has been applied to this obstructive disease [13]. Not uncommonly, stenosis of celiac, mesenteric, and renal arteries is also present. The clinical findings are indistinguishable from coarctation. The obstruction is more diffuse than in juxtaductal coarctation; it was diagnosed by aortography, but could probably be identified now by ultrasound study. Aortic obstruction in the abdominal portion of the descending aorta has been encountered in children with Williams syndrome.

Principles of management

Aortic arch interruption

The initial management of infants with arch interruption is concerned with correction of acidemia and treatment of cardiac failure. In addition, because DiGeorge syndrome is commonly associated, serum calcium concentrations should be carefully monitored and hypocalcemia treated. PGE_1 should be administered by intravenous infusion to dilate the ductus arteriosus, thus increasing descending aortic pressure and blood flow and reducing the risks of acidemia and the risk of renal complications. Prior to infusion of PGE_1, the administration of high percentages of oxygen in inspired air is not recommended, because the high Po_2 that results may cause increased constriction of the ductus arteriosus. For treatment of cardiac failure, diuretic agents should be administered. These procedures will improve metabolic disturbances, but the cardiac failure from the associated lesions frequently does not respond and, as mentioned above, may become worse as a result of reduction of pulmonary vascular resistance by PGE_1. Surgery is indicated to establish communication between the segments of the aorta. In early surgical attempts to correct aortic interruption, mortality was very high. Various surgical techniques were attempted. One technique that was developed for type A interruption was to sever the left subclavian artery and anastomose the proximal end to the descending aorta (Blalock–Park anastomosis). Although it was often successful, it could not be performed if the left subclavian artery was small or if the aorta was interrupted above the left subclavian artery. In type B interruption, some suggested connecting the left common carotid artery by an end-to-side anastomosis to the descending aorta. Although there is concern that the procedure may interfere with blood supply to the brain, it has been performed successfully. However, little information is available regarding long-term neurological effects or intellectual development. In recent years techniques have been modified to avoid sacrificing either the left carotid or subclavian artery; instead surgeons perform an end-to-side anastomosis of the descending aorta to the inferior surface of the arch proximal to the interruption. This is now being performed in many centers with little mortality and establishment of excellent communication with no residual obstruction.

After correction of the interruption, a decision has to be made about the associated lesions. Past experience was that additional surgical procedures were associated with a very high mortality. The tendency has been to limit additional surgery to what was considered necessary to palliate the infant and to delay intracardiac repair until the infant was older. Thus in infants with ventricular septal defects, pulmonary arterial banding has been performed to limit the size of the left-to-right shunt and thus reduce the likelihood of left ventricular failure. It is often difficult to gauge the degree to which the pulmonary artery should be constricted, particularly in the neonatal period, when pulmonary vascular resistance is still elevated. Frequently, the band is found to be inadequate after the infant has recovered from the procedure. However, the main concern is that significant left ventricular outflow obstruction becomes manifest within 1–2 months after surgery in 40–50% of these individuals. The likelihood for significant subaortic stenosis can, to some extent, be predicted by assessing the degree of posterior deviation of the ventricular septum and estimating the subaortic diameter prior to surgery. Relief of the subaortic stenosis can prove to be difficult (see Chapter 10). It has therefore become practice to close the ventricular septal defect and resect subaortic tissue at the same time as the interruption is corrected. Although the surgical procedure is formidable, in recent years excellent results have been achieved with relatively low mortality.

With some lesions such as truncus arteriosus and aortopulmonary transposition, it is also now the practice to attempt to achieve repair of the other defects at the time the interruption is corrected. The repair of truncus arteriosus and interrupted arch is associated with a high mortality, almost 50% with the procedure itself and about 66% by 6 months [14]. About 20% of the infants have associated truncal valve insufficiency and about 10% have truncal valve stenosis. If the infant has features suggestive of DiGeorge syndrome, or has a 22q11 deletion, it may be necessary to treat hypocalcemia related to hypoparathyroidism and, depending on the severity of immunodeficiency, to treat this disorder appropriately.

Juxtaductal coarctation

The infant who presents with decreased flow to the lower body and with acute cardiac failure should be treated with appropriate measures. If necessary, hypoglycemia and hypocalcemia should be corrected; although it was common practice to administer sodium bicarbonate if there was metabolic acidemia with reduction of pH to less than 7.2, this is not considered to be beneficial and could be harmful [11,12]. Diuretic agents should be administered for treatment of cardiac failure. Administration of digoxin was widely recommended, but in recent years the benefit of digitalis preparations has been questioned and they are not frequently used. Inotropic agents such as dopamine, dobutamine and milrinone have been used in treatment of circulatory failure, but their effectiveness is now also being questioned. Intravenous infusion of PGE_1 should be started promptly to attempt to dilate the ductus arteriosus. The action of PGE_1 on the ductus varies somewhat depending on postnatal age; it is usually very effective within the first week, but becomes less so after 10–14 days. However, it is advisable to administer PGE_1 even as long as 4–6 weeks after birth, because occasionally it may have an effect. Nevertheless, if it is evident that it is not being effective, as evidenced by improved perfusion of the lower extremities and improvement of cardiac failure, the infusion should be stopped. These measures are instituted to improve the baby's metabolic and circulatory status prior to surgery.

In past years, the mortality from surgery to correct aortic coarctation in infants was extraordinarily high. It was therefore common practice to try to treat the infant actively for cardiac failure and delay surgery beyond the first year, often to the age of 3–4 years. Although treatment in the neonatal period was often effective, a number of the infants succumbed during the first year as a result of persistent cardiac failure, frequently associated with a respiratory infection. With improvement in surgical and anesthetic techniques, the mortality in infants has fallen dramatically, but there is a high incidence of so-called re-coarctation when the procedure is performed in early infancy.

Controversy exists about the mechanisms for the restenosis following surgery. The procedure that was first used was end-to-end anastomosis of the two ends of the aorta after excising the coarcted segment. One concern was that if an adequate segment of aorta was not removed, some ductus tissue may have remained and this constricted and caused the obstruction. Another explanation was that anastomosis of the ends of the aorta by means of a continuous suture technique did not permit circumferential growth. Therefore the surgery was modified so that a continuous suture was used in the posterior portion of the anastomosis and interrupted sutures anteriorly. However, despite more extensive removal of the aorta and modification of suture technique, the incidence of postoperative obstruction was still substantial. The main concern was that a narrowed isthmus or more extensive tubular hypoplasia of the arch was an important contributor to postoperative obstruction. Several other surgical techniques have been developed. Patch repair was in vogue for some time; it allowed for more extensive opening along a greater length of the aorta that could extend onto a narrowed arch. It was important to excise the posterior shelf and heterograft material such as Teflon or Gore-Tex was used anteriorly. Although this procedure was readily accomplished, it is now rarely performed because there is a high incidence of subsequent aneurysm formation either opposite the patch or along its edge. In some centers the incidence of aneurysm has been almost 40% in patients in whom patch aortoplasty has been used for repair of aortic coarctation.

The subclavian flap technique was designed to relieve isthmus narrowing as well as juxtaductal coarctation. The left subclavian artery was severed and a longitudinal incision was made on the undersurface of the proximal segment and extended through the isthmus and coarctation to the descending aorta. The subclavian artery was then turned down and its edges sutured to the edges of the aortic incision. The vertebral artery was ligated to avoid a steal syndrome. It was hoped that this technique would be more successful than end-to-end anastomosis in avoiding re-coarctation. However, it has not been very successful in doing so and, in addition, some children have poor development and weakness of the left arm as a result of ligation of the subclavian artery. The technique is still used in some infants, but is not generally favored.

Great interest has been generated in attempting to relieve coarctation of the aorta by balloon angioplasty. The gradient across the obstruction can be successfully reduced, thus avoiding surgery in acutely ill infants. However, the initial enthusiasm for the procedure has not persisted, because a relatively high incidence of aneurysm formation has been observed several months to 2–3 years after the procedure. Furthermore, the incidence of recurrent coarctation is very high in infants with patent ductus arteriosus in whom the coarctation was relieved by balloon angioplasty. The use of balloon angioplasty as the first procedure in infants is now not genarally recommended.

Because the results of surgery in infants have been suboptimal, some pediatric cardiologists attempted to avoid surgery until a later age. If cardiac failure could be controlled by medical therapy, it was recommended that surgery be delayed to the age of 3–5 years. The aortic diameter reaches about 50–60% of adult diameter by 3–4 years of age. Based on acute studies which showed that a significant gradient did not develop until aortic diameter was reduced by 50%, it was hypothesized that even if the aorta did not grow after surgery, its diameter would be adequate even in adult life. There are several concerns about this approach. Even though the infant may respond to medical measures, past experience has shown that a number of these infants die during the first year as a result of worsening of cardiac failure in association with a respiratory infection. If the infant manifests significant upper body hypertension, left ventricular hypertrophy may be marked and myocardial fibrosis will possibly develop.

A recent surgical approach has achieved more successful results in neonates with coarctation. The aortic arch and its major branches are mobilized, as is the cranial portion of the descending aorta. The aortic isthmus is ligated beyond the left subclavian artery and the aorta severed beyond the suture. The segment of aorta including the coarctation and ductus tissue is excised. A longitudinal incision is made along the inferior surface of the arch and the distal end of the descending aorta is connected to this incision by end-to-side anastomosis. This procedure has the advantage that it avoids any residual arch narrowing and also is performed using only natural tissue. The results of this approach have been remarkably good; no mortality has been associated and re-coarctation is uncommon [15]. If these results can be achieved generally, it is likely that the majority of individuals with coarctation will be repaired in infancy.

Balloon angioplasty and stenting

Initial percutaneous approaches to relieve aortic coarctation were performed by balloon angioplasty. In early studies, there were many complications, with tears in the aortic wall and the development of aneurysms, particularly in infants. Many of the difficulties were probably related to attempts to achieve complete relief of obstruction with large balloons. In several centers the procedure was abandoned as the original approach for the treatment of native coarctation. However, it was used in relieving obstruction in patients who had developed restenosis after a previous surgical approach. The presence of fibrosis around the aorta appeared to provide protection against tears and aneurysm formation. Subsequently, with the use of intravascular stents, procedures have been more successful.

In a recent review of stenting performed on 588 patients above 4 years of age in 17 institutions, complications including aortic dissection, aortic aneurysm and restenosis due to stent fracture or neointimal growth did occur, but they were fewer than with balloon angioplasty. In this series aortic dissection was significantly more likely to occur in patients above the age of 40 years [16,17]. These procedures were done in older patients and there is still a reluctance to perform procedures in infants. Although ballon dilation could be accomplished in neonates, the incidence of restenosis was very high (as much as 80%), but relief could be obtained by subsequent procedures [18]. In older children and adults, the results achieved with use of stents are superior to those of angioplasty, but their use in infants is not recommended because the diameter will be restricted with growth. A stent consisting of two stent halves connected by resorbable sutures has been developed for use in infants. It is suggested it will be possible to distend the aorta by inserting a new stent if restriction occurs with growth [19]. The success of this device is yet to be demonstrated.

Recommendations and prognosis

I am of the opinion that surgery, using the end-to side anastomosis described above, is still the favored approach for treatment of coarctation of the aorta in infants. It has very low mortality and excellent results, with no significant residual pressure gradient from upper to lower extremities. In older patients, stenting is a reasonable option, but there is still a modest incidence of complications and the long-term success and freedom from complications is yet to be assessed.

Coarctation may be first recognized in older children or adults because they are found to have hypertension or weak or absent lower extremity pulses. In the past, it was recommended that surgery be performed at about 7–8 years of age, because the aorta has attained almost adult size at this age. It was thought that if the anastomosed area did not grow after surgery, no significant obstruction would develop with increasing age. However, with improvement in surgical techniques, there appears to be little reason to delay treatment. Also, with the increasing use of stents, there seems to be little indication to delay relief of the obstruction.

Children and adults who have a small pressure difference between the upper and lower extremities present a difficult problem. This could be due to the fact that although coarctation is severe, a well-developed collateral circulation will reduce upper body hypertension and provide good flow to the lower extremities. The severity of the stenosis can usually be assessed by ultrasound studies. Those individuals who have mild coarctation are not likely to have a well-developed collateral circulation. If the aorta is completely occluded during the surgical reanastomosis, flow to the descending aorta may be severely limited and it has been thought that paraplegia may occur in rare instances. It is not yet known for certain what causes paraplegia following repair of coarctation. One hypothesis is that it results if several intercostal arteries are ligated in an attempt to mobilize the aorta. The intercostal arteries provide anterior spinal arteries to the spinal cord and it is suggested that if several of these arteries are eliminated, paraplegia may result. However, some surgeons recommend placing a temporary shunt in patients with mild coarctation to provide descending aortic flow while the anastomosis is performed. However, with the introduction of percutaneous techniques for stent insertion, this is no longer an issue.

The complications of coarctation surgery are relatively few. Hemorrhage from severed collateral arteries may occur and hemorrhage from the site of the anastomosis may require further surgery to control bleeding. Postoperatively, blood pressure in the upper body usually falls, but occasionally it does not and may actually increase temporarily. Currently, it is recommended that if hypertension persists or becomes more severe after surgery, it should be treated with antihypertensive agents in order to reduce the risk of postoperative bleeding as well as the likelihood for development of so-called post-coarctectomy syndrome. This is an acute intestinal crisis, associated with extensive hemorrhagic necrosis of the small bowel. The actual mechanism of this lesion is not known, but it has been suggested that it may be associated with a sudden release of the obstruction in the aorta and exposure of the mesenteric arteries to the high arterial pressure of the upper body, resulting in arteriolar disruption and hemorrhage into the tissues of the gut. The condition should be suspected if severe abdominal pain, distension, and intestinal obstruction occur soon after surgery. Treatment is directed to reducing blood pressure with antihypertensive drugs and decompression of the gastrointestinal tract. It may be necessary to remove the damaged bowel. Other complications include chylothorax due to damage of the left thoracic duct and hoarseness due to recurrent laryngeal nerve palsy.

In order to avoid postoperative hypertension and its potential complications, recently some have recommended that antihypertensive therapy should be initiated either during surgery or immediately after surgery. The possibility that the renin–angiotensin system may be involved in the development of postoperative hypertension has been proposed. The angiotensin-converting enzyme inhibitor enalaprilat has been administered; although it reduced blood pressure, there is as yet no evidence to indicate it altered postoperative course [20].

The incidence of postprocedural hypertension is considerably less frequent after balloon or stent dilation than after surgery. This difference in response may be related to the fact that a group of patients undergoing surgical repair showed increased plasma catecholamine levels and plasma renin activity, whereas those subjected to balloon angioplasty showed no change in catecholamines or renin activity [21].

Surgical repair of aortic coarctation was initially believed to provide complete relief of systemic arterial hypertension. Residual or recurrent hypertension was thought to be related to incomplete relief of obstruction or to recurrent obstruction. It became apparent that when coarctation is corrected after the age of 20 years, there is a very high incidence of hypertension in later life, even with no demonstrable residual obstruction. Hypertension may persist if the obstruction is relieved in adolescents or adults [22]. Unfortunately, these studies have not related the severity of the coarctation and time of repair to the likelihood of adult hypertension.

From numerous investigations, it is now apparent that although more likely to occur if the repair is beyond childhood, hypertension is present in about 30% of patients who had relief of obstruction in infancy or early childhood. If those who had evidence of obstruction by ultrasound examination were excluded, 20% of these patients had hypertension [23]. However, repair of coarctation does reduce the risk of cerebral hemorrhage or cerebral vascular complications, as well as the risk of aortic rupture. Several reports have indicated that the arterial vessels in the upper extremities show reduced reactivity to endothelium-dependent vasodilation, whereas lower extremity arteries showed normal responses [24]. These arterial abnormalities could account for the persistent hypertension in patients after relief of coarctation. Whether these abnormal arterial responses are the result of the hypertension prior to repair of the obstruction or due to an inherent associated anomaly of the arterial wall is yet to be determined.

Although the effects of relief of coarctation on the risks for infective endocarditis are not known, in the past it was recommended that antibiotic prophylaxis for infective endocarditis be continued after surgery. This was considered important because many of these individuals have bicuspid aortic valves. However, with the changes in the recommendations for use of antibiotic prophylaxis for congenital cardiovascular malformations, prophylaxis for dental or other surgical procedures is no longer indicated [25].

Questions remain regarding prophylaxis after insertion of stents. Some recommend that prophylaxis be practiced for a period of about 6 months after stent introduction, by which time it is felt that endothelium would have covered the stent. There is no evidence to support this recommendation, nor is there any evidence to support use of prophylaxis beyond this time.

References

1 Rosenberg HS. Coarctation of the aorta: morphology and pathogenetic considerations. Perspect Pediatr Pathol 1973;1:339–368.

2 Angelini A, Allan LD, Anderson RH, Crawford DC, Chita SK, Ho SY. Measurements of the dimensions of the aortic and pulmonary pathways in the human fetus: a correlative echocardiographic and morphometric study. Br Heart J 1988;60:221–226.

3 Hornberger LK, Weintraub RG, Pesonen E *et al.* Echocardiographic study of the morphology and growth of the aortic arch in the human fetus. Observations related to the prenatal diagnosis of coarctation. Circulation 1992; 66:741–747.

4 Celoria GC, Patton RB. Congenital absence of the aortic arch. Am Heart J 1959;58:407–413.

5 Rudolph AM, Heymann MA, Spitznas U. Hemodynamic considerations in the development of narrowing of the aorta. Am J Cardiol 1972;30:514–525.

6 Towbin JA, McQuinn TC. Gridlock: a model for coarctation of the aorta? Nat Med 1995;1:1141–1142.

7 Hutchins G. Coarctation of the aorta explained as a branch point of the ductus arteriosus. Am J Pathol 1971;63:203–214.

8 Allan LD, Chita SK, Anderson RH, Fagg N, Crawford DC, Tynan MJ. Coarctation of the aorta in prenatal life: an echocardiographic, anatomical, and functional study. Br Heart J 1988;59:356–60.

9 Hornung TS, Heads A, Hunter AS. Right ventricular dilatation in the fetus: a study of associated features and outcome. Pediatr Cardiol 2001;22:215–217.

10 Stos B, Le Bidois J, Fermont L, Bonnet D. Is antenatal diagnosis of coarctation of the aorta possible? Arch Mal Coeur 2007;100:428–432.

11 Forsythe SM, Schmidt GA. Sodium bicarbonate for the treatment of lactic acidosis. Chest 2000;117:260–267.

12 Weil MH, Tang W. Management of acidosis: the role of buffer agents. Crit Care 1997;1:51–52.

13 Delis KT, Gloviczki P. Middle aortic syndrome: from presentation to contemporary open surgical endovascular treatment. Perspect Vasc Surg Endovasc Ther 2005;17:187–203.

14 Konstantinov IE, Karamlou T, Blackstone EH *et al.* Truncus arteriosus associated with interrupted aortic arch in 50 neonates: a Congenital Heart Surgeons Society study. Ann Thorac Surg 2006;81:214–222.

15 Younoszai AK, Reddy VM, Hanley FL, Brook MM. Intermediate term follow-up of the end-to-side aortic anastomosis for coarctation of the aorta. Ann Thorac Surg 2002;74:1631–1634.

16 Forbes TJ, Garekar S, Amin Z *et al.* Procedural results and acute complications in stenting native and recurrent coarctation of the aorta in patients over 4 years of age: a multi-institutional study. Catheter Cardiovasc Intervent 2007;70:276–285.

17 Forbes TJ, Moore P, Pedra CA *et al.* Intermediate follow-up following intravascular stenting for treatment of coarctation of the aorta. Catheter Cardiovasc Intervent 2007;70:569–577.

18 Rao PS, Galal O, Smith PA, Wilson AD. Five- to nine-year follow-up results of balloon angioplasty of native aortic coarctation in infants and children. J Am Coll Cardiol 1996;27:462–470.

19 Ewert P, Peters B, Nagdyman N, Miera O, Kühne T, Berger F. Early and mid-term results with the Growth Stent: a possible concept for transcatheter treatment of aortic coarctation from infancy to adulthood by stent implantation? Catheter Cardiovasc Intervent 2008;71: 120–126.

20 Rouine-Rapp K, Mello DM, Hanley FL, Mohan Reddy V, Soifer S. Effect of enalaprilat on postoperative hypertension after surgical repair of coarctation of the aorta. Pediatr Crit Care Med 2003;4:327–332.

21 Choy M, Rocchini AP, Beekman RH *et al.* Paradoxical hypertension after repair of coarctation of the aorta in children: balloon angioplasty versus surgical repair. Circulation 1987;75:1186–1191.

22 Hashemzadeh K, Hashemzadeh S, Kakaei F. Repair of coarctation in adults: the fate of hypertension. Asian Cardiovasc Thorac Ann 2008;16:11–15.

23 O'Sullivan JJ, Derrick G, Darnell R. Prevalence of hypertension in children after early repair of coarctation of the aorta: a cohort study using casual and 24 hour blood pressure measurement. Heart 2002;88:163–166.

24 Gardiner HM, Celermajer DS, Sorensen KE *et al.* Arterial reactivity is significantly impaired in normotensive young adults after successful repair of aortic coarctation in childhood. Circulation 1994;89:1745–1750.

25 Wilson W, Taubert KA, Gewitz M *et al.* Prevention of infective endocarditis: guidelines from the American Heart Association: a guideline from the American Heart Association Rheumatic Fever, Endocarditis and Kawasaki Disease Committee, Council on Cardiovascular Disease in the Young, and the Council on Clinical Cardiology, Council on Cardiovascular Surgery and Anesthesia, and the Quality of Care and Outcomes Research Interdisciplinary Working Group. Circulation 2007;116:1736–1754.

13

CHAPTER 13

Total anomalous pulmonary venous connection

Anomalous connection of the pulmonary veins to the systemic venous system instead of to the left atrium may be partial or complete. When one or two veins are connected directly to the systemic veins or the right atrium, the lesion behaves physiologically very much like an atrial septal defect, and it is discussed in Chapter 8.

The early literature on this anomaly was concerned with the anatomical variations of the pulmonary veins and whether they connected directly with the right atrium, with the coronary sinus, through the vertical vein, or with the hepatoportal venous system. Descriptions of the clinical features of total anomalous pulmonary venous return were based largely on whether the connection to the systemic venous system was supradiaphragmatic or infradiaphragmatic. It was generally assumed that when the drainage was supradiaphragmatic, the individual had only mild cyanosis and few if any symptoms in early life. The triad of cyanosis, a small heart, and "pale" lungs in early infancy was widely accepted as being indicative of infradiaphragmatic drainage of the pulmonary veins. Although these anatomical classifications are important in understanding disturbances in embryological development and to the surgical management of these lesions, they do not necessarily explain the clinical features. The physiological effects are largely determined by the presence or absence of an actual or effective obstruction to drainage of the pulmonary veins into the right atrium. The persistence of fetal vascular communications also affects the hemodynamic and clinical presentation during the neonatal period.

Congenital Diseases of the Heart, 3rd edition. By A. Rudolph
 ISBN: 9781405162456

Morphological considerations

There is considerable variation in the manner in which anomalous pulmonary veins connect to the systemic venous system. Only the more common syndromes are discussed in this chapter.

Connection to the superior vena cava

Supracardiac connection of the pulmonary veins occurs in almost half of all patients. They may connect via the vertical vein or directly to the superior vena cava (SVC) [1].

Via the left innominate vein

The pulmonary veins may all drain into the SVC through the left innominate vein. The four pulmonary veins join behind the left atrium and connect to the vertical vein, which sometimes has been designated the persistent left SVC. The vertical vein ascends to join the left innominate vein; it is usually anterior to the left pulmonary artery and the left bronchus and is not commonly obstructed. However, it may be constricted if it passes between the left bronchus posteriorly and the left pulmonary artery anteriorly. Occasionally, the vertical vein and left innominate vein are somewhat narrowed along the whole length; rarely, there may be an obstruction at the junction of the vertical and innominate veins.

Via the right SVC

The pulmonary veins may drain directly into the right SVC. They join behind the heart and a common trunk runs to the posterior aspect of the SVC just above the junction with the right atrium, or it may connect to the right azygous vein. Sometimes the right upper pulmonary vein joins the trunk as it enters the vena cava. The connection of the trunk to the vena cava frequently has a small orifice that may produce considerable obstruction to flow. When the veins drain into the azygous vein, the small size of the vessel may produce obstruction. Obstruction to drainage is present in more than half of these patients. This type of drainage is encountered particularly in individuals with right atrial isomerism or asplenia syndrome. Although almost 90% of patients with asplenia syndrome have total anomalous pulmonary venous return, the connection varies and may be infradiaphragmatic or supradiaphragmatic. The pulmonary veins may be small and not infrequently may be stenosed. The abnormal anatomical connection is usually not of great hemodynamic significance if the pulmonary veins are not obstructed, because usually large atrial or ventricular communications are also present, so that it is relatively immaterial which atrium receives the pulmonary venous blood. However, it becomes very important if the pulmonary venous drainage is obstructed and if surgery is contemplated.

Connection to the heart directly

In about 20% of individuals with total anomalous pulmonary venous connection, the veins may connect to the coronary sinus or directly to the right atrium. The four veins may enter a greatly dilated sac of the coronary sinus behind the right atrium, and this drains through an enlarged coronary sinus orifice. Usually this orifice is widely dilated so that no obstruction exists, but occasionally it is narrow and somewhat obstructed.

When all the veins connect with the right atrium, the four veins may drain independently into the right atrium or the two right or left veins may join just prior to entering the posterior aspect of the atrium. It is most unusual for these veins to be obstructed, but on occasion one or more veins may be narrowed at their junction with the right atrium.

Connection to the hepatoportal system

In about 25% of patients with total anomalous connection, the drainage is infradiaphragmatic. In the usual arrangement, the four pulmonary veins join behind the heart, and from the confluence a single trunk descends anterior to the esophagus and through the esophageal hiatus in the diaphragm. However, in some patients, the upper veins join to form a channel and the lower veins enter as tributaries to this channel, sometimes at different levels. The trunk connects most commonly with the portal vein near the junction of the splenic and superior mesenteric veins, less frequently with the ductus venosus and, rarely, with the left hepatic vein or inferior vena cava (IVC). The common trunk may be wide, but its entrance into the portal or systemic vein may be narrow, and occasionally the whole trunk is quite narrow. It may be compressed where it passes through the diaphragm.

Mixed types

All the pulmonary veins may drain into the systemic venous system, but in about 10% of patients they may not all drain into the same site. Many different types of mixed drainage may be encountered. Thus the left pulmonary veins may drain into the portal vein, whereas the right veins may enter the coronary sinus or the SVC. The left pulmonary veins may enter the left innominate vein through a vertical vein, and the right veins may enter the coronary sinus. Other combinations of mixed drainage may occur; also, drainage to one site may be obstructed, while the other veins may not be obstructed. A rare condition has been described that behaves effectively like total anomalous pulmonary venous drainage. All the pulmonary veins enter the left atrium, mitral atresia is present, and the foramen ovale is closed. A single vein, the levoatriocardinal vein, leaves the left atrium and is connected to the left innominate vein.

Pulmonary venous stenosis

Stenosis of individual pulmonary veins has been noted in association with total anomalous connection of the veins. It is difficult to assess the incidence of these lesions, because many have first been noted after surgery and it is not known whether the stenosis was present prior to the procedure. The pulmonary veins may be narrowed along the whole length, with thickening of the intima and fibrosis of the wall, or only a short segment may be involved. The lesions have been noted in neonates who had not been subjected to surgery, so it is apparent they can develop in the fetus. It is not known what causes stenosis of pulmonary veins, but it is possible that the intimal proliferation is induced by intrauterine pulmonary venous hypertension, which could be the result of severe obstruction of pulmonary venous drainage. The stenoses may involve both the left and right veins but may be unilateral and may involve only one vessel. It is possible that one or more pulmonary veins may be obstructed postoperatively, by being involved in the healing process close to the site of the anastomosis to the left atrium. Pulmonary venous stenosis following surgery is a poor prognostic sign, especially if it is bilateral (see Chapter 13).

Embryological considerations

The embryological disturbances leading to the development of anomalous pulmonary venous connections are still obscure. Normally, the pulmonary vascular bed is derived from the splanchnic plexus, because the lungs develop as an outpouching from the foregut. In the early embryo there is no connection between the primitive pulmonary vascular bed and the heart. The pulmonary segment of the splanchnic plexus is drained by the left and right cardinal and umbilicovitelline systems. A projection grows from the dorsal side of the atrium just to the left of the septum primum and this common pulmonary venous trunk connects to the primitive pulmonary venous system. Later, the common pulmonary venous trunk is absorbed into the left atrium so that the pulmonary veins are connected directly to the left atrium. The left cardinal vein becomes the left side of the sinus venosus and eventually the coronary sinus and left SVC. The right cardinal vein provides the right side of the sinus venosus and subsequently the right SVC and azygous vein. The umbilicovitelline system eventually gives rise to the portal vein, the ductus venosus, and a portion of the IVC.

One hypothesis proposes that the common pulmonary venous trunk becomes atretic before the other connections of the pulmonary circulation to the systemic venous system are obliterated. One or another of these connections enlarges to create the major drainage pathway for the pulmonary veins to the systemic veins. Thus, if the connection to the right common cardinal system becomes dominant, all the pulmonary veins will drain into the SVC or azygous veins. If the left common cardinal vein connection persists, the pulmonary veins will drain into the left innominate vein or the coronary sinus. Persistence of the communication with the umbilicovitelline system will result in drainage into the portal venous system, the ductus venosus or, rarely, the hepatic veins.

Although this hypothesis does provide an explanation, it does not consider why one or another major pathway of drainage may persist.

Hemodynamic considerations

Fetal circulation

Little information is available regarding the influence of total anomalous pulmonary venous return on the fetal circulation. The lesion does not appear to influence fetal development and infants born with the anomaly are usually normally developed at birth. The discussion that follows considers the possible changes in the fetal circulation that may result from this anomaly.

Alteration of Po_2 in arterial blood to upper and lower body

In the normal fetus most of the SVC blood, which has a relatively low oxygen saturation, is directed through the tricuspid valve into the right ventricle and pulmonary artery. The Po_2 of pulmonary arterial blood in the fetal lamb is about 17 mmHg; because the fetal lung is metabolically active and consumes oxygen, the Po_2 of pulmonary venous blood is lower, usually about 14–15 mmHg. Left atrial blood in the fetus is derived largely from umbilical venous blood that passes through the ductus venosus and is then preferentially directed in the IVC through the foramen ovale (see Chapter 1). Distal IVC blood contributes only a small amount of flow through the foramen ovale. In the fetal lamb, foramen ovale flow contributes about two-thirds of blood entering the left atrium, whereas pulmonary venous return contributes somewhat less than one-third. This results in lowering of the Po_2 of left atrial blood, but the Po_2 of blood entering the left ventricle is considerably higher than that of blood in the right ventricle. This accounts for the higher Po_2 in the ascending aorta, which derives its blood from the left ventricle, as compared with the descending aorta, which derives most of its blood from the right ventricle through the ductus arteriosus (see Chapter 1).

The effects of infradiaphragmatic drainage of the portal veins would depend on the vessel to which

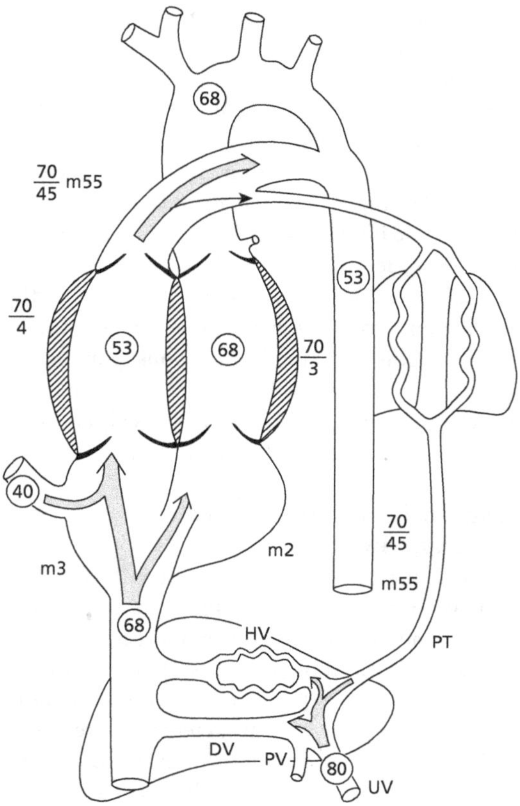

Figure 13.1 Total anomalous drainage of pulmonary veins to the portal vein in a fetus: course of the circulation, oxygen saturations (circled), and pressures. m, mean pressure; DV, ductus venosus; HV, hepatic vein; PT, pulmonary venous trunk; PV, portal vein; UV, umbilical vein.

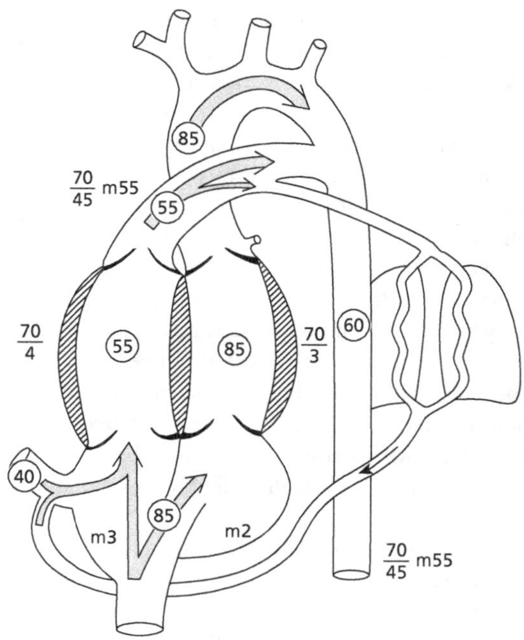

Figure 13.2 Total anomalous drainage of pulmonary veins to the superior vena cava in a fetus: course of the circulation, oxygen saturations (circled), and pressures. m, mean pressure.

they connect (Figure 13.1). If they drain into the ductus venosus, the blood would probably stream preferentially through the foramen ovale to the left atrium. Thus there would be no difference from the normal situation in which pulmonary venous blood enters the left atrium directly. If the pulmonary veins drain into the portal veins, most blood would enter the right lobe of the liver, since right hepatic venous blood streams preferentially through the tricuspid valve. The Po_2 of blood in the pulmonary vein is only slightly lower than that in the pulmonary artery; therefore pulmonary arterial oxygen saturation and Po_2 will not be significantly different from normal.

If all the pulmonary veins drain into the SVC stream, which almost exclusively passes through the tricuspid valve, no pulmonary venous blood would reach the left atrium. Therefore the normal small difference in the Po_2 between the upper and lower body could be exaggerated. Thus, blood with a higher than normal Po_2 could be delivered to the heart muscle and the brain, and blood with a lower than normal Po_2 would reach the lungs and the lower body organs (Figure 13.2). The higher oxygen level in blood distributed to the heart and brain probably has no significant effect. The lower Po_2 of blood in the lungs could induce pulmonary vasoconstriction and possibly increase pulmonary arteriolar smooth muscle development.

Development of the pulmonary circulation

If pulmonary venous return were not obstructed, pulmonary venous pressure would not be increased. Pulmonary blood flow in the fetus is low, so obstruction to pulmonary veins would have to be severe to produce pulmonary venous hypertension. Should this occur, however, reactive pulmonary arteriolar constriction with increased smooth muscle development could possibly result.

The combination of elevated venous pressure and decreased Po_2 of blood perfusing the lung could affect pulmonary vascular smooth muscle development. In a study of infants with total anomalous pulmonary venous connection with obstruction, pulmonary vascular smooth muscle was markedly increased in pulmonary arterioles, and more peripheral vessels also showed increased smooth muscle development [2]. An association between total anomalous pulmonary venous drainage and pulmonary lymphangiectasia has been noted; pulmonary venous hypertension may greatly increase transudation of fluid into the lung parenchyma and lymph flow will increase. Lymphangiectasia is frequently associated with neonatal mortality, because the infant is not able to establish effective ventilation.

Development of the left atrium and left ventricle

The body of the left atrium and the left ventricle are frequently small in infants with total anomalous pulmonary venous return. A lack of pulmonary venous drainage into the atrium has been incriminated as the cause of the underdevelopment. Although in the sheep fetus pulmonary blood flow represents only 15–20% of left ventricular output, in the human fetus it probably provides almost 50% of left ventricular ejection (see Chapter 1). It is possible that if pulmonary venous return to the left atrium were abolished, flow through the foramen ovale would compensate to maintain left ventricular output. However, there is no need for left ventricular output to be maintained, because right ventricular output could be adjusted to maintain adequate aortic flow through the ductus arteriosus. It is thus possible that no compensatory increase in umbilical venous or IVC blood occurs across the foramen ovale and that the abnormal flow dynamics could contribute to the small size of the left atrial and ventricular chambers.

Ultrasound study of fetuses with total anomalous pulmonary venous connection reveals a very characteristic finding of a small left atrial cavity, with inability to identify pulmonary veins entering the atrium. This contrasts with the fetus with tricuspid or pulmonary atresia with intact ventricular septum, in which the total umbilical and systemic venous return must pass through the foramen ovale; these infants have a large foraminal orifice and well-developed left atrium and ventricle after birth. The small size of the left atrium could also result from morphological factors; normally a portion of the left atrium is formed by incorporation of the pulmonary veins into the wall. If the veins drain abnormally, this contribution to the left atrial wall would be lacking. A small left atrium with low compliance could interfere with flow of blood across the foramen ovale and thus result in inadequate left ventricular development. Narrowing of the aortic isthmus and coarctation of the aorta may occur in association with total anomalous pulmonary venous drainage; these lesions could result from reduced left atrial filling and decreased left ventricular output in the fetus (see Chapter 12).

Postnatal adaptations and hemodynamics

When all the pulmonary veins return to the systemic venous system, complete admixture of pulmonary and systemic venous blood occurs at the right atrial level. Pulmonary and systemic arterial oxygen saturations tend to be equal, but saturation differences may result from preferential streaming of IVC blood across the foramen ovale; the effects of this streaming are discussed below. The lack of pulmonary venous return to the left atrium necessitates the presence of blood flow through an adequate atrial, ventricular or aortopulmonary communication to provide systemic blood flow. Because a large ventricular communication is unusual except in those instances in which pulmonary venous drainage anomaly is associated with asplenia or polysplenia syndrome, systemic blood flow is usually maintained through the foramen ovale and sometimes the ductus arteriosus. Flow from the pulmonary artery through the ductus arteriosus into the aorta can occur only if pulmonary arterial hypertension is present, and this would occur only if pulmonary vascular resistance is maintained at high levels.

Relationship between pulmonary and systemic blood flow and pulmonary and systemic arterial oxygen saturation

Complete admixture of pulmonary and systemic venous blood at the right atrial level will result in equal oxygen saturations in pulmonary and systemic arterial blood. The oxygen saturation of arterial blood is determined by the ratio of pulmonary to systemic blood flows (see Chapter 4). However, in the neonatal period, fetal patterns of venous blood flow may modify the oxygen saturations in the pulmonary and systemic arteries. IVC blood is preferentially directed through the foramen ovale to the left atrium, whereas SVC blood is directed through the tricuspid valve. If the pulmonary veins drain to the ductus venosus or portal vein, the oxygen saturation of IVC blood will be higher than that in the SVC. Preferential streaming of IVC blood across the foramen ovale would thus result in higher oxygen saturations in left ventricular and ascending aortic blood than in right ventricular and pulmonary arterial blood. If the ductus arteriosus is open and pulmonary arterial blood flows into the descending aorta, oxygen saturation in the ascending aorta and its branches will be higher than that in the descending aorta.

However, if the pulmonary veins all connect to the left innominate vein or SVC, the better-oxygenated blood would be preferentially distributed through the tricuspid valve; oxygen saturation in the pulmonary artery would be higher than that in the aorta. If the ductus arteriosus is open, flow from the pulmonary artery to the descending aorta will result in a higher oxygen saturation in the descending compared with the ascending aorta. The differences in oxygen saturations are unlikely to be encountered in those infants who also have a large atrial or ventricular communication, because this would further enhance mixing.

During the immediate neonatal period, while pulmonary vascular resistance is still maintained at relatively high levels, pulmonary blood flow will increase only modestly. The pulmonary to systemic blood flow ratio will thus be low, and therefore arterial oxygen saturation and Po_2 would be considerably reduced. The subsequent changes in arterial oxygen saturation vary depending on the hemodynamic developments. If pulmonary venous drainage is severely obstructed, pulmonary blood flow will be reduced and if systemic blood flow is maintained, the pulmonary to systemic flow ratio will decrease further and arterial oxygen saturation will fall to very low levels. This may be exaggerated further by a decrease in pulmonary venous oxygen saturation resulting from pulmonary edema.

In infants with mild or no obstruction to pulmonary venous return, as pulmonary vascular resistance falls, pulmonary blood flow progressively increases after birth, resulting in very large pulmonary to systemic flow ratios and thus relatively high systemic arterial oxygen saturations. Arterial oxygen saturations are frequently 85–88% in infants with unobstructed total anomalous pulmonary venous return and may be as high as 92% in older children and adults.

Restriction of the foramen ovale may occur in infants within the first few weeks after birth (see Chapter 13). This may interfere with flow through the foramen ovale, thus restricting systemic blood flow. Pulmonary blood flow will be very high if pulmonary veins are not obstructed. This will result in a very high pulmonary to systemic blood flow ratio and high arterial oxygen saturation.

Systemic blood flow

Systemic blood flow must be provided from the right side of the heart when all the pulmonary venous blood enters the systemic venous system. In the absence of a ventricular septal communication, it is derived via the foramen ovale or the ductus arteriosus, or both. If flow through the ductus arteriosus contributes to systemic flow, the right ventricle is responsible for providing a portion of the flow and the work of the ventricle is increased. If the foramen ovale provides all the systemic flow, the left ventricle maintains flow. As mentioned above, the left atrium and ventricle are often small and, possibly as a result of diminished flow into the left ventricle *in utero*, left ventricular development could be affected. It is thus possible that left ventricular function may be impaired. Others factors could also influence left ventricular output. The filling pressure of the right ventricle is somewhat higher than that of the left ventricle and ventricular septal displacement by the large volume in the right ventricle could interfere with left ventricular filling. Restriction of the foramen ovale could also be a factor in reducing flow into the left atrium and ventricle. Increases in afterload on the left ventricle, as would occur with systemic vasoconstriction associated with hypoxemia, limit left ventricular output; this would be particularly detrimental if left ventricular function is already somewhat reduced. Postnatally, left ventricular performance appears to be impaired in infants with obstructed pulmonary venous return, but this may reflect poor filling of the ventricle. After relief of obstruction and anastomosis of pulmonary veins to the left atrium, left ventricular function appears to improve, probably because filling is enhanced.

Pulmonary vascular resistance and pulmonary blood flow

The relationships between pulmonary blood flow and pulmonary vascular resistance are important in determining clinical manifestations in infants with obstructed pulmonary venous return. After birth, the increase in pulmonary blood flow associated with the fall in pulmonary vascular resistance results in increased flow in the pulmonary veins; if the veins are obstructed, pulmonary venous pressure becomes elevated. If plasma oncotic pressure is exceeded, increased transudation of fluid into the pulmonary alveoli will occur; when the rate of fluid accumulation exceeds the ability of lymphatic drainage to remove it, pulmonary edema results. This interferes with alveolar ventilation, decreasing the Po_2 to which the pulmonary arterioles are exposed, with resulting pulmonary vasoconstriction. Pulmonary arterial hypertension occurs for several reasons: the high pulmonary venous pressure results in passive pulmonary arterial hypertension, pulmonary vasoconstriction results from alveolar hypoxia, and pulmonary venous hypertension induces pulmonary arteriolar constriction. If there is no communication between the ventricles or between the aorta and pulmonary artery, pressure in the pulmonary artery often exceeds that in the aorta.

It is interesting to speculate on the effects of changes in pulmonary vascular resistance on pulmonary blood flow and pulmonary edema. An increase in pulmonary arterial pressure would tend to increase flow across the pulmonary vascular bed, raise pulmonary venous pressure, and aggravate pulmonary edema. However, pulmonary vasoconstriction would tend to reduce flow through the lungs into the pulmonary veins and thus tend to reduce edema. A balance would be established, but this could readily be upset by changes in pulmonary vascular resistance, such as may result with ventilation after birth or in neonates when assisted ventilation is altered. Also, the ductus arteriosus could have a profound influence on the dynamics of the circulation and on oxygen saturation levels (see Chapter 13).

Pulmonary vascular responses

When obstruction to pulmonary venous drainage is severe, the marked increase in pulmonary venous pressure and the alveolar hypoxia associated with pulmonary edema maintain a high pulmonary vascular resistance (see Chapter 13). Without treatment, these infants do not survive to an age where long-term changes in pulmonary vasculature can be assessed. In those individuals with no obstruction to pulmonary venous return, pulmonary vascular resistance undergoes the normal postnatal changes and pulmonary arterial pressure may be normal, but may show modest elevations to 30–40/15–20 mmHg associated with the marked increase in pulmonary blood flow. The effect of the high blood flow with shear effect on the pulmonary endothelium is similar to that observed in patients with large atrial septal defects (see Chapter 5). The medial smooth muscle layer undergoes normal regression after birth, but the endothelial cells proliferate and encroach on the lumen. As with atrial septal defect, these changes are not usually significant until late adolescence and in many patients do not develop to the extent of causing significant pulmonary vascular obstruction even in adult life. The rare individual develops severe intimal proliferative changes at any time from about 10 to 30 years. This results in progressive decrease in pulmonary blood flow, with increasing cyanosis.

The small pulmonary vessels may show some persistence of the medial smooth muscle layer after birth with moderate obstruction to pulmonary venous return because pulmonary arterial pressure and flow are elevated. The vessels are therefore subject to the development of intimal proliferative changes and pulmonary vascular obstruction (see Chapter 5).

Severe obstruction to pulmonary venous drainage

The degree of obstruction of the pulmonary venous trunk connecting the pulmonary veins to the systemic veins is one of the most important determinants of the hemodynamic effects and clinical manifestations of the anomaly.

Marked obstruction of pulmonary venous drainage was thought to occur only in infants with connection to the umbilicovitelline system. Most infants with infradiaphragmatic drainage do have obstruction; this may occur because the vessel draining the pulmonary venous confluence is narrow, or because it is compressed at its passage through the diaphragm. Narrowing at its junction with the portal vein or ductus venosus may also result in obstruction. If the vessel connects with the portal vein or the ductus venosus, significant obstruction may not become evident for several weeks or months, due to delayed closure of the ductus. The intrahepatic portal circulation may also impose resistance to return of pulmonary venous blood to the IVC. Although in the fetus the intrahepatic vasculature accommodates about 50% of umbilical venous return, in addition to portal venous flow, pulmonary venous flow after birth is considerably greater and may not be accommodated without a rise in venous pressure.

Almost 90% of infants with right atrial isomerism have total anomalous pulmonary venous drainage and one-third to half of these have severe obstruction. The pulmonary veins form a confluence behind the heart and may drain below the diaphragm into the portal venous system, or connect to the right SVC or to the azygous vein. If obstruction occurs with pulmonary venous drainage to the vertical vein, it is usually mild to moderate, but severe obstruction can occur. Severe obstruction is unusual with drainage through the coronary sinus.

Occasionally, with mixed types of drainage, the veins from one lung are obstructed whereas those from the other lung, draining to a different part of the systemic circulation, may be unimpeded. I have encountered one infant with unimpaired drainage of the right pulmonary veins into the coronary sinus, but the left veins drained into a vertical vein, which was obstructed. In another infant, the right veins entered the coronary sinus and the entrance of the coronary sinus into the right atrium was obstructed; the left veins passed infradiaphragmatically and were also obstructed.

Role of the foramen ovale

In the absence of a ventricular communication or a patent ductus arteriosus, systemic blood flow has to be provided by right-to-left shunting through an atrial septal opening, usually a patent foramen ovale. In the absence of pulmonary venous return to the left atrium, right atrial pressure exceeds left atrial pressure and, after birth, flow persists from the right atrium to the left atrium across the foramen ovale. In infants with severe obstruction to pulmonary venous drainage, the foramen ovale is usually large enough to provide adequate systemic blood flow with little elevation of right atrial pressure. Furthermore, the ductus arteriosus is often patent in the first few days and right-to-left shunt from the pulmonary artery to the aorta may contribute to systemic blood flow. Restriction of the foramen ovale is more likely to be encountered in infants with moderate or no pulmonary venous obstruction several weeks after birth (see Chapter 13).

Role of the ductus arteriosus

The ductus arteriosus may profoundly influence the hemodynamic and clinical consequences in infants with severe obstruction to pulmonary venous drainage. Severe obstruction induces pulmonary hypertension by the mechanisms discussed above. Because pulmonary vascular resistance is high, blood shunts from the pulmonary artery to the aorta through the ductus arteriosus; therefore, while the ductus is widely patent, pressure in the pulmonary artery cannot be raised above that in the systemic circulation. The diversion of blood through the ductus reduces flow through the pulmonary circulation. Pulmonary venous flow is reduced, pulmonary venous pressure is lowered, and thus less pulmonary edema is likely to develop. However, the decrease in pulmonary blood flow will restrict oxygen uptake in the lungs and, with the lower pulmonary to systemic blood flow ratio, systemic arterial oxygen saturation will be greatly decreased. This hypoxemia may result in a fall in systemic vascular resistance, which would further facilitate right-to-left shunting through the ductus and reduce pulmonary blood flow. Severe hypoxemia may, through sympathoadrenal stimulation, raise systemic vascular resistance and reduce right-to-left shunt through the ductus, as well as through the foramen ovale. Systemic blood flow would be reduced and tissue oxygen supply would be severely limited (see Chapter 3).

If the ductus arteriosus constricts or closes, the right-to-left shunt would be reduced or eliminated. Pulmonary arterial pressure could now be elevated and perfusion of the lungs would be enhanced. This would increase pulmonary venous flow, raise pulmonary venous pressure, and aggravate pulmonary edema. However, because pulmonary blood flow is increased, the arterial oxygen saturation may improve.

Role of the ductus venosus

When the pulmonary veins drain into the portal venous system, the ductus venosus may play an important role in the circulatory dynamics. During fetal life, a proportion of umbilical blood flow (50% on average) bypasses the hepatic capillary circulation through the ductus venosus. After birth, umbilical blood flow is eliminated and pulmonary blood flow increases. While the ductus venosus is patent, pulmonary venous blood returning to the portal vein can pass through it directly to the IVC, thus bypassing the hepatic circulation (Figure 13.3). If the ductus venosus is widely patent, pulmonary venous drainage may not be obstructed and pulmonary venous hypertension and pulmonary edema would not develop. Closure or inadequate growth of the ductus venosus would necessitate that pulmonary venous blood pass through the hepatic microcirculation; this will result in elevation of portal and pulmonary venous pressures and pulmonary edema may develop (Figures 13.4 and 13.5).

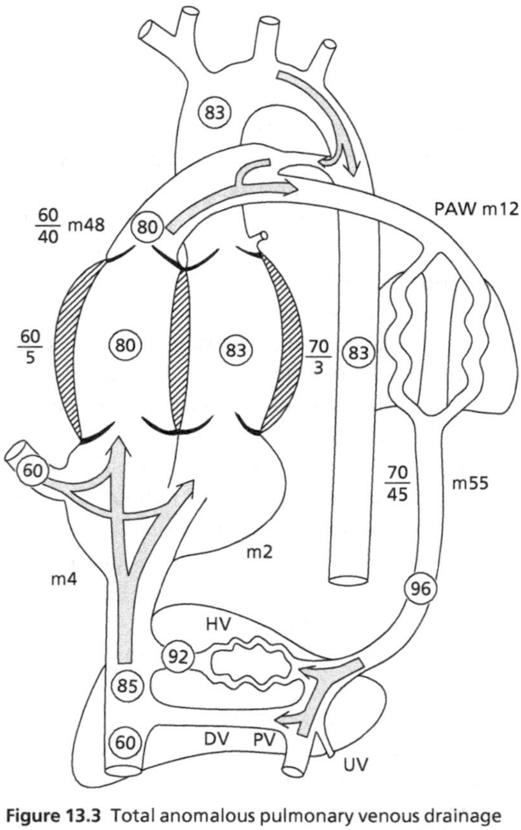

Figure 13.3 Total anomalous pulmonary venous drainage to the portal vein in a newborn infant: course of the circulation, oxygen saturations (circled), and pressures. The patency of the ductus venosus permits pulmonary blood flow to return to the systemic veins with minimal obstruction to flow. m, mean pressure; DV, ductus venosus; HV, hepatic vein; PAW, pulmonary artery wedge pressure; PV, portal vein; UV, umbilical vein.

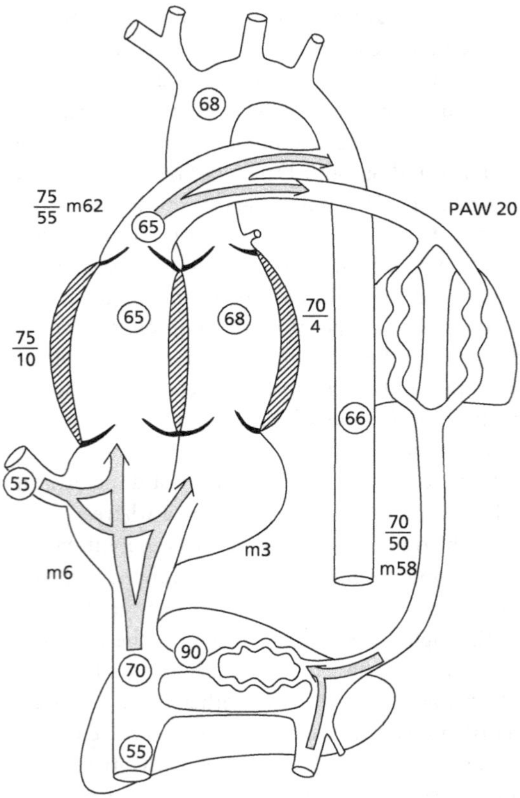

Figure 13.4 Total anomalous drainage of pulmonary veins to the portal vein in a newborn infant: course of the circulation, oxygen saturations (circled), and pressures. The ductus venosus is closed, but the ductus arteriosus is still open (see text for explanation). m, mean pressure; PAW, pulmonary artery wedge pressure.

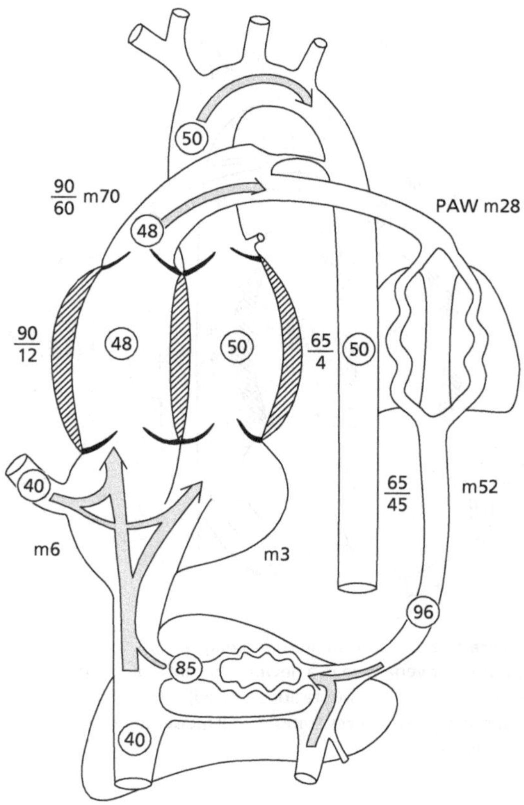

Figure 13.5 Total anomalous drainage of pulmonary veins to the portal vein in a newborn infant: course of the circulation, oxygen saturations (circled), and pressures. The ductus venosus and ductus arteriosus are both closed (see text for explanation). m, mean pressure; PAW, pulmonary artery wedge pressure.

Effect of pulmonary stenosis

Pulmonary stenosis or atresia is frequently one of the cardiac lesions associated with right atrial isomerism (asplenia syndrome) and may influence the clinical presentation of total anomalous pulmonary venous drainage, which is also common in this syndrome. Almost half of these infants also have obstruction to pulmonary venous drainage. With pulmonary atresia or severe pulmonary stenosis, pulmonary blood flow is provided through the ductus arteriosus or aortopulmonary collateral arteries. If pulmonary blood flow is derived mainly from the ductus, constriction of the ductus will decrease flow and cyanosis will be a prominent feature. Even if there is an anatomical obstruction to pulmonary venous drainage, significant pulmonary edema may not develop. The presence of the pulmonary venous drainage anomaly may not be recognized, because attention is directed to the severe hypoxemia. Dilation of the ductus arteriosus by prostaglandin (PG)E_1 infusion may increase pulmonary blood flow and pulmonary edema may develop. Similarly, introduction of a systemic-to-pulmonary arterial shunt may be associated with the appearance of pulmonary edema postoperatively if the obstructed total pulmonary venous connection is not relieved. With the advent of ultrasonography, it is now unusual that total anomalous pulmonary venous connection is not recognized. It is therefore very important to consider the diagnosis and to define pulmonary venous drainage.

Effect of feeding

If the pulmonary veins all drain to the portal vein and the ductus venosus is closed, pulmonary venous, as well as portal venous, blood passes through the hepatic vascular bed to the hepatic veins and IVC. Portal and pulmonary venous pressures are elevated because the microcirculation imposes some resistance to flow. Feeding will result in a considerable increase in gastrointestinal and portal blood flows. Unless hepatic vascular resistance falls, portal and pulmonary venous pressures will rise and pulmonary edema will be aggravated.

Effect of oxygen administration

Oxygen is administered routinely to infants with cyanosis. In the infant with total pulmonary venous anomaly with severe obstruction to drainage, oxygen administration usually increases systemic arterial oxygen saturation. However, there is the risk that oxygen may aggravate the pulmonary edema. Alveolar hypoxemia contributes to the pulmonary vasoconstriction that tends to reduce pulmonary blood flow. Administration of oxygen could cause vasodilatation, with an increase in pulmonary blood flow and pulmonary venous pressure, and aggravate edema. Furthermore, if the Po_2 is increased significantly, the ductus arteriosus could be constricted, raising pulmonary arterial pressure and pulmonary blood flow and thus aggravating pulmonary edema.

Effect of PGE$_1$ infusion

PGE_1 is often administered to infants with cyanotic heart disease to dilate the ductus arteriosus. It has sometimes been given empirically to infants before the specific cardiac anomalies have been identified, in the hope that it will decrease hypoxemia. Potentially, PGE_1 could produce adverse effects in infants with total anomalous pulmonary venous connection with obstruction by two mechanisms. If the ductus arteriosus is constricted, pulmonary arterial pressure is higher than aortic pressure. Dilating the ductus arteriosus may result in an increase in right-to-left shunt and an increase in the degree of cyanosis. Pulmonary arterial pressure will fall and thus pulmonary blood flow may decrease, with a fall in pulmonary venous pressure and reduction in pulmonary edema. However, PGE_1 produces pulmonary vasodilatation and this could result in an increase of pulmonary blood flow. This would tend to accentuate the pulmonary edema, but could improve the cyanosis. The effects on the ductus arteriosus and the pulmonary circulation would thus tend to produce opposing responses. The effect would therefore depend on whether the response is greater in the ductus arteriosus or in the pulmonary vasculature; usually it might be expected that the ductus response to PGE_1 would predominate and cyanosis may be expected to worsen. Another important consideration is that PGE_1 could cause peripheral vasodilatation and reduce systemic arterial pressure; it is therefore very important that pressure is monitored carefully and inotropic support be administered if necessary.

Prostaglandin could have a very beneficial effect in infants with infradiaphragmatic drainage to the portal vein. Constriction of the ductus venosus will result in an increase in portal and thus pulmonary venous pressure and precipitate or aggravate pulmonary edema. PGE_1 relaxes the smooth muscle in the ductus venosus and relieves constriction. This will lower pulmonary venous pressure, with improvement of pulmonary edema.

Little or no obstruction to pulmonary venous drainage

When all the pulmonary veins connect to the left vertical vein and drain through the left innominate vein and SVC, severe obstruction is unusual. Similarly, connection of the pulmonary veins to the coronary sinus is not commonly associated with significant degrees of obstruction. In infants in whom there is mild or no obstruction to pul-

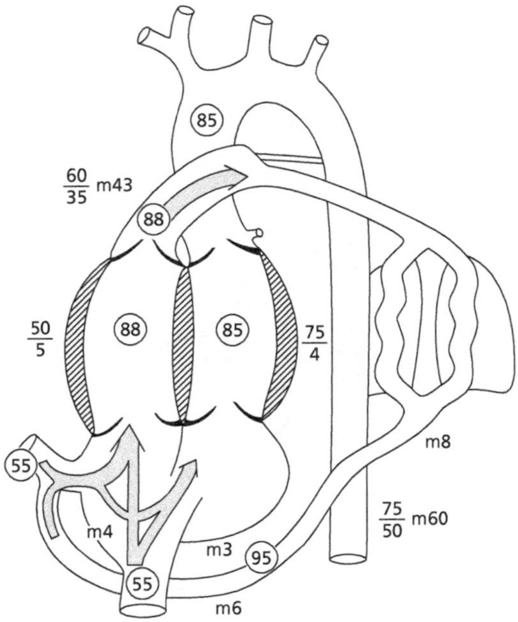

Figure 13.6 Total anomalous drainage of pulmonary veins to superior vena cava in a newborn infant: course of the circulation, oxygen saturations (circled), and pressures. Pulmonary vascular resistance is still moderately increased. m, mean pressure.

monary venous return, pulmonary blood flow progressively increases after birth, in association with the fall in pulmonary vascular resistance (Figures 13.6 and 13.7). Within a few weeks after birth, pulmonary to systemic blood flow ratios may exceed 3:1. Systemic arterial oxygen saturations are usually relatively high, often close to 90%.

The circulatory dynamics in total anomalous pulmonary venous connection with no obstruction to drainage are of considerable interest. Normally, the stroke volumes of the two ventricles are similar; however, the left ventricle is subjected to a higher afterload than the right ventricle and it is somewhat less compliant. To provide similar filling volumes, left atrial is higher than right atrial pressure.

In total anomalous pulmonary venous drainage, a very large volume of blood returns to the right atrium; the proportion destined to systemic blood flow must pass through the foramen ovale. The rest passes through the tricuspid valve to the right ventricle and pulmonary circulation. The volume of blood entering the right ventricle is determined by

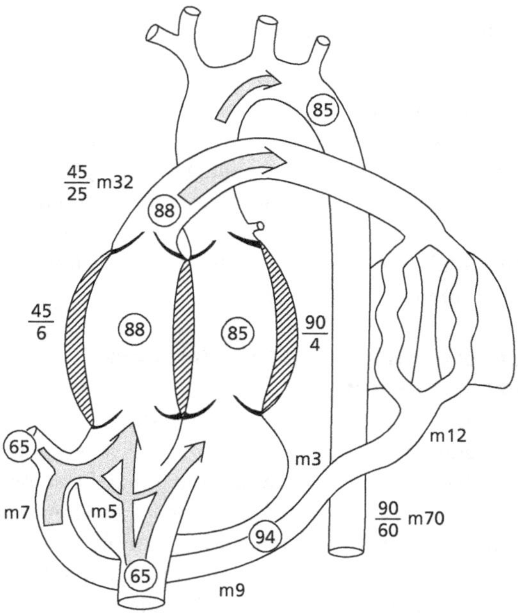

Figure 13.7 Total anomalous drainage of pulmonary veins to the superior vena cava later in infancy: course of the circulation, oxygen saturations (circled), and pressures. Pulmonary vascular resistance has dropped markedly. m, mean pressure.

its end-systolic volume, its compliance, and its filling pressure. If pulmonary vascular resistance has fallen normally after birth, the afterload on the ventricle is reduced, its ejection fraction will be increased, and its end-systolic volume will be low. With total pulmonary venous drainage anomaly, right atrial pressure has to be higher than left atrial pressure to provide adequate systemic blood flow. The high right atrial pressure greatly increases filling of the right ventricle; based on the Frank–Starling relationship, right ventricular contraction is enhanced and stroke volume is increased. Thus the high right atrial pressure drives the output of the right ventricle and increases pulmonary blood flow.

Changes in systemic vascular resistance could have profound effects on the circulation. A decrease in systemic vascular resistance will be associated with an increase in systolic ejection by the left ventricle, resulting in a smaller end-systolic volume and greater flow into the ventricle in diastole. If right atrial pressure does not change, the volume flowing through the foramen ovale would increase to provide a larger systemic blood flow. Pulmonary blood flow would not be affected significantly. However, if right atrial pressure falls, pulmonary blood flow could fall as a result of the reduced filling pressure of the right ventricle. An increase in peripheral vascular resistance would raise the afterload on the left ventricle, limit the stroke volume, and increase end-systolic volume and raise atrial pressure. This will limit flow across the foramen ovale from the right atrium. If right atrial pressure increases, there would be greater filling of the right ventricle and pulmonary blood flow would increase.

The dynamics in total anomalous pulmonary drainage differ from those associated with atrial septal defect. Even with a very large atrial septal defect, in which the pressures in the two atria tend to be equal, right atrial does not exceed left atrial pressure. Thus, unlike in total anomalous pulmonary venous drainage, in which right atrial pressure is higher, the right ventricle is not driven to increase its output by the high filling pressure. This could explain the fact that cardiac failure occurs infrequently in infants with atrial septal defects, but is very common in babies with total anomalous pulmonary venous drainage, because the right ventricle is subjected to a considerably higher volume load.

Influence of the foramen ovale

As mentioned above, the foramen ovale is frequently smaller than normal in the fetus and neonate with total anomalous pulmonary venous return; this is noted in about two-thirds of the infants with no obstruction to pulmonary venous drainage. About one-third has a large fossa ovalis atrial septal defect. The size of the atrial communication has a crucial role in determining the hemodynamic and clinical presentation. If the foramen ovale is large, little pressure gradient would be necessary to provide adequate systemic blood flow, and this could be maintained with a relatively low right atrial pressure. If the foramen ovale is restricted, right atrial pressure would have to be raised to maintain adequate systemic blood flow. As mentioned above, elevation of right atrial pressure drives the right ventricle to increase its output and huge pulmonary blood flows are generated, with the likelihood that right ventricular failure will ensue.

An additional consideration is the effect of the right atrial pressure on pulmonary vascular pressures. Normally, pulmonary venous blood returns to the left atrium, but with total pulmonary venous drainage anomaly it drains to the right atrium, which has a higher pressure than the left atrium. Pulmonary venous pressure is thus higher than normal; foramen ovale restriction would induce even higher right atrial and pulmonary venous pressures. Pulmonary capillary as well as pulmonary arterial pressures will also be increased and pulmonary edema may develop. The rise in pulmonary arterial pressure will add a pressure load to the high volume load on the right ventricle and thus increase the probability that failure will occur.

The finding of a mild reduction in systemic arterial oxygen saturation in asymptomatic individuals who manifest the clinical features of a large atrial septal defect strongly suggests the diagnosis of total anomalous pulmonary venous connection.

Moderate obstruction to pulmonary venous return

Moderate degrees of obstruction of pulmonary veins are usually encountered when drainage is to the left vertical vein or to the coronary sinus (see Chapter 13). The obstruction is not severe enough to cause pulmonary edema and cyanosis in the neonatal period. Postnatally, while pulmonary vascular resistance is still somewhat elevated, pulmonary blood flow will be moderately increased but because the pulmonary to systemic blood flow ratio is only 1.5–2.0:1, moderate cyanosis with arterial oxygen saturations of 80–85% will be evident. As pulmonary vascular resistance falls, pulmonary blood flow will increase to 2.0–2.5:1 and arterial oxygen saturation will increase to 85–88%. Associated with the increase in pulmonary blood flow, the moderate obstruction to pulmonary blood flow becomes manifest. Pulmonary venous pressures increase proximal to the obstruction and a mean pressure gradient of up to 12–15 mmHg between the pulmonary veins and the right atrium develops. The high pulmonary venous pressure may induce pulmonary edema and pulmonary arterial pressure becomes moderately elevated to systolic levels of about 35–45 mmHg. The increased pressure and volume load on the right ventricle may result in failure.

Clinical features

The clinical manifestations of total anomalous pulmonary venous return are largely determined by the severity of obstruction of the pulmonary veins. A clinical spectrum ranging from severe early pulmonary edema in those with severe obstruction to development of right-sided cardiac failure in late adult life in those with no obstruction is encountered.

Severe obstruction to pulmonary venous return

The infant is usually normal at birth but shows moderate to severe cyanosis. Initially, as pulmonary blood flow increases, there may be some lessening of cyanosis. Obstruction of pulmonary venous drainage results in elevation of pulmonary venous pressure with development of pulmonary edema, manifested by increased respiratory effort. This may occur within a few hours after birth, but sometimes not for several weeks depending on the severity and site of the obstruction. In the majority of infants, symptoms are evident within the first week; occasionally, as with drainage into the portal vein, delayed closure of the ductus venosus may postpone the onset of symptoms for several weeks. While the ductus arteriosus is still open, the infant presents predominantly with cyanosis, and pulmonary edema is not severe because pulmonary arterial pressure does not exceed aortic pressure.

In these infants, the Po_2 and oxygen saturation in the ascending and descending aortae may differ. If the pulmonary venous drainage is infradiaphragmatic, oxygen saturation in the ascending aorta may be as much as 10–15% higher than that in the descending aorta, whereas if the veins drain via the SVC saturation in the descending aorta may be higher. With drainage of pulmonary veins into the coronary sinus, there is usually little difference between ascending and descending aortic oxygen saturations. The arterial Po_2 may be reduced to below 30 mmHg and oxygen saturation may be below 60%; Pco_2 may be mildly elevated to 40–45 mmHg and pH may be reduced to 7.2–7.3.

Clinical examination reveals increased respiratory effort, but no retractions. The pulses in both upper and lower extremities are often weak and blood pressure is frequently reduced to 40–50 mmHg systolic and pulse pressure is small. The liver may be slightly enlarged. The heart is not enlarged and there is a normal right ventricular impulse at the lower right sternal border. The first heart sound is normal and the second sound is accentuated but narrow. No murmurs may be heard, but a soft medium-frequency murmur may be heard at the lower sternal level, reflecting tricuspid insufficiency. The chest radiograph shows mild increase of hilar vascular markings, suggesting venous engorgement, but the peripheral lung fields appear poorly vascularized. The electrocardiogram shows right axis deviation and right ventricular hypertrophy. In the majority of infants there is a pure R wave in the right precordial leads and a small or absent R with a dominant S wave in the left precordial leads. The infant may deteriorate rapidly, with increasing cyanosis and metabolic acidemia.

If the hypoxemia and acidemia are not severe, the clinical status may remain unchanged for several days and then, in association with constriction of the ductus arteriosus, the clinical presentation changes. The severity of cyanosis may decrease but respiratory distress becomes more marked, with increase in rate and depth of ventilation, and chest retractions become evident. The difference in oxygen saturation and Po_2 between the upper and lower extremities is no longer apparent. The Po_2 may increase to 35–45 mmHg, the pH to 7.3–7.35, and the Pco_2 to 45–50 mmHg. Air entry into the lung may be decreased and crepitant rales may be heard, indicating clinical pulmonary edema. The liver becomes enlarged to 4–6 cm below the costal margin. The radial and femoral pulses are often only weakly palpable.

The heart is not clinically enlarged, but there is a prominent right ventricular impulse at the lower left sternal border. The first heart sound may be loud at the lower left sternal border, and the second sound is markedly accentuated but narrow at the upper left sternal border. A grade 2–3/6 medium-frequency systolic murmur is commonly present at the lower left sternal border as a result of tricuspid insufficiency. No differences in the electrocardiogram occur, but the chest radiograph shows significant changes. The lung fields show marked hilar vessel enlargement and the lung fields are hazy and stippled due to extensive pulmonary edema. The heart size increases modestly, but it does not show marked enlargement. Without treatment, the infant develops progressive pulmonary edema, with worsening of cyanosis and right heart failure, and succumbs within a few days.

Unobstructed pulmonary venous return

There may be no major clinical symptoms or signs to attract attention to the infant with this lesion. Cyanosis, which may be present at birth, rapidly decreases during the first week. Mild cyanosis, increasing on exertion, may be evident later. Some evidence of right-sided cardiac failure may be present in the first few months, but occasionally no symptoms are noted. These children often do not grow normally and may be underdeveloped and undernourished for their age. As they grow older there is usually some evidence of a decrease in exercise tolerance. However, I have encountered several adolescent patients who have never had any symptoms. An interesting clinical feature that has been reported is so-called dysphonia, an alteration in the cry or the voice. It was noted in about one-quarter of patients with supradiaphragmatic connection without obstruction and it was suggested it is due to compression of the left recurrent laryngeal nerve by the vertical vein [3].

After the first week or two, the patient shows mild or minimal cyanosis. The pulse rate may be slightly increased and blood pressure is normal. There may be slight hepatomegaly. Respirations are usually mildly increased in rate and depth. However, the chest is clear on auscultation. The heart is clinically enlarged and very active, with the major impulse at the lower left sternal border due to increased right ventricular volume overload.

The first heart sound is usually accentuated at the lower left sternal border, probably due to forceful tricuspid valve closure. The second sound is normal in intensity, is widely split, and does not show much variation with respiratory cycles. A third heart sound or, more often, a mid-diastolic low-frequency murmur is heard at the lower left sternal border due to rapid flow of a large volume across the tricuspid valve. Occasionally a fourth heart sound of atrial systolic contraction is also heard.

A systolic ejection murmur of grade 2–3/6 intensity is usually heard at the upper left sternal border due to the increased pulmonary blood flow across the pulmonary valve. In some individuals with a common pulmonary trunk entering the left innominate vein by means of a vertical vein, a high-frequency grade 2–3/6 continuous murmur, without late systolic accentuation, may be heard below the left clavicle. Unlike a venous hum, it is predominantly subclavicular and is not affected by change in head position. It probably originates from turbulence created by the flow from the vertical vein into the innominate system.

In infancy, the electrocardiogram is similar to that described in obstructed pulmonary venous return. In older children there is less rightward deviation. There is prominence of right ventricular precordial voltages and frequently evidence of prolongation of intraventricular conduction in the right ventricle. In older individuals, some left ventricular forces may be seen in the left precordial leads.

The chest radiograph shows a heart that is enlarged, with prominence of the right ventricle and the right atrium. The main pulmonary artery and right ventricular outflow are also large. The pulmonary vessels are dilated and there is a marked increase in pulmonary vascular markings extending to the periphery of the lung fields. When the pulmonary veins drain through the vertical vein into the left innominate vein, the superior mediastinum is enlarged to the left and right of the spine. This classic appearance has been termed a "snowman" or "figure-of-eight." It is usually evident within 6 months after birth, but in early infancy the pulmonary blood flow may not yet have increased enough to cause enlargement of the superior mediastinal vessels. When the pulmonary veins all enter the coronary sinus there is a dilated chamber at the site of confluence, lying behind the right atrium. This may, in an appropriately exposed film, show a double density in the lower region of the cardiac shadow on the right, lower than that seen when the left atrium is enlarged. This may also be seen as a posterior bulge on the lower border of the cardiac shadow in the lateral view.

The subsequent course in these individuals is similar to that of patients with a large atrial septal defect (see Chapter 8). They may manifest some retardation of physical growth and have mild limitation of exercise tolerance. This limitation becomes more marked in adolescence and they become subject to atrial arrhythmias. Although pulmonary vascular obstructive changes may occur, they are not as common as the development of cardiac failure during early adult life. Pulmonary vascular obstruction is evidenced by an increase in the degree of cyanosis, increasing loudness of the second heart sound, and subsequently by the development of right-sided cardiac failure.

Moderate obstruction to pulmonary venous return

Individuals with moderately obstructed pulmonary venous drainage often present in infancy with pulmonary edema and severe right-sided cardiac failure. They have cyanosis postnatally, but as pulmonary blood flow increases only mild to moderate cyanosis persists. Within 2–3 weeks to 3–4 months after birth, they develop increased respiratory effort, sweating, and hepatomegaly.

Peripheral pulse volume may be somewhat decreased and the heart rate is increased to 140–160/min. Respiratory rate may be increased to 60–80/min. The heart is markedly enlarged and there is a prominent hyperdynamic impulse at the lower left sternal border, reflecting right ventricular volume overload. There is often a palpable systolic impulse at the upper left sternal border, produced by systolic expansion of the right ventricular infundibulum and the pulmonary artery.

The first heart sound is accentuated at the lower left sternal border due to forceful tricuspid valve closure. The second sound is well split and does not vary with respiration, and the second component is moderately accentuated. A third heart sound and a short low-frequency mid-diastolic murmur are usually present at the lower left sternal border due to high flow across the tricuspid valve. A grade 2–4/6 systolic ejection murmur is usually heard at the upper left sternal border. A medium-frequency systolic murmur may be heard in the lower xiphoid region due to secondary tricuspid insufficiency.

The electrocardiogram is similar to that described for individuals with obstructed pulmonary veins. The chest radiograph shows a large heart with markedly increased pulmonary vasculature and a prominent right ventricle. The special features described above, depending on the location of drainage, may also be present.

If these infants are not treated, they usually develop progressive failure. Treatment with digitalis and other decongestive measures may produce temporary improvement, but without surgical intervention many succumb during the first year. Some, however, may be reasonably well maintained with digitalis and diuretics and, even though they grow poorly, survive the first 12–18 months.

Total pulmonary venous drainage anomaly with foramen ovale restriction

The infants show cyanosis at birth, which improves as pulmonary blood flow increases. Within a few weeks to 3–4 months after birth, evidence of increasing right heart failure develops. The infant perspires excessively, feeds poorly, and has increased respiratory effort. The pulse rate is increased to 160–180/min. The clinical features relating to restriction of the foramen ovale are pallor, poor peripheral perfusion, and weak pulses. Also, the liver is markedly enlarged to 4–6 cm below the costal margin. Peripheral edema, which is not common in infants with cardiac failure, may occur in these infants. The findings on physical examination of the heart are similar to those in infants with moderate obstruction to pulmonary venous drainage. The radiological features are also similar.

Investigations

Echocardiography

It is now possible to make the diagnosis of total anomalous pulmonary venous drainage accurately in most patients by ultrasound examination using two-dimensional echocardiography, color flow Doppler, and contrast echocardiography. The ultrasound studies should attempt to define:

- site(s) in the systemic venous system to which the pulmonary veins are connected;
- all the individual pulmonary veins, so that one can determine whether all veins are draining into a single confluence, or if drainage is mixed;
- whether the ductus arteriosus is patent;
- if obstruction to drainage is present and the site of obstruction;
- whether any other cardiac lesions are present.

To define the site of drainage of the pulmonary veins, it is advised that each vein should be followed from the hilum to the site of connection.

If the pulmonary veins are all draining below the diaphragm, the common confluence passes caudally through the esophageal hiatus. Ultrasound study reveals the venous channel between the aorta and IVC, slightly anterior and to the right of the descending aorta and posterior and to the left of the IVC. Color flow Doppler study is very helpful, showing fairly continuous flow toward the diaphragm. Flow in the aorta is in the same direction, but is pulsatile; flow in the IVC is toward the heart. The channel can be followed to the portal vein, ductus venosus, or hepatic vein. Any obstruction at the site of passage through the diaphragm, or at the connection with the portal vein, should be assessed. The presence of high-velocity flow through the ductus venosus signifies that it has undergone constriction.

Drainage of veins to the coronary sinus is associated with enlargement of the sinus. It is very important to identify each pulmonary vein, because mixed types of drainage are not unusual when some drain into the coronary sinus. The possible presence of obstruction to drainage should be assessed by examining the ostium through which the pulmonary veins drain, because it is the usual site of obstruction. The left-sided vertical vein is characterized by flow in a cranial direction. It should be followed throughout its course to the left innominate vein and SVC. It should be examined carefully for evidence of obstruction where it crosses in front of the bronchus, as well as along its whole course. The connection of each of the veins to the confluence should be confirmed to exclude mixed types of drainage. When the veins all drain into the SVC or vertical vein, the possibility of obstruction at the site of connection should be examined. With drainage into the azygos vein, the vessel may be obstructive because of its size.

The duration of the ultrasound study may be extended in patients with total anomalous pulmonary venous drainage, because it may be difficult to identify each pulmonary vein and its site of connection. It is therefore important to carefully observe the infant's clinical condition during the study. In some infants, it may not be possible to obtain complete information on the drainage of all the veins. The right atrium and ventricle are enlarged and the ventricular septum is usually noted to bulge toward the left. The left atrium and ventricle are usually noted to be small. The presence of other cardiac lesions should be defined, particularly in patients with right atrial isomerism (asplenia syndrome), in whom atrioventricular septal defects are usual as is pulmonary stenosis or atresia.

Cardiac catheterization and angiocardiography

General considerations

Prior to the introduction of ultrasound examination, cardiac catheterization and angiography were the mainstays of diagnosis; there was significant risk of the procedures when performed in very sick babies with severe cyanosis and pulmonary edema. Two-dimensional echocardiography combined with color flow Doppler study has made it possible to make the diagnosis in most patients. There may still be difficulty in defining the site of drainage of all the veins, but in many centers the information obtained by ultrasound is considered adequate to proceed with surgery. Catheterization is occasionally performed in centers where there is concern about the reliability of ultrasound studies in infants. The following information should be obtained.

- The anatomical arrangement of the pulmonary veins should be delineated, and the site of their connection to the systemic venous system should be defined. If some veins enter the coronary sinus, vertical vein or portal vein, it should not be assumed that all do, because mixed types of connections are not infrequent.
- The presence of obstruction to venous drainage should be addressed and the sites of obstruction determined. It should also be recognized that with mixed types of connections, only some veins might be obstructed.
- The adequacy of the foramen ovale to permit systemic blood flow must be considered. Although there is no reliable method of assessing mild restriction, moderate or severe restriction may be detected from pressure recordings.
- The size of the left atrium and left ventricle should be assessed.
- The pulmonary vascular resistance should be assessed, particularly in older individuals in whom corrective surgery is being considered.
- Other lesions, such as atrioventricular septal defect and patent ductus arteriosus, should be excluded. As indicated below, oxygen saturation measurements may be of little help in diagnosing these lesions in the presence of total anomalous pulmonary venous drainage, because oxygen saturations are similar in all blood samples beyond the right atrial level.

Catheter manipulation

When the pulmonary veins drain through the left vertical vein into the left innominate vein, it is usually possible to pass the catheter from the IVC through the right atrium and the right SVC into the left innominate vein. With further manipulation, it is usually possible to enter the vertical vein and one or more of the pulmonary veins.

Pressure, both phasic and mean, should be recorded distally in the pulmonary vein and then on gradual withdrawal of the catheter to the right atrium. This will demonstrate any localized site of obstruction in the pulmonary venous trunk or the presence of a gradual pressure gradient related to very high flow through a relatively small channel.

If the pulmonary veins enter the coronary sinus, the catheter can usually be passed readily from the right atrium into the coronary sinus and then frequently into the pulmonary veins. In this situation the course of the catheter may not differ from that seen when it is passed from the right atrium through an atrial septal defect or foramen ovale into the left atrium and then into a right or left pulmonary vein.

When the pulmonary veins enter the right atrium directly, the catheter may be passed into one or all of the veins. If the common trunk enters the right SVC or azygos vein, it may be difficult to manipulate the catheter into the trunk, especially if there is obstruction.

When drainage to the portal vein is suspected, the catheter should be manipulated into a hepatic vein, because the presence of a high oxygen saturation in hepatic venous blood almost definitively confirms the diagnosis. The only other condition in which hepatic venous oxygen saturation is high is hepatic arteriovenous fistula. It is not possible to pass a catheter into the pulmonary venous trunk when it enters the portal vein, except possibly in the immediate newborn period. If the pulmonary veins drain into the portal vein, a catheter passed through the umbilical vein could possibly be manipulated into the pulmonary venous trunk from the portal vein; this would be difficult because the portal vein connects with the umbilical vein at an acute angle.

Usually, the left atrium and left ventricle can be readily entered through the foramen ovale. An angiogram in the left atrium will assess the size of the atrium and ventricle, as well as the presence of a left-to-right shunt through an atrial or ventricular septal defect, or a patent ductus arteriosus.

Oxygen saturation

Complete admixture of pulmonary and systemic blood occurs at or before the right atrial level; thus oxygen saturations in the right atrium, the right and left ventricles, the aorta, and the pulmonary artery are similar. However, differences in pulmonary venous drainage may cause some difference in saturations in the left and right ventricles (see above). IVC blood tends to stream preferentially through the foramen ovale, whereas blood from the SVC passes preferentially through the tricuspid valve; this may create differences in oxygen saturation in systemic and pulmonary arteries. These differences are more likely to be greater in infants than in older children because the fetal flow patterns are more prominent soon after birth.

When the pulmonary venous trunk enters the vertical vein or the SVC, oxygen saturation is higher in the SVC than in the IVC and thus saturation in the pulmonary artery may be higher than that in the systemic arteries. In infants, this difference may reach levels of 10–15%, but in older children it is rarely more than 3–5%. The difference in saturation also tends to be larger when pulmonary blood flow is large, as this causes a higher oxygen saturation in the systemic venous channel into which the trunk drains.

Drainage of the pulmonary venous trunk into the infradiaphragmatic veins may be associated with a higher oxygen saturation in the systemic arteries than in the pulmonary arteries. The difference in saturations may be as large as 10–12%, particularly in young infants. It is important to appreciate that this large difference can occur, because the diagnosis of total anomalous pulmonary venous return could otherwise not be considered. When the pulmonary veins enter the coronary sinus or the right atrium directly, the difference between pulmonary and systemic arterial oxygen saturations tends to be small. Since some coronary sinus drainage may flow preferentially across the tricuspid valve into the right ventricle, oxygen saturation may be slightly higher in the pulmonary artery than in the aorta.

It is not possible to measure mixed venous oxygen saturation when all the pulmonary veins enter the SVC or IVC streams. If all the pulmonary veins drain into the coronary sinus or directly into the right atrium, vena cava samples are the best representation of mixed venous blood, although reflux of right atrial blood into the vena cava may also introduce errors in measurement. The oxygen saturation levels of venous blood are determined by the magnitude of systemic blood flow and by the level of systemic arterial oxygen saturation. Mixed venous oxygen saturation is decreased if systemic blood flow is low due to cardiac failure or restriction of the foramen ovale; it may also be low if systemic arterial oxygen saturation is reduced.

Systemic arterial oxygen saturation may range from low levels of 50–60% in infants with obstruction to pulmonary venous return up to as much as 90–92% in patients with no obstruction; this is determined by the ratio of pulmonary to systemic blood flow (see Chapter 3). As mentioned above, if a proportion of systemic blood flow is derived from right-to-left shunting through the ductus arteriosus, differences in oxygen saturation in the ascending aorta and its branches and the descending aorta may be observed (see Chapter 13).

If the diagnosis of total pulmonary venous return to the portal vein is being considered, measuring oxygen saturation in hepatic venous blood may confirm the diagnosis. It is rarely possible to pass the catheter into the portal vein; oxygen saturation in hepatic venous blood is higher than in any other site in the circulation where it is measurable. The importance of this finding was well demonstrated in an extremely cyanotic 1-day-old infant in whom the diagnoses of persistent pulmonary hypertension of the newborn and total anomalous pulmonary venous drainage were considered. Oxygen saturations and pressures were as shown in Table 13.1. The infant had a very low pulmonary blood flow and was maintaining systemic flow largely through the ductus arteriosus, as noted by angiography. Most of the contrast medium injected into the main pulmonary artery passed through the

Table 13.1 Oxygen saturations and pressures in an extremely cyanotic 1-day-old infant.

	Oxygen saturation (%)	*Pressure (mmHg)*
Superior vena cava	32	
Inferior vena cava		
(below hepatic veins)	38	
Hepatic vein	65	
Right atrium	44	12 (mean)
Right ventricle	42	110/16
Pulmonary artery	42	115/80, mean 90
Descending aorta	46	80/55, mean 63
Left atrium	48	8 (mean)
Left ventricle	48	82/10

ductus arteriosus; the pulmonary circulation filled poorly and pulmonary veins were not well visualized. Oxygen saturation in the hepatic vein, although not very high, was consistently higher than that in the descending aorta; this observation allowed the correct diagnosis to be made.

In patients with no obstruction to pulmonary venous drainage, pulmonary venous blood may have an oxygen saturation of 95–96% with a Po_2 of 88–90 mmHg. It has been suggested that the slightly decreased oxygenation is related to the very high pulmonary blood flows; the high velocity of blood flowing through the pulmonary capillaries may not allow adequate time for equilibration with alveolar oxygen.

Pulmonary and systemic blood flows

As mentioned above, the magnitude of systemic and pulmonary blood flow varies greatly, depending on the hemodynamic disturbances. Systemic blood flow is influenced by the size of the atrial septal opening and the size of the ductus arteriosus. Pulmonary blood flow is affected by the degree of pulmonary venous obstruction and the pulmonary vascular resistance.

It is difficult to make accurate measurements of both pulmonary and systemic flow in patients with total anomalous pulmonary venous drainage. The potential errors in measuring systemic blood flow by the Fick method result from inability to obtain a reliable mixed venous sample. Pulmonary blood flow measurements are unreliable in infants with infradiaphragmatic drainage because a pulmonary venous sample cannot be obtained. In the patient with unobstructed pulmonary venous return, the arteriovenous oxygen difference is very small, so that large potential errors may occur in calculation of pulmonary flow (see Chapter 4).

Shunts

The admixture of pulmonary and systemic venous blood makes it difficult to consider vascular shunts in the usual manner as simple left-to-right and right-to-left shunts. The concept of anatomical and physiological shunting has been introduced.

1 The anatomical right-to-left shunt in patients with total anomalous pulmonary venous drainage is the same as total systemic blood flow; it is usually represented by flow across the foramen ovale, unless there also is flow from the pulmonary artery to the aorta through the ductus arteriosus.

2 The anatomical left-to-right shunt is the volume of pulmonary venous blood that enters the systemic circulation and is equal to total pulmonary blood flow.

3 The physiological right-to-left shunt is the volume of mixed venous blood that enters the systemic circulation without passing through the lungs. It is calculated from the equation:

$$\text{Physiological right-to-left shunt} = \dot{Q}s - \dot{Q}ep$$

where $\dot{Q}s$ is systemic blood flow and $\dot{Q}ep$ effective pulmonary flow. $\dot{Q}ep$ is the volume of systemic venous blood that reaches the lungs to be oxygenated (see Chapter 4).

4 The physiological left-to-right shunt represents that portion of pulmonary venous blood that recirculates through the lungs and is calculated from the equation:

$$\text{Physiological left-to-right shunt} = \dot{Q}p - \dot{Q}ep$$

where $\dot{Q}p$ is total pulmonary blood flow.

These calculations are of interest, but are usually unreliable because measurements of pulmonary and systemic blood flows are inaccurate.

It is not possible to detect the presence of left-to-right shunts through a ventricular septal defect or a patent ductus arteriosus by means of oxygen saturation data in the presence of total anomalous pulmonary venous return. Because systemic and pulmonary venous blood mixes almost completely, oxygen saturation of the blood shunted into the right ventricle from the left ventricle or into the pulmonary artery from the aorta is similar to that of the blood in the chamber. Thus, no increase occurs, as is usually noted with left-to-right shunts.

Pressures

Pulmonary venous and pulmonary arterial wedge pressures

With severe obstruction to pulmonary venous return, it is often not possible to measure pulmonary venous pressure directly. Pulmonary arterial wedge pressures provide a good estimate of pulmonary venous pressure; mean wedge pressures may be elevated to as much as 25–30 mmHg.

When the pulmonary veins drain directly into the right atrium, pulmonary venous mean pressure is usually only 2–3 mmHg above right atrial mean pressure. With drainage into the coronary sinus, usually there is also only a slightly higher mean pressure of 2–3 mmHg in the pulmonary veins or the coronary sinus as compared with the right atrium. Occasionally, however, the orifice of the coronary sinus is relatively small, and pressure in the sinus and the pulmonary veins may exceed right atrial pressure considerably.

The pressure difference between the pulmonary veins and the right atrium is quite variable with drainage through the vertical vein. In older children who are asymptomatic, the mean pressure difference may be only 3–4 mmHg. A pressure gradient of as much as 10–15 mmHg may be recorded in the vertical vein at the region where it crosses the left bronchus, particularly if it passes up between the bronchus and the left pulmonary artery. This may produce moderate to severe obstruction and has been termed a "hemodynamic vise."

The contour of the pulmonary venous pressures in veins connected directly to the right atrium is of considerable interest. A dominant *v* wave is recorded when the catheter is advanced well out into a pulmonary vein. This is the pattern seen normally in the pulmonary vein and the left atrium. As the catheter is withdrawn, the *v* wave becomes less prominent and the magnitude of the *a* wave increases. Near the right atrium, a dominant *a* wave and a small *v* wave are noted. This finding supports the view that the dominant *v* wave normally seen in the pulmonary vein and left atrium is not related to left atrioventricular dynamics but to transmission of pressure waves through the pulmonary circulation. It probably represents delayed transmission of the systolic pressure pulse in the pulmonary artery.

Left and right atrial pressures

Invariably there is a higher pressure in the right atrium than in the left atrium. The left atrial pressure contour shows a dominant *a* wave, unlike normally, when the *v* wave is dominant. This is due to absence of pulmonary venous drainage into the left atrium. The actual levels of pressure and the pressure differences between the right atrium and the left atrium vary greatly. In older patients with unobstructed pulmonary venous return and no restriction of the foramen ovale, the right atrial mean pressure is normal or slightly elevated and there is a mean pressure difference of only 1–3 mmHg across the foramen ovale. In infants with cardiac failure, the right atrial mean pressure may be elevated to 10–15 mmHg. If there is obstruction at the foramen ovale, a large mean pressure difference of as much as 8–10 mmHg has been noted between the right and left atrium; however, only a small mean pressure gradient may be observed with moderate restriction of the foramen ovale.

Right ventricular and pulmonary arterial pressures

Right ventricular and pulmonary arterial systolic pressures reflect the degree of pulmonary venous obstruction or increase in pulmonary vascular resistance. In infants with severe pulmonary venous obstruction and high pulmonary vascular resistance, the pressure in the pulmonary artery frequently exceeds that in the systemic arteries. When pulmonary venous obstruction is not severe, pulmonary arterial pressure is usually moderately elevated to 40–60 mmHg systolic, 15–30 mmHg diastolic, and 25–45 mmHg mean pressure. In patients with no pulmonary venous obstruction, pulmonary arterial pressures may be only slightly elevated, with a greater elevation of systolic than diastolic pressure. A systolic pressure gradient across the normal pulmonary valve is common in patients with high pulmonary blood flows. It usually does not exceed 10–15 mmHg, but with very high flows may be as high as 30–40 mmHg. Older children and adults usually have only slightly increased pulmonary arterial pressures. If pulmonary vascular intimal changes develop, pulmonary hypertension occurs.

Right ventricular end-diastolic pressure is usually considerably increased up to 12–15 mmHg in infants with pulmonary venous obstruction and also in infants with high pulmonary blood flow and restricted foramen ovale. It is normal or only slightly elevated in patients with high pulmonary flow without cardiac failure.

Left ventricular and systemic arterial pressures
Left ventricular and systemic arterial pressures are usually normal in older infants and children with total anomalous pulmonary venous return. The pressures may be decreased, and considerably lower than pulmonary arterial pressure in infants with severe pulmonary venous obstruction and a constricted ductus arteriosus. A restricted foramen ovale may also be associated with low systemic ventricular and arterial pressures.

Angiocardiography

This is an essential part of the catheterization procedure, in that it often provides information about the drainage of veins from each lung. It may be difficult to demonstrate the pulmonary veins both when pulmonary flow is increased and when it is decreased. With high pulmonary flows the contrast medium is diluted when it is injected into the pulmonary artery and thus pulmonary venous visualization may be poor. When flow is low in association with obstruction to pulmonary venous return, contrast medium is slow to return to the pulmonary veins and visualization may be poor. Injections into the main pulmonary artery are not usually helpful. If the ductus arteriosus is open, much of the contrast medium is directed to the descending aorta, so little enters the pulmonary circulation. If pulmonary flow is high, the contrast is diluted so much that the pulmonary veins are not well seen. Selective injections should be made in the left and right pulmonary artery and the pulmonary veins identified on the levophase. A useful technique is to use a balloon catheter with an end-hole; the catheter is positioned in the pulmonary artery, the balloon is inflated and contrast is injected, after which the balloon is immediately deflated. This usually provides good visualization of pulmonary veins.

When the pulmonary veins drain into the vertical vein, the catheter can usually be manipulated through the SVC, innominate vein and vertical vein into pulmonary veins. An injection in this site may demonstrate any site of obstruction along the course of the vessels. With drainage of pulmonary veins into the coronary sinus, a density may be seen posteriorly, behind the lower region of the right atrium, but the extent of the chamber is usually not well demonstrated because of dilution of contrast medium and rapid filling of the right atrium. With infradiaphragmatic drainage, the common pulmonary venous trunk can be seen passing down in front of or to the left of the spine, to the region of the portal sinus. Usually there is no visualization of the subsequent course of venous flow, because the contrast medium is further diluted in the liver.

An injection in the left atrium demonstrates the size of the left atrium, the mitral valve annulus, and the left ventricle. Usually this injection is also adequate to exclude the presence of an additional left-to-right shunt at the ventricular level or through a patent ductus arteriosus.

Magnetic resonance imaging

The precise anatomy of the drainage of each pulmonary vein may be difficult to define by ultrasound or cardiac catheterization studies. Magnetic resonance imaging may be extremely useful in delineating the course and connection site of each pulmonary vein.

Differential diagnosis

Problems of differential diagnosis may arise in three different clinical situations.

Newborn infant with pulmonary venous obstruction

The diagnosis of total anomalous pulmonary venous return must be considered in any infant who develops respiratory distress, rales in the lungs, or cyanosis in the first few days after birth. It should also be excluded in infants who have evidence of peripheral circulatory failure, namely weak pulses, low blood pressure, and pallor or mottling of the extremities.

Lung disease and persistent pulmonary hypertension of the newborn

Frequently it is difficult to make a differential diagnosis between total anomalous pulmonary venous connection and either lung disease or persistent pulmonary hypertension of the newborn. Dyspnea and cyanosis, densities in both lung fields on the chest radiograph, and a normal cardiac contour and size are common features. Usually the infant with lung disease has more severe respiratory distress, often with chest retraction, but this can occur with anomalous pulmonary venous drainage if pulmonary edema is severe. Blood gas and oxygen saturation measurements may be helpful. Po_2 is reduced in all three conditions, but Pco_2 is usually considerably higher with lung disease, often above 50 mmHg. With total anomalous pulmonary venous drainage, Pco_2 is usually below 45 mmHg but can be higher if severe pulmonary edema develops. The oxygen saturation may be lower in the lower extremities than in the right arm due to right-to-left shunting through the ductus arteriosus in persistent pulmonary hypertension and respiratory distress syndrome, as well as with infradiaphragmatic total anomalous pulmonary venous drainage. A higher oxygen saturation in the lower extremities than in the right arm cannot be associated with lung disease or persistent pulmonary hypertension; it could be the result of pulmonary venous drainage to the vertical vein or SVC. Other congenital cardiovascular malformations can also account for this (see Chapter 3).

The chest radiograph may be helpful for distinguishing total anomalous pulmonary venous drainage because there is prominence of pulmonary veins and haziness and stippling predominantly in the hilar region, whereas in respiratory distress syndrome the lung densities are more diffuse. However, the differences are not usually conclusive enough to make a definitive diagnosis. In infants with total anomalous pulmonary venous drainage, the electrocardiogram often shows an absence of R waves in the left precordial leads, so if these are present the diagnosis is unlikely.

The differentiation can be made by ultrasound studies. Total anomalous pulmonary venous drainage is a condition that is often not considered by individuals caring for the newborn infant with respiratory distress and cyanosis. It is recommended that an ultrasound study be performed in any infant in whom the diagnosis of respiratory distress syndrome is not definite, and probably in all infants in whom the diagnosis of persistent pulmonary hypertension is being considered in order to exclude the possibility of total anomalous pulmonary venous drainage.

Hypoplastic left heart syndrome

The clinical features of total anomalous pulmonary venous return may be identical to those of aortic atresia. The clinical presentation of dyspnea, cyanosis, respiratory distress, and weak pulses are common to both conditions. Usually the infant with aortic atresia shows less severe cyanosis and greater interference with systemic blood flow. Blood gases may be helpful; with aortic atresia the Po_2 is not usually below 40 mmHg; Pco_2 is usually normal or reduced and pH may be very low. With total anomalous pulmonary venous drainage, Po_2 may be below 40 mmHg, Pco_2 is often increased up to about 45 mmHg, and pH is usually only modestly reduced. Unlike with total anomalous pulmonary venous drainage, in which differences in oxygen saturation between the right arm and lower extremities are not unusual, no differences are noted with aortic atresia. The electrocardiogram usually shows absence of R waves in the left precordial leads in both conditions. The chest radiograph usually shows prominence of the pulmonary arteries in infants with hypoplastic left heart syndrome, but pulmonary edema may also be present, as in total anomalous pulmonary venous drainage. The differential diagnosis is readily made by ultrasound examination.

Other congenital cardiac lesions

In early infancy, while the ductus arteriosus is patent and there is little pulmonary edema, total anomalous pulmonary venous drainage may be confused clinically with lesions with reduced pulmonary blood flow and with aortopulmonary transposition. Severe cyanosis is the dominant feature of all these conditions. The diagnosis is usually readily established by ultrasound studies

Older infants with cardiac failure

The diagnosis of total anomalous pulmonary venous return should be considered in the infant who develops cardiac failure within the first few months after birth, in association with mild cyanosis. Lesions such as Ebstein anomaly, atrioventricular septal defect, truncus arteriosus, aortopulmonary transposition with ventricular septal defect, single ventricle and other cardiac lesions should be considered, but the diagnosis is readily made by ultrasound examination.

Older children with unobstructed pulmonary venous return

The main lesion that may create confusion with total anomalous pulmonary venous return in older children is atrial septal defect.

Atrial septal defect with or without partial anomalous pulmonary venous return

The large volume overload on the right side of the heart that occurs in total anomalous pulmonary venous drainage produces many of the clinical features usually ascribed to atrial septal defect. When pulmonary blood flow is very large, cyanosis may be minimal so that it may not be detected clinically. The presence of a hyperactive right ventricular impulse, a widely split second sound, and a diastolic flow murmur or prominent third sound at the lower left sternal border are signs common to both lesions. The electrocardiogram may not be dissimilar, although absence of R waves in the left precordial leads is more likely with anomalous pulmonary venous return. The radiological features of cardiomegaly, predominantly involving the right ventricle and outflow region, an enlarged pulmonary artery, and markedly increased pulmonary markings are similar in both lesions. The typical superior mediastinal shadow of total anomalous pulmonary venous return to the vertical vein, or the enlarged coronary sinus when the veins drain to this region, may be helpful in diagnosis. The differential diagnosis is readily made by ultrasound study.

Principles of management

The infant with total anomalous pulmonary venous drainage with obstruction to venous return requires urgent surgery. Respiratory support should be provided with assisted ventilation; this may be helpful in providing some relief of pulmonary edema. However, high positive inspiratory pressures should not be used and continuous positive-pressure ventilation should be avoided, particularly in very cyanotic infants, because pulmonary blood flow could be further reduced by these maneuvers. Oxygen should be administered, especially in the infant who has very low systemic arterial Po_2 and oxygen saturation levels. As mentioned above, it is possible that pulmonary edema may be exaggerated by oxygen in infants with severe pulmonary edema. However, oxygen should be administered and the infant should be observed carefully for evidence of progression of pulmonary edema. If peripheral circulation is poor and systemic arterial pressure reduced, inotropic agents such as dobutamine or dopamine have been recommended in an attempt agents such as dobutamine or dopamine have been recommended to improve cardiac output. Infusion of dopamine in doses higher than 5 μg/kg per min should be avoided, because this may induce peripheral vasoconstriction and the increased systemic vascular resistance may limit flow into the systemic circulation. The value of the use of these agents has recently been questioned.

In infants with pulmonary venous drainage to the portal vein, PGE_1 infusion should be given because it could dilate the ductus venosus and relieve obstruction to venous drainage. There is little reported experience with the use of PGE_1; however PGE_1 does relax the ductus venosus in lambs, so it likely is effective in human infants. As mentioned above, the actions of PGE_1 on the ductus arteriosus and the pulmonary circulation could have opposing effects. There is at present no good evidence contraindicating the use of PGE_1 in infants with obstructed pulmonary venous drainage. However, it is important that tracheal intubation and assisted ventilation as well as attention to fluid administration be provided prior to starting PGE_1 infusion.

As mentioned above, attempts should be made to identify the course and site of drainage of each pulmonary vein prior to surgery, but it may be difficult to visualize all the veins during ultrasound examination. The examination should not be so prolonged as to delay surgery, because the surgeon should be able identify all the pulmonary veins.

Surgery

Although early in the surgical experience, mortality in infants was very high, it has fallen dramatically in recent years. The results of surgery are related to the presence of associated defects. The presence of a functional single ventricle was associated with a high incidence of pulmonary venous obstruction and a significantly poorer prognosis. In one series in which about 33% of patients had a single ventricle, survival to 1 month was only 65% compared with 90% for those with two ventricles [4]. In a report of patients with single ventricle and total anomalous pulmonary venous connection, about 30% had pulmonary venous obstruction. Survival was approximately 50% at 6 months and about 25% at 5 years [5]. Many of the patients with single ventricle had right atrial isomerism (asplenia syndrome). Because survival could have been related to the intracardiac anomalies, it is difficult to assess the contribution of the anomalous pulmonary venous connection to the poor survival.

Results have improved considerably in recent years, with a 95% or better survival [1]. Infants with obstructed pulmonary venous drainage have a poorer prognosis; this is the result of associated pulmonary venous stenosis, as well as changes in the pulmonary microcirculation with elevated pulmonary vascular resistance. There is now little mortality in infants with drainage to a vertical vein, to the coronary sinus, or directly to the right atrium. The mortality in infants with infradiaphragmatic drainage is somewhat higher because a large percentage have stenosis of the pulmonary venous trunk or of individual veins. Attempts have been made to treat these stenoses by various surgical techniques, but the results have been only fair in most centers. Attempts have also been made to dilate the veins by balloon angioplasty with, in some cases, introduction of stents. The results have generally been disappointing, but recently some limited success has been reported with aggressive attempts.

A recent surgical approach has been to marsupialize the stenosed pulmonary veins to a space created between the posterior aspect of the heart and the pleural surface. Sutures are placed from the lateral aspect of the epicardium to the pleura, thus creating a space that communicates with the left atrium. This avoids placing sutures in pulmonary veins and it is thought this will reduce the incidence of postoperative pulmonary venous stenosis.

The outlook following successful surgery is excellent. Stenosis of the anastomotic site between the pulmonary veins and the left atrium occurred in as many as 15–20% of infants following surgery, but with recent improvements in technique the incidence of this complication has been reduced considerably. However, a number of infants develop progressive obstruction of preexisting pulmonary venous stenosis.

In infants with lesser degrees of pulmonary venous obstruction who develop evidence of cardiac failure and pulmonary edema several weeks or months after birth, it had been common practice to delay surgery, if possible, to beyond 12–18 months because the risks of surgery in early infancy were high. For this reason, it was recommended that atrial septostomy by balloon and if necessary blade technique be used to improve cardiac failure and thus make it possible to delay surgery. This was successful in a relatively high proportion of infants, probably those with foramen ovale restriction, but it did not result in improvement in those with moderate obstruction to pulmonary venous drainage. Also, even in those who did improve, some degree of cardiac failure persisted and some infants succumbed to respiratory infection. It is now strongly recommended that surgery be performed in these infants without much delay, because the risks of surgery in infancy are very low.

There is some concern that infants who have survived after surgical repair of total anomalous pulmonary venous connection may demonstrate neurodevelopmental concerns. Kirshbom *et al.* [6] studied 30 patients 6–19 years after surgery, six of whom had pulmonary venous obstruction; all had circulatory arrest. Microcephaly was present in 28% and impairments of attention, fine motor skills, and visuomotor coordination were noted. Although these findings are disappointing, it is difficult to assess whether the neurodevelopmental disturbances were related to the surgical procedure or to genetic factors associated with the cardiovascular malformation.

References

1 Karamlou T, Gurofsky R, Al Sukhni E *et al.* Factors associated with mortality and reoperation in 377 children with total anomalous pulmonary venous connection. Circulation 2007;115:1591–1598.

2 Haworth SG, Reid L. Structural study of pulmonary circulation and of heart in total anomalous pulmonary venous return in early infancy. Br Heart J 1977;39:80–92.
3 Shankargouda S, Krishnan U, Murali R, Shah MJ. Dysphonia: a frequently encountered symptom in the evaluation of infants with unobstructed supracardiac total anomalous pulmonary venous connection. Pediatr Cardiol 2000;21:458–460.
4 Hancock Friesen CL, Zurakowski D, Thiagarajan RR *et al.* Total anomalous pulmonary venous connection: an analysis of current management strategies in a single institution. Ann Thorac Surg 2005;79:596–606.
5 Gaynor JW, Collins MH, Rychik J, Gaughan JP, Spray TL. Long-term outcome of infants with single ventricle and total anomalous pulmonary venous connection. J Thorac Cardiovasc Surg 1999;117:506–501.
6 Kirshbom PM, Flynn TB, Clancy RR *et al.* Late neurodevelopmental outcome after repair of total anomalous pulmonary venous connection. J Thorac Cardiovasc Surg 2005;129:1091–1097.

14

CHAPTER 14

Pulmonary stenosis and atresia with ventricular septal defect (tetralogy of Fallot)

A congenital cardiac anomaly characterized by right ventricular outflow obstruction, ventricular septal defect, right ventricular hypertrophy, and dextroposition of the aorta was recognized by a British physician, Thomas Peacock, in 1846. Etienne-Louis Fallot, a French physician, appreciated that the condition could be diagnosed in patients and it is now known as the tetralogy of Fallot. Originally it was thought that the cyanosis often present in patients with this complex was due to passage of blood directly from the right ventricle into the dextroposed or overriding aorta. Although aortic overriding may have some influence on flow of blood from the right ventricle into the aorta, the most important determinant of the degree of cyanosis is the severity of right ventricular outflow obstruction. The complex is characterized by anterior and superior (cephalad) deviation of the infundibular portion of the ventricular septum, but the hemodynamic disturbances and clinical manifestations are determined by the size of the ventricular septal defect and the severity of outflow obstruction. Symptoms and signs range from cardiac failure with no cyanosis to severe cyanosis with hypoxemia and acidemia. Ventricular septal defect with mild or moderate pulmonary stenosis is discussed in Chapter 7. This chapter presents the combination of ventricular septal defect with right ventricular outflow tract stenosis severe enough to produce cyanosis. Hemodynamic and clinical manifestations similar to those manifested in this complex can result from conditions in which pulmonary outflow is obstructed and there is a large communication between the ventricles. These include aortopulmonary transposition with ventricular septal defect and pulmonary stenosis, double-outlet right ventricle with pulmonary stenosis, L-transposition with ventricular septal defect and pulmonary stenosis, atrioventricular septal defect with pulmonary stenosis, and single ventricle with pulmonary stenosis. Some of these are discussed in the chapters devoted to the respective lesions.

Congenital Diseases of the Heart, 3rd edition. By A. Rudolph

Anatomical considerations

The heart is usually not greatly enlarged in these patients but the right ventricular wall is hypertrophied with a thickness similar to that of the left ventricle. The inflow portion of the right ventricle is usually of normal size but the outflow or infundibular region is narrow. Increased trabeculation of the right ventricle may be present, and sometimes thick muscle bundles are noted. The left ventricle is also usually normal in size but in some individuals, particularly those with severe cyanosis, the chamber may be somewhat smaller than normal. The ventricular septal defect is almost always large, with a diameter usually at least as great as that of the aortic valve; it is thus unrestrictive, permitting similar pressures between the left and right ventricles. The defect is usually perimembranous, with the upper margin of the defect formed by the aortic valve annulus. The infundibular portion of the septum separates the defect from the pulmonary valve. Occasionally, a subpulmonary or doubly committed subarterial defect (see Chapter 7) is associated with stenosis of the right ventricular outflow tract. It has been suggested that this association should not be designated tetralogy of Fallot, because the outlet septum is not present and therefore cannot show the characteristic deviation or malalignment. However, the hemodynamic features and clinical manifestations are similar to those of tetralogy of Fallot and it is reasonable to include these patients in the group. In some patients, the septal leaflet of the tricuspid valve is partly adherent to the margins of the ventricular septal defect, effectively decreasing the size of the communication and allowing separation of left and right ventricular pressures. Sometimes more than one defect is present, involving both the membranous and muscle portions. Occasionally, in children with Down syndrome with complete atrioventricular septal defect and right ventricular outflow tract stenosis, the outlet septum may be deviated anterosuperiorly, as in tetralogy of Fallot.

The ascending aorta is dilated and occupies a position somewhat more anterior than usual, partly due to the small size of the right ventricular infundibulum and pulmonary artery. The aortic valve is located more cephalad than usual and the position of the valve varies in its relation to the ventricles and the ventricular septal defect. Normally, the right sinus of Valsalva is positioned over the right ventricle, but separated from it by the ventricular septum. When a perimembranous ventricular septal defect is present, it appears that the aorta is positioned to some extent over the right ventricle. In tetralogy of Fallot, the aorta may arise almost completely from the left ventricle, but 10–15% or as much as 90% of the aortic orifice may override the right ventricle. Differentiation between tetralogy of Fallot and double-outlet right ventricle with pulmonary stenosis is often difficult. It has therefore been suggested that if it is estimated the aorta overrides the right ventricle by more than 50%, the diagnosis of double-outlet right ventricle should be applied. This does not seem to be appropriate, because the characteristic feature of double-outlet right ventricle is the absence of the normal contiguity of the mitral and aortic valves. However, the hemodynamic and clinical features of the two conditions are similar. A right aortic arch is a frequent finding in tetralogy of Fallot, occurring in about 25% of patients.

The dilation of the aortic root and ascending aorta has been ascribed to the fact that, prior to correction, blood flow into the aorta is greater than normal. However, it is now apparent that even after repair of the malformations, the dilation may persist and even become progressive into adult life. The role of increased flow has been reviewed by Bhat *et al.* [1] who noted that aortic enlargement was present in all patients with unrepaired tetralogy of Fallot at any age; enlargement increased if an aortopulmonary shunt was introduced. The enlargement persisted into adult life. However, if the lesions were repaired in infancy, the size of the aortic root was normal within 7 years. In adults following repair of tetralogy, about 15% had aortic root diameters greater than 1.5 of normal. Aortic dilation was associated with longer intervals from insertion of an aortopulmonary shunt to time of repair, with the presence of pulmonary atresia and right aortic arch, and with a deletion of chromosome 22q11 [2]. The aortic dilation is of concern in adults, because it may predispose to dissection and rupture [3]. Also, aortic root dilation may lead to aortic insufficiency, requiring aortic valve replacement [4].

Although most reports favor the greater than normal aortic blood flow as the mechanism responsible for aortic dilation, the possibility that an underlying structural defect may be involved must be considered. The aortic wall shows fragmentation of elastic fibers, which interferes with the elastic properties and makes the wall stiffer [5]. It is difficult to resolve whether the structural changes are primarily responsible for the dilation associated with the increased flow, or are the result of the abnormal flow. The fact that the aortic dilation is associated with the presence of a right aortic arch and with chromosome 22q11 deletion strongly suggests that a genetic defect in the aortic wall may underlie the dilation and that the excessive flow is contributory. It is important to examine the incidence and mechanisms involved in the dilation because of the potential for late risks after successful repair of the ventricular septal defect and outflow tract stenosis.

The coronary arteries are usually normal but abnormalities have been noted in 5–15% of patients. A single left or right coronary artery may be present. An anomaly that has important surgical implications is the coursing of a large coronary artery across the right ventricular outflow tract. This may be an anomalous left anterior descending artery arising from the right coronary artery, a right coronary artery originating from the left coronary artery, or a large branch of the right coronary artery supplying the conus region. Although these vessels are usually on the surface of the outflow tract, they may be positioned deeper in the myocardium and thus be severed during surgery, when the outflow tract is incised to relieve obstruction.

The right ventricular outflow obstruction varies greatly in severity and extent. In the majority of patients, infundibular or subpulmonary stenosis is the dominant lesion, but pulmonary valvar stenosis, with a bicommissural pulmonary valve, or a combination of valvar and infundibular stenosis, may be present. The infundibular obstruction is partly the result of the malalignment of the outlet septum, but hypertrophy of muscle bundles in the outflow tract contributes. The parietal band courses from the ventricular septum beneath the right pulmonary valve cusp to the anterior free wall of the right ventricle. The septal band, or septum trabeculomarginalis, extends from the ventricular septum near the apex toward the pulmonary valve; one arm is directed anteriorly and superiorly to the region of the left pulmonary valve cusp, while an inferior arm passes toward the septal origin of the parietal band. The portions of these muscle bands in the region of the infundibulum were previously collectively called the crista supraventricularis. Infundibular stenosis in the tetralogy of Fallot complex may be the result of varying degrees of hypertrophy of any of these muscle bands. Rarely, additional obstruction may occur proximal to the infundibular region due to hypertrophy of the moderator band and the inferior portion of the septal band. The moderator band originates from the septum near the lower end of the septal band and extends to the free wall of the right ventricle, effectively spanning the junction between the inflow and outflow tracts of the right ventricle. This type of obstruction has been referred to as double-chambered right ventricle. It is important to recognize its presence during surgery to relieve the outflow obstruction.

The pulmonary valve annulus is usually narrowed and the valve is often thickened and the leaflets adherent, producing severe valvar obstruction; one to three cusps may be present. The main pulmonary artery also varies greatly in size from almost normal to a very small diameter. Stenosis of the pulmonary artery just above the valve may result from fibrous constriction; stenoses at the origins of the left and right pulmonary arteries from the pulmonary trunk are also commonly encountered. The main left and right pulmonary arteries are usually relatively normal in size, and are almost always confluent. Rarely, the left pulmonary artery may not have a connection to the main pulmonary artery and during infancy may receive its blood supply from a ductus arteriosus. In later life the ductus arteriosus may close and the distal pulmonary artery becomes hypoplastic or atretic. The condition has been described as tetralogy of Fallot with absent left pulmonary artery. Even more rarely, the right pulmonary artery may receive its blood supply from a patent ductus arteriosus, which may arise from the right subclavian artery. More distal stenoses of intrapulmonary portions of the pulmonary arteries may also occur. Although hypoplasia of the whole pulmonary arterial vasculature is more commonly encountered with pulmonary atresia, occasionally it may be observed in infants with severe outflow tract stenosis.

The right ventricular outflow may be completely obstructed, resulting in pulmonary atresia. When atresia is present, the main pulmonary artery is invariably small and is not infrequently completely absent, or may be represented by a fibrous band. The left and right pulmonary arteries may be connected or confluent at their origins and a left-sided ductus arteriosus, often of small diameter, provides pulmonary blood flow. The left and right pulmonary arteries may not be confluent (15–20% of patients) and each may be supplied by a ductus arteriosus. Unlike in tetralogy of Fallot with a patent outflow tract, the left and right pulmonary arteries are frequently hypoplastic, particularly when they are not confluent. The main pulmonary artery and the central portions of its left and right branches may not develop and only the intrapulmonary arteries are present. Blood supply to these vessels varies greatly. Most commonly, arteries arising from the descending aorta at about the level of the left main bronchus connect with the intrapulmonary portions of the pulmonary arteries. There is controversy regarding the origin of these vessels. One view is that these are enlarged bronchial arteries; they have the same site of origin from the aorta and are often tortuous and thick-walled [6]. Others maintain that these arteries probably represent the persistence of the primitive embryological connections between the intrapulmonary vasculature and the dorsal aorta. These vessels normally regress when the pulmonary vasculature develops connections to the main pulmonary arteries (see Chapter 5). In the neonatal period, these arteries usually have a smooth wall and a uniform diameter. They subsequently become tortuous and develop thick walls and often stenoses [7]. They are now referred to as major aortopulmonary collateral arteries (MAPCAs). The condition of tetralogy of Fallot with pulmonary atresia and pulmonary blood flow from MAPCAs has sometimes been referred to as *pseudotruncus arteriosus*. MAPCAs vary considerably in size and number and in their pattern of distribution to the pulmonary circulation. A MAPCA may perfuse one lobe of a lung, or it may be distributed to more than one lobe of the same lung, or supply segments of both lungs. If there is no narrowing in the vessel, the systemic arterial pressure is transmitted to the small pulmonary vessels, creating a risk for the development of early pulmonary vascular obstructive disease. Areas of stenosis are commonly observed in these vessels, either at their origin from the aorta or along their course. This reduces the risk of pulmonary vascular complications, but restricts pulmonary blood flow. Some segments of the lung may have dual arterial supply. True pulmonary arteries may be distributed to a segment that is also supplied by a collateral artery. The true pulmonary artery is usually small and not connected to a central pulmonary artery; it receives its blood flow from anastomoses with neighboring arteries. The artery is sometimes demonstrated by retrograde pulmonary venous angiography (see Chapter 14).

The ductus arteriosus is frequently abnormal in children with tetralogy of Fallot. When the right ventricular outflow tract obstruction is not severe, the ductus arteriosus may be normal in size and connects with the descending aorta at an oblique inferior angle (see Chapter 6). With severe outflow tract stenosis, the ductus is usually narrow and connects with the descending aorta at an acute inferior angle. In patients with pulmonary atresia with absence of the main pulmonary artery, the ductus may arise from the aorta or the left subclavian artery and connect with the left pulmonary artery. It is usually small and often there is a stenosis at the connection with the pulmonary artery. Less frequently, a similar small ductus may be present on the right side and stenosis of the right pulmonary artery just distal to the site of connection with the ductus arteriosus is common. It has been suggested that the stenosis of the left and right pulmonary arteries is related to extension of ductus tissue into the pulmonary artery; following birth, the same mechanisms that result in closure of the ductus will constrict the pulmonary arteries. Not infrequently, and particularly in the presence of large MAPCAs, a ductus arteriosus is not detectable.

Absent pulmonary valve syndrome

Congenital absence of the pulmonary valve is almost always associated with morphological features of tetralogy of Fallot. The valve leaflets are absent, but sometimes a thin rim of valve tissue is evident at the annulus. The valve annulus is usually stenotic to varying degrees, but the stenosis is not usually severe. Subvalvar stenosis in the right ventricular outflow tract is frequently present, but it too is not usually severe. The malalignment ventricular septal defect and overriding aorta characteristic of tetralogy of Fallot are present, associated with the cephalad and anterior deviation of the outflow septum. In a study by Galindo *et al.* [8], 13 of 14 fetuses with absent pulmonary valve had tetralogy of Fallot. Marked dilatation of the main pulmonary artery has been considered a hallmark of the absent pulmonary valve syndrome; the dilatation extends to the right or left pulmonary artery, but occasionally involves both branches. The aneurysmal dilatation most commonly involves the main and right pulmonary arteries, less commonly the main and left arteries, and least often all three vessels. However, in the Galindo study, the pulmonary arteries were dilated and the heart was enlarged in all fetuses observed beyond 22 weeks' gestation, but in the five diagnosed before 22 weeks' gestation, four had a pulmonary trunk of normal size and three had normal heart size.

The ductus arteriosus has been thought to be absent in most patients with absent pulmonary valve syndrome, but a ligamentum arteriosus has been identified in some infants, indicating that the ductus had been present *in utero*. The possibility that pulmonary regurgitation in the fetus may be responsible for closure of the ductus has been considered. Galindo *et al.* found the ductus to be open in 20% of the fetuses, but there was no correlation between the presence of a patent ductus arteriosus and the size of the pulmonary arteries. Patency of the ductus arteriosus in fetuses with absent pulmonary valve may interfere with flow in the systemic circulation as a result of pulmonary regurgitation, as indicated by the presence of reverse end-diastolic flow in the umbilical artery in three fetuses at 10–14 weeks' gestation [9]. The pulmonary regurgitation may result in cardiac failure with hydrops fetalis.

Occasionally, left pulmonary artery hypoplasia may be associated with the marked dilatation of the main and left pulmonary arteries. Abnormalities in the development of intrapulmonary arteries have been noted in patients with the syndrome; they have abnormalities in branching pattern as well as in morphology. The large pulmonary arteries compress the large airways; depending on which arteries are enlarged, the main, left and right bronchi will be involved. Probably as a result of the compression of the airways *in utero*, there are frequently abnormalities in bronchial and alveolar development. The number of bronchial generations may be reduced and alveolar development may be impaired.

It has been noted in infants with absent pulmonary valve syndrome and a left pulmonary artery arising from the ductus arteriosus that the distal pulmonary architecture is usually normal. This suggests that the abnormal structural changes in the pulmonary arteries are related to hemodynamic disturbances, particularly pulmonary regurgitation, rather than to a genetic abnormality of the arterial wall.

Embryological considerations

The embryological disturbances that produce the tetralogy of Fallot complex have not been defined with certainty. Several possible mechanisms have been proposed. It has been suggested that disturbances in the rotation and separation of the bulbus cordis and truncus arteriosus are responsible. The bulbus is positioned over the right ventricle; during the process of separation of the bulbus by the bulbotruncal ridges into the aorta and pulmonary artery, rotation also occurs and the aorta is positioned posteriorly over the left ventricle. Tetralogy of Fallot has been explained as a disturbance in this rotation, combined with unequal separation of the bulbotruncus by the ridges. The latter results in narrowing of the infundibulum and a small pulmonary artery. The disturbance in rotation results in various degrees of aortic overriding of the right ventricle; it will also interfere with positioning of the infundibular portion of the ventricular septum over the trabecular septum, so that a malalignment ventricular septal defect results. Another hypothesis that has been proposed is that there is inadequate development of the right ventricular conus. This would result in a narrow infundibulum, and poor development of the main and branch pulmonary arteries could be secondary. Abnormal development of the conus could interfere with the normal relationship between the trabecular septum and the bulbotruncal septum, which would prevent the union of the two to close the interventricular foramen. What causes interference with right ventricular conus development is not known.

Recently, the concepts that explain tetralogy of Fallot as disturbances in rotation and separation of the bulbus cordis and truncus arteriosus have been challenged. It has been widely accepted that the heart is formed from the primary cardiac tube arising from splanchnic mesoderm; this develops into the ventricles and anteriorly into the conus and truncus arteriosus. There is now evidence indicating that there is a second population of splanchnic mesodermal cells located anteriorly in the pharyngeal mesoderm; these are myocardial precursors unrelated to the primitive cardiac tube. This region, the secondary, or anterior, heart field, provides the cells that form the myocardial wall of the outflow tract. In the chick embryo, the anterior heart field contributes to the outflow tract of the right ventricle but relatively little to the right ventricular wall; however, in the mammalian embryo, the contribution to the right ventricular wall is considerable [10,11]. The concept that disturbances in development of the anterior heart field could have a role in causing malformations of conal and truncal development is very appealing. In chick embryos, ablation of the secondary heart field resulted in overriding aorta and pulmonary atresia, features characteristic of tetralogy of Fallot [12]. It is yet to be determined what genetic or developmental factors interfere with myocardial precursors in the anterior heart field.

Absent pulmonary valve syndrome

The mechanisms involved in the development of absent pulmonary valve syndrome are obscure. The possible relationship between the absent pulmonary valve, the dilated pulmonary arteries, and the ductus arteriosus is of considerable interest. The ductus arteriosus is often absent in these patients, but it is not known whether this is a component of the malformation or the result of the abnormal hemodynamics. If failure of formation of the ductus is primary, blood ejected by the right ventricle into the pulmonary artery cannot pass into the descending aorta. This, together with the high fetal pulmonary vascular resistance that inhibits flow into the lungs, results in severe pulmonary regurgitation. This increases right ventricular stroke volume and results in progressive dilatation of the central pulmonary arteries. The stenosis in the infundibulum or at the annulus may further contribute to the distension by creating poststenotic turbulence. The factors determining which vessels are dilated have not been fully delineated, but the orientation of the right ventricular outflow tract could have a role. In those infants in whom the main and right pulmonary arteries are involved, it appears that the infundibulum points toward the right; this would direct the turbulent jet into the right pulmonary artery and result in distension. Similarly, when the left pulmonary artery is dilated, the infundibulum appears to be oriented toward the left. When both left and right vessels are involved the infundibulum is oriented directly cephalad [13].

The possibility that pulmonary regurgitation in the fetus may be responsible for closure of the ductus has been considered. Patency of the ductus arteriosus was observed in three fetuses at 10–14 weeks' gestation. These fetuses all had reverse end-diastolic flow in the umbilical artery as a result of diastolic flow from the aorta to the pulmonary artery [9]. I propose that in early gestation the ductus is patent and, as reported by Galindo *et al.* [8], the pulmonary arteries are not enlarged. During this period of gestation, because pulmonary vascular resistance is high and only a small proportion of the blood ejected by the right ventricle is accommodated in the relatively low volume of the pulmonary arteries, a substantial amount passes through the ductus arteriosus into the aorta during systole. During diastole blood flows from the aorta to the pulmonary artery as a result of the pulmonary regurgitation. With advancing gestation, the pulmonary arteries dilate and accommodate a progressively larger proportion of blood ejected by the right ventricle during systole. Also, with lung growth, the pulmonary vascular bed enlarges and pulmonary flow increases. Thus the volume of blood passing through the ductus arteriosus progressively decreases and this could explain its eventual closure. An additional factor that may contribute to reducing flow through the ductus is a decrease in right ventricular output resulting from failure. Dilated pulmonary arteries and cardiomegaly were observed in all fetuses beyond 22 weeks' gestation. Right ventricular failure results from the very large increase in volume load on the right ventricle and may result in hydrops fetalis. As mentioned above, the identification of a ligamentum arteriosum in some patients with absent pulmonary valve syndrome is evidence that the ductus arteriosus must have been present in some fetuses. It is possible that closure of the ductus arteriosus in mid to late gestation could reduce the risk of developing hydrops fetalis by reducing the degree of pulmonary regurgitation.

Recently, there has been considerable interest in the genetic aspects of tetralogy of Fallot. The complex occurs in 3–5% of all infants born with congenital cardiac lesions. Children with tetralogy of Fallot are more likely to have noncardiac-associated congenital cardiac anomalies compared to those with most other congenital cardiac defects. Also, although the incidence is not greatly increased, there is a somewhat greater occurrence of conotruncal anomalies in siblings than with other cardiac anomalies. It has now been shown that there is a frequent association of 22q11 deletion in children with tetralogy of Fallot. The congenital anomalies of the CATCH 22 syndrome, which are associated with 22q11 deletion, are not all characteristically observed in children with tetralogy of Fallot. However, many show at least some of the manifestations of the syndrome. In various series, it has been estimated that 15–35% of patients with tetralogy of Fallot have a microdeletion on 22q11; the deletion appears to be at the D22S39 or D22S398 locus. Interestingly, the deletion has been noticed in about 45% of children with tetralogy of Fallot with pulmonary atresia and in about 65% of those with tetralogy of Fallot and absent pulmonary valve.

Hemodynamic considerations

The important features that determine the hemodynamic consequences in patients with ventricular septal defect and pulmonary stenosis are the size of the defect, the severity of the stenosis, and the level of systemic vascular resistance. In most patients, and certainly in almost all infants, the ventricular septal defect is large and produces an equalization of left and right ventricular pressures. In the ensuing discussion it will be assumed that the ventricular septal defect is large, and separate comments will be made in regard to the few instances in which the defect is small.

Fetal circulation

The presence of the lesions does not appear to influence the fetal circulation adversely or to interfere with the umbilical–placental circulation, because the infants usually have no intrauterine difficulties and are well developed at birth. Oxygen saturations in the superior and inferior vena cava blood returning to the heart are probably normal. I have not been able to identify any reports of ultrasound studies in which patterns of blood flow were studied in fetuses with tetralogy of Fallot. The flows across the foramen ovale and the tricuspid valve are also probably normal. However, if there is severe pulmonary stenosis or pulmonary atresia, and especially if peripheral pulmonary arteries are small, pulmonary blood flow could be reduced and venous return to the left atrium would fall. Flow through the foramen ovale might therefore increase. Because most of the ductus venosus stream already flows preferentially through the foramen ovale, any additional flow would be derived from the superior or distal inferior vena cava streams. This would result in increased flow of poorly oxygenated venous blood into the left atrium across the foramen ovale. If pulmonary blood flow is low, the amount of poorly oxygenated pulmonary venous blood returning to the left atrium would decrease. With all these considerations, it is unlikely that oxygen saturation of left atrial blood does not change significantly.

The volume and direction of blood flow in the pulmonary artery will depend on the severity of right ventricular outflow obstruction. If it is of mild or moderate degree, the right ventricle will eject a somewhat reduced amount of blood into the pulmonary artery but a quantity adequate to supply total pulmonary blood flow and also to provide some blood through the ductus arteriosus to the descending aorta. If the obstruction is severe or complete, blood supply to the lungs will be derived from the aorta by flow through the ductus arteriosus to the pulmonary artery. Serial observations in fetuses have shown that the severity of obstruction may progress with advancing gestational age, even to the point of atresia [14,15]. If pulmonary arterial blood flow is derived through the ductus arterioisus, Po_2 in pulmonary arterial blood would be slightly higher than normal and this could reduce pulmonary vascular resistance and possibly reduce normal development of pulmonary vascular smooth muscle. Whether blood flows from the pulmonary trunk to the aorta or in the opposite direction, the total amount of flow through the ductus arteriosus would be reduced considerably. Whereas normally about 50% of combined ventricular output (CVO) traverses the ductus, in the presence of complete pulmonary atresia only the proportion of CVO distributed to the lungs (about 20–25% in the human fetus) would flow through it. In less severe degrees of obstruction, flow across the ductus would be reduced to a variable extent and the ductus diameter would be decreased. If the obstruction is severe, blood will flow through the ductus arteriosus from the aorta to the pulmonary artery and the orientation of the ductus will be changed. Normally there is an obtuse inferior angle between the ductus arteriosus and the aorta, but in newborn infants with tetralogy of Fallot it is frequently noted to be quite acute. As mentioned above, in the presence of pulmonary atresia with absence of the main pulmonary artery, a left-sided and occasionally a right-sided ductus provides flow to the left or right lung. Because each ductus conducts only a small flow to the respective lung (about 10% of CVO at most), it is narrow.

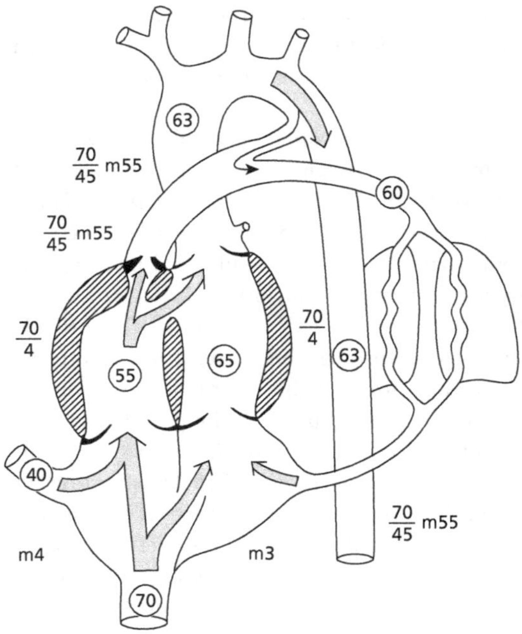

Figure 14.1 Ventricular septal defect and right ventricular outflow obstruction in a fetus: course of the circulation, oxygen saturations (circled), and pressures. m, mean pressure.

The right ventricular outflow obstruction would tend to divert blood away from the pulmonary trunk and through the ventricular septal defect into the ascending aorta (Figure 14.1). The ascending aorta will therefore carry a larger percentage of CVO, depending on the degree of pulmonary stenosis; in the presence of pulmonary atresia, it conducts the total CVO. This explains the fact that the ascending aorta and the isthmus are usually wider than normal in infants with tetralogy of Fallot (see Chapter 14). The normal difference between oxygen saturations of ascending and descending aortic blood will be reduced or eliminated. In the normal fetus, oxygen saturation in the ascending aorta is higher than that in the descending aorta (see Chapter 1). In patients with tetralogy of Fallot, the shunting of right ventricular blood into the aorta through the ventricular septal defect will result in a somewhat lower than normal oxygen saturation and Po_2 in ascending aortic blood. Whereas normally a large percentage of pulmonary arterial blood passes through the ductus arteriosus into the descending aorta, in tetralogy of Fallot less right ventricular blood enters the pulmonary trunk and flow across the ductus arteriosus to the descending aorta is reduced. Therefore the oxygen saturation of descending aortic blood will be somewhat higher than normal. If pulmonary stenosis is severe, no blood from the pulmonary artery passes through the ductus and thus oxygen saturations in the ascending and descending aorta are the same. The lower than normal oxygen content in ascending aortic blood could possibly result in higher than normal cerebral and coronary blood flows in the fetus, because of the vasodilatory effect of hypoxemia. However, whether these changes in ascending and descending aortic oxygen saturations produce any adverse effects in the fetus is not known.

Left and right ventricular output

In the normal human fetus the right ventricle ejects about 55% and the left ventricle about 45% of CVO. The afterload on the right ventricle is relatively low, because it ejects through the large ductus arteriosus into the relatively low-resistance lower body circulation including the umbilical–placental circulation. Left ventricular afterload is higher, because the narrowed aortic isthmus imposes a relatively high resistance (see Chapter 1). In the fetus with tetralogy of Fallot, the pulmonary stenosis increases the resistance to right ventricular output, so flow into the pulmonary artery is reduced. However, because the ventricular septal defect is large and unrestrictive, right ventricular blood can flow readily into the ascending aorta and ascending aortic flow is thus greater than normal; with pulmonary atresia there is no flow from the right ventricle into the pulmonary artery and the total cardiac output is ejected into the aorta. In view of the presence of the large ventricular septal defect and a varying degree of overriding of the aorta, the two ventricles are probably presented with the same afterload and the outputs of the two ventricles are probably similar. I have not been able to obtain any information about the volumes ejected by the left and right ventricle in fetuses with tetralogy of Fallot. As mentioned above, with pulmonary stenosis, the pulmonary venous return to the left atrium would be reduced and this could decrease left ventricular output. However, it is not known whether flow through the foramen ovale increases to maintain left ventricular output.

The electrocardiogram in the immediate neonatal period provides some information about the loading on the ventricles prenatally. In most neonates with tetralogy of Fallot, the electrocardiogram is similar to that in normal infants. However, I have encountered several infants with an ultrasound diagnosis of tetralogy of Fallot who showed dominant left ventricular forces, leading to a clinical diagnosis of tricuspid atresia or pulmonary atresia with intact ventricular septum. It is difficult to explain this finding, but it could possibly be related to the position of the ventricular septum, the size of the ventricular septal defect, and the degree of overriding of the aorta. It would be of great interest to examine these features in relation to the ejection of each ventricle. Another factor that could possibly affect the volumes ejected is filling of the ventricles. If the ventricles eject against the same afterload, it would be expected that the diastolic inflow would be similar. However, venous return to the left ventricle may be altered; with pulmonary atresia it would be dependent on the volume of flow through the ductus arteriosus or the presence of MAPCAs or both. In neonates with large MAPCAs, flow into the lungs is occasionally so large as to cause a volume overload on the left ventricle with failure. MAPCAs have been observed in the fetus, but whether flow is large enough to cause a large volume load on the left ventricle is questionable. The flow pattern in MAPCAs in the fetus shows a peak during systole, with little flow in diastole (similar to that seen in the peripheral pulmonary arteries in normal fetuses), suggesting that pulmonary vascular resistance is high (Lisa Hornberger, personal communication). However, because the pulmonary circulation is being perfused by blood with an oxygen saturation higher that that normally present in pulmonary arterial blood, it is possible that flow is higher than normal in the fetus.

Absent pulmonary valve syndrome

The ductus arteriosus is frequently either atretic or not developed in fetuses with tetralogy of Fallot with absent pulmonary valve. The possible importance of the ductus in inducing the marked dilatation of the pulmonary arteries has been discussed above. The pulmonary regurgitation results in a marked volume overload on the right ventricle; in the fetus, the right ventricular pressure would be similar to aortic systolic pressure because the ventricular septal defect is usually large. In this circumstance, the ventricle would be subjected to a high volume and pressure load. Cardiac failure is a not infrequent association with these cardiac anomalies in the fetus. It is manifested by the development of ascites, pericardial fluid accumulation and generalized edema, or fetal hydrops. The severity of the infundibular or annular stenosis could possibly determine whether fetal cardiac failure would develop. With more severe stenosis, although the afterload on the right ventricle would be higher, the degree of pulmonary regurgitation would be less, and the volume load on the ventricle would be lower; the likelihood for cardiac failure would thus probably be reduced. The presence of marked degrees of pulmonary regurgitation could seriously affect perfusion of the intrapulmonary vessels. In the normal fetus, diastolic pressure in the pulmonary artery is at systemic arterial levels and some perfusion of the pulmonary circulation may occur. However, pulmonary valve regurgitation would greatly lower pulmonary diastolic pressure and limit perfusion. The abnormal development of the intrapulmonary vessels in this syndrome could possibly be related to disturbances in perfusion during fetal life.

Postnatal circulation

Pulmonary blood flow

After birth, with elimination of the placental circulation, the function of gas exchange is transferred to the lung and adequate oxygen supply to the body depends on establishment of ventilation and an adequate pulmonary blood flow. Normally, pulmonary blood flow increases eightfold to tenfold as a result of the decrease in pulmonary vascular resistance associated with ventilation of the lungs with air. In the infant or child with tetralogy of Fallot, several factors determine the magnitude of pulmonary blood flow:

- source of blood flow to the lungs;
- severity and functional behavior of outflow obstruction from the right ventricle;
- level of right ventricular (and systemic arterial) pressure;
- ductus arteriosus.

Source of pulmonary blood flow

In most infants with tetralogy of Fallot with moderate or severe outflow obstruction or pulmonary atresia, pulmonary flow is derived from the right ventricle or through the ductus arteriosus. In those with pulmonary atresia with absence of the main pulmonary artery and confluence of the pulmonary arteries, pulmonary blood flow may be derived through a unilateral or bilateral ductus, but in many of these infants pulmonary blood flow is provided by MAPCAs. The size and number of these collateral arteries determines the course of these infants. In the presence of pulmonary atresia, there is admixture of all systemic and pulmonary venous blood in the ascending aorta, so that the oxygen content of arterial blood distributed to the systemic and pulmonary circulations is essentially similar. The level of oxygen saturation is determined by the ratio of pulmonary to systemic blood flow (see Chapter 4). Immediately after birth, the baby may be moderately cyanosed, but as pulmonary arteriolar resistance falls after birth, pulmonary blood flow may become large.

If MAPCAs are well developed, the degree of cyanosis may decrease, although occasionally evidence of cardiac failure develops as a result of the high volume load placed on the left ventricle. Because MAPCAs arise from the aorta or its major branches, the pressure in these vessels is at systemic levels, unless stenosis occurs either at their origin or along their course. In the absence of stenosis, the pulmonary arterioles are subjected to the high pressures and there is thus a serious risk for development of pulmonary vascular obstructive changes in the segments of lung supplied by the vessels. Although stenoses in MAPCAs do not appear to be significant during infancy, they tend to either develop or progress with advancing age. This would reduce the risk of morphological changes in the pulmonary circulation, but pulmonary blood flow would be reduced and cyanosis becomes more severe.

When pulmonary blood flow is derived predominantly from the ductus arteriosus, as with very severe outflow tract obstruction or atresia, the magnitude of flow is determined by the size of the ductus and its degree of constriction (see discussion in Chapter 15).

Pulmonary blood flow may be derived partly or completely from flow through the right ventricular outflow tract, in which case it is determined by the degree of obstruction. In the absence of MAPCAs or a patent ductus arteriosus, this is the only source of flow through the lungs during infancy. However, with severe outflow stenosis, collateral connections from bronchial arteries to precapillary pulmonary arteries develop with advancing age. These may become quite extensive and provide substantial pulmonary blood flow. The factors responsible for an increase in bronchial flow are not fully understood; it has been shown that bronchopulmonary arterial flow increases when there is an increase in systemic arterial pressure or a decrease in pulmonary arterial pressure. Pulmonary arterial pressure is decreased in patients with tetralogy of Fallot and this may be one of the factors stimulating the development of bronchial flow, but other mechanisms are probably involved. Usually an extensive bronchial circulation is not developed in infancy or early childhood, but large bronchial collateral blood flows may be established over several years to permit survival into adult life.

Right ventricular outflow obstruction

Both the site and severity of the right ventricular outflow tract obstruction are important in affecting the hemodynamic features of tetralogy of Fallot. Stenosis of the infundibular region is usually present and in addition the pulmonary valve annulus is often stenosed; the pulmonary valve leaflets may be thickened and immobile, and stenosis beyond the valve may be present, often at the origin of the branch pulmonary arteries. The outflow resistance from the right ventricle is reflected by the sum of resistances at all these sites plus the pulmonary vascular resistance. In the majority of children the ventricular septal defect is large enough to permit equalization of pressures in the left and right ventricles. With equal ejection pressures, the relative afterloads determine the volume ejected by each ventricle. Thus if the total outflow resistance of the right ventricle exceeds systemic vascular resistance, some right ventricular blood will be diverted through the ventricular septal defect into the aorta (right-to-left shunt), causing cyanosis, and the volume ejected into the pulmonary circulation would be reduced. The more severe the outflow tract stenosis, the greater the right-to-left shunt and the smaller the blood flow to the lung.

If the degree of outflow tract stenosis is such that the resistance is less than systemic vascular resistance, blood flows preferentially through the ventricular septal defect from the left ventricle into the right ventricle and pulmonary artery (left-to-right shunt). Pulmonary blood flow will exceed systemic flow, and no cyanosis will be evident (pink tetralogy). When the outflow obstruction is mild, the pulmonary annulus and valve are often normal and the stenosis is infundibular in location; although deviation of the outlet septum reduces the infundibular channel, hypertrophy of the parietal and septal muscle bands may contribute to the narrowing. When the outflow tract stenosis is mild, the circulatory dynamics and clinical course may be similar to those of patients with large ventricular septal defects (see Chapter 7). During the neonatal period, the infundibular stenosis and high pulmonary vascular resistance may combine to limit left-to-right shunting and may even induce right-to-left shunting with varying degrees of cyanosis (Figure 14.2). As pulmonary vascular resistance

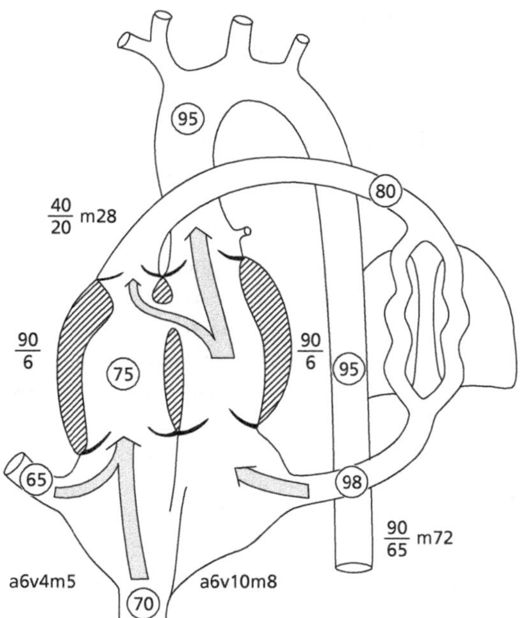

Figure 14.2 Ventricular septal defect with moderate degree of right ventricular outflow obstruction: course of the circulation, oxygen saturations (circled), and pressures. In this case there is a small ventricular left-to-right shunt and pulmonary arterial pressure is increased slightly. m, mean pressure.

falls, the total outflow resistance falls, resulting in left-to-right shunting through the ventricular septal defect. The shunt may be large enough to greatly increase left ventricular volume load and cause cardiac failure, which is not usually severe because the infundibular stenosis limits the size of the left-to-right shunt. The pulmonary arterial pressure is usually only mildly or moderately elevated, in contrast with the child with a large ventricular septal defect with no right ventricular outflow tract stenosis. The risk for development of morphological changes in the pulmonary vasculature is therefore not significant. This risk is further reduced by the tendency for the infundibular stenosis to progress with advancing age, further reducing pulmonary arterial pressure. The increasing severity of the infundibular narrowing results from progressive hypertrophy of the muscle. This increases right ventricular afterload, reducing the left-to-right shunt and the volume loading of the left ventricle. Symptoms of failure disappear and the child appears well. Progression of the infundibular hypertrophy may result in the appearance of cyanosis, which occurs first with exertion, and subsequently persists. The time course for the progression in severity of infundibular hypertrophy varies. It may result in appearance of cyanosis within 6–8 months after birth, but this may be delayed for several years.

Progression of the severity of outflow tract stenosis frequently also occurs as a result of infundibular hypertrophy in patients with cyanosis during infancy. This results in a further decrease in pulmonary blood flow and a larger ventricular right-to-left shunt, with increasing cyanosis.

The functional behavior of the hypertrophied infundibular muscle has been the subject of considerable conjecture. It has been proposed that the muscle in the infundibulum is capable of contracting sufficiently to produce a marked increase in outflow tract stenosis and thus severely reduce pulmonary blood flow. This has been proposed as a possible mechanism for the occurrence of hypoxic spells (see Chapter 14). Although it is difficult to demonstrate that the infundibular region has undergone constriction during a spell, there is some evidence to suggest that this may occur. In one study, acute administration of disopyramide (Norpace), an antiarrhythmic agent that also has a negative inotropic effect on the myocardium, resulted in widening of the infundibular area and an increase in systemic arterial oxygen saturation. Stimulation of myocardial contractility by increased sympathoadrenal activity induced by anxiety, stress or exercise could cause infundibular constriction. Pulmonary blood flow would be reduced and right-to-left shunt increased. It has also been shown that the number of β-adrenoceptors in infundibular muscle is greater in children with tetralogy of Fallot who have suffered hypoxic spells than in those who have not [16]. The infundibular muscle would thus be unusually sensitive to sympathetic nerve stimulation or circulating catecholamines. The concept that infundibular constriction is an important mechanism in causing hypoxic spells forms the basis for the administration of β-adrenoceptor blockers such as propranolol for treatment or prevention of these spells (see Chapter 14).

Right ventricular pressure

Since the ventricular septal defect is large in most patients with tetralogy of Fallot, right and left ventricular pressures are equal. Right ventricular pressure assumes the same contour as left ventricular pressure, with a rapid upstroke, a squared-off top, and a rapid descent; this contrasts with the triangular contour of the right ventricular pressure pulse in the patient with pulmonary stenosis and an intact ventricular septum. Right ventricular pressure closely follows changes in left ventricular pressure so that, even with ectopic beats, pressures are identical; there is also little postectopic potentiation of systolic pressure in either ventricle. A decrease in systemic vascular resistance results in a fall in aortic and left ventricular pressures, with a similar change in the right ventricle.

Administration of anesthetic agents or sedative drugs to patients with tetralogy of Fallot frequently results in peripheral vasodilatation. Systemic vascular resistance and left and right ventricular pressures fall; reduction in cardiac output may contribute further to this fall. The drop in right ventricular pressure reduces the pressure gradient and blood flow across the outflow tract, and pulmonary blood flow falls. This interferes with total oxygen uptake in the lungs, resulting in exaggeration of hypoxemia (see below). In addition, the fall in systemic vascular resistance permits a larger right-to-left shunt.

The volume of systemic venous blood returning to the heart affects the level of right ventricular pressure. Posture is an important determinant of venous return. Quiet standing, or passive tilt with the head up, results in pooling of blood in the lower extremities and abdomen. Associated with the decrease in venous return, right ventricular pressure and pulmonary blood flow fall. It has also been suggested that a reduction in venous return may result in a reduction in right ventricular volume and thereby increase the infundibular narrowing, further contributing to the fall in pulmonary blood flow; however, this has not been documented. A decrease in venous return may also be an important factor in the increased hypoxemia associated with anesthesia and sedation. The infant or child is usually placed on a flat surface and is immobile. Venous dilatation results in pooling of blood and venous return is reduced. The influence of posture on venous return is also important in infants with hypoxic spells and in the response to exercise in children with tetralogy of Fallot.

Elevation of right ventricular pressure may result from the increase in aortic and left ventricular pressure associated with a rise in systemic vascular resistance. Since the right ventricular obstruction is relatively fixed, pulmonary blood flow will be increased by the rise in perfusion pressure. In addition, the increase in systemic vascular resistance will result in a decrease in right-to-left shunt. These responses form the basis for the use of peripheral vasoconstrictor agents such as phenylephrine in the treatment of infants with acute hypoxic spells [17]. An increase in systemic venous return to the right ventricle will also increase right ventricular pressure and thus enhance pulmonary blood flow; this could explain the beneficial effect of posture in raising arterial oxygen content in infants with hypoxic spells or in children after exercise (see Chapter 14). An increase in right ventricular pressure and volume could have additional beneficial effects by distending the infundibular area, thus reducing the outflow tract obstruction.

Although the right and left ventricular pressures are usually equal in patients with tetralogy of Fallot, occasionally the ventricular septal defect is relatively small, and the pressures may separate. This is not usually encountered in infancy and is probably due to acquired partial closure of the defect.

Although the causes of partial closure of the defect are not usually apparent, one mechanism that may be responsible is adherence of the septal leaflet of the tricuspid valve to the margins of the defect. When the defect size is limiting, systolic pressure in the right ventricle may exceed that in the left ventricle and aorta, and the peak of the pressure tracing may assume the triangular shape characteristic of pulmonary stenosis with an intact septum.

Ductus arteriosus

This channel is important in providing pulmonary blood flow after birth when right ventricular outflow obstruction is severe and few or no MAPCAs are present. Because it conducts only a small pulmonary blood flow during fetal life, it is usually considerably smaller than normal. With the fall in pulmonary vascular resistance associated with ventilation, flow through the ductus increases, but it is rarely possible to establish normal postnatal levels of pulmonary flow. However, systemic arterial oxygen saturation increases and occasionally reaches 85–92% (Figure 14.3). The maintenance of oxygen saturation above the fetal level is dependent on continued patency of the ductus arteriosus. The behavior of the ductus in response to oxygen and other constrictor agents in infants with tetralogy of Fallot is not known. Since the ductus is often smaller than normal, the musculature may not be developed normally and its responses could be different. If it does respond normally to oxygen, the higher Po_2 achieved by the increased pulmonary blood flow after birth will tend to constrict the ductus. An intriguing relationship may then exist between systemic arterial Po_2, the degree of constriction of the ductus, and pulmonary blood flow. The increased pulmonary blood flow will result in an increased systemic arterial Po_2, which will in turn tend to constrict the ductus. This will interfere with maintenance of pulmonary blood flow, resulting in decreased arterial Po_2 and subsequent dilatation of the ductus. A variable and unstable condition could develop in which intermittent cyanosis could occur.

The level of systemic arterial pressure could be important in influencing pulmonary blood flow by its effect on blood flow through the ductus arteriosus. Thus a fall in arterial pressure could have an adverse effect by reducing pulmonary blood flow

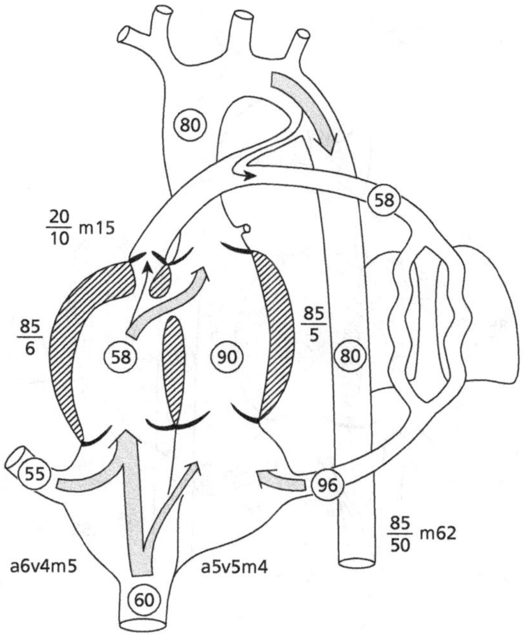

Figure 14.3 Ventricular septal defect with severe obstruction to right ventricular outflow in a newborn infant: course of the circulation, oxygen saturations (circled), and pressures. In this case the ductus arteriosus was still patent. m, mean pressure.

derived through the ductus, as well as across the right ventricular outflow tract. In infants with tetralogy of Fallot, closure of the ductus is often delayed for several days or even weeks. This could be related to abnormalities in either morphological development or functional behavior.

Constriction or closure of the ductus arteriosus will result in a fall in systemic arterial oxygen saturation and Po_2 (Figure 14.4). The degree and rate of fall are determined by the degree of right ventricular outflow stenosis and the time period over which the ductus arteriosus closes. If pulmonary stenosis is severe and the occlusion is rapid, systemic arterial saturation will fall rapidly to as low as 35–40%, Po_2 will drop to 20–30 mmHg, and hypoxia and acidemia may develop. If there has been adequate opportunity for development of a collateral circulation to the lungs, pulmonary blood flow may be maintained when the ductus closes.

In patients with pulmonary atresia, the ductus arteriosus may not be important in providing postnatal pulmonary blood flow, because MAPCAs are

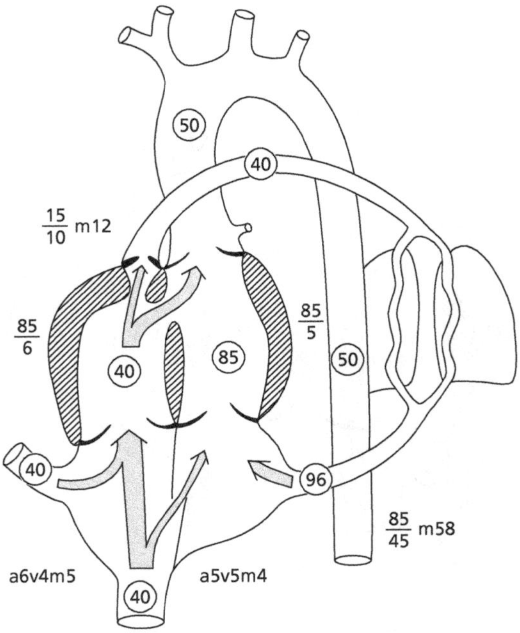

Figure 14.4 Ventricular septal defect with severe obstruction to right ventricular outflow in an infant: course of the circulation, oxygen saturations (circled), and pressures. In this case the ductus arteriosus had closed. m, mean pressure.

frequently present. The ductus may provide some benefit in the early neonatal period, because the fall in pulmonary vascular resistance in the segments of lung supplied by MAPCAs may be delayed by exposure to the high systemic arterial pressure. Closure of the ductus will curtail perfusion of the pulmonary arteries: they will not grow and possibly will become more hypoplastic. When the left and right pulmonary arteries are not confluent and one or both are supplied by a ductus arteriosus, closure of the ductus results in hypoplasia and sometimes atresia of the pulmonary artery.

Oxygen supply to the body

In patients with ventricular septal defect with mild or moderate right ventricular outflow obstruction, pulmonary blood flow is usually normal and oxygen supply to the body is adequate. However, with severe right ventricular outflow obstruction, the main manifestation is hypoxemia and the concern is the adequacy of oxygen supply to the tissues. The roles of pulmonary blood flow, hemoglobin concentration, and the P_{50} of hemoglobin in tissue oxygen supply are discussed in detail in Chapter 3. These factors are reviewed briefly, specifically in relation to tetralogy of Fallot.

Pulmonary blood flow

The amount of oxygen that can be delivered to the tissues is limited by the total amount of oxygen that can be taken up in the lungs, and this is related to pulmonary blood flow. In infancy and early childhood, flow through the pulmonary valve is usually necessary to maintain pulmonary capillary flow. The magnitude of flow is determined by right ventricular pressure and the degree of obstruction. Since systolic pressure in the right ventricle follows that in the left ventricle and aorta, a decrease in systemic arterial pressure, as may occur with peripheral vasodilatation due to anesthetic agents, sedative drugs or exercise, will result in a decrease in pulmonary blood flow. An increase in right and left ventricular pressures and enhancement of pulmonary flow may be induced by peripheral vasoconstrictor drugs. Monitoring blood pressure can readily assess the potential harmful effects of any pharmacological agent, procedure or maneuver in patients with tetralogy of Fallot. A fall in systemic arterial pressure will produce a corresponding fall in right ventricular pressure and place the individual in jeopardy by reducing pulmonary flow. Pulmonary blood flow may also be increased by facilitating venous return, such as by elevating the legs.

Blood oxygen capacity

The amount of oxygen that can be carried by blood is mainly dependent on the hemoglobin concentration, or oxygen capacity. The higher the oxygen capacity of blood perfusing the lungs, the larger the amount of oxygen that can be taken up per unit of blood flow. Oxygen content of blood at any level of Po_2 increases linearly with the rise in oxygen capacity. Thus, blood with a higher oxygen capacity will be capable of providing more oxygen to the tissues for the same flow rate and arterial oxygen saturation. Even though systemic arterial Po_2 and oxygen saturation may be quite low, adequate oxygen may be supplied to the tissues. In the newborn infant hemoglobin concentration is relatively high (15–18 g/dL), as is hematocrit (50–55%). Normally, hemoglobin concentration falls to about

10–12 g/dL by 3–4 months after birth. Persistent hypoxemia after birth results in increased blood erythropoietin concentrations, which stimulates bone marrow production of erythroid cells. In order to maintain or increase hemoglobin levels, iron is required; however, iron stores are limited in infants, and food intake in early infancy provides little iron. Therefore, there is a high incidence of relative anemia in infants with tetralogy of Fallot with moderate to severe hypoxemia [18]. The anemia is considered to be relative, because although the hemoglobin level may be in the range normal for the age of the infant, it is reduced under the circumstances of hypoxic stimulation. The stimulation for red cell formation continues and very high red cell counts of $7–8 \times 10^6/mm^3$ may be achieved, but the cells are microcytic and hypochromic and mean corpuscular hemoglobin concentration and mean corpuscular volume are markedly reduced. Administration of iron to these infants results in a rapid increase in hemoglobin concentration to levels well above normal. Since arterial oxygen saturation usually does not change, the total amounts of both oxygenated and reduced hemoglobin increase. The patient may therefore appear more cyanotic but total oxygen delivery will increase and symptoms of hypoxia may improve.

The administration of iron to hypoxemic patients results in an increase in mean corpuscular hemoglobin concentration and mean corpuscular volume, and a rise in hematocrit. The hematocrit has a marked effect on blood viscosity. The relationship is curvilinear: when hematocrit is raised from 30 to 50%, viscosity increases only slightly; above this level there is a marked increase in viscosity, and at hematocrit above 60–65% viscosity rises steeply. The increased viscosity produces an effective increase in resistance to blood flow through the tissues (see Chapter 4). At very high hematocrit, blood flow may be reduced so that the beneficial effect of the increased oxygen capacity is abolished.

2,3-Diphosphoglycerate

The release of oxygen from hemoglobin is facilitated by the presence of 2,3-diphosphoglycerate (2,3-DPG) in the red cell (see Chapter 3). In infants with tetralogy of Fallot with systemic arterial hypoxemia, 2,3-DPG levels in the red cells increase and thus aid in oxygen delivery to the tissues.

Hypoxemia and hypoxia in tetralogy of Fallot

In infants with severe pulmonary stenosis or pulmonary atresia, constriction or closure of the ductus arteriosus will result in a rapid decrease in systemic arterial oxygen saturation and Po_2. If this occurs rapidly, there will be inadequate time for a compensatory rise in hemoglobin concentration. Inadequate oxygen supply to the tissues will result in increased anaerobic glycolysis, with production of lactic acid and progressive metabolic acidemia (see Chapter 3). The decreased pH and Po_2 stimulate peripheral and central chemoreceptors, with a resultant increase in respiratory depth and rate (see Chapter 2). Since alveolar ventilation is increased and pulmonary blood flow is reduced, the ventilation–perfusion ratio is markedly increased. Pulmonary venous Po_2 may be raised to 110–115 mmHg, Pco_2 reduced to 15–20 mmHg, and pH increased to 7.48–7.50, in an attempt to compensate for the metabolic acidemia. However, the reduced pulmonary blood flow does not permit adequate correction of systemic arterial blood gases and Po_2. Systemic arterial Pco_2 may be maintained at normal levels or may be reduced. This is partly due to the reduction in pulmonary venous carbon dioxide content, but is also related to the reduced production of carbon dioxide; this is related to the fact that lactate accumulates and is not metabolized to carbon dioxide and water. Significant increases in Pco_2 to levels above 40 mmHg are unusual and are usually related to the presence of pulmonary disease. Po_2 may fall to 20–25 mmHg and pH to 7.0 or less.

Hypoxic spells

Many infants do not have serious hypoxemia in the neonatal period but develop symptoms about 2–6 months after birth. The factors responsible for the onset of symptoms may be closure of the ductus arteriosus, development of relative anemia, growth with relative increase in right ventricular outflow tract stenosis, and increased activity with increased oxygen requirements. The infant may be only mildly hypoxemic at rest but episodes of severe hypoxemia with hypoxia and acidemia, known as *hypoxic* or *tetralogy spells*, occur. The actual mechanisms responsible for these attacks are not known. Guntheroth *et al.* [19] have presented the view that spells are precipitated by any stimulus producing hyperventilation. They suggest that increased ventilation enhances venous return to the right atrium and ventricle and thus increases right ventricular output. Since the proportion of blood passing to the pulmonary circulation would be limited by the fixed pulmonary stenosis, the amount of venous blood ejected into the aorta increases, thus lowering arterial oxygen saturation. I do not believe that this can be an important mechanism in the spell syndrome, because the effect of increased venous blood flow into the aorta on arterial oxygen saturation could be only temporary. As mentioned above, the increase in venous return will raise right ventricular pressure and pulmonary blood flow will increase to some extent, because the pressure gradient across the narrowed outflow tract increases. Even if pulmonary blood flow did not change, the total amount of oxygen taken up in the lungs would not be influenced and thus oxygen availability to the tissues would not be affected. It is likely that the hyperpnea associated with spells does not precede the episode, but develops as a chemoreceptor-induced response to exaggeration of hypoxemia.

However, prolonged crying may have a deleterious effect on systemic arterial oxygen saturation, because the increased pulmonary vascular resistance developed by prolonged expiration, particularly during the Valsalva maneuver, may result in a decrease in pulmonary blood flow. If, during crying, the infant also has periods of breath-holding, the combined effects of inadequate ventilation and decreased pulmonary blood flow may markedly reduce systemic arterial oxygen saturation.

A reduction in pulmonary blood flow could also result from functional contraction of the right ventricular infundibulum; this has been claimed to be an important cause of hypoxic spells. Although there is as yet no convincing evidence that infundibular spasm is a frequent mechanism, the hypothesis has received support from evidence that β-adrenoceptor inhibitors, which decrease myocardial contractility, may relieve the spells and decrease their incidence (see Chapter 14).

There is a good deal of evidence to suggest that changes in venous return to the heart and in peripheral vascular resistance may have important roles in the production of spells. Infants immobilized for cardiac catheterization after having received certain types of premedication frequently develop hypoxic spells. It is quite likely that this is due to a decrease in systemic vascular resistance, with a decrease in systemic arterial pressure and thus in right ventricular pressure and pulmonary blood flow. Furthermore, a decrease in venous return to the heart, which could result from peripheral venous pooling, would facilitate a further reduction in right ventricular pressure. The ensuing decrease in pulmonary blood flow could precipitate a hypoxic episode. Many attacks of hypoxic spells occur in infants in the early morning after waking; the reason for occurrence of the spells at this time is not clear. Factors that could possibly account for this relationship are decreased systemic venous return associated with standing in the crib, increased activity with an increased requirement for oxygen, and a reduction in circulating volume due to relative dehydration because of lack of fluid intake overnight.

Effects of oxygen administration

Oxygen administration to the normal individual results in an increase in systemic arterial Po_2 to 500–600 mmHg. In patients with tetralogy of Fallot, the effects of 100% oxygen inhalation are related to the magnitude of pulmonary blood flow. While breathing room air, hemoglobin is usually fully saturated; the dissolved oxygen content in pulmonary venous blood is 0.3 mL/dL. With 100% oxygen breathing, the amount of dissolved oxygen can increase to about 1.5 mL/dL. If pulmonary blood flow is not greatly reduced, the oxygen will increase systemic arterial oxygen saturation and Po_2 by moderate amounts. However, if pulmonary flow is very low, the total amount of extra oxygen that can be taken up in the lungs is limited and thus there would be little increase in systemic arterial saturation and Po_2. Therefore, inhalation of oxygen is least effective in those individuals who require it most (see Chapter 3).

Effects of exercise and postural change

During exercise oxygen requirements in various body tissues and organs increase. To provide this increased oxygen requirement, pulmonary blood flow must increase. The increased venous return associated with exercise would tend to increase pulmonary blood flow by raising right ventricular pressure. However, the decrease in systemic vascular resistance will tend to decrease systemic arterial as well as right ventricular pressure. Pulmonary blood flow may remain constant, decrease or increase slightly but not enough to provide the amount of oxygen required. This will result in increasing hypoxemia and tissue hypoxia, with increased anaerobic glycolysis and acidemia. Patients with tetralogy of Fallot are frequently limited in their ability to perform exercise and often squat when they become tired. The squatting posture is important in assisting in recovery from hypoxia. I have studied the effects of exercise on systemic arterial oxygen saturation in several patients with tetralogy of Fallot. The saturation falls rapidly during a 2-min exercise period. If the patient is allowed to squat immediately, saturation rises rapidly and reaches baseline levels within 3–5 min. However, if the child is kept in the standing position, arterial oxygen saturation recovers very slowly and may not reach control levels for 10–15 min.

The beneficial effect of squatting in these patients may be related to two factors.

- Compression of muscles in the lower extremities will increase venous return to the heart and thus increase right ventricular stroke volume and pressure and improve pulmonary blood flow.
- The posture may produce an increase in systemic vascular resistance by compression of the vessels in muscles in the lower extremities and thus raise arterial and right ventricular systolic pressures. It has also been suggested that the femoral arteries may be kinked in the groin and this raises systemic vascular resistance. Possibly reduction in flow to the lower extremities may decrease the area of the body to which systemic blood flow is distributed and thus limit the area to which oxygen is distributed.

The effects of postural changes in patients with tetralogy of Fallot have been well documented. If patients are tilted with the head up, arterial oxygen saturation falls dramatically and syncope often occurs; tilting with the head down results in a rapid increase in oxygen saturation. If compression bandages are placed on the lower limbs or if venous compression is produced by immersion of the lower extremities in a tub of water with a high hydrostatic pressure, arterial oxygen saturation is maintained even though the legs are below the level of the head. The improvement in arterial oxygen saturation and in symptoms of hypoxia produced by postural changes has been recognized for some time. Infants with hypoxic spells often improve rapidly when placed in the knee–chest position or when placed prone with the head down.

Tetralogy of Fallot with absent pulmonary valve

Infants with tetralogy of Fallot with absent pulmonary valve will have a right-to-left shunt through the ventricular septal defect during the immediate postnatal period, because the combination of right ventricular outflow tract stenosis and high pulmonary vascular resistance imposes a high afterload. The subsequent hemodynamic changes are determined by the pulmonary vascular resistance and the degree of infundibular stenosis. As pulmonary vascular resistance falls after birth, the right-to-left shunt will decrease and, depending on the degree of infundibular stenosis, left-to-right shunt will develop. Milder degrees of stenosis will not only permit a large left-to-right shunt but will also allow a greater degree of pulmonary valve regurgitation. The combined left and right ventricular volume overload may result in early cardiac failure. Associated with the increasing left-to-right shunt after birth, the dilated pulmonary arteries may be further distended, causing bronchial compression. A large left-to-right shunt may also cause left atrial enlargement and this may contribute to bronchial compression. The combination of ventilatory disturbances with a left-to-right shunt is likely to result in pulmonary edema. When infundibular stenosis is more severe, both the magnitude of the left-to-right shunt and the degree of pulmonary regurgitation will be considerably less.

Clinical features

The clinical features of tetralogy of Fallot vary greatly; they are influenced by the specific cardiac anomalies as well as by the severity of the individual lesions. Thus infants with pulmonary atresia, as well as those with tetralogy of Fallot with absent pulmonary valve, are likely to develop symptoms soon after birth. They often have rapid progression of symptoms, and without therapy almost half of the infants in these two groups will not survive beyond a year of life. Although many patients with tetralogy of Fallot have no other developmental anomalies, recently the association of a chromosome 22q11 deletion with conotruncal anomalies has been recognized; about 25% of patients with tetralogy of Fallot have this abnormality. Some of the features of CATCH 22 syndrome may therefore be noted in those individuals who have the deletion. These include thymic hypoplasia, hypoparathyroidism, cleft palate, and craniofacial dysmorphism (hypertelorism, small palpebral fissures, small mouth, open at rest, low nasal bridge, malformed ears). Also, tetralogy of Fallot may be associated with esophageal atresia, tracheoesophageal fistula, hemivertebrae, anal atresia, and radial abnormalities (VACTERL syndrome).

The clinical aspects are presented in four categories: mild to moderate right ventricular outflow tract obstruction, moderate to severe right ventricular outflow tract obstruction, pulmonary atresia, and tetralogy of Fallot with absent pulmonary valve.

Mild to moderate right ventricular outflow obstruction

When right ventricular outflow tract obstruction is mild, the infant shows no cyanosis after birth. As pulmonary vascular resistance falls, left-to-right shunt increases and the clinical presentation is similar to that of the infant with a ventricular septal defect. The magnitude of the left-to-right shunt is determined by the degree of outflow tract stenosis in addition to the pulmonary vascular resistance. In some infants, the shunt may be so large that the infant develops all the features of cardiac failure, with sweating, respiratory distress, hepatomegaly, and failure to thrive. If the outflow tract stenosis is more prominent, the left-to-right shunt will be smaller and the infant does not develop any symptoms. With advancing age, the outflow tract stenosis frequently becomes more severe. This is probably the result of hypertrophy of infundibular muscle. When the stenosis becomes sufficiently severe that the outflow resistance exceeds systemic vascular resistance, right-to-left shunting occurs with cyanosis. This first occurs with exercise, but later becomes persistent. The rate of progression of this process varies greatly. In some patients, cyanosis is noted during the first year, but in others it may not appear until several years later.

With large left-to-right shunts, the precordium is hyperactive with prominence of both left and right ventricular impulses. The first sound is usually normal and the second sound is prominent at the mid-left sternal border due to aortic displacement. Unlike in patients with severe stenosis, the second sound is split, although the pulmonary component may be soft. A loud harsh pansystolic murmur is audible along the whole left sternal edge; it is of even intensity throughout systole. At the upper left sternal border, the murmur may assume the qualities of a stenotic murmur, with crescendo–decrescendo characteristics. If the left-to-right shunt is large, a short mid-diastolic murmur may be audible at the cardiac apex. Small left-to-right shunts are not associated with cardiac enlargement and the right ventricular impulse at the lower left sternal border predominates. The second heart sound is best heard at the mid-left sternal border and is single. A systolic murmur, stenotic in character, is best heard at the mid to upper left sternal border.

The chest radiograph reflects the degree of infundibular stenosis. With a large left-to-right shunt, the heart is enlarged, with prominence of both left and right ventricles. The main pulmonary artery segment is prominent and pulmonary vascular markings are increased. When there is little or no left-to-right shunt, the heart size is usually normal and the pulmonary arteries are usually of normal size. The electrocardiogram also reflects the hemodynamic changes. With a large left-to-right shunt, both left and right ventricular enlargement are reflected by right axis deviation and prominent R waves in all precordial leads. With small shunts, the electrocardiogram usually shows right axis deviation with large R waves in the right precordial leads.

Moderate to severe right ventricular outflow obstruction

Neonatal period

With moderate to severe stenosis of the right ventricular outflow, the infant is usually only mildly cyanotic in the immediate postnatal period, but with constriction of the ductus arteriosus increasing cyanosis develops. The rate of progression of cyanosis is quite variable, depending on the severity of the obstruction and the size of the pulmonary arteries. Infants with very small pulmonary arteries usually have severe outflow tract obstruction and may be very cyanosed within days after birth, particularly because the ductus arteriosus is also usually very small. Other infants become severely cyanosed within a few weeks after birth; arterial oxygen saturation may fall to 50–60% with a Po_2 of 20–25 mmHg: the Pco_2 is usually normal or decreased to about 35 mmHg. The baby is irritable, does not feed well, and has hyperpnea and tachypnea. The infant's behavior is often very trying on the parents, who become frustrated with their inability to pacify the baby. Tachycardia is usually present and the pulses are full. Blood pressure is well maintained until severe acidemia develops, when it may fall rapidly. The liver edge is often palpable 2–3 cm below the right costal margin and this, in association with the increased respiration, may suggest the infant has cardiac failure. However, the liver is not enlarged but is displaced downward by the hyperventilation. The chest is often hyperresonant and is clear on auscultation. Persistent severe cyanosis is associated with progressive acidemia, with arterial blood pH falling to 7.00 or lower. The infant becomes pale and mottled and blood pressure falls.

The heart is not clinically enlarged and the precordium is not very active, but the impulse is maximal at the lower left sternal border, indicating right ventricular dominance. The first heart sound is usually accentuated at the lower left sternal border; the second sound is single and is heard well at the lower to mid-left sternal border but is soft or absent at the upper left sternal border. No murmurs may be heard, but often there is a short, grade 2–3/6, rough systolic murmur, starting immediately after the second sound, at the mid-left sternal border; the murmur occupies only one-third to half of the systolic cycle. A grade 2–3/6 continuous murmur may be heard at the upper left sternal border when the ductus arteriosus is still open.

The chest radiograph shows a heart of normal size with prominence of the right ventricle. The pulmonary artery segment is deficient so that the upper mediastinal shadow is narrow in both the frontal and lateral projections. The upturned apex and small pulmonary artery segment creates a typical cardiac contour in the anteroposterior projection, often described as a "sheep-nose" or "wooden shoe" (*coeur en sabot*). The hilar lung vessels are narrow and there are few peripheral vascular markings. The aortic arch is frequently on the right and it displaces the superior vena cava shadow to the right.

The electrocardiogram shows right axis deviation and right ventricular hypertrophy, but often it is difficult to distinguish the tracing from that of a normal newborn infant; a persistent upright T wave in the right precordial leads may be the only evidence of right ventricular hypertrophy. As mentioned above, occasionally a dominance of left ventricular forces may be noted.

Clinical course

Although palliative or corrective procedures are now performed even in premature infants, the clinical course of untreated infants has been derived from past experience. With growth, oxygen requirements increase and the cyanosis becomes more severe and physical activity is increasingly limited. Physical development is impaired in some children, but because other genetic disturbances are often associated, it is difficult to know whether the delayed growth is related to the hypoxemia. The child reacts adversely to infection and may develop increased cyanosis, hypoxia and acidemia due to the increased oxygen requirements and may succumb. Following a severe and prolonged spell, or associated with infection and dehydration, cerebral injury with neurological sequelae, with a variety of manifestations including hemiplegia, may occur. It has been suggested that neurological involvement is due to embolic phenomena associated with the right-to-left shunt, or to cerebral venous thrombosis resulting from the high hematocrit. It is more likely that it is due to severe hypoxemia, because it may occur following a spell, even when the hematocrit is not increased. In fact, it is much more likely to occur in those individuals who have relative anemia due to iron deficiency (see Chapter 14). Another important complication is the development of brain abscess; this is unusual in children under 2 years of age and is discussed in Chapter 14. Infective endocarditis, which is not infrequent in older children, is unusual during infancy. Many infants succumb to infection or hypoxia, but some survive and present with the features discussed.

Older infants and children

When the stenosis is not very severe, hypoxic symptoms usually do not occur in the newborn period.

Mild cyanosis that increases on straining or crying may be present; it is not unusual for the infant to progress favorably, with normal development. Symptoms may not appear for 2–6 months or even longer. The earliest evidence of the lesion may be the onset of hypoxic spells (see Chapter 14), which creates great anxiety for parents. The infant may be only mildly cyanotic most of the day but suddenly develops an episode of marked cyanosis with pallor, hyperventilation and flaccidity, and consciousness may be lost. The spells frequently occur when, after a prolonged bout of crying, the child suddenly stops crying and becomes limp and pale and breathes very deeply. Spells may also occur with breath-holding. However, they may occur apparently unrelated to crying, particularly early in the morning soon after waking. The episodes usually last only a few minutes and recovery is spontaneous; at first, they occur infrequently but increase in severity and frequency and may be noted every day or several times a day. Some spells are more prolonged and may even result in death.

Between spells, the child may be quite well and often has only mild cyanosis at rest, with underlying pallor. Relative anemia is quite common 3–4 months after birth if iron intake has not been supplemented. Hemoglobin concentration is often 8–12 g/dL. It is of interest that hypoxic spells are most common in infants who do not usually appear to be markedly cyanotic in the periods between the spells. Often the arterial oxygen saturation is in the range 85–90%. This relatively high resting oxygen saturation may not provide a stimulus to increase the hemoglobin concentration; this would make the infant more vulnerable to any incident that might reduce pulmonary blood flow and oxygen delivery. Iron administration results in a rapid increase in hemoglobin concentration; in patients with arterial oxygen saturations below 70%, levels of 22–24 g/dL are common. The frequency and severity of spells usually decreases but the cyanosis increases, often to alarming degrees; this is due to the increase in the amount of reduced hemoglobin. The hematocrit also rises to as much as 85–90%; when it reaches above 75–80%, the improvement in symptoms may not be sustained (p. 359). This could be due to the dramatic increase in blood viscosity, which may interfere with perfusion of the lungs, the heart, and other organs.

If the infant has adequate iron intake, development may be fairly normal and the degree of cyanosis, as well as the level of activity, is related to the severity of the right ventricular outflow obstruction. Even though cyanosis is prominent, patients may survive even into adult life, but are quite limited in their physical activities. Patients with persistent marked cyanosis often have poorly developed dental enamel and the teeth are soft, discolored, and subject to severe caries. Petechiae may be noted all over the body and there is an increased bleeding tendency. Blood fibrinogen levels may be decreased and the platelet count is often moderately reduced, with large dysfunctional platelets. Clubbing of the fingers and toes is not seen in early infancy but develops during the first year when cyanosis is persistent. Usually the fingers and toes are warm and the peripheral veins are prominent, probably due to the presence of multiple peripheral arteriovenous anastomoses.

If right ventricular outflow obstruction is less severe, spells may not be noted during infancy and the child may develop normally, manifesting only mild cyanosis, which increases on crying or with exertion. The earliest symptoms may occur when the child begins to walk, when it is noted that exercise tolerance is markedly limited. With exertion, cyanosis increases and the child hyperventilates. The assumption of the squatting position is a very characteristic response to tiring with exercise (see Chapter 14). In severely affected patients, the squatting position may be assumed for most of the day, and the child may sleep in the knee–chest position. Sometimes parents do not appreciate that children have exercise limitation and insist that they play normally, but detailed questioning indicates that movements are intermittent and that there is an inability to perform sustained activities.

The pulses in these patients are usually prominent and pulse pressure may be slightly increased. There is no evidence of cardiac failure and the lungs are clear on auscultation. The heart is not clinically enlarged and there is a prominent right ventricular impulse at the lower left sternal border. The first heart sound is usually loud at the lower left sternal border. The second sound is single or narrowly split; it is very soft at the upper left sternal border but is accentuated at the lower left sternal border. These characteristics of the second sound are useful in differentiating tetralogy of Fallot from pulmonary stenosis with intact ventricular septum, because the intensity of the second sound is decreased over the whole precordium in the latter complex. A systolic murmur is usually heard, loudest at the mid or lower left sternal border, but when valvar or supravalvar stenosis predominates, it is most prominent at the upper left sternal border and may radiate to the infraclavicular area and the lung fields. The murmur originates from the outflow tract stenosis; the ventricular septal defect does not create a murmur because it is large and flow through it (right-to-left shunt) is relatively low. The murmur varies greatly in intensity and duration; it is loud and rough and extends throughout systole and is of about equal intensity (so-called plateau-shaped) when the stenosis is not very severe. In more severe obstruction, the intensity of the murmur may be only grade 2–3/6 and the murmur may occupy only the first half to two-thirds of systole; it usually commences immediately after the first sound and is also of even intensity. During hypoxic spells, the intensity and duration of the murmur may be markedly decreased, indicating decreased flow across the stenosed area. A decrease in the intensity of the murmur may also be noted when the hematocrit is greatly increased, and is probably related to the increased viscosity and decreased turbulence that results. A high-pitched continuous murmur due to the presence of a small patent ductus arteriosus may be heard at the upper left sternal border. In older children a very high-pitched, distant, continuous murmur can sometimes be heard on either side of the spine, related to the development of large bronchial collateral arteries.

The response of the systolic murmur to peripheral vasodilatation induced by inhalation of amyl nitrite was used to differentiate between patients with tetralogy of Fallot and those with pulmonary stenosis and an intact ventricular septum. In tetralogy of Fallot, the murmur decreases because systemic and right ventricular systolic pressures fall and flow across the stenotic area decreases. In patients with intact ventricular septum, the murmur increases because flow across the stenosis is increased by the augmented venous return. Inhalation of amyl nitrite may aggravate hypoxemia and there may be some risk in using it. The test is no longer used, but is of interest because it demonstrates differences in circulatory dynamics between the two lesions.

The chest radiograph shows a heart of normal size, often with a *coeur en sabot* contour (see above). The pulmonary conus and artery segment are deficient, so that the upper mediastinum is narrow. A right aortic arch is frequently present, and the superior vena cava shadow is displaced to the right. The pulmonary arterial shadows in the lungs are decreased and the peripheral vascular markings in the lungs are deficient. When the bronchial collateral circulation is well developed, diffuse fine vascular markings may be noted throughout the lung. The electrocardiogram shows right axis deviation and right ventricular hypertrophy of variable degree.

Clinical course

Many children with marked cyanosis survive into adult life. Ability to exercise is limited to varying degrees. Some are able to live reasonably normal lives, but others are severely restricted and sedentary. As with infants, infection presents a serious problem because fever increases oxygen requirements. Respiratory infections are particularly poorly tolerated because they may interfere with oxygen uptake in the lungs. During infancy and childhood, death is usually the result of hypoxia and infection. The presence of unexplained persistent fever is cause for concern, because it may represent the early manifestation of cerebral abscess or infective endocarditis. As mentioned above, cerebral abscess is unusual before the age of 1.5–2 years in patients with tetralogy of Fallot. The manifestations are varied and initial symptoms may be subtle. Changes in behavior, minor neurological symptoms or signs, or unexplained fever should suggest that the lesion be seriously considered. Acute neurological complications may result from cerebral embolic events; these may follow intravenous procedures such as cardiac catheterization. The risk of emboli is also high in patients in whom intravenous cannulation is maintained for prolonged periods. Infective endocarditis is an important cause of death in patients with tetralogy of Fallot who have not had complete repair. The risk of endocarditis is high, not only in those who have had no surgery but also in those who have had palliative shunt procedures and those with residual lesions after attempted complete repair.

Few individuals with untreated tetralogy of Fallot are likely to survive beyond the age of 25 years. If they do not die from one of the complications mentioned above, they commonly develop cardiac failure; it has been suggested this may be the result of myocardial fibrosis, but this has not been documented. In late adolescence and early adult life, ventricular arrhythmias are prone to occur, probably also as a result of myocardial damage.

Pulmonary atresia

The clinical features of infants with tetralogy of Fallot with pulmonary atresia are determined by the size of the pulmonary arteries, the ductus arteriosus, and the number and size of MAPCAs. The prognosis is generally poor, with fewer than 50% of untreated infants surviving beyond 1 year of age. In the infant with small pulmonary arteries and insignificant MAPCAs, cyanosis is present at or soon after birth. The ductus arteriosus is patent postnatally but is usually small, so that it does not provide adequate pulmonary circulation. Ductus closure appears to be delayed in these infants; however, within a few weeks, ductus constriction results in progressive increase in cyanosis and without intervention the baby succumbs to hypoxia and acidemia. Irritability, tiring with feeding, and tachypnea and hyperpnea are manifestations of progressive hypoxemia. The heart is not clinically enlarged and a lower left sternal border impulse, normal for an infant, is palpable. The first heart sound is prominent and occasionally a systolic ejection click is heard; it probably reflects high flow into the ascending aorta. The second sound is well heard at the mid-left sternal border and is single; it arises from the displaced aortic valve. Usually no murmurs are audible, but a soft continuous murmur may be heard in the left infraclavicular area, arising from the ductus arteriosus. If a right-sided ductus is present, the continuous murmur may be heard on the right side. As the ductus constricts, this murmur will disappear. The radiological and electrocardiographic features are similar to those described above for infants with severe right ventricular outflow tract stenosis. The prognosis in these infants is particularly poor.

The presentation varies in the infants with MAPCAs, depending on their size and number. In most infants MAPCAs are small and relatively few in number, providing only modest pulmonary blood flow; the clinical features will not differ much from those described above. On occasion large MAPCAs may provide an abundant pulmonary blood flow. The high flow may not be established immediately after birth, because pulmonary vascular resistance is maintained at greater than normal levels by exposure to systemic arterial pressure. The infant may have moderate cyanosis at birth, but as pulmonary blood flow rises, the degree of cyanosis will decrease. Within several weeks, pulmonary blood flow may become so large as to present a volume overload of the left ventricle with resultant failure. The large runoff from the aorta into the pulmonary circulation may result in a wide arterial pulse pressure, with bounding peripheral pulses. The heart is enlarged and a prominent left ventricular impulse is palpable at the apex. The first heart sound is normal; the second sound is single and prominent at the mid-left sternal border. A systolic ejection click, which arises from the aorta, may be heard at the mid-left sternal border. Murmurs may not be audible over the precordium, but a short mid-diastolic murmur may be heard at the apex. Continuous murmurs may be heard parasternally on the left, right, or both sides of the chest. The chest radiograph shows varying degrees of cardiomegaly depending on the magnitude of pulmonary blood flow. The apex is directed caudad, reflecting left ventricular enlargement. The pulmonary conus region is deficient, but the pulmonary vascular markings are increased to varying degrees. The electrocardiogram shows right axis deviation and prominent R waves in the right precordial leads indicating right ventricular hypertrophy, as well as varying degrees of prominence of left ventricular forces. Exposure of the pulmonary arterioles to systemic arterial pressure makes them prone to development of progressive vascular obstruction and increased pulmonary vascular resistance. This causes a progressive fall in pulmonary blood flow, with improvement in symptoms of cardiac failure and loss of clinical signs of increased pulmonary blood flow. In addition, increasing cyanosis results.

As mentioned above, stenoses of MAPCAs either at their origin from the aorta or along their course are frequent. Stenosis at the origin of MAPCAs, common within a few months after birth, limits the magnitude of pulmonary blood flow. The infants are thus moderately cyanotic, but also do not develop evidence of cardiac failure. Also, the stenosis decreases pressure in the MAPCAs, reducing the risk for pulmonary vascular obstructive changes. Stenoses either at the origin or along the course are prone to develop at any time after birth in arteries that have no evidence of obstruction at birth. Multiple sites of stenosis may develop in a single artery. The obstructions tend to increase in severity with age and result in progressive increase in cyanosis. Many of the patients with MAPCAs with moderate obstruction survive into adult life, albeit with marked cyanosis and exercise limitation.

Tetralogy of Fallot with absent pulmonary valve

In the immediate postnatal period, the infant is usually mildly or moderately cyanosed, but over the course of a few days the cyanosis lessens or disappears. Within a variable period of a few days to several weeks, respiratory symptoms occur in many of the infants, related to airway compression. The walls of the airways are soft in the infant and are easily compressed by the large main and left or right pulmonary arteries. The arteries are large at birth, but become more distended by the high volume related to the left-to-right shunt. Initially, hyperinflation of lung segments may result from predominant obstruction of expiration, but later atelectasis develops. Severe respiratory distress is a major feature in many of these infants, and respiratory failure is a common cause of death. Any respiratory infection is very poorly tolerated. Those infants with moderately severe infundibular stenosis are usually less symptomatic in infancy, but tend to show mild to moderate cyanosis. The stenosis is usually not severe enough to cause severe cyanosis.

The heart is clinically enlarged, with a prominent lower left sternal border impulse. The first heart sound is often accentuated at the lower left sternal border; the second sound is loud at the mid-left sternal border but is single. The murmur is almost diagnostic of this syndrome; a loud harsh crescendo–decrescendo systolic murmur, followed by a loud decrescendo diastolic murmur, is heard at the mid and upper left sternal border. The murmurs are not continuous but are separated by a short interval and have been described as "seesaw" or "to and fro" in character. Findings in the chest vary, depending on whether there is hyperinflation or atelectasis.

Few conditions cause a prominent diastolic murmur in the neonate; they include aortic–left ventricular tunnel, sinus of Valsalva fistula, and truncus arteriosus valve insufficiency. In those infants who develop a large left-to-right shunt, the heart is often greatly enlarged, and both ventricles are prominent. A mid-diastolic low-pitched murmur may be heard at the apex, associated with the high flow across the mitral valve.

Investigations

Echocardiography

The morphological features of tetralogy of Fallot can now usually be identified with reliability in most patients with two-dimensional echocardiography and color flow Doppler examination. Many centers proceed with surgery based on ultrasound examination in a high proportion of infants and children with the anomaly. The ventricular septal defect can be readily imaged and the overriding of the aorta assessed. Some pediatric cardiologists have suggested that if the degree of overriding is greater than 50%, the diagnosis of double-outlet right ventricle should be entertained. This is quite arbitrary, because some patients with more than 50% overriding have all the other characteristic features of tetralogy of Fallot and it is inappropriate to label them otherwise. The anterior and superior displacement of the outlet septum is usually readily evident. The size of the defect should be estimated to ensure it is not restrictive. A careful search for the presence of other ventricular septal defects should be made by both two-dimensional assessment and color flow Doppler examination. In addition the possibility that the child has an atrioventricular septal defect with right ventricular outflow tract stenosis should be considered.

The right ventricular outflow tract and main and branch pulmonary arteries should be evaluated for the severity of obstruction at various sites. It is important to note if the infundibulum is completely obstructed; color flow Doppler study is helpful in determining whether there is flow through the infundibulum. The size of the pulmonary valve annulus and the presence and severity of valvar stenosis should be determined. Because the stenosis of the infundibulum usually has some length and is not discrete, it has been said that the pressure gradient across the right ventricular outflow tract obtained from estimates based on peak velocity may not be reliable. However, comparison of pressure gradients measured at cardiac catheterization with those estimated by ultrasound shows reasonably good correlation. Main pulmonary arterial and left and right pulmonary arterial diameters should be measured and the presence of confluence of the branch arteries confirmed. Doppler flow study in the infundibulum and main pulmonary artery may be very useful in deciding whether pulmonary atresia is present. Evidence of either forward flow or regurgitation through the pulmonary valve confirms the presence of an opening. It is also helpful in demonstrating the presence of flow into the pulmonary artery through the ductus arteriosus. The left and right pulmonary artery diameters should be measured just beyond their origin from the main pulmonary trunk, because many observers consider it important in making decisions about operability of the patient and the type of procedure to perform (see Chapter 14). Although the left and right pulmonary arteries can usually be imaged, their more distal portions and the intrapulmonary arteries cannot be readily assessed. Also, some MAPCAs may be identified, but it is not possible to ensure that all the collateral arteries have been defined. Recently, cardiac magnetic resonance imaging (MRI) has been found to be useful in defining the anatomy of the pulmonary arterial arborization and the origin of MAPCAs from the descending aorta, as well as their course and distribution.

The position of the aortic arch should be determined, because right aortic arch is present in about 25% of individuals with tetralogy of Fallot and in an even higher percentage of those with pulmonary atresia. The first branch arising from the right aortic arch is the innominate artery, which provides the left carotid and subclavian arteries. This information may be important to some surgeons in making decisions about introducing a systemic-to-pulmonary artery shunt. It is very important to attempt to define the origins of the left and right coronary arteries and to follow their course, so that the presence of a major coronary artery passing across the right ventricular outflow tract can be excluded. This information is essential to the surgeon, because the coronary artery could be severed during the procedure to relieve outflow tract obstruction.

A detailed examination should also be made to exclude other lesions. Drainage of the left superior vena cava into the coronary sinus is not infrequently noted in patients with tetralogy of Fallot, particularly in association with right aortic arch. A large coronary sinus opening would lead one to suspect this anomaly. A patent foramen ovale or a fossa ovalis defect in the atrial septum is frequently noted in tetralogy of Fallot patients.

Tetralogy of Fallot is one of the congenital cardiac lesions most frequently diagnosed prenatally. The presence of the large malalignment ventricular septal defect with aortic overriding has been identified as early as 10–14 weeks' gestation by transvaginal ultrasound examination. The main pulmonary trunk is often of normal size at 18–20 weeks' gestation; the size may not change with advancing gestation, but several observers have noted a progressive relative decrease in diameter in some fetuses. The left and right pulmonary arteries are usually normal in mid-gestation, but with severe right ventricular outflow obstruction or pulmonary atresia, the branch arteries as well as the trunk show a progressive relative decrease in diameter. When the outflow tract stenosis is relatively mild, forward flow into the pulmonary trunk and through the ductus arteriosus into the descending aorta may be demonstrable by Doppler examination. However, retrograde flow in the ductus from the aorta to the pulmonary artery signifies severe pulmonary stenosis or atresia. The ductus venosus may be patent prior to about 25 weeks' gestation, and subsequently becomes progressively smaller and then completely occluded.

Findings on ultrasound examination of patients with tetralogy of Fallot with absent pulmonary valve are characteristic. The main pulmonary trunk and left or right, or both, pulmonary arteries are dilated; Doppler examination shows varying degrees of increased velocity of forward flow and considerable pulmonary regurgitation, with enlargement of the right ventricle. Stenosis of the infundibulum is usually of mild to moderate severity; frequently the pulmonary annular area is narrowed and rudimentary valve leaflet tissue may be apparent. The ventricular septal defect is typical of that seen in tetralogy of Fallot, with malalignment, and overriding of the aorta. Also, the outlet septum is deviated cranially and anteriorly.

Tetralogy of Fallot with absent pulmonary valve is one of the congenital heart lesions most readily diagnosed *in utero*. The dilated right ventricle and large pulmonary arteries, with marked pulmonary regurgitation, associated with a large ventricular septal defect are features that are diagnostic of the condition. With severe pulmonary regurgitation, the right ventricle is markedly dilated and hydrops fetalis may be noted. The presence of a patent ductus arteriosus is variable; most infants do not have a patent ductus arteriosus, but this is not infrequently observed in fetuses. A large patent ductus in the fetus may have adverse effects by allowing flow from the aorta through the ductus and thus aggravate the magnitude of pulmonary regurgitation.

Cardiac catheterization and angiocardiography

General considerations

Although the diagnosis of pulmonary stenosis and ventricular septal defect can frequently be made with reasonable confidence by clinical examination, radiography and electrocardiography, cardiac catheterization with angiocardiography was performed previously. This was done to both confirm the diagnosis and obtain information about the detailed abnormal anatomy, essential in making surgical decisions. It was also performed to exclude lesions that may produce a clinical picture similar to that of tetralogy of Fallot, such as aortopulmonary transposition with ventricular septal defect and pulmonary stenosis, double-outlet right ventricle with pulmonary stenosis, and atrioventricular septal defect with pulmonary stenosis. Advances in ultrasound techniques have now made it possible to make an accurate diagnosis of tetralogy of Fallot and to differentiate it from other lesions. Also, most of the features important to making decisions about surgery, such as the site and severity of stenosis, the size of the pulmonary arteries, the laterality of the aorta, and abnormal coronary artery course over the infundibulum, can be defined by ultrasound study. Therefore, many centers are subjecting patients to surgery without catheterization procedures. Cardiac catheterization with angiocardiography is still considered necessary to provide additional information in some patients. If the major coronary arteries cannot be imaged adequately, angiography will be required to define the vessels. Particularly in infants with pulmonary atresia, it may be difficult to assess whether there is confluence of the pulmonary arteries. It is also difficult to image all MAPCAs, and it is difficult to determine whether there is stenosis in MAPCAs. However, the introduction of MRI has made it possible to resolve many of these issues, so that catheterization and angiography are becoming increasingly unnecessary. Recently, catheterization has been performed in an attempt to partly relieve right ventricular outflow tract obstruction by balloon angioplasty, thus enhancing pulmonary blood flow until surgery is performed. This is discussed below.

Cardiac catheterization of infants with tetralogy of Fallot is associated with a significant risk because hypoxic spells occur frequently. The probable contributing factors are the combined effects of sedation and immobilization, which may reduce arterial and right ventricular systolic pressures and decrease venous return (see Chapter 14). The usual practice of withholding oral intake, not only of solid food but also liquids, may result in some degree of dehydration, which may further contribute to the decrease in arterial blood pressure.

In newborn infants with severe hypoxemia, it is useful to insert a catheter into the umbilical artery to monitor pH, blood gases, and blood glucose concentration. Glucose should be given to correct hypoglycemia. The use of sedatives or hypnotics that tend to reduce blood pressure should be avoided. Morphine has proved to be useful in these infants, because it reduces irritability and does not cause hypotension if given in doses of 0.1 mg/kg body weight; this dose can be repeated after 1–2 hours if necessary. In those institutions where the procedures are done routinely using general anesthesia, it is advisable to select agents that have little tendency to cause hypotension. Also, the anesthesiologist should carefully monitor blood pressure. In the older infant or if an umbilical arterial catheter has not been placed, it is advisable to cannulate the femoral artery early in the procedure; continuous monitoring of blood pressure will help to recognize the onset of hypotension, which usually presages onset of hypoxia. Should hypotension develop, peripheral vasoconstrictor agents, such as phenylephrine, should be administered to maintain arterial pressure.

Catheter approach and manipulation

The venous approach is made from the groin. After catheterizing the superior vena cava, the catheter is withdrawn into the right atrium and may then be manipulated across the foramen ovale into the left atrium and into a pulmonary vein or the left ventricle. If the position and size of the ventricular septal defect and the presence of additional defects have been clearly defined by ultrasound examination, an angiogram in the left ventricle is not necessary. If there are any questions about these features, it should be performed. Although it is possible to manipulate a balloon-tipped catheter into the ascending aorta from the left ventricle, in small infants it is usually more readily accessed from the right ventricle through the ventricular septal defect.

If the catheter passes into the right ventricle, it is preferable to perform an angiogram before attempting to manipulate it into the outflow tract or through the ventricular septal defect into the aorta, particularly in infants. This delineates the anatomy of the right ventricular outflow and aids in further manipulation. In young infants with severe infundibular stenosis, it is not advisable to attempt to pass the catheter into the pulmonary artery because no particularly important information will be derived and considerable risk is involved. During manipulation in the infundibular region, multiple ventricular ectopic beats may be induced and a hypoxic spell may follow. Also, if the catheter is passed through a very narrow orifice, its presence may make the obstruction critical and severe hypoxemia may occur (see Chapter 14). A further risk, particularly if a stiff catheter is used, is that the right ventricular infundibulum may be perforated, especially in infants. It has further been suggested that manipulation in the infundibulum may stimulate constriction and thus aggravate hypoxemia. The infundibulum and pulmonary arteries can usually be visualized adequately from the right ventricular injection. In order to optimize visualization of the pulmonary arteries and define whether they are confluent, it is helpful to perform the angiogram with a posteroanterior projection and a craniocaudal angulation of 20–30°.

The catheter can usually be manipulated into the aorta from the right ventricle by passing the tip to the right of the crista supraventricularis in the frontal projection, and an aortogram can be performed just above the valve. This will define the laterality of the aorta and the arrangement of the arteries arising from the arch. It may also provide adequate visualization of the coronary arteries in order to determine whether there is an abnormal vessel coursing across the right ventricular outflow. If this is not clear, additional aortic angiograms should be obtained. A very useful technique in infants is to use a balloon-tipped catheter with the catheter lumen opening proximal to the balloon. The catheter is positioned in the ascending aorta, the balloon is inflated to occlude or partially occlude the aorta, and the contrast injection is done immediately. The balloon is then rapidly deflated. This procedure usually provides excellent views of the coronary arteries. If this maneuver cannot be accomplished and the coronary arterial pattern is not clear from one of the ventricular injections, a retrograde arterial catheter can be passed to the root of the aorta. For optimal visualization of the coronary arteries, it is useful to use a balloon catheter with the lumen distal to the balloon. The balloon is inflated in the ascending aorta a short distance above the valve, the contrast injection made, and the balloon is then rapidly deflated.

There is a high incidence of persistent left superior vena cava in patients with tetralogy of Fallot and the catheter often enters this vessel through the coronary sinus. This course should not be confused with entrance into the left atrium.

Oxygen saturation data

In infants with severe hypoxemia, the mixed venous oxygen saturation is markedly reduced, often to about 20%. The saturations in the right atrium, right ventricle, and pulmonary arteries are similar to those in the vena cava. Pulmonary venous blood has an oxygen saturation of 98–99% and, if there is marked hyperventilation, Po_2 may be raised to 112–115 mmHg, $P\text{co}_2$ reduced to 15–20 mmHg, and pH raised to 7.48–7.50. Often there is some degree of atrial right-to-left shunt through the foramen ovale, so that left atrial oxygen saturation is decreased. Oxygen saturation in the left ventricle reflects that in the left atrium. Systemic arterial oxygen saturation may be markedly reduced to 30–40% with a $P\text{o}_2$ of 20–25 mmHg; when acidemia is severe, pH may be below 7.0. $P\text{co}_2$ is usually normal or slightly increased. Arterial oxygen saturation is higher than that in the body of the right ventricle, but lower than that in the left ventricle. Oxygen saturation in the aorta or systemic arteries is higher than that in the right ventricle and lower than that in the left ventricle. If the ductus arteriosus is patent, oxygen saturation in the pulmonary artery may be higher than that in the right ventricle.

In patients with less severe stenosis, venous oxygen saturations are normal. A small increase in oxygen saturation may be noted at the right ventricular level due to minor degrees of shunting through the ventricular septal defect. Blood oxygen saturations, gases, and pH in pulmonary venous and left atrial samples are usually normal but left ventricular oxygen saturation may be slightly decreased. Aortic and peripheral arterial saturation is variable, depending on the magnitude of pulmonary blood flow. In many instances of moderate stenosis, the systemic arterial oxygen saturation varies during the procedure and large changes of 15–20% may be observed occasionally, particularly in infants and children who are restless or excited.

Blood flows and shunts

Systemic blood flow is usually normal, but when hypoxemia is marked it may be increased to 5–6 L/min per m^2. In the calculation of systemic blood flow by the Fick method, it should be appreciated that the flow represents systemic venous return to the heart and not necessarily the volume ejected into the ascending aorta. If there are MAPCAs or large bronchial collateral vessels supplying blood to the lungs, this flow is excluded when the usual equation for calculating systemic blood flow is applied.

Calculation of pulmonary blood flow may also be subject to considerable error in patients with tetralogy of Fallot who have MAPCAs or large bronchial collateral flows. The equation used for calculating pulmonary blood flow is as follows:

$$\dot{Q}\text{p} = \frac{\dot{V}\text{o}_2}{\begin{matrix}\text{Pulmonary venous} \\ \text{oxygen content}\end{matrix} - \begin{matrix}\text{Pulmonary arterial} \\ \text{oxygen content}\end{matrix}}$$

MAPCAs or bronchial arterial blood is derived from the aorta and has a higher oxygen saturation than pulmonary arterial blood; thus blood entering the pulmonary capillaries and participating in oxygen uptake would have a higher oxygen saturation than that used in the above equation. The arteriovenous difference calculated using pulmonary arterial oxygen saturation would be larger than the actual arteriovenous difference and pulmonary capillary blood flow would therefore be underestimated. Since the magnitude of collateral versus pulmonary arterial flow is not known, it is not possible to estimate total flow across the pulmonary capillary bed. In patients with pulmonary atresia, it is possible to calculate pulmonary blood flow, because it can be assumed that all flow to the lung is from collateral arteries derived from the aorta. The following equation provides an estimate of pulmonary flow:

$$\dot{Q}\text{p} = \frac{\dot{V}\text{o}_2}{\begin{matrix}\text{Pulmonary venous} \\ \text{oxygen content}\end{matrix} - \begin{matrix}\text{Systemic arterial} \\ \text{oxygen content}\end{matrix}}$$

Patients with severe right ventricular outflow tract stenosis do not have significant left-to-right shunting within the heart but may have shunting through a patent ductus arteriosus. Also, flow through the collateral circulation must be considered to be an anatomical left-to-right shunt, as it represents blood flowing from the aorta to the pulmonary circulation. The right-to-left shunt can be calculated from the usual equation:

$$\text{Right-to-left shunt} = \dot{Q}\text{s} - \dot{Q}\text{ep}$$

where $\dot{Q}$s represents systemic blood flow and $\dot{Q}$ep effective pulmonary blood flow. Right-to-left shunts may be large in patients with marked hypoxemia, and pulmonary to systemic flow ratios may be reduced to as low as 0.5:1. In patients with milder stenosis, bidirectional shunting may occur at the ventricular level. At different phases of the cardiac cycle, left-to-right and right-to-left shunting may occur. Although the quantities of blood shunted may be calculated from the equations presented in Chapter 4, these represent net physiological shunts. Greater quantities of blood may actually be shunted because some blood shunted left to right may also then be shunted right to left.

Pressures

Right atrial mean pressure is usually normal but the *a* wave may be slightly increased to about 8–10 mmHg. Left atrial pressure is usually normal but the mean pressure may be slightly decreased and the *a* wave is lower than that in the right atrium. If pulmonary blood flow is markedly decreased, the left atrial *v* wave may be less prominent than normal and similar to the *a* wave.

Right ventricular end-diastolic pressure may be slightly increased, corresponding to the increased *a* wave in the right atrium. Systolic pressure in the right ventricle is usually identical to that in the left ventricle and aorta. This can be demonstrated by inducing ectopic beats by pushing the catheter against the wall of the right ventricle while monitoring right and left ventricular pressures simultaneously. The pressures both fall equally with the ectopic beat and rise equally with the postectopic beat; little postectopic potentiation of the pressures occurs in patients with tetralogy of Fallot. The pressure contour in the right ventricle is similar to that normally seen in the ventricles; there is a rapid upstroke, a rather square top, and a rapid descent. Infrequently, when the ventricular septal defect is small or functionally closed during systole, right ventricular pressure exceeds left ventricular pressure and systolic pressures may exceed 200 mmHg. In this event, the right ventricular pressure contour may be triangular, similar to that observed in patients with pulmonary stenosis with intact ventricular septum. In some of these patients, the right ventricular pressure tracing has a notch on the upstroke that probably coincides with the moment of closure of the ventricular septal defect.

The pressure in the pulmonary artery may be normal or even increased if the stenosis is mild, but when hypoxemia is present it is reduced and has a low pulse pressure. Often it has the appearance of an almost flat line with little systolic and end-diastolic excursion, and the mean pressure may be only 6–8 mmHg. When the pressure is at these low levels, it is important to recognize that it is not possible to detect stenosis beyond a severe proximal stenosis from pressure recordings. This is noted frequently in patients with severe infundibular stenosis, in whom the pressures just beneath the pulmonary valve, in the main pulmonary artery, and in the left and right pulmonary arteries are similar. This finding does not exclude the possibility that various degrees of branch stenosis or valvar stenosis are present in addition to the infundibular stenosis. Flow across the narrowed areas may be so small that additional pressure reductions are not observed. The site of the stenosis in the right ventricular outflow tract may be identified by slow withdrawal of the catheter from the pulmonary artery to the right ventricle. The flipping of the catheter tip into the right ventricle may make it difficult to define the site of stenosis. Use of a catheter with the lumen 2–3 cm proximal to the tip is helpful in defining the stenotic sites during withdrawal of the catheter. When the infundibular stenosis is long and narrow, the catheter has to be withdrawn a long distance from the valve to the body of the right ventricle before the pressure change is noted. Occasionally, no pressure gradient is noted across the pulmonary valve. The pressure tracing in the infundibulum sometimes suggests that a well-formed chamber is present; the contour is similar to that of the right ventricle, but systolic pressure is lower and diastolic pressure may be slightly higher. The pressure withdrawal tracing should not be relied on to determine the actual level of stenosis or the presence of multiple stenoses; detailed angiocardiographic studies are more reliable in defining the anatomy of the right ventricular outflow and pulmonary arteries.

Angiocardiography

Prior to the introduction of sophisticated ultrasound techniques, angiocardiography was essential for diagnosis and delineation of the detailed abnormal anatomy. An injection into the right ventricle usually demonstrates the cavity to be of normal size, but rarely it may be hypoplastic. It is important to observe if there are any constant filling defects, which may be due to large muscle bundles in the body of the ventricle. The amount of contrast medium entering the aorta is variable, but the relation of the aortic valve to the upper border of the ventricular septum can be examined and the degree of overriding assessed. The major proportion of contrast medium may enter the aorta when the outflow tract stenosis is severe. In the aorta, the stream of left ventricular blood, which does not contain contrast medium, can be seen mixing with the right ventricular stream. This sign is useful in confirming the presence of a ventricular septal defect.

The right ventricular outflow tract varies greatly. The whole length of the infundibular region, as well as the pulmonary valve annulus, may be severely narrowed; the diameter of the main pulmonary artery may be markedly decreased. Marked narrowing of the infundibulum may be noted well below the pulmonary annulus, and an infundibular chamber is seen between the stenosis and the annulus. Occasionally, the pulmonary valvar stenosis predominates and the main and left pulmonary arteries may be dilated. In most patients, the pulmonary valve annulus is narrowed and the leaflets are thickened and have limited mobility. Particularly in older infants and children who have developed progressive cyanosis, muscular hypertrophy of the infundibulum may result in severe constriction during systole, but with relaxation during diastole the outflow tract widens considerably. No contrast material can be seen to pass from the right ventricle through the pulmonary valve with pulmonary atresia. It is important to define the distance between the cavity of the right ventricle and the pulmonary artery, particularly if balloon opening of the outflow tract is being considered. If this cannot be assessed reliably from the right ventricular angiogram alone, it may be helpful to insert a catheter retrogradely into the aorta and position the tip in the ascending aorta or in the arch. Simultaneous injections into the aorta and right ventricle often show the main pulmonary artery filling from a ductus arteriosus and the right ventricular cavity, permitting assessment of the degree of separation.

The main pulmonary artery and its branches may be normal but often the main pulmonary trunk is small and there may be stenosis at the origin of one or both major branches. Stenoses may also be observed in the left or right pulmonary arteries. In infants with pulmonary atresia, it is important to demonstrate the size of the pulmonary arteries; this can be done best by injecting contrast medium into the ascending aorta just above the ductus arteriosus, which is often patent.

The left ventricular angiogram usually demonstrates a normal cavity but on occasion it is rather small. If the coronary arteries are not well visualized, an aortic angiogram should be performed, and it has been suggested that coronary arteriograms should be performed if there is any question about abnormal coronary vessels crossing the right ventricular outflow tract. However, direct coronary arteriography may be difficult and possibly dangerous in small infants. Almost invariably, excellent coronary arterial filling can be accomplished with the use of balloon catheters, as mentioned above. The ascending aorta is large and the aortic arch and isthmus are wider than normal. A right aortic arch with a left descending aorta is present in about 25% of patients with tetralogy of Fallot, and it is important to visualize the main branches of the aortic arch should a systemic-to-pulmonary shunt be considered. The aortogram will also demonstrate filling of the pulmonary arteries from a ductus arteriosus; the ductus arises from the aorta at an acute inferior angle. In patients with pulmonary atresia, one or several MAPCAs are seen to arise from the aorta; their distribution to the lung segments is variable. In older children or adults, large bronchial arteries are sometimes seen to arise from the descending aorta and provide blood flow to precapillary pulmonary arteries. It is important to demonstrate the origin and course of MAPCAs and to assess the presence of stenoses at their origin from the aorta or along their course. If they are not well visualized from an aortogram, it may be necessary to perform injections of contrast medium directly into these vessels.

In making decisions about repair by the unifocalization procedure (see Chapter 14), it may be helpful to know whether lung segments are perfused by true pulmonary arteries, by MAPCAs, or both. Since the intrapulmonary portions of the true pulmonary arteries cannot be catheterized, other means of visualization are necessary, Sometimes a pulmonary artery may be demonstrated from a contrast injection into a MAPCA. Another means of filling the pulmonary artery is by pulmonary venous wedge angiography. An end-hole catheter is manipulated through the foramen ovale into the left atrium and into various pulmonary veins. The catheter is wedged into a pulmonary vein and contrast medium is injected carefully at low pressure, best accomplished by manual injection. The pulmonary artery may fill by retrograde passage of contrast medium. Manipulating a balloon-tipped catheter with a distal lumen into the pulmonary vein, inflating the balloon to occlude the pulmonary vein, and then injecting contrast medium into the pulmonary vein manually may examine a larger area of retrograde flow of contrast medium.

Tetralogy of Fallot with absent pulmonary valve

In patients with tetralogy of Fallot with absent pulmonary valve, there is usually little indication to perform a cardiac catheterization study, because most of the morphological features can be readily defined by ultrasound examination. It may be indicated if surgery is contemplated and there is concern about the presence of branch pulmonary stenosis; also the presence of an anomalous course of a coronary artery across the right ventricular outflow tract should be excluded.

Mixed venous oxygen saturation is usually normal but may be decreased if systemic arterial saturation is reduced either by right-to-left shunting through the ventricular septal defect or by ventilatory disturbance. The oxygen saturation is increased at the right ventricular level by left-to-right shunting. Left atrial and pulmonary venous oxygen saturations may be reduced if ventilation is disturbed by bronchial compression. Oxygen saturation in the left ventricle and aorta may be reduced below that in the left atrium by right-to-left shunting through the ventricular septal defect. Right atrial and right ventricular end-diastolic pressures may be elevated to varying degrees by right ventricular failure. Right ventricular systolic pressure is at the same level as left ventricular and aortic systolic pressures, which are usually normal. A systolic pressure difference is noted between the right ventricle and the pulmonary trunk; the level of stenosis may be maximal at the lower infundibular level or at the pulmonary valve annulus. Pulmonary arterial diastolic pressure is very low and may be at or slightly higher than end-systolic pressure in the right ventricle. It may be difficult to manipulate the catheter into branch pulmonary arteries, but a small systolic pressure gradient may be observed at the origins of the left or right pulmonary artery. An angiogram performed in the right ventricle shows considerable dilation of the chamber; infundibular or annular stenosis, or both, are noted. The pulmonary trunk is markedly dilated and the distension extends into the left or right pulmonary artery and occasionally into both branches. An angiogram performed in the pulmonary artery shows marked pulmonary regurgitation. To demonstrate the possibility of branch stenosis, the pulmonary arteriogram should be performed with a 30° craniocaudal projection. As mentioned above, if surgery is planned, an aortogram should be performed to define the course of the coronary arteries because it may be necessary to make an incision across the outflow tract.

Differential diagnosis

In infants with severe hypoxemia, several conditions could be confused with tetralogy of Fallot. These include aortopulmonary transposition, pulmonary stenosis with intact ventricular septum and atrial right-to-left shunt, tricuspid atresia, atrioventricular septal defect with pulmonary stenosis, double-outlet right ventricle with pulmonary stenosis, and rarer lesions such as single ventricle with severe pulmonary stenosis. The physical examination is not often helpful, because any of the lesions associated with pulmonary stenosis may be associated with a similar systolic murmur. Usually, aortopulmonary transposition is differentiated by the more prominent pulmonary vasculature on radiography; however, in infants who are hyperventilating, the lung vascular markings may not appear to be increased because the lungs are hyperexpanded. The superior mediastinal shadow may be narrow in the infant with transposition because the pulmonary artery is posterior to the aorta; it is often narrow in tetralogy of Fallot because the pulmonary artery segment is small or absent. Tricuspid atresia can usually be differentiated by the findings of left axis deviation and dominant left ventricular forces in the electrocardiogram. However, as mentioned on p. 353, dominant left ventricular forces have been noted occasionally. Also, in the unusual association of tetralogy of Fallot with hypoplastic right ventricle, left axis deviation may be present. In the child with atrioventricular septal defect with pulmonary stenosis, the electrocardiogram shows left axis deviation or an indeterminate axis, as well as right ventricular hypertrophy.

The diagnosis is usually readily made by ultrasound studies. However, the differentiation between tetralogy of Fallot and double-outlet right ventricle with pulmonary stenosis may be difficult. As mentioned on p. 346, some have recommended that the diagnosis of double-outlet right ventricle be made if there is greater than 50% of aortic overriding. However, it is advisable to attempt to define whether mitral–aortic valve contiguity is present. If it is, the child should be considered to have tetralogy of Fallot; if there is clearly separation between the valves, the lesion should be named double-outlet right ventricle. Unfortunately, it is sometimes difficult to resolve whether there is mitral–aortic valve separation. The same quandary often exists after angiographic study; therefore, if the question is not resolved by ultrasound, it is not recommended that cardiac catheterization be performed for this purpose alone.

In older infants and children several lesions can be confused with tetralogy of Fallot. Pulmonary stenosis with an intact ventricular septum and a patent foramen ovale or atrial septal defect may also result in cyanosis that occurs late in infancy or in early childhood. The differential diagnosis is discussed in detail in Chapter 13. Cyanosis may not be evident if right ventricular outflow tract stenosis is mild or moderate, and the diagnosis of isolated ventricular septal defect may be considered. The presence of a loud systolic murmur at the upper left sternal border should suggest the possible association of outflow tract stenosis. Also, ventricular septal defect with a large left-to-right shunt is associated with a loud pulmonary component of the second sound, whereas with tetralogy of Fallot the pulmonary component is soft or absent.

Tetralogy of Fallot with absent pulmonary valve is rarely confused with other lesions because the loud to-and-fro murmur is characteristic. A similar murmur may be heard with sinus of Valsalva fistula or aortic–left ventricular tunnel, but these lesions would also be associated with a wide systemic arterial pulse pressure. Ultrasound study will usually provide the diagnosis.

Complications

Cerebrovascular incidents

Infants with severe cyanosis have a tendency to develop neurological signs, particularly within the first 18 months after birth. The infant may be apparently well and suddenly develop convulsions and, after recovery, have hemiplegia. The cause of this complication is not known, but it has been suggested that it may be due to cerebral venous thrombosis associated with severe polycythemia. Some episodes occur during hot weather or in association with an infection and it is assumed that the infant has become dehydrated. However, neurological complications may develop in infants who have relative anemia and it is assumed that the insult is related to severe cerebral hypoxia.

Cerebral abscess

This is a rare complication in infants during the first year but is not unusual after this age. The development of personality changes, neurological signs, or unexplained fever or leukocytosis in a child with tetralogy of Fallot should make one suspect this diagnosis and all attempts should be made to confirm or exclude it.

Infective endocarditis

This is an important complication; the lesion occurs most frequently in the region of the ventricular septal defect. In patients who have had systemic-to-pulmonary shunts, the vegetations frequently occur in the pulmonary artery around the margin of the shunt and may extend into the pulmonary arteries. The diagnosis should be entertained in a patient with tetralogy of Fallot who has unexplained fever, petechiae, microscopic hematuria, or evidence of embolic phenomena.

Principles of management

Background

Tetralogy of Fallot was the first cyanotic congenital cardiac lesion that was palliated by surgery. Recognizing that the predominant factor contributing to the cyanosis was inadequate pulmonary blood flow, Taussig and Blalock designed the procedure to connect a subclavian artery to a pulmonary artery by an end-to-side anastomosis. Dramatic results were achieved in individuals of all ages. Although the procedure did not abolish the cyanosis, systemic arterial oxygen saturation increased considerably, often to about 90%. Ability to exercise and to perform normal daily activities improved and hemoglobin and hematocrit fell toward normal values. Early in the experience with the procedure, which was usually performed on the right side, several difficulties were encountered. Kinking and obstruction of the subclavian artery was noted when a right aortic arch was present (almost 25% of patients with tetralogy of Fallot). This was due to the acute angulation of the artery when it was turned inferiorly to connect to the pulmonary artery. It was recognized that the subclavian artery originating from the innominate artery is the preferred vessel because it can be anastomosed with a gentler curve; thus with a right aortic arch the procedure should be performed on the left side. Technical difficulties were also encountered in performing the anastomosis in infants because of the small size of the vessels. Furthermore, thrombotic obstruction of the small vessels sometimes occurred. For these reasons, procedures to connect the descending aorta to left pulmonary artery (Potts) and ascending aorta to right pulmonary artery (Waterston) were developed.

The Potts and Waterston shunts have several disadvantages compared with the Blalock–Taussig shunt. The size of the subclavian artery limits the diameter of the orifice of the systemic–pulmonary communication, and the length of the artery also provides some resistance to flow. The increase in pulmonary blood flow is therefore limited and it is not usually large enough to cause cardiac failure. Also, pulmonary arterial pressure is increased only modestly, so there is little risk of pulmonary vascular damage. Potts and Waterston anastomoses are both side-to-side communications, which create an orifice between the aorta and the pulmonary artery. It is difficult to select the diameter of the orifice that should be created; a small difference in diameter has a major influence on the resistance. Thus the 1-mm difference in communications with diameters of 3 and 4 mm will be associated with a 1.7-fold difference in cross-sectional area. Another problem is that the size of the orifice after healing may not be the same as that created at the time of surgery. Because of the concern that a small anastomosis may become occluded by thrombosis, the tendency is to create a somewhat larger communication than is appropriate. The increase in pulmonary blood flow is more likely to be excessive with these anastomoses than with Blalock–Taussig shunts, and cardiac failure was a not infrequent complication. Also, because larger communications resulted in elevated pulmonary arterial pressures, the combination of increased flow and pressure quite commonly resulted in pulmonary vascular damage with obstructive changes, which developed over a variable period of months to years (see Chapter 5). The progressive increase in pulmonary vascular resistance reduced pulmonary blood flow; cyanosis increased and ability to exercise again became limited.

A serious disadvantage of the Potts and particularly the Waterston procedure is the development of distortion at the anastomotic site associated with growth. This occasionally reduced the size of the shunt, but the main concern is that the pulmonary artery often became kinked and obstructed, so that the right or left pulmonary artery required reconstruction at the time of corrective surgery. Although some degree of narrowing of the pulmonary artery may occur after a Blalock–Taussig anastomosis, it is not usually severe and the pulmonary artery is not distorted. Because of these concerns about the Potts and Waterston shunts, a procedure was developed to produce a shunt by connecting a short tubular graft of woven fabric such as Teflon or GoreTex from the aorta to the main pulmonary artery (central shunt). There are two important advantages of this type of shunt: the size of the communication could be controlled by selecting a tube with a diameter appropriate for the patient; and the branch pulmonary arteries are not disturbed so that reconstruction is not required at the time of corrective surgery.

One disadvantage of the Blalock–Taussig shunt is that the subclavian arterial supply to the upper extremity is interrupted. Although arterial anastomoses around the shoulder provide adequate flow to the extremity, interference with growth commonly occurs and muscular power may be impaired. It has therefore become common practice to avoid sacrificing the subclavian artery by interposing a tubular graft of woven or knitted Teflon or GoreTex between the left or right subclavian and pulmonary arteries. Whereas the communications using native tissues have the ability to enlarge with growth of the child, both the central and interposition grafts are of fixed diameter and length, so that their size becomes inadequate after a varying time. Although this was a disadvantage in the past, it is now not usually a concern because corrective surgery is being accomplished at an early age.

Surgery to correct the anomalies by closure of the ventricular septal defect and relief of the right ventricular outflow tract obstruction was introduced by Lillehei almost 50 years ago. In the early experience the mortality was quite high, particularly when the procedure was performed in infants and young children under the age of 3–4 years. However, in recent years, with improvements in surgical technique and perioperative management, results have improved dramatically. Corrective surgery can now be performed with low mortality on infants during the neonatal period in a number of pediatric cardiac centers. The ability to perform corrective surgery, even in young infants, has introduced controversy regarding the optimal time for surgical repair. Some contend that total correction should be performed as the initial procedure in all infants; the age for repair will depend on the severity of the outflow tract obstruction, but supporters of this approach maintain it should be done by 6–9 months in all patients. Others advise that an initial palliative procedure should be used in some circumstances, because it may improve the results achievable by delaying the performance of complete repair. The various recommendations are discussed below, as well as the advantages and disadvantages of early correction.

Medical management

In considering the management of patients with tetralogy of Fallot, it is convenient to divide them into three groups based on the clinical presentation: newborn infants with severe cyanosis; older infants with moderate cyanosis; infants and children with mild or no cyanosis.

Newborn infants with severe cyanosis

Infants with severe right ventricular outflow obstruction or pulmonary atresia develop severe cyanosis when the ductus arteriosus closes. Metabolic acidemia soon ensues and without therapy the infant will succumb. Administration of 100% oxygen should be instituted immediately; although it may not be very effective when pulmonary blood flow is greatly reduced, it may have some beneficial effect (see Chapter 3). Infusion of prostaglandin (PG)E_1 should be started as soon as intravascular access is achieved to attempt to dilate the ductus arteriosus and increase pulmonary blood flow. If the child is not in a center with pediatric cardiology services, PGE_1 should be given and the infant transported with a continuous infusion. Also, because there is a risk of apnea associated with PGE_1 infusion, particularly in the preterm infant, the trachea should be intubated prior to transportation to provide assisted ventilation. The initial infusion rate usually advised is 0.1 μg/kg per min; if a favorable response is achieved, the rate can be reduced to 0.05 μg/kg per min and even lower if still effective. Although the favorable response is predominantly due to the effect of PGE_1 on the ductus, some improvement may occur even in infants with pulmonary atresia with no ductus arteriosus. It has been suggested that the increase in arterial oxygen saturation that may occur is the result of decreased pulmonary vascular resistance and increased pulmonary blood flow. The infant with severe metabolic acidemia may also be treated by administration of alkali such as sodium bicarbonate. If improvement results, the decision about the timing of surgery and the procedure to be performed can be delayed, but if the infant continues to manifest severe hypoxia and acidemia, this decision has to be made promptly.

Infants and children with moderately severe stenosis

In those infants in whom hypoxemia is not severe enough to result in hypoxia and acidemia in the neonatal period, the first symptoms may appear at 2–3 months after birth and manifest as hypoxic spells.

Acute treatment of hypoxic spells

The objectives of therapy are to attempt to increase oxygen supply to the tissues and to reduce oxygen demands. It is important to advise the parents about the possibility of hypoxic spells and what procedures should be adopted if they occur. If an infant has had a spell, it is advisable to have oxygen available at home. Administration of 100% oxygen may provide some increase of oxygen uptake but, as mentioned above, this is of limited value when pulmonary blood flow is very low.

Morphine is very effective in quieting the distressed infant and improving oxygen saturation; its benefit is probably the result of reduction of oxygen consumption. It should be administered in a dose of 100 μg/kg; it is most effective when given slowly by intravenous injection, but can be used intramuscularly.

The most effective means of increasing oxygen supply is to enhance pulmonary blood flow. In the home setting, much can often be accomplished by improving venous return by postural means. When an infant is distressed, the parents usually hold the baby with the head up and the legs dependent; this tends to enhance pooling of venous blood in the lower body. They should be advised to hold the baby in the knee–chest position; this can be done readily by lying supine and holding the baby on the chest and abdomen. This serves to both pacify the infant and improve venous return. If oxygen administration and postural change do not result in rapid improvement, the infant should be transported to a facility where further measures can be instituted. Raising peripheral vascular resistance with vasoconstrictors increases systemic arterial and right ventricular pressures and thus improves pulmonary flow. Use of catecholamines that have significant β-adrenoceptor stimulant effects, such as dopamine, dobutamine or epinephrine, are not advised because they could possibly cause infundibular contraction and further reduce pulmonary blood flow. Although these drugs can be given as a single dose, in general it is preferred to use a continuous infusion. Methoxamine (Vasoxyl) has almost no β-adrenoceptor effect; it is administered as a single dose of 100 μg/kg intravenously by slow injection or 250 μg/kg intramuscularly. Phenylephrine (Neo-Synephrine) has predominantly α-adrenoceptor stimulant effects and produces marked peripheral vasoconstriction, with minor β-adrenoceptor stimulant effects. The single intravenous dose is 20 μg/kg and the intramuscular dose 100 μg/kg. The preferred method of administration is to infuse phenylephrine initially at 1 μg/kg per min and to gradually increase to 5 μg/kg per min if necessary, as indicated by level of oxygen saturation and systemic arterial blood pressure.

It has been recommended that administration of propranolol may be effective in treating spells acutely, by relieving constriction of the right ventricular outflow tract and thus increasing pulmonary blood flow. I have serious concerns about the use of β-adrenoceptor blockade during an acute hypoxic period. Studies in newborn lambs with induced severe hypoxia showed that propranolol markedly reduced the tachycardia and increased cardiac output response to hypoxia; this drastically reduced oxygen delivery and resulted in severe metabolic acidemia.

If the above procedures do not result in improvement in hypoxia, transfusion of whole blood or red cells may be effective. This raises hemoglobin concentration and increases oxygen uptake in the lungs. Recently, success has been achieved in increasing pulmonary blood flow by balloon dilatation of the pulmonary annulus (see Chapter 14). This would be a useful approach in the infant who has persistent hypoxia despite the measures mentioned above.

Continuing management of spells

Frequently the onset of spells is associated with relative anemia (see above). It is therefore important to provide supplemental iron as ferrous sulfate soon after birth; if iron has not been administered at an earlier age, treatment should be started promptly. The increase in hemoglobin concentration often results in dramatic improvement of symptoms. If there is no anemia and spells become more severe and frequent, the decision must be made regarding oral administration of propranolol, a β-adrenoceptor blocking agent. I do not recommend the use of propranolol for prevention of spells; if the other means of therapy are not effective, I consider it preferable to attempt balloon dilatation of the pulmonary valve annulus or to proceed with surgery. If catheter intervention or surgery is not available, it is reasonable to consider the use of propranolol in doses of 0.5–1.0 mg/kg given every 6 hours; it has been effective in either completely relieving spells or reducing their frequency and severity. This approach was frequently used in the past in centers in which palliative shunt procedures could not be performed with a high success rate in small infants. It was also sometimes used to avoid performing a palliative shunt procedure prior to planning corrective surgery some months in the future. The actual mechanism by which propranolol relieves the symptoms is not known. It is generally believed that the beneficial effect may be due to the myocardial depressant action, which relieves contraction of the infundibulum and thus improves pulmonary blood flow. Other possible mechanisms of action could explain the beneficial effect. Propranolol shifts the blood oxygen dissociation curve to the right and thus could increase the release of oxygen from hemoglobin at the tissue site. β-Adrenoceptor stimulation causes peripheral vasodilatation; blockade of β-adrenoceptors could result in vasoconstriction and increase peripheral vascular resistance, thus elevating systemic arterial pressure, or preventing reductions of pressure. This would help to maintain pulmonary blood flow. There are potential risks with administration of propranolol for prolonged periods in infants with tetralogy of Fallot; several instances of sudden death have been reported with the doses used.

Infants and children with mild stenosis

Hypoxia is not a problem in these individuals. Occasionally, the left-to-right shunt is large and symptoms and signs of cardiac failure develop. This may require therapy as discussed in Chapter 7.

Surgical considerations

The corrective surgical procedure for tetralogy of Fallot consists of closing the ventricular septal defect and relieving the right ventricular outflow obstruction. Closure of the ventricular septal defect is accomplished with a patch of flexible synthetic material. Some surgeons attempt to close the defect from an atrial incision, through the tricuspid valve; this is technically difficult to perform in small infants. Others approach the defect by making an incision in the anterior wall of the right ventricle. Relief of right ventricular outflow tract obstruction may require only removal of hypertrophied muscle in the infundibulum. In older infants and children, this can sometimes be accomplished from incisions in the right atrium and pulmonary artery. With more severe infundibular stenosis, an incision over the outflow tract is necessary; if adequate relief of obstruction cannot be achieved by excising muscle, it may be necessary to insert a patch over the incision. In the past, pericardium was often used as the patch, but because aneurysms over the outflow tract sometimes occurred it is no longer considered acceptable; a synthetic cloth is now preferred. If the pulmonary valve annulus is very narrow, it may be necessary to open the annular region and to extend the patch to the main pulmonary artery. It may also be necessary to enlarge the main pulmonary artery and the junction of the branch pulmonary arteries with the patch.

Adequate relief of right ventricular outflow obstruction is an important determinant of a successful outcome. If it is inadequate and the ventricular septal defect is closed, blood flow through the pulmonary circulation may not be large enough to provide adequate systemic output; this will be manifested by hypotension and poor perfusion postoperatively. The ratio of right to left ventricular systolic pressure at the time of surgery has been used as an indicator of the adequacy of relief of outflow tract obstruction. A right to left ventricular ratio greater than 0.8 was considered an indication to attempt further relief of outflow obstruction. Previously, if there was concern about the ability to adequately relieve right ventricular outflow obstruction, it was recommended that the ventricular septal defect should be left at least partly open to allow for maintenance of systemic output by right-to-left shunting, if necessary. The practice subsequently was to place a nonvalved conduit between the right ventricle and the pulmonary artery, but more recently a valved prosthesis was recommended. Aortic homografts as well as pulmonary homografts have been used extensively, but it is becoming apparent that many develop degeneration and valve insufficiency over a period ranging from several months to several years. Replacement is then necessary and recently, rather than using another homograft, some surgeons have used the Contegra Pulmonary Valved Conduit, a prosthesis made from a segment of bovine jugular vein that includes a tricuspid valve. Some reports suggest it is preferable to the pulmonary homograft [20]. However, experience is still limited but a considerable incidence of stenosis at the junction of the prosthesis and the pulmonary arteries has been reported.

Inadequate opening of the outflow tract was frequently associated with the coursing of an anomalous coronary artery across the outflow tract, because it was necessary to avoid cutting the artery.

Surgical problems

The two main concerns relating to closure of the defect are the potential for creating heart block by damaging the conduction bundle, and interference with aortic valve function by placing a suture through a cusp. With the knowledge that conduction tissue courses along the posterior and inferior margins of the defect, heart block is now an unusual complication, even in infants. Postoperative aortic insufficiency occasionally occurred due to aortic valve damage, but this also is now a rare complication.

Several problems may be related to the incision in the right ventricle. An extensive incision may interfere with right ventricular function; this may be a serious concern if there is a postoperative load on the ventricle due to incomplete relief of the obstruction or to pulmonary insufficiency. The right ventricular incision almost always creates right ventricular conduction disturbance with complete right bundle-branch block. It is thought that the incision may contribute to the development of postoperative ventricular arrhythmias.

If a patch has been placed across the pulmonary valve annulus, varying degrees of pulmonary insufficiency will develop. It was thought that pulmonary insufficiency was not an important concern, but recent experience suggests that serious long-term effects may result. If the insufficiency is mild, the right ventricle will probably tolerate the increased volume load for many years without evidence of failure. However, severe insufficiency will result in marked dilatation of the right ventricle; the ability to exercise becomes increasingly limited and failure then ensues. The time after surgery that right ventricular dysfunction becomes evident varies; with severe insufficiency in infants it may progress rapidly over 1–3 years, whereas with mild insufficiency difficulties may not become apparent for several decades. In addition to the size of the pulmonary valve annulus, other factors will influence the severity of regurgitation. A reduced pulmonary vascular bed, small pulmonary arteries, or stenosis in branch pulmonary arteries will all increase distal resistance and thus accentuate the degree of regurgitation.

Marked right ventricular dilatation may result in stretching of the tricuspid valve annulus, resulting in superimposed tricuspid regurgitation that further contributes to the development of right ventricular failure. For many years, the presence of postoperative pulmonary insufficiency did not create serious concern. However, there is considerable unease that moderate to severe insufficiency may result in myocardial fibrosis of the right ventricle over the course of several months to years, depending on the severity. It is therefore recommended that a pulmonary valve, or a conduit that incorporates a valve, be inserted before severe right ventricular dysfunction occurs. The indications for inserting a valve are not yet well defined, but evidence of significant right ventricular enlargement and reduced ejection fraction on ultrasound examination are indications to consider this procedure. Another important indication is the occurrence of arrhythmias. It is now also becoming evident that even if considerable right ventricular enlargement and dysfunction have already occurred, providing a functioning pulmonary valve improves ventricular function and performance and may also be helpful in reducing the incidence of arrhythmia [21]. It may also be effective in delaying progression of the right ventricular functional deterioration.

It is important to recognize the abnormal course of a coronary artery across the right ventricular outflow tract. If the artery is only a small branch, cutting it may create only minor disturbance of cardiac function, but incision of a major vessel, such as a left anterior descending artery arising from the right coronary artery, could seriously impair ventricular performance and the individual may not survive. In the presence of an abnormal coronary artery, it is therefore important to avoid making an extensive incision across the outflow tract to relieve the stenosis. Some have recommended that a transatrial and transpulmonary approach be used to close the defect and relieve the obstruction. This is often successful, but it may be necessary to make a limited incision into the infundibulum to relieve stenosis adequately, avoiding damage to the coronary artery. If the pulmonary annulus is very small and the coronary artery is close to the annulus, it may not be possible to relieve the stenosis. In this event, it will be necessary to use an external conduit or graft between the ventricle and the pulmonary artery.

The size of the pulmonary arteries is an important consideration in determining the success of surgical correction. If the main pulmonary artery is hypoplastic, it is important to extend the patch into the artery to relieve obstruction. The left and right pulmonary arteries are not commonly very small in patients with tetralogy of Fallot with an open right ventricular outflow tract, but they are often diminutive in patients with pulmonary atresia. If a complete repair is attempted, the branch pulmonary arteries may not be large enough to accommodate an adequate pulmonary blood flow. Right ventricular pressure would be maintained at or exceed systemic arterial levels and postoperative hypotension and poor cardiac output would result. As with inadequate relief of the right ventricular outflow tract, the ventricular septal defect would have to be left open to maintain systemic blood flow by right-to-left shunting. Numerous measurements have been reported in attempts to predict, prior to surgery, whether the pulmonary arteries are large enough to accommodate an adequate blood flow and lower right ventricular pressure if the ventricular septal defect is closed.

The Nakata index is the sum of the cross-sectional areas of the left and right pulmonary arteries at their pre-branching points, as related to body surface area. The measurement was originally made on angiograms, but can also be done by ultrasound. A normal value is about 300 mm^2/m^2; in tetralogy of Fallot with outflow tract stenosis, the index is below 150 mm^2/m^2 in 10–15% of patients, but is 50–100 mm^2/m^2 in most patients with pulmonary atresia. Although criteria vary, it was generally considered that an index below 150 mm^2/m^2 should raise concerns. The McGoon ratio expresses, as the numerator, the sum of the pre-branching diameters of the left and right pulmonary arteries and, as the denominator, the diameter of the descending aorta at the level of the diaphragm. The normal ratio is about 2.0; it varies greatly in tetralogy of Fallot, but a level below about 1.3 is considered cause for concern. Because the descending aortic diameter is often below normal levels in patients with tetralogy of Fallot, the ratio tends to exaggerate the size of the pulmonary arteries. As mentioned below, the value of these assessments of pulmonary artery size has recently been questioned.

Current approaches

In recent years, with improvements in surgical technique and perioperative management, results have improved dramatically. Because excellent results are achievable in infants, some recommend the following guidelines for corrective surgery. Infants with very severe right ventricular outflow tract stenosis and those with pulmonary atresia, with systemic arterial oxygen saturations below 70%, should have surgery within a few weeks after birth. Infants with moderately severe stenosis and marked cyanosis (oxygen saturation 70–90%) should have corrective surgery by 2–4 months. Corrective surgery should be performed in all other infants with tetralogy of Fallot by 6 months. However, other surgeons recommend that, other than those corrected in the neonatal period, all patients should have surgical correction by 2 months of age.

The ability to perform surgery in infants with a low mortality has introduced controversy about the optimal time for surgical repair. Some contend that total correction should be performed as the initial procedure in all infants; others advise that an initial palliative procedure should be used in some circumstances, because it may improve the results achievable by delaying the performance of complete repair.

Advantages of early total correction

- Elimination of hypoxia will prevent neurological complications of cerebral hypoxia and hematological changes.
- Closure of the ventricular septal defect and elimination of the right-to-left shunt will reduce the risk of cerebral complications resulting from embolus and abscess.
- Decreasing right ventricular pressure will prevent persistent myocardial hypertrophy and probably reduce the risk of fibrosis of the right ventricle.
- Providing adequate pulmonary blood flow will optimize the opportunity for normal growth of the main and branch pulmonary arteries. In addition, during infancy and early childhood, while new alveolar units are being generated, normal pulmonary circulation may be important for lung development.
- The tendency for progressive hypertrophy of the right ventricular infundibular region is largely abolished by early repair.
- If MAPCAs are separated from the aorta early and connected to the pulmonary arterial system, the risk of pulmonary vascular obstructive changes would be reduced. Also, the development of stenoses in the MAPCAs may possibly be avoided.

Early correction would also be advantageous in avoiding the complications that may result from palliative systemic-to-pulmonary arterial shunts.

- The potential risk for pulmonary vascular obstructive disease due to large communications is abolished.
- Pulmonary arterial stenosis and distortion would not present a problem.
- The risk of left ventricular failure due to a large shunt will be eliminated.
- The possible development of left ventricular fibrosis due to chronic volume overload resulting from the shunt will be prevented.

Arguments against early total correction

The pulmonary arteries may be too small to accommodate an adequate pulmonary blood flow. It is suggested that introducing an arteriopulmonary shunt will increase their size so that complete repair would be better tolerated. It has been shown that pulmonary arteries do enlarge modestly after shunting; the dilatation occurs soon after the surgery but is usually no more than about 20%. No further significant change occurs after about 2–6 weeks. In recent years, balloon angioplasty of the pulmonary valve annulus has been quite successful in increasing pulmonary blood flow, with resultant modest increase in the diameter of the pulmonary arteries. There is the risk of a marked increase in pulmonary blood flow after angioplasty if the pulmonary arteries are normal or increased in size, because relief of outflow tract stenosis may permit a large left-to-right shunt through the ventricular septal defect. This may be severe enough to precipitate the onset of cardiac failure.

The presence of a major coronary artery crossing the right ventricular outflow may make it difficult to relieve the outflow tract stenosis in a small heart by a combined transatrial and transpulmonary approach. This would increase the likelihood that an external conduit or homograft would be necessary; when inserted in infants, the long-term outlook without development of stenosis or insufficiency is poor.

Corrective surgery during early infancy, when the pulmonary annulus is markedly stenotic, frequently requires the insertion of a long and wide transannular patch. This greatly increases the likelihood that marked pulmonary insufficiency may result. It is especially likely to be severe in the infant who has small pulmonary arteries. As mentioned above, this is not well tolerated. Because of these concerns, the surgeon may elect to use an extracardiac bypass across the outflow tract. Limited information is available suggesting that an arteriopulmonary shunt procedure early in infancy may result in enlargement not only of the pulmonary arteries but also of the annulus; this also appears to result after balloon angioplasty of the annulus. It has therefore been suggested that a palliative procedure may reduce the need for an extensive transpulmonary patch, or a conduit, when corrective surgery is performed later. There is as yet no documentation of this supposition.

My view is that a careful trial of the various techniques should be instituted and the immediate and long-term outlook in infants undergoing complete correction in early infancy should be compared with those who first have a palliative procedure. It seems to me that balloon angioplasty of the pulmonary valve annulus is preferable to a shunt procedure: it is less traumatic, it avoids a thoracotomy, and also reduces the likelihood that distortion of the pulmonary arteries will develop.

Surgery for tetralogy of Fallot with pulmonary atresia

Most individuals with these lesions have small pulmonary arteries and frequently many lung segments receive blood supply from collateral arteries. The recognition that these collateral arteries provide pulmonary capillary blood flow led to attempts at surgical correction. The procedure is complicated and consists of connecting as many as possible of the MAPCAs, as well as the small native pulmonary arteries, to one source of blood flow from the right ventricle via a conduit such as an aortic allograft; this is called a *unifocalization procedure*. In the first attempts, the procedure was done in older patients and often in a staged approach. Some of the MAPCAs on one side of the chest were anastomosed to each other and to pulmonary arteries, and at one or more later procedures the unifocalization was completed. The success rate was not high; many older patients had significant pulmonary vascular obstructive changes in the segments supplied by the MAPCAs and stenoses in the MAPCAs were common. Because the pulmonary vascular resistance was high, it was sometimes not possible to close the ventricular septal defect.

Recently, the unifocalization procedure has been performed successfully as a one-stage procedure in early infancy, with a high success rate. MAPCAs and pulmonary arteries are connected using native tissues, without inserting foreign graft material. These vessels are then connected to an aortic valved allograft that forms the conduit from the right ventricle. The advantage of performing the procedure early is that development of pulmonary vascular obstructive changes, as well as stenoses in the MAPCAs, is largely avoided. If the pulmonary vascular morphology and resistance are such that adequate pulmonary blood flow can be accommodated, right ventricular pressure after correction will be low enough to close the ventricular septal defect. To assess whether this is likely, surgeons at the University of California in San Francisco perfuse blood from the perfusion system through the pulmonary artery at a rate of 2.5 L/min per m^2. If pulmonary arterial mean pressure is below 25 mmHg, it is considered safe to close the ventricular septal defect. If it is not closed, the patient is followed; the pulmonary vascular resistance may decrease over time, allowing later closure. Also, if stenoses in pulmonary vessels are noted, relief by balloon angioplasty, with stenting if necessary, may permit right ventricular pressure to fall and permit closure of the defect. Current experience is that the defect can be closed in about two-thirds of infants at the time of first surgery. The immediate results that can be achieved are remarkably good considering the high mortality of tetralogy of Fallot with pulmonary atresia during the first year. Survival is about 80–85%; with improvements in technique and selection of younger infants, the surgical mortality should decrease further. One major concern is that pulmonary arterial pressure is frequently still elevated after the corrective procedure; this greatly aggravates pulmonary insufficiency and may result in decrease in function with right ventricular failure. Also, persistent elevation of pulmonary arterial pressure may result in pulmonary vascular obstructive changes.

Prior to performing a unifocalization procedure on infants with pulmonary atresia, it is very important to determine by either ultrasound or angiocardiography if the main pulmonary artery and the left and right branches are present. Recently, it has been observed that if these vessels are present, even though very small (diameter 3 mm), they are capable of considerable enlargement if blood flow through them is increased. In several infants with this anatomy, construction of an aortopulmonary window between the aorta and main pulmonary artery early in infancy has resulted in sufficient enlargement of the pulmonary arterial tree to later perform successful repair using the normal pulmonary arteries and thus avoiding a unifocalization procedure.

Tetralogy of Fallot with absent pulmonary valve

The most serious symptoms of this complex are related to airway compression. If the ventricular left-to-right shunt is large, left and right ventricular failure may develop. Also, if pulmonary regurgitation is severe, right ventricular enlargement and failure may occur. Treatment with diuretics and perhaps digitalis is indicated if there is evidence of failure. The respiratory distress may be severe enough to require intubation with assisted ventilation. There has been some reluctance in the past to initiate mechanical ventilation because, once started, it is difficult to wean the infant. However, this view was held at a time when surgery in early infancy was attended with a very high mortality. Some improvement in spontaneous ventilation was achieved by placing the infant in the prone position with the head elevated; this was thought to reduce some of the pressure by the aneurysmal pulmonary arteries on the airways.

The early surgical approaches were largely directed to attempts to reduce pulmonary arterial size by plicating the dilated pulmonary arteries, or to reduce pulmonary arterial pressure by banding the pulmonary artery. Another procedure that was conceived was to attempt to relieve pressure on the airways by using a sling to displace the enlarged pulmonary artery toward the anterior chest wall. None of these procedures were particularly successful. Recently, surgery has been directed toward attempts to perform a complete correction. In the past, it was shown that good results could be achieved in some patients by closing the ventricular septal defect without attempting to correct pulmonary insufficiency; this reduced the left-to-right shunt, as well as pulmonary arterial pressure. If there was adequate residual infundibular or annulus stenosis, the pulmonary insufficiency was not severe and thus did not present a serious problem.

Recently, the tendency is to be more aggressive in attempting to completely correct the lesions. The procedure consists of closing the ventricular septal defect and inserting a valved allograft between the right ventricle and pulmonary artery. Some surgeons have also reduced the size of the dilated pulmonary arteries in the process of attaching the pulmonary arterial end of the graft. The experience with this procedure is still limited, but it seems that excellent results are achievable. One concern is that, as mentioned above, abnormalities in the morphology of both the pulmonary microvasculature and alveolar pattern may interfere with adequate pulmonary perfusion and with ventilation. It remains to be seen whether these will improve with growth if the lesions are corrected in early infancy.

Results of surgery

Prior to the advent of surgery, only a small percentage of patients with tetralogy of Fallot survived beyond the age of 25–30 years. Following corrective surgery, most patients experience what has been considered to be right ventricular failure. It is not surprising that this will occur if there is pulmonary insufficiency, inadequate relief of outflow tract stenosis, high resistance in the pulmonary vasculature, or residual ventricular septal defect with significant left-to-right shunt. However, even without these associations, hepatomegaly and edema of the lower extremities is common. It is thought to be related to reduced compliance of the right ventricle and possibly due to some disturbance in right ventricular function related to the incision in the anterior wall. Whether the transatrial and transpulmonary approach reduces the likelihood of these postoperative complications has yet to be evaluated. The manifestations of failure are usually not severe and persist for 2 weeks to about 3 months. They respond well to diuretic treatment, but digoxin may also be required. If the ventricular septal defect has not been fully closed, a left-to-right shunt develops which, if large, can result in cardiac failure. If the shunt is large, reoperation is indicated to close the defect completely.

Electrocardiographic changes are common after surgery. Although complete heart block was not an unusual complication in the early experience with complete repair, it is now uncommon; usually, a pacemaker is required if this does occur. Right bundle-branch block is noted in almost all patients who have had a right ventricular incision. This finding does not seem to be associated with any long-term adverse effects. Not uncommonly, left axis deviation, indicating the presence of left anterior hemiblock, is noted. Concern was expressed about this association with right bundle-branch block, because it was thought that the bifascicular block would predispose the individual to complete heart block. However, there does not appear to be any significant long-term adverse effect of the bifascicular block. Ventricular premature beats are occasionally noted after surgery; most of these are benign, but it is now thought that the occasional occurrence of sudden death some years after surgery is due to ventricular arrhythmia. The presence of frequent or multifocal ventricular premature beats is considered cause for concern and treatment with antiarrhythmic drugs is recommended. Residual right ventricular hypertension, with pressures more than half systemic levels, due to inadequate relief of outflow tract obstruction is thought to be an important factor in inducing ventricular arrhythmia. It is recommended that, if possible, further procedures be considered to reduce right ventricular pressure.

Moderate to severe pulmonary insufficiency, with right ventricular enlargement is not uncommon after surgery, particularly if a large patch has been placed in the right ventricular outflow tract. This may contribute to the development of ventricular arrhythmisas. It may be treated as outlined on p. 380.

References

1 Bhat AH, Smith CJ, Hawker RE. Late aortic root dilatation in tetralogy of Fallot may be prevented by early repair in infancy. Pediatr Cardiol 2004;25:654–659.

2 Niwa K, Siu SC, Webb GD, Gatzoulis MA. Progressive aortic root dilatation in adults late after repair of tetralogy of Fallot. Circulation 2002;106:1374–1378.

3 Kim WH, Seo JW, Kim SJ, Song J, Lee J, Na CY. Aortic dissection late after repair of tetralogy of Fallot. Int J Cardiol 2005;101:515–516.

4 Niwa K. Aortic root dilatation in tetralogy of Fallot long-term after repair. Histology of the aorta in tetralogy of Fallot: evidence of intrinsic aortopathy. Int J Cardiol 2005;103:117–119.

5 Chong WY, Wong WH, Chiu CS, Cheung YF. Aortic root dilation and aortic elastic properties in children after repair of tetralogy of Fallot. Am J Cardiol 2006;97: 905–909.

6 Nørgaard MA, Alphonso N, Cochrane AD, Menahem S, Brizard CP, d'Udekem Y. Major aorto-pulmonary collateral arteries of patients with pulmonary atresia and ventricular septal defect are dilated bronchial arteries. Eur J Cardiothorac Surg 2006;29:682–687.

7 Hanley FL. MAPCAs, bronchials, monkeys and men. Eur J Cardiothorac Surg 2006;29:633–644.

8 Galindo A, Gutiérrez-Larraya F, Martínez JM *et al.* Prenatal diagnosis and outcome for fetuses with congenital absence of the pulmonary valve. Ultrasound Obstet Gynecol 2006;28:32–39.

9 Berg C, Thomsen Y, Geipel A, Germer U, Gembruch U. Reversed end-diastolic flow in the umbilical artery at 10–14 weeks of gestation is associated with absent pulmonary valve syndrome. Ultrasound Obstet Gynecol 2007;30:254–258.

10 Mjaatvedt CH, Nakaoka T, Moreno-Rodriguez R *et al.* The outflow tract of the heart is recruited from a novel heart-forming field. Dev Biol 2001;238:97–109.

11 Zaffran S, Kelly RG, Meilhac SM, Buckingham ME, Brown NA. Right ventricular myocardium derives from the anterior heart field. Circ Res 2004;95:261–268.

12 Ward C, Stadt H, Hutson M, Kirby ML. Ablation of the secondary heart field leads to tetralogy of Fallot and pulmonary atresia. Dev Biol 2005;284:72–83.

13 Lakier JB, Stanger P, Heymann MA, Hoffman JIE, Rudolph AM. Tetralogy of Fallot with absent pulmonary valve: natural history and hemodynamic considerations. Circulation 1974;50:167–174.

14 Hornberger LK, Sanders SP, Sahn DJ *et al.* In utero pulmonary artery and aortic growth and potential for progression of pulmonary outflow tract obstruction in tetralogy of Fallot. J Am Coll Cardiol 1995;25:739–745.

15 Pepas LP, Savis A, Jones A, Sharland GK, Tulloh RM, Simpson JM. An echocardiographic study of tetralogy of Fallot in the fetus and infant. Cardiol Young 2003; 13:240–247.

16 Sun LS, Du F, Quaegebeur JM. Right ventricular infundibular beta-adrenoceptor complex in tetralogy of Fallot patients. Pediatr Res 1997;42:12–16.

17 Shaddy RE, Viney J, Judd VE, McGough EC. Continuous intravenous phenylephrine infusion for treatment of hypoxemic spells in tetralogy of Fallot. J Pediatr 1989; 114:468–470.

18 Rudolph AM, Nadas AS, Borges WH. Hematologic adjustments to cyanotic congenital heart disease. Pediatrics 1953;11:454–464.

19 Guntheroth WG, Morgan BC, Mullins GL. Physiologic studies of paroxysmal hyperpnea in cyanotic congenital heart disease. Circulation 1965;31:70–76.

20 Brown JW, Ruzmetov M, Rodefeld MD, Vijay P, Darragh RK. Valved bovine jugular vein conduits for right ventricular outflow tract reconstruction in children: an attractive alternative to pulmonary homograft. Ann Thorac Surg 2006;82:909–916.

21 Discigil B, Dearani JA, Puga FJ *et al.* Late pulmonary valve replacement after repair of tetralogy of Fallot. J Thorac Cardiovasc Surg 2001;121:344–351.

CHAPTER 15

Pulmonary stenosis and atresia with intact ventricular septum

Pulmonary stenosis is a common congenital anomaly that may occur as an isolated lesion or be associated with a large variety of other cardiac defects, the simplest being persistent patency of the foramen ovale. Pulmonary stenosis or atresia is frequently found in association with ventricular septal defect (tetralogy of Fallot) and may occur with aortopulmonary transposition, double-outlet right ventricle, atrioventricular septal defect, Ebstein malformation, and many other anomalies. I have separated pulmonary stenosis lesions into two main groups, pulmonary stenosis with ventricular septal defect and pulmonary stenosis with intact ventricular septum, because there are important embryological and hemodynamic differences between them. Pulmonary stenosis or atresia in aortopulmonary transposition, double-outlet right ventricle and endocardial cushion defect is discussed either in the specific chapters devoted to these lesions or in the chapter on pulmonary stenosis with ventricular septal defect (Chapter 14). Although the vast majority of cases of pulmonary stenosis with intact ventricular septum are confined to the pulmonary valve itself, there may be stenosis of the main or branch pulmonary arteries, most commonly in association with rubella syndrome, or of the subvalvar region of the right ventricle. In this chapter I present a description of valvar pulmonary stenosis or atresia and refer only briefly to the other types.

The spectrum of severity of pulmonary stenosis ranges from minor abnormalities of the pulmonary valve with minimal pressure gradient between the right ventricle and pulmonary artery, to complete atresia. Most classifications of severity have been based on the pressure gradient across the right ventricular outflow tract. Generally, pressure gradients below about 40 mmHg have been considered to represent mild stenosis, gradients of 40–80 mmHg moderate stenosis, and gradients above 80 mmHg severe stenosis. Similarly, degree of severity has been based on the relation between right ventricular systolic pressure and systemic systolic pressure. The stenosis has been considered mild when right ventricular systolic pressure is less than half systemic systolic pressure, moderate when it is above half but less than systemic, and severe when it is greater than systemic systolic pressure. Although these criteria are reasonable in children, they may not be appropriate in infants, because the high right ventricular pressures noted with severe stenosis in older infants and children may not be developed in neonates. Also, significant tricuspid regurgitation or reduced cardiac output may limit the levels of right ventricular systolic pressures achieved, even with severe stenosis. Furthermore, as discussed below, the gradient may be markedly altered by changes in heart rate and systolic ejection time.

Therefore, it is probably more reliable to base the classification on valve orifice area in patients with valvar stenosis. Normally, the pulmonary valve orifice diameter is about 2.0 cm/m^2 body surface area and pulmonary valve area is about 2.5–3.0 cm^2/m^2. Experimentally, the pulmonary artery has to be constricted to less than one-third its diameter to produce a significant pressure gradient. Mild pulmonary stenosis can be considered to be present when the valve area is 0.75–1.0 cm^2/m^2 and valve diameter is 8–10 mm/m^2. Stenosis is severe when pulmonary valve area is less than 0.3 cm^2/m^2 or valve diameter is less than 3 mm/m^2. Values

Congenital Diseases of the Heart, 3rd edition. By A. Rudolph
© 2009 Blackwell Publishing, ISBN: 9781405162456

between these ranges are considered to represent moderate stenosis.

Morphological and embryological considerations

The mechanism of embryological development of pulmonary stenosis is not known. The pulmonary and aortic valve leaflets develop from endocardial cushions in the truncus arteriosus. If anomalous development of the cushions were responsible for pulmonary stenosis, it might be expected that aortic valve anomalies would be commonly associated. Although both aortic and pulmonary valvar stenosis may occur in the same individual, this is rare. Questions have been raised as to whether pulmonary stenosis is a true developmental anomaly, because in many instances the pulmonary valve cusps, the pulmonary valve annulus, and the sinuses of Valsalva and main pulmonary trunk are well formed. Only rarely is it possible to distinguish two or, on occasion, four cusps. Furthermore, in serial observations of human fetuses by ultrasound, progression of the stenosis from mild to moderate or severe has been observed in occasional fetuses [1]. It has been suggested that the pulmonary valve anomaly has developed after the ventricular septum has closed in the embryo and that pulmonary stenosis and atresia with intact ventricular septum is not a true embryological anomaly.

It has been proposed that pulmonary stenosis or atresia may be the result of fetal endocarditis, caused by either viral or other organisms. In the rubella syndrome, it is well known that the pulmonary arteries, the ductus arteriosus, and other vessels may be involved in an inflammatory and degenerative process when fetal infection occurs. In rubella vasculitis, the main pulmonary trunk and the left and right branches are affected most severely, and the pulmonary valve mechanism is usually involved only as an extension of the process. However, it is quite possible that other viruses or mycoplasma organisms may have a predilection for the pulmonary valve.

Pulmonary valve and artery

The pathology of the pulmonary valve varies greatly. In the mildest forms of pulmonary stenosis, there are three normal cusps with three well-defined raphae that are not complete, so that the leaflets are not able to open completely during systole. In more severe forms there is less clear separation of the leaflets and the cusps are thickened and immobile. There may be no separation into distinct cusps, and the pulmonary valve is formed from a thick tough membrane projecting convexly into the pulmonary artery with a small orifice a few millimeters in diameter. Although in older children the pulmonary valve annulus is usually normal or only slightly reduced in size, it is not uncommon to find variable degrees of annulus narrowing in infants; this is the usual finding in atresia of the pulmonary valve. The size of the annulus is an important consideration with regard to surgery. When the annulus is narrowed, the valve is often dysmorphic; it may be grossly deformed, being thick and immobile, without distinct cusps. However, in some instances, there may be a perfectly well-formed valve with three cusps and adherent raphae. The morphology also varies greatly with pulmonary atresia and appears to reflect the development of the right ventricle. In those infants in whom the right ventricle is very hypoplastic, the annulus is often narrow and the valve primitive in appearance with poor differentiation into cusps. In those with a well-developed right ventricle, the annulus is wider and there is a thickened but still pliable valve with raphae formation but no orifice. In infants under 3 months of age with severe pulmonary stenosis or atresia, the valve is often thickened and dysmorphic, with a myxomatous appearance.

The size of the pulmonary trunk beyond the stenosis varies greatly. In most children, the pulmonary trunk is considerably dilated and the dilatation often extends into the left pulmonary artery; in infants, the pulmonary artery may be dilated but is usually of fairly normal size. In infants with pulmonary atresia, the size of the pulmonary trunk varies; it may be small but is usually normal in size. In lambs in which the pulmonary trunk was banded, marked poststenotic dilatation of the pulmonary artery beyond the band sometimes developed. On occasion this extended into the branch pulmonary arteries, and sometimes into the ductus arteriosus.

Stenosis of the branches of the pulmonary artery or of the main pulmonary artery distal to the valve occurs most commonly in association with infundibular stenosis in tetralogy of Fallot or in infants in whom there was fetal infection with rubella. However, pulmonary branch stenosis may occur in the absence of any other lesions. Most commonly, the stenoses are bilateral and often multiple, affecting secondary and tertiary divisions of the pulmonary artery. Poststenotic dilatations beyond the obstructions are noted commonly; sometimes the poststenotic dilatation is marked and the dilated segment may compress airways.

In experimental pulmonary stenosis in fetal lambs, the pulmonary arterioles exhibit decreased thickness of the medial muscle layer [2]. This could be related to the change in oxygen saturation of blood perfusing the fetal pulmonary circulation (Chapter 5). It could be the result of decreased flow or alteration in pressure contour in the large pulmonary arteries (see Chapter 15). Similar changes have been noted in these vessels in neonatal infants with pulmonary atresia.

Right ventricle and tricuspid valve

The right ventricle may appear to be normal in patients with minor degrees of pulmonary stenosis. In moderate degrees of stenosis, the right ventricular myocardium as well as the septum and papillary muscles are diffusely hypertrophied. The trabeculation is increased, but the cavity is usually either normal or somewhat reduced in size. The ventricular septum often bulges into the left ventricle in patients with more severe degrees of stenosis. In some patients there is marked localized hypertrophy of the muscle in the infundibulum involving the crista supraventricularis and its parietal and septal bands. The marked degree of obstruction that this imposes during life in association with ventricular contraction may not be fully appreciated in the relaxed heart at autopsy. The tricuspid valve is usually normal in size and morphology. In patients who develop cardiac failure, an unusual event in infancy and early childhood but more common in adults, the right ventricle is enlarged, the tricuspid annulus diameter is increased, and tricuspid valve insufficiency is evident.

In infants with severe pulmonary stenosis, the right ventricular wall is also markedly thickened, and cavity size and the tricuspid valve orifice are usually normal. Hypertrophy of the outflow tract, with subvalvar obstruction in addition to the valvar stenosis, not infrequently develops with advancing age. It is important to recognize the presence of this subvalvar stenosis, because if it is not relieved at the time that the pulmonary valve is opened surgically, it may produce critical postoperative obstruction (see Chapter 15).

The size and morphology of the right ventricle vary considerably in patients with pulmonary atresia. In some infants, the right ventricle has a similar appearance to that in severe pulmonary stenosis. The wall is markedly hypertrophied, but the inlet, trabecular and infundibular portions are all developed. The tricuspid valve and orifice are also normal. This group has the best prognosis of all types of pulmonary atresia.

In about two-thirds of infants, the right ventricular cavity is small. In this group, either the inlet portion alone or the inlet and trabecular portions of the right ventricle have developed, but the outflow tract, or infundibulum, is not identifiable; this results in considerable separation between the cavity of the right ventricle and the pulmonary artery. This is an important consideration when treatment is aimed at establishing a communication from the ventricle to the pulmonary artery (see Chapter 15). The small ventricle is associated with a correspondingly small tricuspid valve orifice and a small pulmonary valve annulus with a thick valve. Frequently, the tricuspid valve leaflets are abnormally thickened and the chordae tendineae are short and stiff. The ventricular wall is markedly thickened. This thickening may be so severe that the infundibulum and even the trabecular portion of the ventricle have only a very narrow lumen. It is important to appreciate this, because if it is thought that only an inlet portion of the ventricle is present, the decision may be made to forgo an attempt to perform a two-ventricle repair (see Chapter 15).

In the remaining infants, all three portions of the right ventricle are developed (tripartite ventricle). The pulmonary valve usually has three cusps, but in infancy is thick and often myxomatous in appearance. Ventricular size is markedly increased; although the wall is not thickened, total muscle mass is increased. The size of the tricuspid valve orifice is greatly increased and the leaflets are abnormal, creating marked insufficiency. In some infants, the anterior leaflet is voluminous and sail-like; the septal leaflet may be displaced into the right ventricle, characteristic of Ebstein malformation. Although the proportion of individuals with pulmonary atresia with intact ventricular septum who have associated Ebstein malformation varies in different series, it appears to be 10–15%. This group has a particularly poor prognosis. In these patients, the right atrium is markedly enlarged and the wall of the inlet portion of the right ventricle is very thin, as in Ebstein anomaly. A patent foramen ovale or fossa ovalis defect in the atrial septum is present. In some of these infants, the large tricuspid valve leaflet may encroach on the infundibular region of the right ventricle and cause intraventricular obstruction. The leaflet may even create a complete obstructive membrane in the right ventricle and an opening in the membrane is the only communication from inlet to infundibular regions.

Some infants with severe tricuspid insufficiency, diagnosed as having pulmonary atresia based on both ultrasound and cardiac catheterization studies, are found either at surgery or autopsy to have normal pulmonary valves. This phenomenon of functional pulmonary atresia is discussed on p. 397.

The variations in the morphology of the right ventricle and the tricuspid valve are most important in decisions regarding surgical management of infants with pulmonary atresia. An important question is whether a hypoplastic ventricle and narrow tricuspid valve will accommodate a flow adequate to provide sufficient pulmonary blood flow. Various criteria have been used. Right ventricular volume in relation to body surface area has been calculated by ultrasound study, but because of the irregular shape of the ventricle these measurements are not reliable. Furthermore, as mentioned above, the marked hypertrophy of the ventricle may occlude the cavity and create an impression of severe hypoplasia. Recently, the sizes of the ventricle and tricuspid valve have been expressed as Z-scores or standard scores. This represents the number of standard deviations that an observed value is away from the mean:

$$Z\text{-score} = \frac{\text{Observed number} - \text{Mean}}{\text{Standard deviation}}$$

The mean values for ventricular size and tricuspid orifice diameter have been determined for different ages or body surface areas. A negative Z-score indicates that the observed value is smaller than the mean. The Z-score has been used by some pediatric cardiologists and cardiovascular surgeons to make decisions about surgical approach in patients with pulmonary atresia or severe stenosis (see Chapter 15).

The wide spectrum of morphological features of the pulmonary valve and right ventricle has yet to be explained. It could be related to the severity of the initial insult. Experimental studies in fetal lambs suggest that the period of gestation at which pulmonary valve obstruction is induced may be a factor in determining right ventricular and tricuspid valve development. The later in gestation the stenosis is induced, the better the development of the ventricle and valve, because they have already had the opportunity to grow to a reasonable size.

We produced pulmonary stenosis in a series of fetal lambs by banding the pulmonary artery at about 60 days' gestation (0.4 gestation) in an attempt to define the factors affecting ventricular growth [1]. At about 120 days' (0.8) gestation, many animals demonstrated marked reduction in right ventricular cavity size and tricuspid valve diameter. However, several lambs developed moderate enlargement of the right ventricle, with a large tricuspid orifice and apparent tricuspid insufficiency. Thus in the experimental model, we observed the same spectrum that has been reported in human infants. It is proposed that blood flow handled by the right ventricle is an important determinant of the size of its cavity. Obstruction to outflow of the right ventricle in the fetus interferes with filling, and superior vena cava (SVC) and inferior vena cava (IVC) blood will preferentially pass through the foramen ovale into the left atrium and ventricle. The volume of blood ejected by the right ventricle is greatly reduced and therefore the cavity does not develop normally. If the tricuspid valve becomes insufficient, the right ventricle ejects a greater volume of blood during systole; diastolic filling may be normal or increased, facilitating achievement of normal or increased ventricular size. In some of the lamb fetuses that developed severe tricuspid insufficiency, the right ventricle became greatly enlarged and the fetuses developed hydrops, suggesting the occurrence of cardiac failure. Pericardial effusion, indicating the onset of cardiac failure, has been reported in two human fetuses with severe pulmonary stenosis or atresia and large right ventricles [3]. Thus although pulmonary atresia alone does not appear to have an adverse effect on normal fetal development *in utero*, when associated with tricuspid regurgitation it is not well tolerated. No adequate explanation has been proposed regarding the development of tricuspid insufficiency in only some fetuses with pulmonary stenosis.

The tricuspid valve orifice is small when ventricular cavity size is reduced, but is normal or large with increased cavity size. Although it is likely that tricuspid valve is determined by ventricular growth, the concept that abnormal tricuspid valve development may be the primary anomaly and ventricular development a subsequent result cannot yet be discarded.

Left ventricle, aorta, and ductus arteriosus

The left side of the heart is usually normal in patients with mild or moderate pulmonary stenosis. In children with moderate to severe stenosis, the ventricular septum is displaced into the left ventricle and the cavity may be somewhat restricted. In infants with pulmonary atresia or severe pulmonary stenosis, the left ventricle is enlarged and myocardial mass is increased, because during fetal life all or most of the venous blood returning to the heart is directed through the foramen ovale into the left ventricle. Infants with pulmonary atresia have also been reported to show changes in left ventricular myocardial morphology suggesting ischemia and some also have increased collagen content, suggesting myocardial fibrosis. This could be related to the coronary vascular anomalies occurring in many of these individuals (see Chapter 15).

The ascending aorta is wider than normal in infants with pulmonary atresia. In those with a hypoplastic right ventricle, the aortic isthmus does not show the usual reduction in diameter compared with the ascending or descending aorta. In this group the ductus arteriosus is narrow and arises from the descending aorta at an acute inferior angle (see Chapter 5). In those with a normal or large right ventricle, the aorta and ductus arteriosus are usually normal.

Myocardial morphology

During fetal life, normal myocardial growth is achieved almost exclusively by increase in numbers of myocytes or *hyperplasia* (see Chapter 1). Recent studies by Jonker *et al.* [4] indicate that, in later gestation (beyond about 120 days in fetal lambs), some increase in myocyte size and maturation of some cells becomes evident. Postnatally, myocardial muscle mass increases largely by increase in myocyte size, or *hypertrophy*, with negligible hyperplasia. Increased pressure loading of the heart in the adult results in an increase in muscle mass, which is accomplished almost exclusively by hypertrophy, with minimal increase in cell numbers. Everett *et al.* [5] produced pulmonary stenosis in adult dogs and found a marked increase in protein synthesis with an increased mass of the right ventricular wall, suggesting that hypertrophy was induced.

In fetal lambs in which we simulated pulmonary stenosis by banding the main pulmonary artery at 60 days' gestation, right ventricular wall thickness and muscle mass had doubled by 120 days. Myocyte diameter did not increase, indicating that the abnormal growth of the right ventricular myocardium was accomplished exclusively by hyperplasia. However, Barbera *et al.* [6] noted that simulation of pulmonary stenosis in fetal lambs induced some enlargement as well as increased maturation of right ventricular myocytes, as evidenced by an increase in the number of binucleate cells. Whereas we induced pulmonary stenosis at 60 days' gestation, Barbera *et al.* induced it in late gestation. Thus it appears that the increase in right ventricular muscle mass induced by pulmonary stenosis in earlier gestation, when normal growth is exclusively by hyperplasia, is accomplished by exaggeration of the normal hyperplastic process, with no increase in differentiation. However, in later gestation, when some differentiation and increase in myocyte size has begun to appear normally, induction of pulmonary stenosis may enhance the differentiation of muscle cells. In association with the increased volume load presented to the left ventricle, its muscle mass also increased modestly. Although this was also largely due to hyperplasia in our studies in early-gestation fetuses, there was a small increase in myocyte diameter. This suggests that myocardial growth responses may differ with pressure versus volume loading.

Of considerable interest were the observations on myocardial capillaries. The number of capillaries per unit area in the section of myocardium was considerably reduced in the right ventricles of the lambs with pulmonary stenosis. Because myocyte diameter did not change significantly, this indicated that the ratio of capillaries to myocytes fell. Furthermore, capillary diameters were increased in the right ventricular myocardium, suggesting that capillaries had dilated to maintain adequate myocardial blood flow. Similar but less marked changes in capillary development were observed in the left ventricular myocardium. These findings of relatively reduced coronary capillary numbers in the right ventricular myocardium are of considerable interest, because disturbances in coronary vascular development have been observed in infants with pulmonary atresia and severe stenosis. They may explain the presence of areas of myocardial ischemia that have been reported in some infants with severe pulmonary stenosis.

These observations in fetal lambs are important because it has been suggested that the left ventricular myocardium may not be normal in some patients with pulmonary valve obstruction. Thus Akiba and Becker [7] noted left ventricular hypertrophy with evidence of ischemia and increased collagen content in hearts with pulmonary atresia with intact ventricular septum. Abnormalities of both right and left ventricular myocardium, as well as of coronary arteries, were also noted histologically by Beçu *et al.* [8] in patients with pulmonary stenosis.

Hemodynamic considerations

Fetal circulation

Acute pulmonary artery obstruction

In the normal fetal lamb, the right ventricle ejects about 66% of the combined ventricular output (CVO) into the pulmonary artery and about 55–60% of CVO passes through the ductus arteriosus to the descending aorta. Acute compression of the pulmonary trunk results in a decrease in stroke volume of the right ventricle and, associated with diversion of blood through the foramen ovale, an increase in left ventricular stroke volume. In studies we performed in fetal lambs, acute constriction of the pulmonary artery resulted in a considerably greater fall in CVO compared with constriction of the ascending aorta. In the fetus the right ventricle appears to be more sensitive to an increase in afterload than the left ventricle and thus its output falls to a greater degree. With mild to moderate degrees of compression, the CVO is maintained. The proportion of descending aortic blood flow derived through the ductus arteriosus is decreased, but a greater proportion is derived across the aortic isthmus. More severe obstruction results in a marked reduction of right ventricular output, blood flow to the lungs, and flow through the ductus arteriosus to the descending aorta. Although there is an increase in left ventricular output, it is not adequate to compensate and CVO falls. Umbilical–placental blood flow also falls and progressive fetal hypoxemia supervenes. Right ventricular systolic pressure increases from resting levels of about 60 mmHg to about 80 mmHg at 75 days' gestation, and from resting values of 70–80 mmHg to 100–110 mmHg at 120 days' gestation.

Chronic pulmonary artery obstruction

When the stenosis develops more gradually the right ventricle undergoes hyperplasia, the degree depending on the severity of the stenosis. If mild, the changes in fetal circulation may be insignificant. With moderate degrees of stenosis, the increase in right ventricular mass may be capable of maintaining a normal output. When pulmonary stenosis is severe, there is a marked decrease in right ventricular output. In experimental pulmonary stenosis in fetal lambs, right ventricular pressures are only 10–40 mmHg higher than left ventricular pressures. This is related to the reduction in stroke volume, with a greater residual volume and thus higher end-diastolic pressure. Right ventricular compliance may also be reduced by the increased wall thickness associated with increased muscle mass; a greater diastolic filling pressure will be required to maintain diastolic volume. However, increase in right atrial pressure is limited because the foramen ovale acts as a relief from the right to the left atrium. Progressive stenosis results in further decreases in right ventricular filling and output. Because blood is diverted through the foramen ovale to the left atrium and ventricle, left ventricular output increases. Unlike with acute obstruction to right ventricular outflow, slowly developing pulmonary stenosis allows the left ventricle to undergo hyperplasia and thus provide an increase in left ventricular output to compensate fully or almost completely for the fall in right ventricular output in order to maintain a relatively normal CVO. Because CVO is well maintained, umbilical–placental blood flow would be relatively normal and fetal growth and development is not disturbed.

Blood flow patterns

Normally, in the sheep fetus, about 25% of CVO, or about 125 mL/min per kg, traverses the foramen ovale to enter the left atrium. In the fetus with pulmonary atresia, only pulmonary venous return does not have to flow through the foramen ovale. All the blood returning to the heart from the SVC and IVC and the coronary sinus must cross the foramen ovale to reach the systemic and pulmonary circulation (Figure 15.1). In the sheep fetus, this represents about 90% of CVO, or about 450 mL/min per kg. The foramen ovale is thus quite large to accommodate this markedly increased flow. Venous inflow into the left atrium and ventricle is thus increased and flow through the ascending aorta is increased. Normally, left ventricular output and ascending aortic blood flow constitutes about 33% of CVO in the lamb and about 45% in the human fetus. In the fetus with pulmonary atresia,

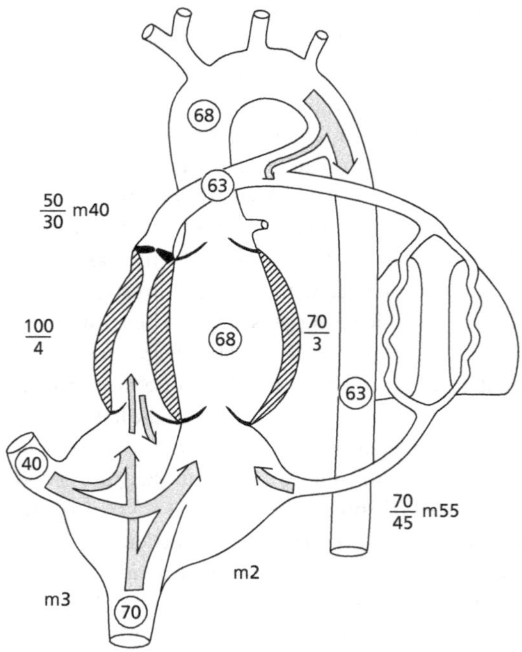

Figure 15.1 Pulmonary atresia in a fetus: course of the circulation, oxygen saturations (circled), and pressures. m, mean pressure.

the left ventricle has to eject the total cardiac output, so that the ascending aorta will carry two to three times its usual flow. The aortic isthmus normally conducts a flow of about 10% of CVO, but in pulmonary atresia all the blood distributed to the lower body, including the placenta, and to the lungs passes across the isthmus. In those fetuses in which pulmonary atresia has been present from early in gestation, in contrast with the normal infant in whom the isthmus is only about 0.7 of descending aortic diameter, the isthmus is as wide as the rest of the aorta (see Chapter 12). The pressure in the pulmonary arteries in fetuses with pulmonary atresia is determined largely by the size of the ductus arteriosus, but could also be influenced by pulmonary vascular resistance. If the ductus has a normal diameter, pressure in the pulmonary artery would be similar to that in the aorta and pulmonary blood flow will be determined by pulmonary vascular resistance. The main factor that would modify pulmonary vascular resistance is oxygen saturation of pulmonary arterial blood (see Chapter 15). If the ductus diameter is decreased, pulmonary arterial and aortic pressures could separate. Unless pulmonary vascular resistance increased markedly, pulmonary arterial pressure would be lower than aortic pressure. This lower pulmonary arterial pressure could contribute to the lesser development of smooth muscle in the media of the pulmonary arterioles (see Chapter 15). It is also possible that even if pulmonary arterial pressure was normal for the fetus, exposure of the pulmonary arterioles to a higher than normal oxygen saturation could explain the reduced smooth muscle development.

When the stenosis is not complete, the effects are related to the severity of the obstruction and to gestational development. If obstruction is severe, the circulation will be altered in a manner similar to that noted in atresia. However, because some blood is ejected by the right ventricle, the chamber is usually reasonably well developed (Figure 15.2). In our studies of experimental pulmonary stenosis in fetal lambs, we noted that right ventricular systolic arterial pressure may increase to 80–110 mmHg whereas systemic arterial pressure is normal at about 70 mmHg near term. The pulmonary trunk beyond the obstruction often developed marked poststenotic dilatation. Pulmonary arterial pressure would be similar to aortic pressure if the

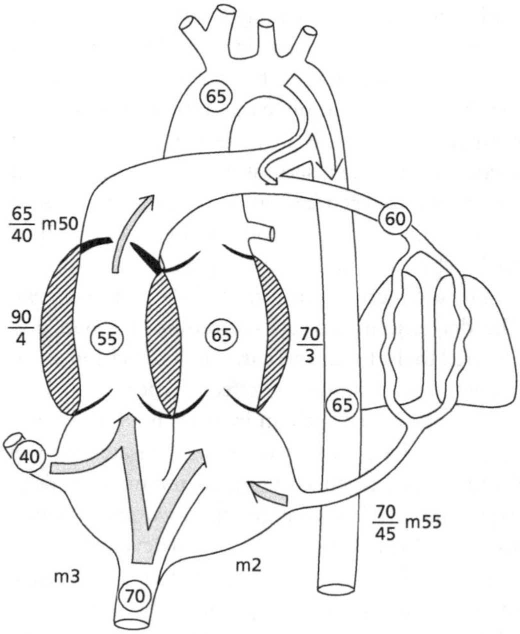

Figure 15.2 Severe pulmonary stenosis in a fetus: course of the circulation, oxygen saturations (circled), and pressures. The right ventricular cavity is larger than in the fetus with pulmonary atresia and the pulmonary artery is dilated. m, mean pressure.

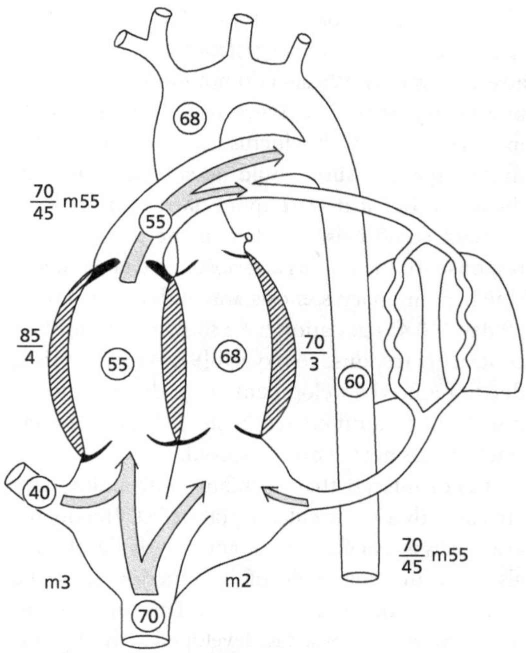

Figure 15.3 Mild pulmonary stenosis in a fetus: course of the circulation, oxygen saturations (circled), and pressures do not differ greatly from the normal. m, mean pressure.

ductus arteriosus is, as is usual, normally developed. However, a small ductus could affect pulmonary arterial pressure and pulmonary vascular development as in pulmonary atresia.

If the stenosis is mild, the effects on fetal circulation will be less dramatic. There may be some decrease in right ventricular output and therefore some reduction in flow across the ductus arteriosus, with some compensatory increase in left ventricular output and aortic isthmus flow (Figure 15.3). Right ventricular muscle and cavity size will probably be normal.

Ductus arteriosus

In the fetus with pulmonary atresia, the ductus arteriosus provides blood flow to the fetal lung. Unlike in the normal fetus in which a major proportion of right ventricular output passes through the ductus to the descending aorta, with pulmonary atresia only pulmonary blood flow passes through the ductus from the aorta to the pulmonary arteries. This represents only about 8–10% of CVO in the fetal lamb and about 20% of CVO in the human fetus. In infants with pulmonary atresia and intact ventricular septum, the size of the ductus arteriosus and its junction with the descending aorta vary. It may be relatively normally developed in diameter and wall thickness, and connect to the aorta at the normal oblique inferior angle. In some patients with a very small right ventricle, the diameter of the ductus is decreased and it joins the descending aorta at an acute inferior angle. This could reflect the stage during gestation that the pulmonary valve becomes obstructed. If the atresia develops during late gestation, blood would normally flow through the ductus from the pulmonary artery to the aorta prior to the onset of pulmonary valve occlusion. However, if it occurs early in gestation, blood flow through the ductus would be reversed and also reduced, causing the ductus to decrease in size and join the aorta at an acute inferior angle.

The reduced blood flow through the ductus arteriosus could also influence the development of the ductus smooth muscle, but we have no information about the morphology of the ductus arteriosus related to the time during gestation that pulmonary atresia develops. We also do not know the level of pulmonary arterial pressure in fetuses with pulmonary atresia. If the ductus arteriosus were relatively large, pressure would be similar to that in the aorta, but if it were quite narrow, a pressure gradient could exist. Studies of the physiological responses of the ductus arteriosus in fetal lambs in which pulmonary stenosis was induced at about 70 days' (0.45) gestation have shown a diminished contractile response to oxygen [9]. Whether this is due to reduced development of the ductus smooth muscle or to a difference in smooth muscle contractility has not yet been resolved.

It is of interest that in infants with pulmonary atresia with a ventricular septal defect, the ductus arteriosus is usually narrow and poorly developed; also, the inferior angle of its junction with the descending aorta is usually acute. This suggests that the pulmonary atresia had developed early in gestation and points to different etiological mechanisms for development of atresia in pulmonary atresia with ventricular septal defect and pulmonary atresia with intact ventricular septum. It also appears that there is a functional difference. The ductus arteriosus appears to remain patent for a longer period after birth, usually several weeks, in infants with pulmonary atresia with ventricular septal defect compared to those with pulmonary atresia with intact ventricular septum, in whom it is usually open for only a few days. However, in some infants with pulmonary atresia with intact ventricular septum, the ductus is patent for many weeks. It would be interesting to correlate the time of closure with size of the ductus and the inferior angle of its junction with the aorta. Thus the narrower ductus may have less smooth muscle development with less contractility and remain patent longer.

Blood oxygen saturation

In the fetus with pulmonary atresia, blood returning from the SVC and IVC streams will mix completely in the left atrium, so oxygen saturations in blood distributed to the ascending and descending aortae, and also to the pulmonary circulation, will be similar (see Figure 15.1). Oxygen saturation of blood entering the ascending aorta will be lower than normal, whereas that in blood distributed to the lower body and the lungs would be higher than normal. Although the changes would not be large, their potential influence has not been assessed. In the sheep fetus, complete admixture of all venous returns would result in a decrease in ascending aortic blood oxygen saturation from about 65% to about 55%. Oxygen saturation of descending aortic blood would increase from about 52% to about 55%, whereas pulmonary arterial oxygen saturation would increase from about 50% to about 55%. The decrease in oxygen saturation of blood distributed to the brain and coronary circulation is not likely to have a significant effect. Hypoxemia in the fetus is associated with an increase in cerebral and coronary blood flow, which compensates for the decrease in oxygen content, to maintain normal oxygen supply. The changes in flow would be small and probably not influence normal development.

The fetal pulmonary circulation is sensitive to small changes in Po_2, particularly as gestation advances (see Chapter 5). In the fetus with pulmonary atresia, the higher oxygen saturation in blood perfusing the lungs could reduce constriction of the arterioles and limit the development of the medial muscle layer (see Chapter 5). As mentioned on p. 388, both in experimental pulmonary stenosis in fetal lambs and in human infants with pulmonary atresia, the smooth muscle layer in the media of the small pulmonary arteries (30–50 μm diameter) is thinner than normal. Whether this is related to a higher oxygen saturation, or to other factors, has not been resolved. Altered development of the pulmonary circulation could have an important influence on postnatal circulatory changes, resulting in a more rapid decrease in pulmonary vascular resistance than occurs normally.

Ventricular–coronary artery communications (coronary sinusoids) and coronary arteries

An interesting finding in many infants with pulmonary atresia with intact ventricular septum is the presence of communications between the right ventricular chamber and coronary arteries by means of large sinusoidal connections. These connections may be to the right or left anterior descending coronary arteries, and rarely to the left circumflex branch. Ventricular–coronary artery communications are not encountered in infants who have either normal or enlarged right ventricles, but are common when the ventricle is hypoplastic, particularly when only the inlet portion has developed. It appears that they are most likely to occur when pulmonary atresia develops early in gestation. The coronary circulation first develops in the embryonic myocardium as an isolated plexus of vessels; communications first develop to the ventricular cavity and only later do coronary arteries develop and connect with the aorta. It is suggested that when pulmonary atresia develops before the coronary arterial connection to the aorta has developed, the high pressure in the right ventricle maintains flow into the sinusoids to the coronary arteries and maintains their patency with subsequent enlargement.

The patterns of blood flow in the sinusoids are of considerable interest. If they connect with the coronary arterial system, it might be anticipated that flow would tend to occur from the high-pressure right ventricle into the sinusoids during systole, thus providing blood with venous oxygen saturations to the coronary circulation. However, during diastole, pressure in the right ventricle would be low and this could result in blood flowing preferentially from the coronary arteries to the right ventricular cavity, rather than perfusing the left ventricular myocardium. This has been referred to as *coronary artery steal*. A concern is that if there is a large anastomosis of sinusoids to coronary arteries, reduction of right ventricular pressure may interfere with systolic perfusion of the coronary arterial system, with resultant left ventricular failure. The concept of coronary artery steal has prompted some centers to eliminate the abnormal flow pattern by occluding the tricuspid valve and thrombosing the right ventricle to occlude the entry of the sinusoids into it. However, some question remains as to the clinical importance of coronary artery steal in patients with pulmonary atresia.

A more significant problem is the association of abnormal connections or stenoses of the coronary arteries. Stenoses frequently occur in the coronary arteries in the region of the ventricular–coronary artery communications; multiple sites of stenosis may be present. The left or right coronary artery may have no connection to the aorta, and perfusion is provided exclusively from the sinusoid connecting to it from the right ventricle. Perfusion of the myocardium supplied by this artery will be dependent on the pressure generated by the right ventricle, so that any attempt to reduce the pressure by opening the pulmonary outflow could result in onset of myocardial hypoperfusion with reduced performance and possibly infarction. However, if there are collateral anastomoses from other coronary arteries, adequate myocardial blood flow could be provided even though right ventricular pressure is reduced. Thus, even if it is determined that a portion of myocardium appears to be perfused from the right ventricle, it is possible that opening the right ventricular outflow tract will have no adverse effect. It has been suggested that if multiple sites of coronary artery stenosis are demonstrable on angiography, reducing right ventricular pressure may not be tolerated. This could be explained by the inability of collateral coronary arteries to develop. An important question to consider is how effectively the pressure in the right ventricle can perfuse the coronary circulation. During systole, when right ventricular pressure is high, the ventricles are contracting and intramyocardial pressure would be high, so that coronary perfusion would be limited. During diastole, when most coronary blood flow occurs, right ventricular pressure is low and therefore ineffective in providing much flow.

Inadequate perfusion of the myocardium could occur during fetal life if myocardial perfusion is provided exclusively by the ventricular–coronary artery anastomoses, but may be limited because flow would occur only during systole, when ventricular pressure is high. This may account for the subendocardial fibroelastosis and areas of myocardial ischemia and fibrosis that have been reported in association with pulmonary atresia.

In addition to the influences of the ventricular–coronary artery communications on coronary blood flow, they are also associated with morphological changes in the large as well as the intramural arteries. Intimal hyperplasia with smooth muscle cell migration is prominent, resulting in endothelial prominence and medial thickening; this may result in considerable narrowing of the lumen. These changes are probably caused by the stress on the vessels due to the high systolic pressure of the right ventricle. These changes are similar to those observed in the coronary arteries in patients with supravalvar aortic stenosis, in whom the coronary arteries are also subjected to very high pressures.

Circulatory adjustments after birth

The course of the circulation after birth depends on the severity of the pulmonary stenosis, the degree of development of the right ventricle, and tricuspid valve function.

Pulmonary atresia and severe pulmonary stenosis

When there is no communication or only a very small opening between the right ventricle and the pulmonary artery, the establishment of adequate pulmonary blood flow postnatally depends almost entirely on the diameter of the ductus arteriosus (Figure 15.4). The venous blood returning to the heart enters the right atrium. There may be some flow into the right ventricle and if there is a small opening in the pulmonary valve, a small amount may enter the pulmonary artery. With complete atresia, the right ventricular blood usually returns to the right atrium through an insufficient tricuspid valve. In infants in whom coronary sinusoids are well developed, blood will be ejected into them during systole and enter the coronary arteries (see Chapter 15). When the tricuspid valve annulus is small, there is often also immobility of the valve leaflets with a combination of stenosis and insufficiency. In these infants, the right ventricular cavity is invariably quite small and the volume of blood that enters the ventricle and ejected back into the atrium is quite small; the circulation is very similar to that in tricuspid atresia (see Chapter 16). When the tricuspid valve orifice is large there is free regurgitation from the right ventricle to the right atrium during systole; in view of the greater volume entering the right ventricle, its cavity is considerably larger.

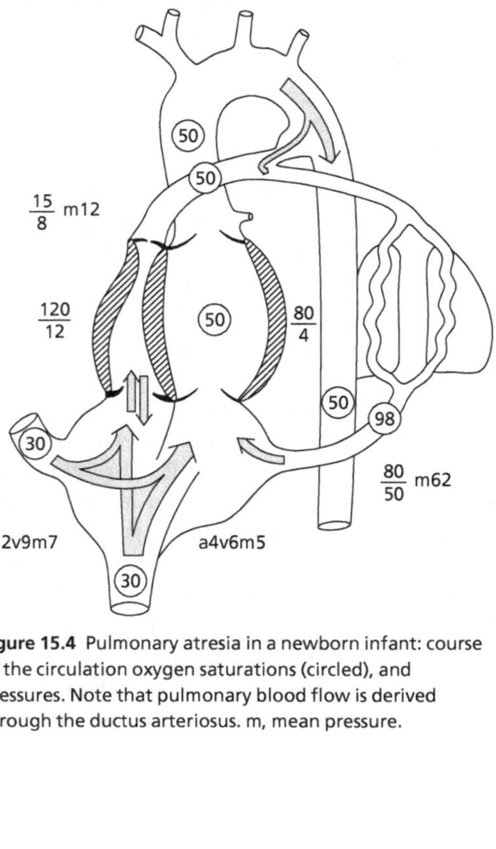

Figure 15.4 Pulmonary atresia in a newborn infant: course of the circulation oxygen saturations (circled), and pressures. Note that pulmonary blood flow is derived through the ductus arteriosus. m, mean pressure.

Whatever occurs at the tricuspid valve level, eventually all systemic venous blood crosses the atrial septum through the foramen ovale or a fossa ovalis defect. Much discussion has arisen as to the adequacy of the size of the foramen ovale in permitting the total venous return to enter the left atrium and it has been suggested that in some infants the foramen may be too small. It is most unlikely that this is a problem in the neonatal period. Before birth, the foramen ovale is large enough to carry the total systemic venous return as well as umbilical venous return. After birth, removal of umbilical venous return would produce a reduction of about 40% of the flow that is conducted prenatally in the lamb and of about 30% in the human fetus. However, difficulty may arise after pulmonary blood flow has been established and pulmonary venous return to the left atrium is increased. While pulmonary blood flow is low, there will be no interference with flow from the right atrium. If pulmonary blood flow increases, left atrial filling will be greater and this will increase left atrial pressure, thus tending to close the foramen ovale, and right atrial pressure would have to be increased to maintain flow of systemic venous return to the left atrium.

The magnitude of pulmonary blood flow is determined by the size of the ductus arteriosus. Since there is complete admixture of pulmonary and systemic blood flows in the left atrium, the systemic arterial oxygen saturation is determined by the pulmonary to systemic flow ratio (see Chapter 4). If the ductus arteriosus is patent, the pulmonary to systemic flow ratio will be higher and arterial oxygen saturation may be high enough to permit adequate oxygen supply to the tissues. However, when the ductus constricts, pulmonary blood flow falls and arterial oxygen saturation will decrease, producing all the consequences of hypoxemia; if the hypoxemia is severe, tissue hypoxia will ensue (see Chapter 3). The behavior of the ductus arteriosus is therefore very important in determining the clinical features in these infants.

As mentioned on p. 394, the constrictor response of the ductus to oxygen is reduced in fetal lambs with induced pulmonary stenosis. However, a delicate balance between ductus constriction, pulmonary blood flow, and systemic arterial Po_2 develops after birth. If the ductus is widely patent, this could permit a large pulmonary flow and a rise in arterial Po_2. If Po_2 rose to levels above about 40 mmHg, the ductus would begin to constrict, pulmonary blood flow would be reduced, and arterial Po_2 would drop, resulting in relaxation of the ductus. It is interesting that in those babies with pulmonary atresia who do survive for several days or weeks, the arterial Po_2 is usually in the range 35–40 mmHg. It is not known whether it is related to this physiological balance or whether it is due to poor development of the ductus, so that it cannot accommodate a higher flow. It has been suggested that administration of oxygen to infants with pulmonary atresia may be inadvisable, as it may tend to constrict the ductus arteriosus and decrease pulmonary blood flow. However, this is not a serious risk in the infant with markedly reduced arterial Po_2. Since pulmonary flow is quite low there would be only a small additional amount of oxygen taken up in the lungs, about 1.5 mL/dL of pulmonary blood flow; this represents the additional oxygen that will be physically dissolved when 100% oxygen is administered (see Chapter 3). The lower the pulmonary blood flow, the less the total additional oxygen that can be taken up and thus the less the benefit. It is unfortunate that administration of oxygen is least effective in those infants who have the most severe degrees of hypoxia because their pulmonary blood flow is so low. Even the small additional amount of oxygen will provide some benefit, but it is unlikely that the Po_2 will be raised enough to affect the ductus arteriosus.

The majority of infants with pulmonary atresia have small right ventricles and present within a few days after birth with increasing hypoxemia related to the decrease in pulmonary blood flow associated with ductus arteriosus constriction. The tricuspid valve annulus is small and thus inflow into the ventricle is limited. Right ventricular pressure is increased to varying degrees, often exceeding systemic arterial pressure. The blood that enters the right ventricle is either regurgitated into the atrium or passes through the ventricular–coronary artery communications during systole. Much of it returns to the right atrium through the sinusoids during diastole, or traverses the coronary circulation and coronary sinus to the right atrium. If the coronary arteries are atretic or stenosed on the aortic side of the anastomosis with the sinusoids, perfusion of some or all of the coronary circulation will be dependent on a high right ventricular pressure. Even though right ventricular pressure is maintained at high levels, coronary perfusion may be inadequate. Although some myocardial blood flow occurs during ventricular systole, most flow occurs during diastole, when the ventricles are relaxed. If the right ventricle were responsible for perfusion, myocardial blood flow would occur only during systole because, during diastole, the pressure would be too low to provide perfusion. Disturbances in myocardial blood flow may be responsible for the areas of myocardial infarction and fibrosis frequently encountered in these infants, as well as for the reduced cardiac output and peripheral circulation they sometimes manifest.

In infants with normal or large right ventricles, significant tricuspid regurgitation is usually associated and an Ebstein anomaly of the tricuspid valve is frequently present. The right atrium is also enlarged and right atrial pressure is increased with a prominent *v* wave. Right ventricular systolic pressure does not usually exceed systemic arterial pressure because the insufficiency of the valve does not permit development of higher pressures. When tricuspid regurgitation is severe, pressure in the right ventricle is frequently lower than that in the left ventricle or aorta; if the ductus arteriosus is widely patent, pulmonary arterial pressure may exceed right ventricular pressure. The enlarged right ventricle may produce septal displacement into the left ventricular cavity, thus interfering with left ventricular filling and output. This, combined with tricuspid regurgitation, may seriously compromise systemic blood flow and result in shock. In the infant with severe pulmonary stenosis or atresia, in whom pulmonary blood flow is dependent on the ductus arteriosus, the decrease in systemic arterial pressure may interfere with ductus flow and thus aggravate the hypoxemia.

Moderate to severe pulmonary stenosis

The hemodynamic changes associated with moderate stenosis are depicted in Figure 15.5. When the valve orifice is large enough to permit an adequate pulmonary flow after birth, closure of the ductus arteriosus is of no consequence. Not uncommonly, cyanosis is not evident in the infant with severe stenosis in the neonatal period, because the ductus arteriosus permits augmentation of pulmonary blood flow. After it closes within a few days, cyanosis may become manifest; this results from the increase in right-to-left shunt associated with the decrease in pulmonary venous return to the left atrium, with a lowering of left atrial pressure. This shunt may increase considerably with crying or as the infant becomes more active.

Right ventricular systolic pressure does not fall normally but is maintained at or somewhat above fetal levels. The pressure is determined by the degree of stenosis, but in the neonatal period it rarely exceeds about 120 mmHg. The increased afterload on the right ventricle may interfere with emptying during systole. In addition, the thickened wall of the right ventricle may reduce its compliance and result in increased right atrial pressure, with a high *a* wave. Beyond the neonatal period, right ventricular pressure increases in association with increased demands for pulmonary blood flow and closure of the ductus arteriosus (Figure 15.6).

Changes with growth

The course beyond the neonatal period is related to the severity of the stenosis and the increased requirements for cardiac output associated with increase in body size and activity. With growth after birth there is an increase in body oxygen requirements and an increase in cardiac output related to body surface area. The cross-sectional area of the pulmonary valve is about 2.0 cm^2/m^2 body surface area; the orifice of the normal pulmonary valve increases in proportion to surface area from infancy to adulthood. The growth of the orifice of

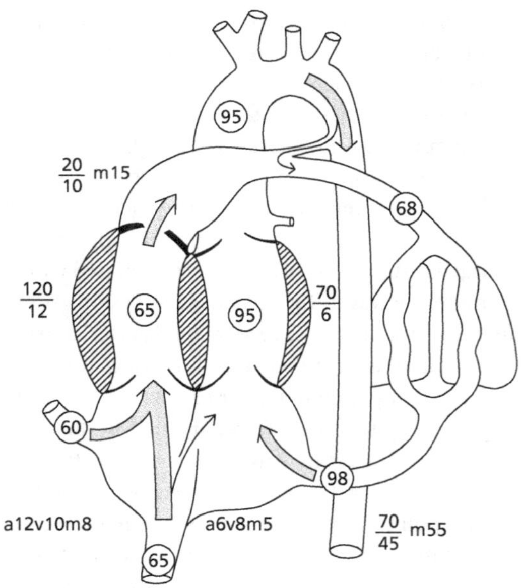

Figure 15.5 Severe pulmonary stenosis in a newborn infant: course of the circulation, oxygen saturations (circled), and pressures. The right ventricle is hypertrophied and maintains a normal output. m, mean pressure.

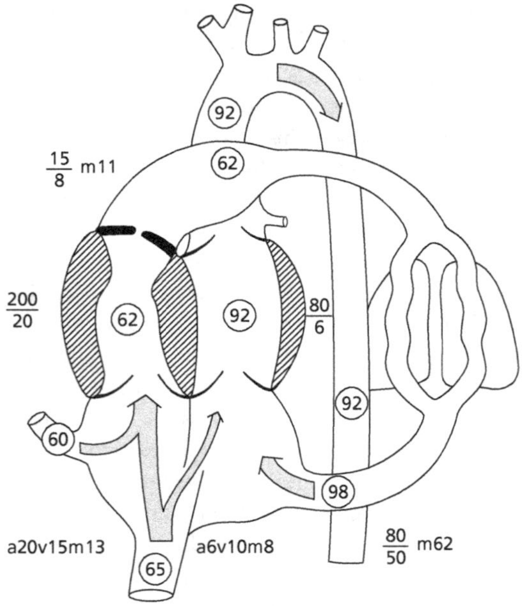

Figure 15.6 Severe pulmonary stenosis in an older infant: course of the circulation, oxygen saturations (circled), and pressures. Right ventricular pressure is markedly increased, end-diastolic pressure is very high, and early failure is present. m, mean pressure.

the pulmonary valve varies in children with pulmonary stenosis. In some, particularly with milder degrees of stenosis, the valve orifice increases in proportion with body surface area and little change is required in right ventricular pressure to maintain flow across the valve at rest. However, changes in heart rate with age may influence this. However, if the valve orifice does not enlarge relative to the increase in cardiac output, a higher right ventricular pressure would be required to effect the same flow if other factors, such as heart rate, did not change.

Gorlin and Gorlin have shown that flow across a stenosed pulmonary valve is related to the square root of the mean systolic pressure difference across it (see Chapter 4).

$$A = \frac{\dot{Q}}{44.5\sqrt{\Delta P}} \text{ or}$$

$$A \times 44.5\sqrt{\Delta P} = \dot{Q}$$

$\dot{Q}$ (flow) varies as the square root of ΔP. Thus if valve area, A, does not change and mean systolic flow, $\dot{Q}$ increases by a factor of 2, the mean pressure gradient across the valve will increase by a factor of 4; a threefold rise in blood flow would be associated with a ninefold increase in the mean pressure gradient across the valve. The effects of modifying flow on right ventricular pressure in the presence of a fixed pulmonary stenosis are shown graphically in Figure 15.7.

During postnatal development, several changes occur that are important in determining the right ventricular pressure required to maintain flow across the stenosed valve. Cardiac output increases from about 1.0 L/min after birth to about 5.0 L/min in adolescence (see Chapter 2). However, since heart rate drops from a postnatal level of 120–140/min to about 70/min, the stroke volume increases by about tenfold. Using the equation above, I have calculated the mean pressure difference required to produce flows ranging from 1 to 5 L/min across pulmonary valves with four assumed orifice areas of 0.1, 0.2, 0.3, and 0.5 cm^2, equivalent to orifice diameters of 3.6, 5.1, 6.1, and 7.7 mm, respectively. In making these calculations, I have used a value of 25 s/min for the systolic ejection period and assumed that it did not change with the increase in total cardiac output. Figure 15.7 shows

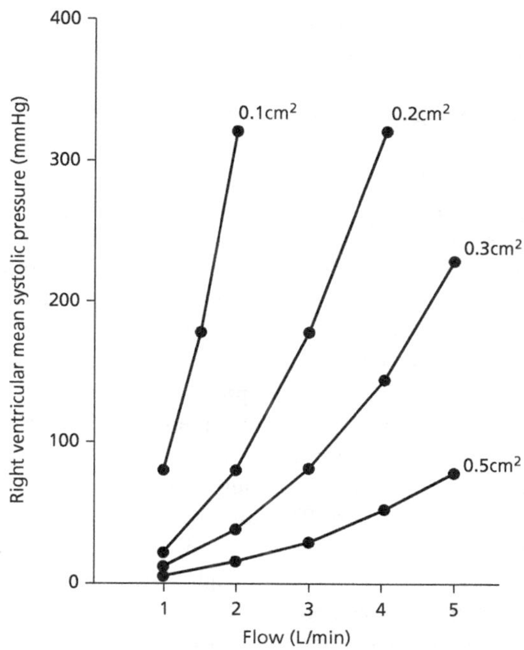

Figure 15.7 Relationship between mean right ventricular systolic pressure and flow across a stenotic pulmonary valve for orifice sizes of 0.1, 0.2, 0.3, and 0.5 cm^2. This has been calculated using the Gorlin and Gorlin formula as described in the text.

the mean pressure difference required to produce varying flows through the different valve orifices.

The pulmonary valve area is normally about 2.0 cm^2/m^2 body surface area. Thus, at birth, the orifice has an area of about 0.5 cm^2 and there is no gradient or a negligible gradient across it. If the valve did not undergo normal growth but remained the same size as at birth, it can be seen from Figure 15.7 that the mean pressure difference across the valve in adolescence would be about 78 mmHg. If the valve diameter were 1.6 mm less, with an area of 0.3 cm^2 at birth, there would be only a small gradient of 9 mmHg at birth. However, if the valve area did not change with age, a mean pressure difference of 233 mmHg would be required to produce a flow of 5 L/min. With marked stenosis and a valve area of 0.1 cm^2 the pressure gradient at birth would be 81 mmHg, and excessively high levels would have to be accomplished to produce a flow of only 2 L/min.

The levels of pressure presented in Figure 15.7 are mean pressure differences; peak right ventricular systolic pressures would be much higher. In infants under the age of about 6 months, peak right ventricular systolic pressures greater than 150–200 mmHg are unusual, but in older children and adults pressures may reach 250–300 mmHg. I have encountered an adolescent patient with a pressure of 320 mmHg. It is not known why higher pressures cannot be achieved. It could be related to several factors, including a limit to the degree of myocardial hypertrophy, inability to maintain coronary blood flow to sustain greater myocardial work, and an architecture of the right ventricle that is unable to generate higher pressures.

Certain changes in the dynamics of ventricular contraction with advancing age are advantageous in achieving an adequate output at a lower right ventricular pressure. The duration of systolic ejection increases with age. This is not related to the decrease in heart rate, although systolic ejection time increases as heart rate decreases. However, even at the same heart rates, systolic ejection time is greater in older children than in infants. At a heart rate of 100/min, for example, systolic ejection time is about 240 ms in a 2-year-old child but 320 ms in a 12-year-old child, so that systolic ejection periods are 24 and 32 s/min respectively. Although at first glance this would not appear to be of particular importance, a simple calculation indicates that it can have a striking effect on right ventricular pressure. Assuming a pulmonary valve area of 0.3 cm^2 and a cardiac output 4 L/min, mean systolic flow would be 4000/24 = 167 mL/s if the systolic ejection period is 24 s/min and 4000/32 = 125 mL/s if the systolic ejection period is 32 s/min. If these figures are now applied to the Gorlin formula (see Chapter 4), when systolic ejection is 240 ms

$$\sqrt{\Delta P} = \frac{167}{44.5 \times 0.3} = 12.5 \text{ and } \Delta P = 156 \text{ mmHg}$$

When systolic ejection time is 320 ms

$$\sqrt{\Delta P} = \frac{125}{44.5 \times 0.3} = 9.4 \text{ and } \Delta P = 88 \text{ mmHg}$$

Thus it is evident that the longer systolic ejection time associated with growth could provide a great advantage by allowing higher flows at lower peak systolic pressures in the right ventricle.

Because resting heart rate is higher in the young infant than in the child, the resting systolic ejection periods (heart rate × systolic ejection time) are similar. Thus, in a 1-year-old infant with a heart rate of 120/min and an ejection time of 186 ms, the systolic ejection period is 22.3 s/min. In a 12-year-old child with a heart rate of 85/min and an ejection time of 270 ms, the systolic ejection period is 23.0 s/min.

Coronary blood flow

Since the increased right ventricular pressures developed in patients with pulmonary stenosis require increased energy utilization, coronary blood flow is an important consideration in providing adequate oxygen and substrate supply to the myocardium. Normally, the myocardial blood flow to the left ventricle occurs mainly during diastole and is negligible during systole when left ventricular pressure equals aortic pressure. In view of the pressure gradient from the inner to the outer layers of the ventricle during systole, some flow may occur to the outer myocardium. The right ventricular myocardium normally receives flow throughout the cardiac cycle, since aortic pressure always exceeds right ventricular pressure.

In the presence of pulmonary stenosis, the systolic flow to the right ventricular myocardium will be reduced, and the higher the right ventricular pressure, the less the systolic flow. Since intramyocardial pressure is greater in the inner layers, there would be a more severe interference with flow to the subendothelial layers. The chronic reduction in flow to the subendothelial myocardium could result in the develoment of subendocardial fibrosis of the right ventricle in older patients with moderate to severe pulmonary stenosis.

Effect of exercise

When an individual exercises there is increased oxygen utilization and increased demand on the circulation to provide a greater oxygen supply. In the normal individual, this is accomplished by increasing cardiac output, partly by increasing stroke volume but largely by increasing heart rate. If the increase in cardiac output is inadequate, there is also increased oxygen extraction by the tissues, so that mixed venous oxygen saturation falls and arteriovenous oxygen difference increases.

In the patient with pulmonary stenosis, the ability of the right ventricle to increase stroke volume is limited by the high afterload placed on it by the obstruction. The increase in heart rate will achieve an increase in cardiac output if stroke volume is maintained. However, because systolic ejection time decreases as heart rate increases, right ventricular systolic pressure would have to increase in order to eject the same stroke volume at the higher heart rate. The more severe the stenosis, the greater the increase in right ventricular pressure.

Associated with the increased heart rate, the diastolic filling time of the ventricle will be reduced because even though systolic ejection time is decreased, the total time for diastole is reduced. This would have two potentially deleterious effects. First, if right ventricular compliance is reduced because of severe hypertrophy and possibly fibrosis, right ventricular filling would be impaired and this could interfere with maintenance of stroke volume. A compensatory increase in right atrial contraction with a large *a* wave would help to maintain adequate filling. Second, because myocardial blood flow occurs only during diastole when pulmonary stenosis is severe, a reduction in diastolic filling time could interfere with myocardial blood flow and thus with the ability of the right ventricle to increase its systolic pressure. This would limit the ability of the ventricle to maintain stroke volume at higher heart rates and thus the main adjustment to exercise will be an increased arteriovenous oxygen difference.

Effect of arrhythmias

Arrhythmias producing either marked bradycardia or marked tachycardia are poorly tolerated in patients with pulmonary stenosis. When heart rate falls, it is necessary to increase stroke volume in order to maintain cardiac output. When severe pulmonary stenosis is present, stroke volume cannot be increased adequately because of the high afterload on the right ventricle, even though right ventricular systolic pressure is increased.

When supraventricular tachycardia develops, right ventricular filling time is decreased and synchronous contraction of the atrium and ventricle is also lost, thus further disturbing ventricular filling. These events result in a decrease in cardiac output, a reduction in aortic pressure and coronary blood flow, and thus impairment of right ventricular function.

Changes in valve orifice

Several studies have shown that right ventricular systolic pressure increases with growth in some individuals. The more dramatic increases have been noted during the period of infancy, usually in babies with moderately severe stenosis, with pressure gradients across the valve greater than 50 mmHg [10,11]. I have observed an infant in whom right ventricular pressure was 80–90 mmHg 2 days after birth but which increased to 210 mmHg at 13 months. Beyond infancy, less dramatic changes have been recorded. Beyond infancy, pressure gradients below about 40 mmHg do not usually increase with age [12]. When pressure gradients are greater than 50 mmHg in early childhood, the pressure gradient tends to increase and calculated valve area to decrease, relative to body surface area. It is difficult to assess whether right ventricular pressure has increased as a result of inadequate growth of the valve orifice, because changes in heart rate and cardiac output have to be considered.

One of the difficulties in evaluating possible changes in orifice size relates to the development of muscle hypertrophy of the right ventricular outflow tract, which may produce secondary obstruction. It is difficult to distinguish between the amount of stenosis imposed by the valve itself and by the hypertrophied infundibulum. The factors influencing the development of infundibular hypertrophy are not known, nor is the time course of its occurrence. Little or no hypertrophy occurs in some individuals but others develop very marked changes. The more severe degrees of infundibular hypertrophy are usually observed in patients with marked valvar stenosis. There may be diffuse narrowing of a long length of the infundibulum but usually there is a more localized area, involving the crista supraventricularis with its parietal and septal bands. The infundibular stenosis is dynamic in nature, being manifest primarily during ventricular systole, when the subvalvar region may narrow to an extreme degree; however, during diastole a wide channel is evident.

Some patients with moderate degrees of stenosis show no change in right ventricular systolic pressure over many years of observation, suggesting that the valve orifice is increasing commensurate with the rise in cardiac output. The course of individuals with very high ventricular pressures is quite variable. Some patients have been known to maintain systolic pressures over 150 mmHg for years without developing any symptoms, but in others cardiac failure develops. Right ventricular end-diastolic pressure and right atrial *a* wave are increased in patients with marked pulmonary stenosis, presumably because a higher pressure is required to fill the thick-walled right ventricle. With the onset of failure, these pressures increase further, and venous congestion with hepatomegaly occurs. Once right ventricular failure is manifest it progresses rapidly, because right ventricular output and thus systemic output are decreased and this places coronary perfusion in jeopardy. When cardiac failure develops, right ventricular systolic pressure falls, interfering with flow into the pulmonary and systemic circulation; this causes a fall in systemic pressure, further affecting coronary flow and right ventricular performance and resulting in progressive deterioration.

The failure of the right ventricle may be related to the inability of the right ventricular myocardium to maintain an adequate cardiac output when progressive right ventricular obstruction occurs. An additional factor that could contribute to the production of cardiac failure is the development of myocardial fibrosis. Although it has been proposed that this may occur in older children and particularly in adults, there is no reliable documentation of its occurrence. The fibrosis would not only affect systolic performance of the ventricle but would almost certainly decrease ventricular compliance and filling, particularly if the heart rate is increased.

In a number of patients with moderately severe stenosis, the foramen ovale may remain patent beyond infancy and childhood. Frequently, no cyanosis is evident in infancy or early childhood, but if right ventricular systolic pressure increases with growth, the end-diastolic pressure in the ventricle and the right atrial *a* wave also become elevated. Right-to-left shunting can then occur through the foramen ovale, particularly during atrial systole. The cyanosis may occur first during exercise, due to a decrease in systemic vascular resistance and an increase in systemic venous return to the right atrium, which will result in an increase in right ventricular end-diastolic pressure since right ventricular emptying is restricted.

Mild pulmonary stenosis

Mild pulmonary stenosis may be associated with a small pressure difference of only 5–30 mmHg across the pulmonary valve. The slight elevation in right ventricular systolic pressure does not appear to interfere with normal right ventricular function. In the newborn period, only a small pressure difference across the pulmonary valve may occur (Figure 15.8), but with growth it may increase somewhat. The right ventricle shows little or no hypertrophy, but poststenotic dilatation of the pulmonary artery usually occurs (Figure 15.9). Idiopathic dilatation of the pulmonary artery, which was thought to occur independently of associated lesions, could be related to the presence of mild pulmonary valve stenosis with poststenotic dilatation.

There are numerous reports of individuals with mild pulmonary stenosis who have survived to late adult life with no evidence of any serious hemodynamic or clinical disturbance. However, some have questioned whether persistent slight elevation in right ventricular pressure may, over many years, cause fibrosis of the right ventricular myocardium, resulting in cardiac failure in the fourth or fifth decade. It is difficult to assess whether this is due

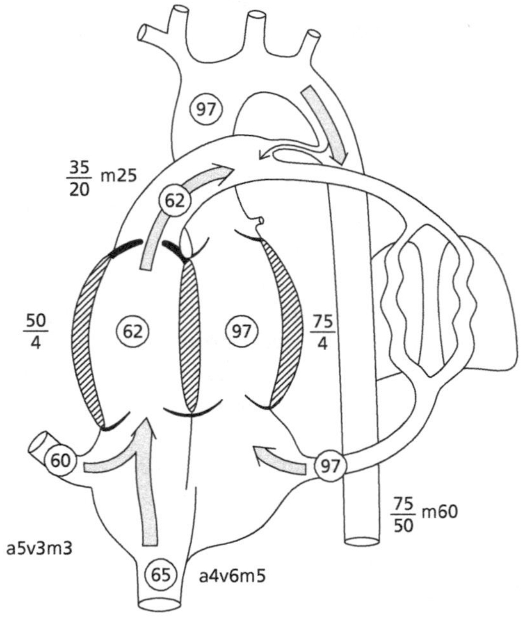

Figure 15.8 Mild pulmonary stenosis in a newborn infant: course of the circulation, oxygen saturations (circled), and pressures. m, mean pressure.

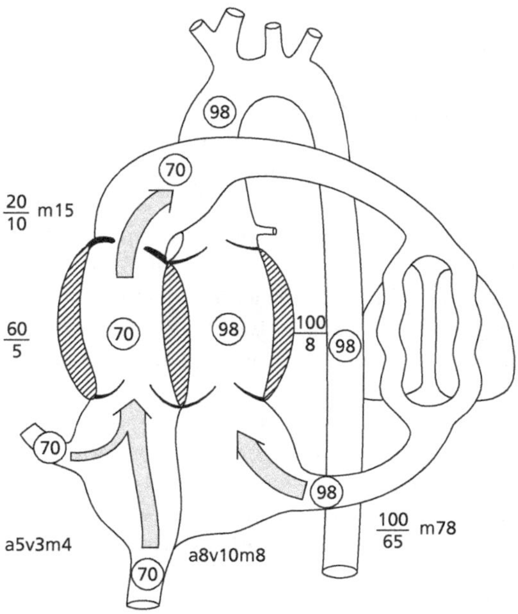

Figure 15.9 Mild pulmonary stenosis in a child: course of the circulation, oxygen saturations (circled), and pressures indicate that there is little effect on cardiovascular dynamics. m, mean pressure.

to the pulmonary stenosis or to coronary artery disease.

Clinical features

The onset of symptoms in patients with pulmonary stenosis and atresia is related to the severity of the obstruction. Infants with pulmonary atresia or severe pulmonary stenosis may present with serious difficulties within 24–48 hours after birth but patients with mild stenosis may never have symptoms. The clinical features are also markedly affected by the presence of tricuspid regurgitation.

Pulmonary atresia and severe pulmonary stenosis

Neonatal period

Infants with pulmonary atresia or severe stenosis are usually normal and well developed at birth. Cyanosis may be present at birth, but even with pulmonary atresia it may be mild, because pulmonary blood flow is provided by the ductus arteriosus. Cyanosis may increase progressively during the first 7–10 days, but may suddenly become severe if the ductus closes rapidly. Apart from the cyanosis, the baby is usually asymptomatic. Only when hypoxemia is severe, with arterial Po_2 usually below 25 mmHg and arterial oxygen saturation below 45%, do symptoms occur. Metabolic acidemia develops due to tissue hypoxemia and increased anaerobic glycolysis. Stimulation of carotid chemoreceptors causes tachypnea, but particularly hyperpnea. With progressive acidemia, pallor due to peripheral vasoconstriction ensues and the skin becomes mottled and cold. Urgent treatment of the hypoxia is indicated (see Chapter 15).

In infants with little or no tricuspid insufficiency, the precordial impulse is not hyperactive and it is thus difficult to assess whether the right or left ventricle is prominent. In the presence of tricuspid insufficiency, the cardiac impulse is hyperactive over the whole precordium. The first heart sound is usually normal, but may be soft if tricuspid regurgitation is present. In infants with pulmonary atresia, the second sound is not heard or is soft at the upper left sternal border, but may be normal in intensity and single at the lower left sternal border (due to aortic valve closure). In infants with severe pulmonary stenosis, the second sound in the pulmonary area is of low intensity but may be widely split. A prominent atrial or fourth sound may also be heard at the mid-left sternal border in infants with severe stenosis, and also in those who have associated Ebstein malformation.

In infants with pulmonary atresia, ejection murmurs are not audible at the upper left sternal border, but a systolic murmur of grade 2–3/6 intensity and blowing in character may be heard over the lower portion of the sternum, probably due to the presence of tricuspid regurgitation. A medium-frequency continuous murmur may be present at the upper left sternal border due to flow from aorta to pulmonary artery through a narrow patent ductus arteriosus, but this is unusual. In infants with severe pulmonary stenosis, a systolic ejection murmur may be heard at the upper left sternal border. The murmur is of variable duration, sometimes occupying about two-thirds of systole and occasionally the whole of systole. It may appear to extend into diastole, because it extends beyond the second sound. This is explained by the fact that only the aortic component of the second sound is heard and the murmur extends to the end of right ventricular systole, but the pulmonary component of the second sound is inaudible. The absence of an ejection murmur does not exclude the possibility that stenosis rather than atresia is present. Blood flow through the valve may be so reduced that no murmur is audible. Systolic ejection clicks are not heard in infants with pulmonary atresia, but are occasionally heard at the lower left sternal border in infants with severe stenosis.

In infants with tricuspid regurgitation, no ejection murmur is usually audible over the upper left sternal border, but a decrescendo medium-frequency systolic murmur is heard at the lower left sternal border, with radiation to the right side of the sternum.

The main presenting feature in the newborn period is hypoxemia; cardiac failure does not occur in infants with normal or small right ventricles. In infants with marked tricuspid regurgitation, in addition to the hypoxemia, hepatomegaly, weak pulses, pallor, and mottling are common. Generally, the prognosis is poor in these infants.

Child and adult

With less severe stenosis, the infant may be asymptomatic. If the foramen ovale remains patent, cyanosis may be evident with crying. With growth, cyanosis, not present at rest, may appear with exercise. The age at which cyanosis appears varies considerably: 10–20% have cyanosis at or soon after birth, 30–40% develop cyanosis within a year, and 60–70% manifest cyanosis by about 5 years of age. Individuals who have cyanosis also develop limitation of exercise tolerance; this becomes progressively more severe as cyanosis increases with age. However, unlike patients with tetralogy of Fallot, these individuals rarely squat with exertion (see Chapter 14).

If the foramen ovale closes, cyanosis does not occur. No symptoms are usually evident during childhood, even with stenosis severe enough to induce pressures greater than 200 mmHg. Although some limitation of exercise may be noted, many patients have no exercise intolerance. There is little information regarding the clinical course of patients with severe pulmonary stenosis beyond childhood. It has generally been assumed that the right ventricular myocardium develops progressive fibrosis and that increasing limitation with eventual cardiac failure will occur, but this has not been well documented. Some adults with severe pulmonary stenosis have been observed to develop cardiac failure, and this has been the basis for relieving the stenosis at an early age.

In the patient who does not have cardiac failure, the heart is not clinically enlarged but there is a prominent right ventricular impulse at the lower right sternal border. Because there is no volume overload on the right ventricle, the impulse is tapping rather than heaving. No chest deformity is evident. In older children a prominent *a* wave may be noted in the jugular pulse. The arterial pulses are normal. A systolic thrill is often palpable at the upper left sternal border.

The first heart sound is usually normal but may be moderately accentuated at the lower left sternal border. A systolic ejection click is frequently heard along the left sternal border. The ejection click tends to be louder in patients with less severe degrees of stenosis; in those with severe stenosis with a thick immobile valve, a click may not be heard. The disappearance of an ejection click over several months or years may indicate the development of secondary infundibular stenosis. The time interval between the first heart sound and the ejection click or between the Q wave of the electrocardiogram and the ejection click has been shown to be related to the severity of pulmonary valve stenosis. The interval tends to be shorter with more severe degrees of stenosis.

The aortic component of the second heart sound is usually normal but the intensity of the second, or pulmonary, component is decreased. The loudness of the pulmonary sound is related to the severity of the stenosis; it is absent, or very soft, in severe stenosis. The second sound is also split more widely than normal in patients with pulmonary stenosis, and the width of splitting of the sound is related to the severity of the stenosis. In severe stenosis, the second sound is very widely split, but this may not be appreciated because the pulmonary component may be so soft that it is difficult to hear, particularly in the presence of the loud murmur.

A systolic murmur of ejection or crescendo–decrescendo configuration and grade 4–6/6 intensity is heard at the upper left sternal border; it radiates to the left infraclavicular area, the suprasternal region, and often both lung fields. The loudness of the murmur does not correlate well with the severity of the stenosis, but usually the peak intensity of the murmur occurs later in the systolic cycle with more severe degrees of stenosis. Because right ventricular ejection is prolonged when stenosis is severe, the systolic murmur may extend beyond the aortic second sound. This may give the impression that there is an early diastolic murmur at the upper left sternal border, but the murmur does not extend beyond the pulmonary component of the second sound.

Mild and moderate pulmonary stenosis

Patients with mild or moderate degrees of pulmonary stenosis do not manifest symptoms. They usually have normal exercise tolerance during childhood, but with moderate stenosis and a patent foramen ovale mild cyanosis may appear with exertion and exercise tolerance may be limited. This progresses with age. As with severe stenosis, it has been assumed that moderate stenosis may induce right ventricular myocardial fibrosis over years, and that cardiac failure may develop in adult life. As mentioned above, there is little documentation of this with severe stenosis, and even less with mild and moderate stenosis.

The clinical findings are similar in infants and children. The heart is not clinically enlarged. An increased right ventricular impulse may be palpated at the lower left sternal border and a systolic thrill may be detected at the upper left sternal border. The first sound is normal. The second sound is normal with mild stenosis, but the second component may be delayed and soft with moderate stenosis. A systolic ejection click is commonly heard along the left sternal border in children and adults, but is less frequently noted in infants. A systolic crescendo–decrescendo murmur of grade 3–5/6 intensity is heard maximally at the upper left sternal border. The murmur radiates to the infraclavicular area and may be transmitted to the right chest.

Investigations

Electrocardiography

The electrocardiographic findings vary depending on the severity of the pulmonary stenosis and the size of the right ventricle. With mild pulmonary stenosis, the electrocardiogram may be normal, although frequently there is delayed right ventricular conduction, with an rsr′ pattern in the right precordial leads, with no increase in voltage. More severe stenosis is associated with right axis deviation to 90–150° and right ventricular hypertrophy. The P waves in limb leads II and III, aVR, and the right precordial leads may be peaked and the amplitude may be increased slightly.

In infants with severe stenosis, the T waves in the right precordial leads are upright, reflecting right ventricular hypertrophy, but in children and adults the T waves are often deeply inverted in these leads. It has been suggested that this reflects myocardial ischemia, but there is no reliable evidence supporting this concept. R-wave amplitude in V4R and V1 is increased to 10–35 mm. In children and adolescents in whom there is an R wave with minimal S wave in the right precordial leads, the level of right ventricular systolic pressure is roughly correlated with the amplitude of the R wave. When the electrocardiogram is calibrated so that 1 mV equals 10 mm of deflection, multiplying the R-wave amplitude in millimeters by 5 provides an estimate of right ventricular systolic pressure. Thus an R wave of 15 mm indicates a right ventricular systolic pressure of 75 mmHg. This relationship may not be applicable in infants or adults. The S wave in the left precordial leads is often prominent. When Ebstein malformation is associated with pulmonary atresia, right ventricular conduction is delayed, but the amplitude of the R wave is not usually greatly increased.

In infants with pulmonary atresia, the electrocardiographic changes are related to the size of the right ventricle. With a large ventricle, the changes are similar to those seen with severe stenosis. If the ventricle is markedly hypoplastic, the electrical axis is often 0–30° and may be slightly negative. The right precordial R waves may be markedly increased in infants with large right ventricles, but may be in the normal range for neonates. In infants with pulmonary atresia with small right ventricles, there may be dominance of left forces with small or absent R waves in the right precordial leads. The degrees of axis deviation and right ventricular hypertrophy are not reliable indicators of the size of the right ventricle.

Chest radiography

Radiographic changes are influenced by the severity of the lesion and age. In infants with pulmonary atresia or severe stenosis and a large right ventricle, the cardiac shadow is large; the right atrium may be prominent and the right ventricle enlarged. In those with a hypoplastic ventricle, the heart is not enlarged and occasionally appears to be small. The pulmonary artery segment is not prominent in infants with atresia, but may show mild post-stenotic dilatation in those with severe stenosis. Pulmonary vascular markings are determined by the patency of the ductus arteriosus. While the ductus is open, pulmonary vascular markings appear to be normal or slightly reduced, but they become reduced when the ductus constricts.

Infants with mild or moderate stenosis have hearts of normal size, but with more severe stenosis the right ventricle may be prominent. Poststenotic dilatation of the main pulmonary artery may be noted in infants, but it is usually mild in degree. Children and adults with mild or moderate stenosis also have hearts of normal size, but right ventricular prominence may be evident. Poststenotic dilatation of the main pulmonary artery is a prominent feature; it is not related to severity of the stenosis. Some patients with small pressure gradients of 10–15 mmHg across the valve may have marked poststenotic dilatation. In adolescents and adults with severe stenosis, the heart may demonstrate enlargement, with right ventricular prominence. This probably represents the onset of right ventricular failure.

Echocardiography

Ultrasound has greatly facilitated the diagnosis, as well as the assessment of severity, of pulmonary stenosis. It has been invaluable in differentiating the various congenital cardiac lesions causing cyanosis in the newborn infant. The combined use of two-dimensional echocardiography and color flow Doppler ultrasound has made it possible to evaluate most of the features necessary for making decisions about management of infants with severe pulmonary stenosis or atresia.

Infant with cyanosis

The morphology of the pulmonary valve should be assessed to determine whether the valve is membranous and domes during systole, or if it is thickened, dysplastic and immobile; whether there is any flow through the valve from the right ventricle; and the diameter of the valve annulus. In neonates the valve is frequently myxomatous and thickened and the annulus may be small, especially when the ventricle is monopartite. The right ventricle should be assessed to determine its size and whether it is tripartite, bipartite, or monopartite. The degree of separation between the right ventricular cavity and the pulmonary valve should be examined. The size of the tricuspid valve should be measured and the presence and magnitude of insufficiency assessed. In addition, the morphology of the valve should be defined to exclude the presence of Ebstein malformation.

Ventricular–coronary communications connecting with the right ventricular cavity can be identified. Although it has been noted that blood in the sinusoids flows away from the right ventricle during systole, it has not usually been possible to assess whether there is constriction or obstruction of distal coronary arteries, and thus whether coronary flow is right ventricular dependent. It is therefore still necessary to perform angiography to define coronary blood flow patterns more precisely.

The pressure in the right ventricle can be assessed from the velocity of a tricuspid valve insufficiency jet. Right-to-left flow across the foramen ovale and left-to-right shunt through the ductus arteriosus should also be assessed by color flow Doppler study. The position of the atrial septum may be helpful in deciding whether to perform balloon atrial septostomy. If the septum shows significant bulging into the left atrium, it is likely that the foramen ovale is somewhat restrictive. If it is decided to introduce an aortopulmonary arterial shunt, left atrial pressure could increase sufficiently to further restrict flow from the right to the left atrium and result in right-sided congestion. A balloon atrial septostomy would therefore be indicated prior to introducing the shunt.

The diagnosis of pulmonary atresia may be made inappropriately under circumstances when right ventricular function is poor and the ductus arteriosus widely patent. The pressure in the pulmonary artery is raised by the open ductus, and the right ventricle is not capable of generating a pressure high enough to open the valve. Therefore no flow through the valve is recorded in Doppler study of the right ventricular outflow or pulmonary artery. It is important to recognize the occurrence of functional pulmonary atresia in some infants with Ebstein malformation, because morphological pulmonary atresia is occasionally associated with Ebstein malformation. The possibility of functional atresia should be considered when the pulmonary valve is thin and membranous and is flat during systole, rather than doming into the pulmonary artery.

Older infant and child

Before the use of Doppler techniques for assessing blood flow patterns, M-mode and even two-dimensional echocardiography were not always totally reliable in diagnosing pulmonary stenosis. Normally, the pulmonary valve leaflets are thin and during systole are not visible because they are flattened against the wall of the pulmonary artery. In the presence of stenosis, the pulmonary valve leaflets do not open fully and are visible in systole, showing doming into the pulmonary artery. With mild stenosis, the valve motion may not be restricted greatly and the presence of stenosis may not be appreciated; also, the pulmonary valve leaflets are not always well visualized. For these reasons, in the past, pulmonary stenosis was not recognized in almost 25% of patients with pulmonary stenosis. With better imaging and the use of Doppler techniques, the diagnosis is now made routinely.

Although the pulmonary valve leaflets are frequently thick and immobile in newborn infants, in older infants and children they are usually membranous but sometimes quite thick. Very thickened dysplastic pulmonary valves may be observed in those patients with Noonan syndrome who have pulmonary stenosis.

The size of the right ventricle should be determined and its wall thickness measured to assess right ventricular pressure, as an indication of the degree of hypertrophy and severity of stenosis. The right ventricular cavity should be examined for evidence of abnormal muscle bands and for the presence of muscle hypertrophy causing stenosis in the outflow tract. The size of the pulmonary artery should be determined, but the degree of post-stenotic dilatation is not a useful index of the severity of stenosis. Mild stenosis may be associated with marked dilation of the pulmonary artery and, particularly in infants, little dilation may occur with severe stenosis.

Doppler ultrasound has greatly enhanced the evaluation of patients with pulmonary stenosis. Applying the Bernoulli equation, it is possible to estimate the pressure gradient across the valve from the flow velocity recording. The relationship of pressure gradient (P) to peak flow velocity is expressed by the equation P (mmHg) $= 4V^2$, where V represents peak velocity (m/s). Although the pressure gradients estimated by this method compare favorably with those measured by catheterization techniques, they tend to be somewhat higher. This is related to the fact that peak velocity measured by Doppler techniques occurs early in systole and provides an instantaneous measure of the pressure gradient at that moment. However, the pressure gradient measured by catheter techniques is the difference between the peaks of pressure, which occur later in systole and not usually simultaneously. The differences in transvalvar pressure gradients measured by the two techniques are relatively small in patients with pulmonary stenosis, but are greater in those with aortic stenosis. It should be appreciated that the Doppler technique cannot be applied to measuring the pressure gradient reliably if stenosis of the subvalvar region is present.

Ventricular–coronary artery communications can be identified by ultrasound techniques. Blood can be seen to flow from the ventricular cavity into large sinusoids, but it is not possible to obtain precise information about myocardial perfusion or about the presence of stenoses or other anomalies in the smaller arteries. It is therefore necessary to perform cardiac catheterization and angiography to define coronary blood flow patterns and coronary artery stenoses.

Cardiac catheterization and angiocardiography

General considerations

Cardiac catheterization and angiocardiography were essential for confirming the diagnosis of pulmonary atresia in the cyanotic newborn infant and for defining the size of the right ventricle, tricuspid valve, pulmonary valve annulus, and pulmonary arteries. It was also important in defining the distance between the right ventricular cavity and the pulmonary artery. In older infants and children, cardiac catheterization was the only method for accurately determining the severity of pulmonary stenosis. Since the introduction of ultrasound techniques, the morphological features of the right ventricle, tricuspid valve, and pulmonary valve and arteries can be defined, and the right ventricular pressure and gradient across the pulmonary valve estimated, so that the indications for catheterization have changed. If it is planned to perform a systemic-to-pulmonary artery shunt in the cyanotic newborn infant, catheterization is not indicated. The main indications for catheterization and angiography currently are to define the presence of ventricular–coronary communications, delineate the pattern of coronary blood flow, and perform therapeutic procedures to relieve obstruction.

Pulmonary atresia and severe pulmonary stenosis in infants

Catheterization was performed as an emergency in the cyanotic infant before the availability of prostaglandin (PG)E_1. It is now advisable to delay the procedure and administer PGE_1 to improve oxygenation and relieve metabolic acidemia. The infant should be placed in an optimal environmental temperature, and glucose administered to correct hypoglycemia.

Approach and catheter manipulation

From the groin approach, the catheter is passed through the IVC to the right atrium. Often the catheter passes preferentially across the foramen ovale into the left atrium. It may be difficult to maneuver the catheter through the tricuspid valve into the right ventricle, particularly when the ventricle is hypoplastic or when there is marked tricuspid regurgitation. The cardiac rhythm should be carefully monitored during manipulations to enter the right ventricle because serious cardiac arrhythmias, predominantly supraventricular tachycardias, may result. These are especially likely to occur if there is associated Ebstein malformation. However, entering the right ventricle is desirable, particularly in the infant with a small right ventricle, because ventricular–coronary communications are likely to be present and it is important that flow patterns be determined. An angiogram should be performed in the right ventricle to confirm the ultrasound assessment of its size and the distance from the cavity to the region of the pulmonary valve. If it is evident that the ventricle has no infundibular region, no attempts should be made to pass the catheter to the pulmonary valve. If the ventricle is tripartite, an attempt can be made to place the catheter just beneath the valve, where an angiogram with a small amount of contrast material can be done to determine whether the valve is atretic or severely stenosed.

Prior to the availability of PGE_1 there was considerable risk in passing the catheter across a severely stenotic pulmonary valve, because even the small area occupied by the catheter was sufficient to accentuate the obstruction and induce rapidly progressive hypoxemia. Providing pulmonary blood flow by dilating the ductus arteriosus has overcome this risk.

A catheter can be passed across the foramen ovale into the left atrium and left ventricle. The pulmonary arteries will fill from flow through the ductus arteriosus when an angiogram is performed in this site, and the position of the valve in relation to the right ventricular cavity will be further defined. However, it is important to perform an angiogram in the ascending aorta to define the left and right coronary arteries. This can be accomplished by manipulating a flow-directed (balloon) catheter passed from the vein, through the left ventricle, and across the aortic valve. The balloon is inflated to occlude the ascending aorta; injection of contrast medium proximal to the balloon provides excellent filling of the coronary vessels. Simultaneous injections of contrast medium into the right ventricle and the aorta close to the ductus arteriosus have been recommended to provide precise information about the degree of separation of the right ventricular cavity from the pulmonary artery. If it is not possible to pass the venous catheter into the aorta, a retrograde arterial catheter should be passed into the aorta either via the umbilical artery or from the femoral artery. Prior to the use of PGE_1, passing the arterial catheter across the ductus arteriosus was contraindicated, because the ductus could possibly be stimulated to constrict and thus limit pulmonary blood flow. Even with the use of PGE_1, it is probably not advisable to attempt to manipulate the catheter through the ductus; entering the pulmonary artery does not provide additional useful information in these infants.

Oxygen saturation and partial pressure

The SVC, IVC, right atrial, and right ventricular oxygen saturations are similar and decreased. Levels below 30% are quite common when systemic arterial oxygen saturation is very low. Oxygen saturations in the left atrium, left ventricle, and aorta also are similar, although there may be small differences between left atrial and left ventricular oxygen saturations due to streaming of pulmonary venous blood and blood shunted through the foramen ovale in the left atrium. Pulmonary venous oxygen saturation is high, usually above 95%; if the infant is receiving oxygen, it is 100%. Pulmonary venous blood gases reflect the decrease in pulmonary blood flow. When the infant is breathing air, pulmonary venous $P\text{O}_2$ is often above 100 mmHg, sometimes reaching 110–115 mmHg. Pulmonary venous $P\text{CO}_2$ is reduced to 15–20 mmHg and pH raised to 7.45–7.48. These blood gas values are related to the relative hyperventilation associated with reduced pulmonary blood flow but normal or increased alveolar ventilation (see Chapter 4).

Systemic arterial $P\text{CO}_2$ is usually normal or slightly decreased, sometimes to 30–35 mmHg. This is related to reduced carbon dioxide production if hypoxia is severe (see Chapter 3). Arterial pH may be normal if oxygenation is adequate, but is reduced, sometimes to below 7.0, if hypoxemia is severe. The levels of arterial oxygen saturation and $P\text{O}_2$ are determined by the magnitude of pulmonary blood flow; a $P\text{O}_2$ of 20–25 mmHg is not unusual.

With complete pulmonary atresia, the oxygen saturation in pulmonary arterial blood is similar to systemic arterial oxygen saturation; this is helpful in calculation of flows and shunts.

Blood flows and shunts

Systemic blood flow is normal or increased in most infants with pulmonary atresia or severe pulmonary stenosis, whereas pulmonary blood flow is reduced considerably, sometimes to as low as 0.5 L/min per m^2. Infants who have marked tricuspid regurgitation often have low systemic blood flows. Calculation of systemic blood flow by the Fick method is usually possible, but there may be difficulty in calculating pulmonary blood flow. If samples cannot be obtained, pulmonary venous oxygen saturation will have to be assumed, because there is right-to-left shunting at the atrial level. Oxygen saturation in the pulmonary artery is the same as that in the aorta if pulmonary atresia is present. However, with severe pulmonary stenosis, it is difficult to estimate pulmonary arterial oxygen saturation, because the contribution from flows through the pulmonary valve and the ductus arteriosus varies. Passing the catheter distally into the left or right pulmonary artery may not provide a mixed pulmonary arterial blood sample, because blood flowing through the ductus may be distributed preferentially to the left pulmonary artery.

In infants with pulmonary atresia, pulmonary and systemic blood flows may be calculated using the following equations:

$$\dot{Q}\text{p} = \frac{\dot{V}\text{O}_2}{\begin{matrix}\text{Pulmonary venous}\\ \text{oxygen content}\end{matrix} - \begin{matrix}\text{Systemic arterial}\\ \text{oxygen content}\end{matrix}}$$

$$\dot{Q}\text{s} = \frac{\dot{V}\text{O}_2}{\begin{matrix}\text{Systemic arterial}\\ \text{oxygen content}\end{matrix} - \begin{matrix}\text{Systemic mixed venous}\\ \text{oxygen content}\end{matrix}}$$

where $\dot{Q}\text{p}$ indicates pulmonary blood flow and $\dot{Q}\text{s}$ systemic blood flow. Because complete admixture of pulmonary and systemic blood flows occurs in the left atrium, the ratio of pulmonary to systemic blood flow determines the level of oxygen saturation in the systemic arterial circulation (see Chapter 4).

The anatomical right-to-left shunt represents the total volume of blood that passes from the right atrium to the left atrium and is equal to the systemic blood flow. The anatomical left-to-right shunt is the volume of blood passing from the aorta to the pulmonary artery through the ductus arteriosus, and in pulmonary atresia it represents pulmonary blood flow.

Physiological left-to-right shunt is the proportion of oxygenated blood that recirculates through the lungs and is calculated from:

$$\dot{Q}_{\text{L–R}} = \dot{Q}\text{p} - \dot{Q}\text{ep}$$

where $\dot{Q}\text{ep}$ indicates effective pulmonary blood flow. Physiological right-to-left shunt represents the volume of venous blood that enters the systemic arterial circulation without passing through the lungs and is calculated from:

$$\dot{Q}_{\text{R–L}} = \dot{Q}\text{s} - \dot{Q}\text{ep}$$

Pressures

The right atrial pressure usually shows a tall *a* wave, which may reach 15–20 mmHg, but right atrial mean pressure may be only moderately increased to 8–10 mmHg. Left atrial mean pressure is usually 2–3 mmHg lower than right atrial mean pressure; the dominant *v* wave usually noted in the left atrial pressure pulse is not present if pulmonary venous return is decreased, in which case *a* and *v* waves are equal. Left ventricular and systemic arterial pressures are in the normal range. Right ventricular systolic pressure is markedly elevated to above systemic systolic levels, and may reach 120–160 mmHg. The pressure contour is usually triangular in shape, with a relatively slow upstroke and downstroke. Right ventricular end-diastolic pressure is raised to 15–20 mmHg.

Infants with tricuspid insufficiency usually have right ventricular systolic pressures below left ventricular and systemic arterial systolic pressures: they usually range from 40 to 60 mmHg, but occasionally are lower. Also, these infants often have systemic arterial hypotension, related to decreased cardiac output. In infants with tricuspid regurgitation, it is important to consider the possibility that the apparent pulmonary atresia is functional.

Functional pulmonary atresia is not infrequently encountered in infants with Ebstein malformation. The right ventricle is unable to achieve a systolic pressure similar to that in the systemic circulation, either because a major portion of the wall is very thin or because there is marked tricuspid regurgitation. If the ductus arteriosus is patent, aortic pressure is transmitted to the pulmonary artery. The aortic pressure then exceeds right ventricular pressure and the pulmonary valve does not open during systole. Infusion of PGE_1 may induce the phenomenon by opening the ductus widely. It may also occur in infants with Ebstein malformation when the displaced tricuspid valve leaflet obstructs the right ventricular outflow, thus reducing pressure proximal to the pulmonary valve. It is important to recognize that the atresia is functional, so that no attempt is made to open the outflow tract. The condition should be suspected when the pulmonary valve annulus is wide and the pulmonary valve is identified as a thin membrane. In organic atresia, the valve is often dysmorphic and thickened and the annulus narrowed. Also the region just proximal to the valve should be examined carefully by ultrasound and angiography to detect regurgitation.

Angiocardiography

Angiograms are most important in providing details of the precise anatomy of the right ventricle and the pulmonary arteries. A right atrial angiogram is not usually helpful, because a large amount of contrast medium crosses the foramen ovale. Occasionally it is performed when it is difficult to pass the catheter into the right ventricle and the diagnosis of tricuspid atresia is being considered. The right ventricle usually fills, but the procedure is not completely reliable in excluding the possibility of tricuspid atresia, because a small ventricle may not fill. If Ebstein anomaly is associated, a large atrial chamber and atrialized portion of the ventricular chamber is seen. With severe tricuspid regurgitation, contrast medium may not be ejected from the right ventricle into the pulmonary artery because, as mentioned above, there may be functional pulmonary atresia. The right ventricular injection demonstrates chamber size and the diameter of the tricuspid valve and whether there is any opening between the right ventricle and the pulmonary artery. The size of both the right ventricular cavity and the tricuspid valve should be assessed and the distance between the right ventricular cavity and the pulmonary artery measured. In some infants, particularly those with severe stenosis, the ventricular size is normal, the three portions of the chamber are present, and tricuspid valve diameter is normal. Only a small amount of tricuspid regurgitation is evident.

In the majority of infants with pulmonary atresia, the right ventricular cavity is quite small and the diameter of the tricuspid valve orifice is reduced. Right ventricular volume and tricuspid valve diameter should be calculated. Ventricular–coronary communications fill with contrast medium injected into the right ventricle; the large sinusoids are seen to connect with coronary arteries, usually the right or left anterior descending vessels, but rarely to the left circumflex artery. Contrast material usually then flows retrograde in the artery to fill the aorta. If the aorta does not fill, it should be suspected that the proximal connection of the artery to the aorta is missing or is stenosed and the filling of vessels from the aortic angiogram should be examined carefully.

An attempt should also be made to evaluate perfusion of the myocardium from the ventricular–coronary artery communications. A left ventricular injection is not especially helpful; before the availability of ultrasound, it was useful in excluding a ventricular septal defect. The left ventricular chamber is somewhat enlarged but otherwise normal.

As mentioned above, a contrast injection into the aorta is important in defining the coronary arteries. Excellent visualization of the coronary arteries can usually be obtained by passing a flow-directed catheter from the femoral vein through the foramen ovale into the left atrium and through the left ventricle to the ascending aorta. The balloon on the catheter is inflated to occlude the aorta distal to the coronary artery origins; contrast injected proximal to the balloon produces excellent definition of the coronary arteries. It should be determined if both coronary arteries are filled from the aorta and they should be examined carefully for areas of stenosis. When the balloon is deflated contrast medium will be seen to pass from the aorta through the ductus arteriosus to the pulmonary artery. The main pulmonary artery is usually smaller than normal, as are the left and right branches.

If the right ventricular cavity is small, it is often helpful to perform angiograms simultaneously in the right ventricle and the aorta just proximal to the connection of the ductus arteriosus. Simultaneous visualization of the right ventricular cavity and the pulmonary artery, which fills through the ductus, will define the distance between them.

Pulmonary stenosis in older infants and children

Before the advent of ultrasound techniques, cardiac catheterization was frequently performed in children and adults with pulmonary stenosis to confirm the diagnosis, assess the severity of the lesion, and define the site(s) of obstruction. These features can now usually be defined by ultrasound study. Cardiac catheterization is now performed mainly for purposes of treatment by balloon angioplasty. Occasionally diagnostic procedures are still indicated to clarify sites of intraventricular and peripheral pulmonary arterial obstruction.

Approach and catheter manipulation

An approach is made percutaneously through the femoral vein; the catheter is advanced through the IVC to the right atrium, right ventricle, and pulmonary artery. The site(s) of obstruction are identified by continuous pressure monitoring as the catheter is advanced or withdrawn. If right ventricular pressure is markedly elevated and there is a history of cyanosis, the child's condition should be carefully monitored when the catheter is advanced through the pulmonary valve. Restlessness, anxiety, or increasing cyanosis may indicate critical obstruction of the valve orifice; the catheter should be withdrawn promptly to the right ventricle. The foramen is patent in a number of infants and children with pulmonary stenosis, and the venous catheter can be passed into the left atrium and ventricle.

Oxygen saturation

The oxygen saturations in the right heart chambers are usually similar, indicating the absence of shunts. Mixed venous oxygen saturation may be reduced in infants with pulmonary atresia with large right-to-left shunts through the foramen ovale resulting in systemic arterial hypoxemia. It may also be reduced in patients who have severe pulmonary stenosis with cardiac failure, due to increased oxygen extraction associated with reduced cardiac output. When the foramen ovale is widely patent or a fossa ovalis atrial septal defect is present and the pulmonary stenosis is mild, an increase in oxygen saturation may occur at the right atrial level due to left-to-right shunting. Oxygen saturation in the left atrium and ventricle and in the aorta may be reduced by right-to-left shunting through the foramen ovale.

Blood flows

The cardiac output is usually in the normal range in children with pulmonary stenosis unless cardiac failure is present, in which case it is reduced. Pulmonary blood flow is usually normal. Exercise in patients with mild pulmonary stenosis results in a normal rise in cardiac output and an increase in stroke volume. In severe stenosis, the rise in cardiac output is restricted and stroke volume is limited to the resting level or frequently it decreases.

Pressures

The right atrial pressure is normal in the presence of mild pulmonary stenosis; with severe stenosis there is a prominent *a* wave reaching pressures of up to 15–20 mmHg and mean pressure may be increased to 8–10 mmHg. Right ventricular systolic pressure is related to the severity of the stenosis; with mild stenosis, it may be as low as 25–30 mmHg, with a pressure drop of as little as 5–10 mmHg across the pulmonary valve. Right ventricular pressure may be elevated to 280–300 mmHg in patients with severe pulmonary stenosis. Characteristically, there is a slow upstroke and slow descent of the pressure, producing a rather triangular contour of the pressure tracing. In patients with severe stenosis, alternans of the right ventricular pressure may occur, with systolic pressure differences of as much as 20–30 mmHg. When ectopic beats occur or are induced there is a striking postectopic potentiation of right ventricular systolic pressure; in patients with mild stenosis, this may be only 5–10 mmHg above the control, but with severe stenosis it may be as high as 30–50 mmHg. Right ventricular end-diastolic pressure is normal in individuals with mild stenosis but elevated up to 15–20 mmHg in severe stenosis.

In patients with severe valvar pulmonary stenosis, secondary hypertrophy of the right ventricular outflow may develop, resulting in a pressure difference between the body of the right ventricle and the infundibular region. The exact site of the stenosis may be difficult to appreciate on the pressure tracing because the pulmonary arterial and infundibular pressures are quite low and do not have contours characteristic of normal pressure tracings. One helpful point is to carefully examine the diastolic portion of the pressure pulse; when the catheter is in the right ventricle, the pressure falls sharply in early diastole and then rises to the *a* wave, whereas in the pulmonary artery, pressure falls slowly through diastole. However, the exact site of the stenosis should always be confirmed by right ventricular angiography.

Pulmonary arterial mean pressure is usually normal, but there is often a reduction in the pulsatile pressure contour and a dicrotic notch is not well seen. In patients with moderate or severe stenosis, a reduction in systolic pressure or an actual negative pressure may be recorded just distal to the pulmonary valve as the catheter is withdrawn from the pulmonary artery into the right ventricle; this is due to the Bernoulli phenomenon (see Chapter 4). Pressures in the left atrium, left ventricle, and systemic artery are normal in children with pulmonary stenosis.

Valve area

The normal pulmonary valve area is about 2 cm^2/m^2 body surface area. In patients with mild stenosis, the calculated valve area ranges from 1 to 2 cm^2/m^2. When stenosis is severe, the pulmonary valve area may be reduced to as little as 0.2 cm^2/m^2. Application of the Gorlin formula to calculate valve area cannot be considered valid when all or part of the pressure difference across the right ventricular outflow is due to subvalvar stenosis. The formula was derived for flow across an orifice, and it cannot be used when there is a long area of stenosis or when there is more than one site of obstruction.

Angiocardiography

The most useful information is obtained from injections of contrast medium into the right ventricle. The cavity is usually of normal size and has prominent trabeculations. In patients with severe stenosis, the cavity may be smaller than normal and the wall of the ventricle is markedly thickened. In the rare instances in which cardiac failure is present, the ventricle is moderately enlarged, end-diastolic volume is increased, and ejection fraction is decreased.

In patients with severe stenosis, the pulmonary valve is often thickened and its motion may be restricted. During systole, it domes into the pulmonary artery and a jet of contrast medium is noted to flow through the orifice during the whole of systole; the jet is usually central in position, but may be peripheral. The main pulmonary artery and often the left branch are dilated, and contrast medium is often seen to swirl as the jet enters the dilated vessel. It is important to assess the size of the pulmonary annulus; the diameter is usually normal and the sinuses of Valsalva are well developed. However, in young children with severe stenosis, the annulus may be narrow and the sinuses poorly developed. In rare instances, the valve may be markedly thickened and irregular due to myxomatous degeneration.

When mild stenosis is present, the valve leaflets are also observed to be thickened and do not have a full range of motion in systole. A jet is not observed during systole when stenosis is very mild, and it may be difficult to document any abnormality of valve function or thickening of the valve. Often the only evidence of abnormality is a jerky motion of the valve.

The infundibular region of the right ventricle should be examined carefully in both the frontal and lateral projections. In patients with mild stenosis, the action of the infundibular region is quite normal, but in some patients with severe stenosis the infundibulum contracts actively and frequently almost completely occludes the lumen during systole. The systolic narrowing of the infundibulum is usually best observed in the lateral projection. The narrowing may be so severe as to produce a very small string-like channel during peak systole. The extent of infundibular narrowing varies considerably, from a long area extending from the body of the ventricle to the subvalvar area to a short segment in the immediate subvalvar region. The behavior of the infundibulum during diastole varies. In milder degrees of stenosis, it usually opens to provide a wide channel, but in severe grades of valvar stenosis, especially in older children, the muscle hypertrophy is marked and the infundibulum is narrowed even during diastole.

Left ventricular angiograms usually show normal left ventricular appearance and behavior and normal aortic anatomy. In cases of severe stenosis, the ventricular septum may bulge into the left ventricular cavity.

Differential diagnosis

Although pulmonary stenosis may be confused with several cardiac lesions, three clinical situations in which pulmonary stenosis with intact ventricular septum must be considered in the differential diagnosis are presented.

Infants with marked cyanosis

The diagnosis of pulmonary stenosis or atresia with intact ventricular septum must be considered in any infant who has cyanosis. When atresia is present, a murmur may not be audible, and the lesions that must be considered are aortopulmonary transposition, pulmonary atresia with ventricular septal defect, tricuspid atresia, total anomalous pulmonary venous drainage with obstruction of pulmonary venous drainage, and more complicated conditions such as atrioventricular septal defects, double-outlet right ventricle and single ventricle with severe pulmonary stenosis or atresia.

Since the introduction of ultrasound, the differential diagnosis of the cardiac lesions causing cyanosis in the newborn infant can be made readily, but clinical assessment is often useful. A prominent second heart sound at the upper left sternal border is not heard with pulmonary stenosis or atresia, but is usually audible in infants with aortopulmonary transposition and total pulmonary venous return. Although systolic murmurs are often not heard with pulmonary atresia, the presence of tricuspid regurgitation may be associated with a systolic murmur over the lower precordium. Many of the other lesions may or may not be associated with systolic murmurs. Chest radiographs help to distinguish between lesions with normal or increased pulmonary blood flow and those with reduced flow. With aortopulmonary transposition, the heart size is usually normal, but there is often a narrow superior mediastinum and pulmonary vascular markings are normal or increased. With total anomalous pulmonary venous connection and obstructed venous return, the heart is usually of normal size, but pulmonary vascular markings are prominent and pulmonary edema is often evident. Pulmonary atresia with intact ventricular septum with no significant tricuspid regurgitation is associated with normal heart size and reduced pulmonary vascular markings. Similar findings occur with pulmonary stenosis or atresia with ventricular septal defect and with tricuspid atresia without ventricular septal defect. When Ebstein malformation is associated, the heart is enlarged, often markedly. The electrocardiogram is often helpful; in infants with atrioventricular septal defect with pulmonary stenosis, there is left axis deviation and usually marked right ventricular hypertrophy. Left axis deviation is often present in infants with tricuspid atresia, but it may also occur in infants with pulmonary atresia with intact ventricular septum. Other lesions are usually associated with right axis deviation in infancy, but if right ventricular hypoplasia complicates other lesions, such as aortopulmonary transposition, left axis deviation may result. In the precordial leads, there are prominent right forces in infants with most of the lesions mentioned above. Exceptions are infants with tricuspid atresia and those with pulmonary atresia with intact ventricular septum with very hypoplastic right ventricles. Although ultrasound studies usually readily distinguish between the lesions, occasionally it may be difficult to identify the small tricuspid valve and flow through it into the ventricle in the infant with a hypoplastic ventricle, and the diagnosis of tricuspid atresia is considered.

Differentiation between pulmonary stenosis with intact ventricular septum and patent foramen ovale and pulmonary stenosis with ventricular septal defect in older infants and children

Patients with pulmonary stenosis may be cyanotic if there is a right-to-left shunt through either a ventricular septal defect or an atrial septal defect or patent foramen ovale. It is important to distinguish between patients with and without a ventricular septal defect, because the management is different.

Although the infant with pulmonary stenosis and ventricular septal defect (tetralogy of Fallot) usually manifests cyanosis in early infancy, it may not appear for several months or even years after birth. The onset of cyanosis may also be delayed in the child with moderate pulmonary stenosis and a patent foramen ovale. Squatting is unusual when the ventricular septum is intact but is common in children with tetralogy of Fallot. The heart is not enlarged in either group and there is a prominent lower left sternal impulse in both. The second heart sound is usually narrowly split or single with tetralogy of Fallot; it is soft at the upper left sternal border but is heard accentuated at the lower left sternal border. With intact ventricular septum, the second sound is soft throughout the precordium and is widely split, although the pulmonary component may be difficult to hear. A systolic ejection click is usually heard at the mid-left sternal border in patients with pulmonary stenosis with intact ventricular septum but is rare in tetralogy of Fallot. The systolic murmur is crescendo–decrescendo in quality and occupies the whole of systole in patients with intact ventricular septum, whereas in those with ventricular septal defect the murmur starts immediately after the first sound, is of even intensity, and often ends some time before the second sound. Although the effect of peripheral vasodilation is no longer examined in these patients, the response is interesting because it indicates the physiological differences. Inhalation of amyl nitrite results in a reduction in intensity and shortening of the duration of the murmur in patients with tetralogy of Fallot, but an increase in intensity of the murmur in patients with pulmonary stenosis and intact ventricular septum. The peripheral vasodilatation produced by amyl nitrite produces a decrease in both systemic arterial and right ventricular pressures in patients with large ventricular septal defects; this results in a decrease in ejection from the right ventricle and thus a decrease in the murmur. The increase in cardiac output associated with amyl nitrite inhalation produces increased venous return to the right atrium and right ventricle (in the patient with intact ventricular septum), the right ventricular end-diastolic and systolic pressures are raised, and stroke volume is increased, resulting in a louder murmur. This test is interesting but no longer used because amyl nitrite causes a disturbing sensation in children and is also potentially risky.

The radiograph may be helpful; in most patients with tetralogy of Fallot, the pulmonary artery segment is small and the pulmonary vasculature often decreased. The aortic arch is right-sided in about 25%, and persistence of the left SVC may be observed. When the ventricular septum is intact, the pulmonary artery is usually prominent due to poststenotic dilatation and the peripheral pulmonary vessels are normal. The size of the pulmonary artery is largely related to the site of the stenosis rather than to the presence or absence of a ventricular septal defect. When the stenosis is predominantly infundibular, as in tetralogy of Fallot, the pulmonary artery is usually not prominent, but valvar or immediate subvalvar stenosis occurring in patients with tetralogy of Fallot may cause pulmonary arterial enlargement.

Usually, the electrocardiogram is not conclusive. Right ventricular hypertrophy is present in both lesions. Right atrial hypertrophy reflected by tall peaked P waves in leads II and III is more frequent when the ventricular septum is intact. Severe degrees of right ventricular hypertrophy with R waves greater than 30 mm in the right precordial leads are more common when the ventricular septum is intact; however, in patients in whom the ventricular septal defect is restrictive (see Chapter 14), very tall R waves may be observed.

Ultrasound studies are usually conclusive in demonstrating the ventricular septal defect and the infundibular stenosis in the right ventricle in children with tetralogy of Fallot. The stenosis is usually valvar when the ventricular septum is intact, but secondary subvalvar stenosis can develop in children with severe pulmonary stenosis and intact ventricular septum.

Cardiac catheterization is currently not necessary to differentiate the two lesions. However, the features are presented because they demonstrate interesting differences in physiology. Patients with pulmonary stenosis and patent foramen ovale, who have right-to-left shunting, will demonstrate a decrease in oxygen saturation in the left atrium. Most patients with tetralogy of Fallot shunt at the ventricular level; however, the patient with tetralogy of Fallot may have a patent foramen ovale with shunting through it as well as through the ventricular septal defect. The right atrial *a* wave is usually more prominent when the ventricular septum is intact. In tetralogy of Fallot, systolic pressure in the right ventricle is equal to that in the left ventricle or aorta and has a rapid upstroke, a rather squared-off top, and a rapid descent. If ectopic beats are induced by advancing the catheter against the wall of the ventricle, the left and right ventricular pressures remain equal with all increases and decreases, and it is also noted that there is little postectopic potentiation of right ventricular systolic pressure. When the ventricular septum is intact, right ventricular systolic pressure may be considerably lower or higher than left ventricular or aortic pressure, unless there is a small ventricular septal defect. Frequently, the left and right ventricular pressures are quite similar at rest, but they separate when ectopic beats are induced; right ventricular pressure shows marked postectopic potentiation, not observed in the left ventricle. The right ventricular pressure contour is also different, showing a slow rise and descent, giving it a triangular appearance.

Differentiation between pulmonary stenosis and ventricular septal defect

A loud systolic murmur at the mid-left sternal border may be due to either pulmonary stenosis or ventricular septal defect. Differentiation is usually not difficult because the locations of the murmurs are typical; the murmur of ventricular septal defect is usually most prominent at the lower left sternal border and xiphoid region. The murmur of pulmonary stenosis is most prominent at the upper left sternal border and left infraclavicular area. However, confusion may arise, especially with a doubly committed subarterial (subpulmonary) ventricular septal defect, because the murmur in this lesion is heard best at the mid and upper left sternal border. The murmur of pulmonary stenosis has a crescendo–decrescendo configuration, whereas the murmur of ventricular septal defect is of even intensity. The second heart sound is usually soft at the upper left sternal border with pulmonary stenosis, but is normal or increased in intensity at this site with ventricular septal defect. The radiograph may show poststenotic dilatation of the pulmonary artery with pulmonary stenosis. Also, pulmonary vascular markings may be increased with ventricular septal defect if there is a moderate or large left-to-right shunt, but are normal if the shunt is small; they are normal with pulmonary stenosis. The electrocardiogram shows right ventricular hypertrophy in pulmonary stenosis, but may show combined ventricular hypertrophy with ventricular septal defect. However, with either mild pulmonary stenosis or a small ventricular septal defect, the electrocardiogram is often normal.

Differentiation between mild pulmonary stenosis and atrial septal defect

It may be difficult to distinguish between mild pulmonary stenosis and atrial septal defect. With both lesions a systolic crescendo–decrescendo murmur is heard at the upper left sternal border. It is usually harsher in quality in patients with pulmonary stenosis. The second heart sound at the upper left sternal border is well split with atrial septal defect, and does not narrow significantly during expiration. With pulmonary stenosis, the sound is also often split, but does narrow or become single during expiration. The presence of a prominent ejection click is supportive of the diagnosis of pulmonary stenosis. The chest radiograph may be helpful; with atrial septal defect, cardiomegaly may be present if the left-to-right shunt is large. The heart is not usually enlarged with pulmonary stenosis. The pulmonary vascular markings may be increased with atrial septal defect, but are normal with pulmonary stenosis. Right ventricular hypertrophy may be present on electrocardiography with both lesions, but with atrial septal defect the right precordial voltages are not usually greatly increased and right ventricular conduction delay is usually present. However, with small atrial septal defects and with mild pulmonary stenosis, the electrocardiogram may be normal. Some children with large atrial left-to-right shunts have been found at cardiac catheterization to have a systolic pressure difference of up to 30–40 mmHg across the pulmonary valve in the absence of evidence of pulmonary valve disease. It is related to high flow across the orifice, and results in a murmur with all the characteristics of pulmonary stenosis.

Principles of management

Pulmonary stenosis in the fetus

The ability to recognize the presence of pulmonary stenosis in the fetus by ultrasound examination has raised questions about attempts to relieve the obstruction *in utero*. There are only a few published reports of balloon dilation of the pulmonary valve by transabdominal approach in fetuses with valvar pulmonary stenosis with intact ventricular septum. The procedures were performed for perceived cardiac failure at 28–30 weeks' gestation and were successful. Cardiac failure was relieved and right ventricular size increased after the procedure [3,13]. As discussed in Chapter 11, several centers have been performing aortic balloon valvuloplasty to attempt to prevent the development of hypoplastic left ventricle in fetuses with aortic stenosis. Interest is now being directed to relieving pulmonary stenosis *in utero*, in the hope that prenatal relief of the stenosis may allow the right ventricle to grow and improve the likelihood that there will be two functional ventricles after birth. No published reports of this procedure are available, but verbal reports of the procedure in a small number of fetuses have come to my attention. The indications for performing dilation of the pulmonary valve in the fetus are not yet defined. Several studies have examined the influence of morphological findings in the fetus with pulmonary stenosis on the likelihood of achieving a biventricular heart after birth. A small tricuspid valve orifice, a small pulmonary valve annulus, and the presence of coronary sinusoids were all indicators of the unlikelihood of achieving a functional right ventricle postnatally [14,15]. Whether balloon angioplasty of the pulmonary valve in the fetus will improve the chances of achieving a biventricular circulation is yet to be explored.

Infants with cyanosis

The presence of severe cyanosis in the newborn infant with suspected pulmonary stenosis or atresia is an indication for urgent treatment. The infant should be maintained in a neutral thermal environment to minimize oxygen consumption (see Chapter 3). Oxygen should be administered; although it may not be particularly beneficial when pulmonary blood flow is markedly reduced, it will still result in some improvement in arterial oxygen content (see Chapter 3). If possible, an umbilical arterial catheter should be inserted to monitor blood gas status. Also, because it is very likely that PGE_1 will be indicated, it is advisable to intubate the trachea to provide assisted ventilation if necessary. If the umbilical artery cannot be catheterized, an arterial sample should be obtained by radial artery puncture. Arterial blood pH, Po_2, Pco_2, and glucose levels should be measured. Acidemia and hypoglycemia should be treated promptly and electrocardiography, echocardiography, and chest radiography obtained as soon as possible. Prior to the introduction of prostaglandin treatment, urgent surgery to improve pulmonary blood flow was indicated, but opening the ductus arteriosus with PGE_1 infusion has eliminated the urgency for operation.

The important decision will have to be made regarding the administration of PGE_1 to dilate the ductus arteriosus, particularly in the infant who is to be transported to a cardiac center. PGE_1 infusion would be contraindicated in only few cyanotic congenital cardiac lesions; it could possibly produce adverse effects in some infants with total anomalous pulmonary venous drainage (see Chapter 13) or with aortopulmonary transposition (see Chapter 18). It is also not indicated in infants who have lung disease as the primary cause of cyanosis. Lung disease causing severe cyanosis would be associated with marked respiratory distress, including chest retraction. Also, the arterial Pco_2 would most likely be elevated. Therefore, if the Po_2 is very low and the Pco_2 normal, and particularly if the pH is reduced, it would be reasonable to administer PGE_1 prior to making a definitive diagnosis. As soon as the studies have been obtained, the situation can be reassessed. If the infant is already in a tertiary care center, it would be reasonable to delay PGE_1 therapy until the results of diagnostic studies can be performed, unless metabolic acidemia is evident from blood gas measurements.

PGE_1 may be administered by intravenous infusion or through an umbilical arterial catheter. The recommended initial infusion rate is 0.05 μg/kg per min. This dose is usually effective and results in improvement in arterial oxygen saturation and metabolic acidemia, but the dose can be increased if necessary to 0.1 μg/kg per min. After 2–3 hours, if blood pH has returned to normal, the dose can be reduced progressively to 0.002–0.005 μg/kg per min. The infant's blood oxygen status should be carefully monitored while the dose is being reduced; should there be any deterioration, the infusion rate should be increased promptly. The important immediate adverse effects of PGE_1 are respiratory depression leading to apnea, particularly in premature infants, and systemic arterial hypotension. It is thus recommended to intubate the trachea, especially in preterm infants, and to be prepared to provide mechanical ventilation. Reduction in infusion rate often eliminates the need for assisted respiration. Similarly, reducing the infusion rate usually allows blood pressure to return to normal levels, but if necessary catecholamines such as dopamine or dobutamine can be added. Other adverse effects include flushing due to peripheral vasodilatation; fever due to a central hypothalamic effect; and irritability, sometimes with myoclonic jerks, also due to a central nervous system effect.

The lower the arterial oxygen saturation and Po_2, the more dramatic the effects of PGE_1 in raising arterial oxygen levels. This is explained by the relationship between the pulmonary to systemic blood flow ratio and arterial oxygen saturation when complete mixing of pulmonary and systemic blood flow occurs (see Chapter 4). If arterial Po_2 is above about 40 mmHg, PGE_1 has little effect in further increasing the level.

Considerations for surgery or interventional procedures

The mortality and morbidity following surgery for pulmonary atresia and severe stenosis has varied considerably in different centers, but in general has been very high. In a number of reports, mortality was greater than 50%. It is often difficult to compare results of various approaches in different series because of the many factors influencing survival and success of procedures, including (i) size of the right ventricle and tricuspid valve orifice; (ii) morphology of the pulmonary valve; (iii) presence of coronary sinusoids; (iv) dependence of coronary perfusion on right ventricular pressure; and (v) tricuspid valve anomalies.

The options available include the following.

- Surgical opening of the pulmonary valve and, if necessary, the right ventricular outflow tract.
- Introducing a systemic arterial to pulmonary arterial shunt surgically.
- A combination of the above two procedures.
- Transcatheter opening of the pulmonary valve.
- Maintaining ductus arteriosus patency.
- Introducing a systemic venous to pulmonary arterial shunt.
- Closing the tricuspid valve.
- Inserting a shunt from the aorta to the right ventricle.

Although there is currently no consensus on the specific procedures recommended for these infants, I present what seem to be the most rational approaches in different circumstances.

Severe pulmonary stenosis or pulmonary atresia with well-developed right ventricle and mild or no tricuspid regurgitation

This group of infants is the most favorable with regard to achieving relief of obstruction and a right ventricle with normal size and function. The right ventricle is usually tripartite in these infants; the right ventricle and pulmonary artery are separated by the valve tissue. The tricuspid valve orifice is normal or may have a somewhat increased diameter. Until the advent of balloon valvuloplasty by transcatheter approach, the pulmonary valve was opened surgically from an incision in the pulmonary artery. It was often difficult to define the anatomy of the valve because it was dysplastic. In addition, the valve annulus was often small, so that stenosis could not be adequately relieved by the procedure. It was therefore common practice to make an incision across the annulus and insert a patch extending from the right ventricular outflow tract to the main pulmonary artery across the annulus. Experience indicated that if a transannular patch was not inserted at the original procedure, it would be required within 2–3 years in a high percentage of infants.

Following this procedure, in many infants adequate pulmonary blood flow was established, right ventricular pressure decreased, and arterial oxygen saturation increased to near normal levels. However, in some, mild to moderate cyanosis persisted. It was noted that although the pulmonary stenosis was relieved and right ventricular systolic pressure was quite low, the end-diastolic pressure was increased; this was thought to be related to decreased right ventricular compliance resulting from myocardial hypertrophy or fibrosis. The high diastolic pressure resulted in elevated right atrial pressure, with right-to-left shunt through the foramen ovale.

Over the past 15–20 years, the pulmonary valve has been opened successfully by transcatheter techniques. With severe pulmonary valve stenosis, a wire and then a balloon angioplasty catheter can be manipulated through the orifice. With complete atresia, it is necessary to create an opening. This has been achieved by both laser and radiofrequency techniques. The laser technique consists of placement of an end-hole catheter just beneath the pulmonary valve. A fiberoptic guidewire attached to a laser is passed through the catheter to the tip and after making an opening in the valve, a guidewire is passed through it, followed by balloon angioplasty to 6–8 mm. A 2F ring-tipped radiofrequency catheter (Coe) has been developed. It is passed to the valve and after an opening is made, a guidewire can be passed through the end-hole of the catheter to be used for balloon angioplasty.

Following balloon angioplasty of the pulmonary valve, the infant may continue to have moderate to severe hypoxemia. In a few patients, the ductus arteriosus has been kept open by inserting a stent into its lumen by transcatheter techniques. In my opinion, it is preferable to maintain patency by means of PGE_1 because the infant may tolerate closure of the ductus within days or a few weeks. If a stent has been inserted, another procedure will be required to close the ductus arteriosus.

If the obstruction is not adequately relieved, it may be necessary to provide additional pulmonary blood flow. In the past, the only means available was to introduce a systemic artery to pulmonary artery shunt. Various shunt techniques have been used, including Blalock–Taussig (subclavian artery to pulmonary artery), Potts (descending aorta to left pulmonary artery), and Waterston (ascending aorta to right pulmonary artery) shunts). Because relief of the right ventricular outflow obstruction was not pursued aggressively, a second surgical procedure to introduce a shunt was often necessary. It therefore became common practice to perform a shunt procedure at the same time as the relief of stenosis was attempted. It is now evident that, even with good relief of obstruction, adequate pulmonary blood flow may not be achieved for several days or weeks, probably because establishment of normal right ventricular function is delayed. It would be unfortunate if a shunt was introduced unnecessarily in this situation.

Recently, therefore, it has become common practice to continue PGE_1 administration in a low dose to maintain ductus patency for some days. The infusion is gradually reduced and stopped if the baby does not show increasing cyanosis. Should cyanosis become more severe, the infusion can be restarted. Only in those infants in whom it appears that adequate pulmonary blood flow cannot eventually be attained through the pulmonary valve is an aortopulmonary shunt introduced. The Potts and Waterston shunts are currently not favored, because it is difficult to judge their size and excessive pulmonary blood flow with cardiac failure may result. Either a Blalock–Taussig or a modified Blalock–Taussig shunt is performed. The Blalock–Taussig shunt has the disadvantage that the subclavian artery is disconnected from its supply to the upper extremity and impaired growth and decreased power have occasionally resulted. The modified procedure consists of interposing a tube graft (such as GoreTex) between the subclavian and pulmonary arteries. It has the advantage that the subclavian artery is not separated, but the disadvantage that it does not grow. Some have preferred to introduce a tube graft between the aorta and the main pulmonary artery.

Pulmonary atresia with well-developed right ventricle and marked tricuspid regurgitation

As mentioned on p. 410, this combination of defects is frequently associated with Ebstein malformation of the tricuspid valve. These infants are difficult to manage and have a high mortality. Several approaches have been recommended. Systemic arterial to pulmonary arterial shunts may relieve cyanosis, but the combination of increased left ventricular volume load and high right ventricular volume load often induces cardiac failure. Opening the pulmonary valve by balloon valvuloplasty may reduce right ventricular pressure and thus reduce the severity of tricuspid regurgitation. However, if the ductus arteriosus is still patent, the high pulmonary arterial pressure may result in severe pulmonary regurgitation, which could aggravate the tricuspid regurgitation and precipitate right ventricular failure.

One is confronted with a difficult decision regarding the use of PGE_1 in the early neonatal period. Infusion would be indicated to provide adequate pulmonary blood flow through the ductus arteriosus in the presence of pulmonary valve obstruction. However, if ballon valvuloplasty achieves excellent relief of pulmonary stenosis, the patent ductus arteriosus could have an adverse effect by increasing tricuspid regurgitation, as discussed above. Under these circumstances, it may be advisable to administer indomethacin or ibuprofen to close the ductus and, if necessary, to attempt to reduce pulmonary vascular resistance (by nitric oxide inhalation or other agents). However, if the pulmonary valve cannot be opened sufficiently to provide adequate pulmonary blood flow, PGE_1 infusion could be continued and, if necessary, an aortopulmonary shunt could be introduced. Beyond the age of about 3 months, it is suggested that an SVC to pulmonary artery communication (bidirectional Glenn procedure) be performed. In addition to providing adequate pulmonary blood flow, this may relieve some of the volume load on the right ventricle by reducing the total volume entering the right ventricle. At a later stage, the tricuspid valve can be closed and the IVC can be connected to the pulmonary artery to complete the Fontan type of procedure.

Pulmonary atresia with hypoplastic right ventricle and tricuspid valve

It is important to assess the size of the right ventricle and tricuspid valve in considering the approach to management. It is desirable to retain the right ventricle in the circulation if it is capable of maintaining the total, or even part of, pulmonary blood flow. Numerous indices have been proposed to decide whether the tricuspid valve and right ventricle are of adequate size to accommodate the total cardiac output. Unfortunately, none of these is totally predictable and thus different values have been used in various centers. A right ventricular volume of less than 35–40% has been considered unlikely to sustain total cardiac output, but because estimates of right ventricular volumes are not very reliable in infants, particularly those with pulmonary atresia, I recommend that tricuspid valve size be used in decision-making. It is very likely that if the tricuspid valve is too small, one can assume that no significant benefit will be derived from opening the pulmonary outflow. Values that have been considered inadequate include:

- tricuspid valve diameter less than 8 mm in a newborn infant;
- tricuspid to mitral valve diameter ratio less than 0.7;
- tricuspid valve diameter *Z*-scores of −3 or smaller.

Another factor important in the decision to recommend a particular approach is the morphology of the ventricle, i.e., whether it is tripartite, bipartite, or monopartite. The degree of separation of the pulmonary artery from the right ventricular cavity is also a consideration. If the ventricle is tripartite and the pulmonary artery is separated from the right ventricle by a short distance, usually the right ventricular outflow is opened. If the ventricle is monopartite, consisting only of a small inlet portion, and there is a wide separation between the ventricular cavity and the pulmonary artery, attempts to provide an adequate output by the right ventricle are usually not successful. Instead, either a systemic-to-pulmonary arterial shunt is introduced or PGE_1 is infused until such time as a bidirectional Glenn procedure is performed. However, as mentioned above, a false impression of the potential size of the right ventricular cavity can be obtained from both echocardiographic and angiographic studies. Marked hypertrophy of the right ventricular wall may obliterate the cavity in the trabecular, and especially the infundibular, regions. It is therefore probably advisable to seriously consider attempts to maintain the right ventricle in the circulation.

Based on the fact that it is occasionally possible to achieve adequate output by a small ventricle after opening the outflow, I recommend that an attempt be made in all patients to relieve the obstruction as effectively as possible, unless there are other contraindications (see section on coronary sinusoids Chapter 15). The pulmonary valve is opened by balloon valvuloplasty; following the procedure, PGE_1 is infused. If it appears from ultrasound study that there is reasonably good flow across the right ventricular outflow and there is not a large flow across the foramen ovale, an attempt can be made to stop the infusion. The dose is gradually reduced while systemic arterial oxygenation is monitored closely. If arterial oxygen saturation falls significantly, the dosage should be immediately increased. If the infant cannot tolerate cessation of PGE_1 infusion, two options are available. As mentioned above, a systemic-to-pulmonary arterial shunt can be introduced or PGE_1 can be continued until 3–4 months of age, at which time a cavopulmonary anastomosis (bidirectional Glenn procedure) is performed.

Chronic intravenous infusion of PGE_1 does create problems. The infant requires hospitalization and technical difficulties may arise with venous access. Although oral administration of PGE_1 has been used successfully, it also usually requires hospitalization because it must be given frequently. In addition, persistent and often severe diarrhea may prevent administration via this route. It has also been suggested that it may result in morphological changes in the ductus arteriosus, but no consequences have been noted, and the ductus closes normally after PGE_1 is discontinued. Prolonged infusion has also been noted to cause cortical hyperostosis, but this bone complication has not had any long-term adverse effects. It is unfortunate that PGE_1 is not available as a long-acting or intramuscular/subcutaneous preparation.

A systemic venous to pulmonary artery connection is not generally recommended before the age of 3–4 months, because adequate pulmonary blood flow is not usually established. This is probably because the postnatal changes in the pulmonary circulation have not progressed to the point where resistance is low enough for adequate perfusion to occur at low venous pressures. It is for these reasons that an arterial shunt is frequently performed. A disadvantage of arterial shunts is that distortion of the pulmonary artery at the site of the anastomosis may result in obstruction, which will complicate later attempts to introduce a venous shunt. If an arterial shunt is performed, as mentioned above, currently a modified Blalock–Taussig procedure (interposition of a tube graft between the suclavian artery or aorta and the pulmonary artery) is recommended.

Venous to pulmonary arterial shunts include the following.

- Glenn procedure: end-to-end anastomosis of the SVC to the left pulmonary artery.
- Cavopulmonary anastomosis or bidirectional Glenn procedure: anastomosis of the SVC to the pulmonary artery so that both lungs can be perfused by SVC blood.
- Atriopulmonary connection or Fontan procedure: anastomosis of the right atrial appendage to the pulmonary artery to divert all venous return into the pulmonary artery.
- Modified Fontan procedure: SVC–pulmonary anastomosis and extracardiac conduit connection of IVC to the pulmonary artery.

None of these procedures are recommended in early infancy, as pulmonary perfusion is likely to be inadequate because pulmonary vascular resistance may not have fallen sufficiently.

The Glenn procedure has not generally been recommended before the age of 2–3 years, because direction of total SVC flow into one lung may not create adequate perfusion. SVC pressure may be markedly elevated and adequate relief of cyanosis may not occur. A distinct disadvantage of the procedure is that, after a variable period, pulmonary arteriovenous fistulae are likely to develop in the right lung, This will result in a progressive increase in cyanosis.

The Fontan procedure is also not usually well tolerated in infancy. It was generally not performed before the age of 4 years, although recently, with better selection and improvement in technique, some success has been achieved at younger ages, but not usually below 2 years of age. Systemic venous pressure may increase to 15–20 mmHg or higher for several reasons, including pulmonary vascular resistance above 2 mmHg/L per min per m^2, pulmonary arterial mean pressure above 15–18 mmHg, and poor left ventricular function. This may be associated with persistent ascites, chylothorax, protein-losing enteropathy, or a combination of these problems. Protein-losing enteropathy is associated with a high mortality of near 50%.

Cavopulmonary anastomosis (bidirectional Glenn shunt) is now generally considered the procedure of choice. Initially it was recommended that it be performed beyond the age of 6 months and it is usually well tolerated at that age. Usually arterial oxygen saturation increases to 85–88% and the infant is mildly cyanosed, but otherwise asymptomatic. Recently, the procedure has been performed in infants as young as 1 month of age, but results are not consistently as favorable and often oxygen saturation does not increase to more than 75–78%; also, the infant may show alarming cyanosis with crying. Currently, I consider 3 months of age the lower limit for performing the procedure.

The caval to right pulmonary artery and bidirectional caval to pulmonary artery anastomoses are associated with the development of pulmonary arteriovenous fistulae in the right lung, or with the bidirectional shunt in both lungs. When the caval to right pulmonary arterial connection is done in early childhood, the fistulae are not usually evident for several years. However, the bidirectional shunt may be associated with significant development of pulmonary arteriovenous fistulae within a few months. This results in a progressive increase in the degree of cyanosis. The early onset of pulmonary arteriovenous fistulae is much more likely to occur in early infancy, and the impression is that they are more likely to occur in infants with atrial isomerism. This requires further analysis to assess whether this is related to associated venous anomalies, such as absence of the IVC.

The mechanism responsible for these fistulae has not been defined, but it appears to be related to exclusion of direct perfusion of the lung by blood from the IVC, which includes hepatic venous blood. It has been shown that after development of pulmonary arteriovenous fistulae, considerable improvement can be achieved by redirecting some hepatic venous blood into the pulmonary artery. Therefore, in infants with pulmonary atresia, if it is possible to open the right ventricular outflow to provide some pulmonary blood flow from the IVC return, the likelihood for fistula formation should be reduced. If the fistulae can be well localized by catheterization and angiography, it may be possible to occlude them by embolization. However, it may be advisable to complete the systemic venous connection to the pulmonary artery by connecting the IVC with an extracardiac conduit and thus provide hepatic venous blood to the pulmonary circulation.

An important issue in those infants in whom prolonged PGE_1 infusion is administered, or a systemic-to-pulmonary arterial shunt is introduced, is whether balloon atrial septostomy should be performed to maintain patency of the foramen ovale. Increasing pulmonary blood flow may increase left atrial pressure sufficiently to tend to close the foramen ovale if the valve is competent. This would result in an increase in right atrial pressure, because all or most of the systemic venous blood has to pass across the foramen ovale, and venous congestion could result. Also, total output from the left ventricle could possibly be reduced. If it is evident from the ultrasound examination prior to introducing the shunt that there is considerable bulge of the atrial septum into the left atrium and that the foramen ovale appears to be small, then atrial septostomy should probably be performed prior to the shunt procedure. If this is not obvious, it would be reasonable to first perform the procedure and assess the need for atrial septostomy subsequently.

In those patients in whom a shunt has been introduced or long-term PGE_1 administered, in addition to opening the pulmonary outflow, there is an argument against routinely performing atrial septostomy. If the right ventricle is hypoplastic, it is hoped that increasing blood flow by opening the valve would enhance its growth. A somewhat restrictive foramen ovale would facilitate blood flow through the right ventricle, whereas atrial septostomy may favor flow across the atrial septum and thus limit development of the right ventricle.

Pulmonary atresia with hypoplastic right ventricle and coronary sinusoids

The presence of coronary sinusoids may drastically influence decisions regarding management. If small, sinusoids will not significantly affect hemodynamics, but if large they could influence myocardial perfusion. The presence of large sinusoids dramatically decreases survival of infants with pulmonary atresia. It is therefore important to assess the patterns of flow in the sinusoids before instituting any procedures; this is accomplished by right ventricular and aortic angiography. As mentioned above, the sinusoids may be the only or dominant source of coronary blood flow to some areas of the left ventricular myocardium and perfusion is dependent on maintaining a high right ventricular pressure. Therefore, attempts to open the outflow tract, thus possibly reducing right ventricular pressure, are contraindicated. In the neonatal period, a systemic-to-pulmonary arterial shunt or prolonged PGE_1 infusion is recommended. After the age of 3–4 months, cavopulmonary anastomosis could be performed. Tricuspid regurgitation of significant degree would have a deleterious effect on these individuals because it could affect the level of systolic pressure achieved by the right ventricle. A procedure that has been performed to assure coronary perfusion by the right ventricle is to close the tricuspid valve and introduce a tube graft from the aorta to the right ventricular cavity.

If it is evident that the flow pattern in the sinusoids is from the coronary arteries to the right ventricular cavity during diastole, perfusion of the left ventricular myocardium could be impaired, with eventual development of left ventricular ischemia and failure. Successful opening of the right ventricular outflow tract could reduce right ventricular systolic and diastolic pressures and aggravate runoff from the coronary circulation into the right ventricle via the sinusoids. Introducing a systemic-to-pulmonary arterial shunt could also have adverse effects because it may reduce systemic arterial diastolic pressure and thus interfere with coronary perfusion. Furthermore, it creates a greater demand for left ventricular coronary blood flow, because it increases left ventricular volume load. Beyond the age of 3–4 months a cavopulmonary anastomosis can be performed, but in the early neonatal period either prolonged PGE_1 infusion or a systemic-to-pulmonary arterial shunt would be necessary to provide adequate pulmonary blood flow. The likelihood for left ventricular failure increases progressively with age, with few surviving beyond 3–4 years of age. It has been suggested that this may be due to the fact that the coronary sinusoids divert a large volume of blood away from the left ventricular myocardium. It has therefore been recommended that the procedure of closing the tricuspid valve, with thrombo-occlusion of the right ventricular cavity, should be performed before the age of 10–12 months. Another approach that has been reported in a few infants is to attempt to close the sinusoids. The pulmonary outflow was opened and the sinusoids ligated; some good results were achieved, but the procedure needs to be studied more carefully with regard to feasibility and success. There is no convincing evidence to support the effectiveness of these procedures. The problem of left ventricular dysfunction could possibly be related to intrinsic abnormalities in coronary vascular development rather than to coronary steal (see Chapter 12).

Pulmonary valvar stenosis in older infants and children

These patients may have presented in early infancy with evidence of mild stenosis or of moderate stenosis with mild degrees of cyanosis during crying. The infant may develop increasing cyanosis over the first few months associated with a rise in the pressure gradient resulting from an increase in cardiac output. Relief of valvar obstruction is recommended in those infants with intermittent or persistent cyanosis.

Prior to the introduction of transcatheter procedures for relieving pulmonary valve obstruction, valvar stenosis could be treated surgically with low mortality and morbidity. The right ventricle is usually well developed in these infants, and the procedure involved opening the pulmonary valve through an incision in the pulmonary artery. If the stenosis was not severe enough to produce cyanosis, the child was carefully followed with repeated ultrasound studies, first at 3-monthly and then at 6-month intervals, to monitor changes in pressure gradient across the valve. A systolic pressure gradient across the pulmonary valve of greater than 80 mmHg at rest was considered an indication for surgery. Surgery was not recommended for those with pressure gradients at rest of less than about 60 mmHg. Recommendations varied for those with gradients of 60–100 mmHg.

As mentioned on p. 388, in older children who have had moderate to severe stenosis, infundibular or subvalvar stenosis may develop. In some of these individuals, relief of pulmonary valvar stenosis was associated with no reduction, or even a rise, in right ventricular pressure due to severe contraction of infundibular muscle. This resulted in decreased right ventricular output with reduction in left ventricular filling and poor systemic perfusion. Also, right-sided failure with congestion occurred. This development after surgery has been referred to as "suicidal right ventricle." It was often difficult to decide whether hypertrophied infundibular muscle should be resected or whether the infundibular area should be widened with a patch. If the angiogram showed a moderate degree of narrowing of the infundibulum during systole with complete relaxation during diastole, there was little indication to resect any muscle in the infundibulum. However, when there was marked hypertrophy with persistent narrowing throughout the cardiac cycle, the need for removal of some infundibular muscle through the pulmonary valve was reassessed. After closing the pulmonary artery and allowing the circulation to be reestablished, right ventricular systolic pressure was measured. If it was below about 70–80 mmHg when systemic arterial systolic pressure was at least 70–80 mmHg, the patient usually did not require infundibular resection. However, if right ventricular systolic pressure was very high, resection of infundibular muscle was recommended. If this did not adequately open the outflow tract, a patch was inserted. If the patient survived the surgical procedure without the need for infundibular resection, the hypertrophy resolved spontaneously over several months and right ventricular pressure fell to near normal levels.

Surgery has now been largely replaced by transcatheter balloon angioplasty. Because the procedure does not require major surgery with thoracotomy, there has been a considerable change of opinion regarding indications for relief of stenosis. Currently, the consensus is that balloon valvuloplasty should be performed in all infants who have a systolic pressure gradient above 80 mmHg, or who have cyanosis due to atrial right-to-left shunting. If the infant has a gradient less than 80 mmHg, the procedure can be delayed until about 9–12 months. Ultrasound studies should be repeated every 3 months to ensure that the stenosis does not become more severe with growth. The advantage of delaying the procedure is that the valve may be myxomatous and thickened in early infancy, and valvuloplasty may not be as effective as when performed later, when the valve may have become more membranous. Not infrequently, a second procedure is required at a later age when it is first performed in early infancy.

In children above about 1 year of age, many centers are recommending that balloon valvuloplasty should be performed if the resting systolic pressure gradient is above 50 mmHg. The rationale for relieving obstruction is to prevent the development of right ventricular infundibular hypertrophy with secondary stenosis and to avoid myocardial fibrosis in later life. However, there is no convincing evidence to indicate that this is a significant problem. In fact, the recommendations are based largely on the impression that myocardial fibrosis may develop, rather than on authentic factual information. There is some evidence that a slow mild increase in right ventricular pressure may occur when pressure is above 50 mmHg [10], but this does not appear to be associated with clinical deterioration. Although I was inclined to recommend relief of stenosis if right ventricular pressure at rest is 50–80 mmHg, I am now of the opinion that these children be observed and a procedure performed only if there is a significant increase in the pressure with repeat observations or if there is evidence of right ventricular enlargement.

Some centers now advise balloon valvuloplasty in children with peak systolic pressure gradients, measured by ultrasound, below 40 mmHg at rest or even less, but there is no evidence that the stenosis progresses in these individuals [11,12] nor is there evidence for the development of myocardial fibrosis. It is difficult to decide at what level of pressure gradient balloon valvuloplasty should be performed. Because the procedure has a low morbidity and few late adverse effects, the tendency has been to perform it at lower pressure gradients. If the peak systolic pressure gradient is below 40 mmHg, isoproterenol or dobutamine infusion has been used to increase cardiac output and valvuloplasty has been recommended if the pressure gradient reaches 40–50 mmHg during the infusion. As mentioned above, altering heart rate and cardiac output will influence the gradient. Basing the decision for the procedure on the gradient during isoproterenol infusion is not justified, because all studies of natural history have been based on studies at rest. Currently, my recommendation is that valvuloplasty should not be considered if the resting gradient is below 50 mmHg.

Prognosis and long-term results after procedures

Infants with well-developed right ventricles who have the pulmonary valve opened surgically usually have immediate improvement of cyanosis, but it is not unusual that some degree of cyanosis persists for several days or even weeks after surgery. This is related to persistence of some right-to-left shunt at the atrial level and is probably the result of reduced compliance of the hypertrophied right ventricle, with a high atrial *a* wave. The cyanosis disappears in association with regression of right ventricular hypertrophy. Balloon valvuloplasty performed in the neonatal period may not be as effective in relieving stenosis, because the valve is often dysplastic during this period. Thus cyanosis is likely to persist and repeat valvuloplasty may be necessary within 6–9 months.

Infants with pulmonary atresia and hypoplastic right ventricles who have had surgical opening of the outflow tract frequently do not immediately develop adequate pulmonary blood flow and require either PGE_1 infusion or a systemic-to-pulmonary arterial shunt procedure. Although flow through the right ventricular outflow may improve, so that the PGE_1 infusion can be stopped, mild to moderate degrees of cyanosis persist because the hypoplastic right ventricle, as well as the small tricuspid valve, are associated with elevated right atrial pressures. An important issue in these patients is whether closure of the atrial communication will eliminate the cyanosis, increase flow into the right ventricle, and promote its growth. However, closure of the atrial communication could result in marked increase in right atrial and systemic venous pressures and reduce systemic blood flow. If closure of the atrial communication is considered, an attempt should be made to assess the ability of the tricuspid valve and right ventricle to accommodate total systemic venous return by closing the atrial septal opening. A balloon catheter is passed across the defect into the left atrium and the inflated balloon is pulled against the septum to close the defect. Atrial and systemic arterial pressures should be monitored for a period of at least 15 min to determine whether closure of the communication can be tolerated. If systemic arterial pressure falls and does not quickly recover, or if right atrial mean pressure rises to more than 10 mmHg, the balloon should be deflated. It would then be advisable to perform SVC to pulmonary connection at 4–6 months of age. At a later date, balloon closure of the atrial communication can be attempted again. It is quite possible that it could be well tolerated because SVC return passes directly into the pulmonary artery. Only IVC blood would have to be accommodated by the tricuspid valve and right ventricle.

Residual pulmonary valve insufficiency

The development of pulmonary valve insufficiency after surgical opening of the pulmonary valve is common. When the procedure is performed in older infants and children and the valve alone is opened without incision into the outflow tract or annulus, insufficiency is usually only mild and infrequently results in significant right ventricular enlargement. However, in infants who have had surgical opening of the right ventricular infundibulum and the annulus of the valve, marked insufficiency may ensue. In fact, because it was thought that pulmonary insufficiency was not a serious problem, many surgeons created a wide opening and sometimes even excised a dysplastic pulmonary valve. We now know that even though severe pulmonary insufficiency is well tolerated for some years, the large volume load results in marked right ventricular enlargement and progressive right cardiac failure. Furthermore, when failure occurs, pulmonary valve replacement does not usually result in much improvement, presumably because severe right ventricular dysfunction has resulted from myocardial fibrosis.

The presence of pulmonary insufficiency after balloon valvuloplasty is also common. Long-term observations in several series showed that 30–90% of patients exhibited pulmonary insufficiency [16–18]. Although in most individuals the insufficiency was mild and not associated with significant right ventricular enlargement, in a considerable proportion the insufficiency was moderate or severe. The younger the child at the time of balloon valvuloplasty, the more likely moderate to severe insufficiency developed. However, even in older children and adolescents, pulmonary insufficiency was noted. Also, the insufficiency on some occasions increased progressively over time. These observations are disturbing and provide further support to the recommendation that patients with peak systolic pressure gradients below 40–50 mmHg should not be subjected to the procedure, because potentially the treatment could be worse than the disease.

If marked pulmonary insufficiency does develop, the size of the right ventricle and its contractility should be assessed at first every 3 months and then every 6 months by ultrasound techniques. No specific criteria have been developed regarding indications for pulmonary valve replacement, but if there is progressive right ventricular enlargement and reduced contractility, surgery should not be delayed. Some attempts to construct a pulmonary valve from pericardium or other materials have been made, with varying success. Currently, the recommended approach is to insert a valved aortic homograft between the right ventricle and pulmonary artery, but recently considerable success has been achieved by percutaneous implantation of a pulmonary valve in patients with severe pulmonary insufficiency [19].

Right ventricular development

Although attention has largely been directed toward ventricular development, of equal importance is the capacity for tricuspid valve growth. Hypoplasia of the tricuspid valve is usually proportionate to ventricular size. However, occasionally the tricuspid valve orifice appears to be larger than might be expected in relation to the ventricular size. It is likely that this occurs when the chamber size is reduced by marked hypertrophy. Tricuspid valve diameter may therefore be a better index of capacity for development of the right ventricle after relief of obstruction. Currently, the predominant view is that the tricuspid valve grows only in proportion with body size, i.e., that the *Z*-score does not change with age, even if obstruction is relieved. However, more extensive long-term studies are crucial.

Growth of the right ventricular chamber has received most attention, but little thought has been given to right ventricular function. If the ventricle is small, the total number of myocytes at birth will be reduced, unless there is marked increase in myocardial thickness. Because postnatal increase in muscle mass is accomplished largely by hypertrophy of individual myocytes, rather than by increase in cell numbers, development of the right ventricle may be restricted and functional capacity limited. Furthermore, the hypoplastic right ventricle has been shown to have considerable disarray of muscle fibers and abnormality of relationships between capillaries and myocytes [8]. Whether these abnormalities can be resolved by early postnatal relief of obstruction has yet to be determined. Relief of pulmonary stenosis during fetal life is most likely to be beneficial in those fetuses in whom the pulmonary valve obstruction is acquired fairly late in gestation. If pulmonary atresia is acquired early in gestation, major technical hurdles would have to be overcome to relieve obstruction in very small fetuses.

References

1 Hsiao SM, Wu MH, Shih JC, Hsieh FJ. In utero progressive pulmonary stenosis successfully treated with transcatheter intervention after delivery. J Formos Med Assoc 2001;100:347–349.

2 Levin DL, Heymann MA, Rudolph AM. Morphological development of the pulmonary vascular bed in experimental pulmonic stenosis. Circulation 1979;59:179–182.

3 Tulzer G, Arzt W, Franklin RC, Loughna PV, Mair R, Gardiner HM. Fetal pulmonary valvuloplasty for critical pulmonary stenosis or atresia with intact septum. Lancet 2002;360:1567–1568.

4 Jonker SS, Zhang L, Louey S, Giraud GD, Thornburg KL, Faber JJ. Myocyte enlargement, differentiation, and proliferation kinetics in the fetal sheep heart. J Appl Physiol 2007;102:1130–1142.

5 Everett AW, Taylor RR, Sparrow MP. Increased protein synthesis during right ventricular hypertrophy following pulmonary stenosis in the dog. Recent Adv Stud Cardiac Struct Metab 1976;12:35–38.

6 Barbera A, Giraud GD, Reller MD, Maylie J, Morton MJ, Thornburg KL. Right ventricular systolic pressure load alters myocyte maturation in fetal sheep. Am J Physiol 2000;279:R1157–R1164.

7 Akiba T, Becker AE. Disease of the left ventricle in pulmonary atresia with intact ventricular septum. The limiting factor for long-lasting successful surgical intervention? J Thorac Cardiovasc Surg 1994;108:1–8.

8 Beçu L, Somerville J, Gallo A. "Isolated" pulmonary valve stenosis as part of more widespread cardiovascular disease. Br Heart J 1976;38:472–482.

9 Mahony L, Clyman RI, Heymann MA. Decreased contractility of the ductus arteriosus in experimental pulmonic stenosis. Circulation 1984;70:695–699.

10 Danilowicz D, Hoffman JI, Rudolph AM. Serial studies of pulmonary stenosis in infancy and childhood. Br Heart J 1975;37:808–818.

11 Anand R, Mehta AV. Natural history of asymptomatic valvar pulmonary stenosis diagnosed in infancy. Clin Cardiol 1997;20:377–980.

12 Drossner DM, Mahle WT. A management strategy for mild valvar pulmonary stenosis. Pediatr Cardiol 2008;29: 649–652.

13 Arzt W, Tulzer G, Aigner M, Mair R, Hafner E. Invasive intrauterine treatment of pulmonary atresia/intact ventricular septum with heart failure. Ultrasound Obstet Gynecol 2003;21:186–188.

14 Peterson RE, Levi DS, Williams RJ, Lai WW, Sklansky MS, Drant S. Echocardiographic predictors of outcome in fetuses with pulmonary atresia with intact ventricular septum. J Am Coll Cardiol 2008;51:1299–1308.

15 Roman KS, Fouron JC, Nii M, Smallhorn JF, Chaturvedi R, Jaeggi ET. Determinants of outcome in fetal pulmonary valve stenosis or atresia with intact ventricular septum. Am J Cardiol 2007;99:699–703.

16 Rao PS, Galal O, Patnana M, Buck SH, Wilson AD. Results of three to 10 year follow up of balloon dilatation of the pulmonary valve. Heart 1998;80:591–595.

17 Poon LK, Menahem S. Pulmonary regurgitation after percutaneous balloon valvoplasty for isolated pulmonary valvar stenosis in childhood. Cardiol Young 2003;13: 444–450.

18 Garty Y, Veldtman G, Lee K, Benson L. Late outcomes after pulmonary valve balloon dilatation in neonates, infants and children. J Invasive Cardiol 2005;17: 318–322.

19 Khambadkone S, Coats L, Taylor A *et al.* Percutaneous pulmonary valve implantation in humans: results in 59 consecutive patients. Circulation 2005;112:1189–1197.

16

CHAPTER 16

Tricuspid atresia and hypoplastic right ventricle

Tricuspid atresia represents complete absence of an opening between the right atrium and right ventricle. An associated ventricular septal defect is very common with tricuspid atresia, being present in about 90% of these individuals during infancy. The cardiac morphology in some patients is very similar to that described for one form of single ventricle: in the so-called Holmes heart, generally classified as single ventricle, the atrioventricular connection to the ventricles is that of a double-inlet left ventricle and a rudimentary chamber, which has some of the features of a right ventricle, gives rise to the pulmonary artery. There has been considerable controversy about whether tricuspid atresia should be considered one of the forms of single ventricle, but this has not been resolved. Functionally, the hemodynamic disturbances are the same and the therapeutic approach is the same, whatever the eventual decision regarding classification.

Morphological considerations

The morphology of the tricuspid valve varies considerably. Usually there is no vestige of a tricuspid valve and the portion of the right atrium overlying the right ventricle is purely muscular in composition. Occasionally, the tissue separating the atrium and ventricle is membranous, or partly membranous and partly muscular. Less frequently there is a small structure that has features of a valve with a pit or depression but no orifice.

The size of the right ventricle varies. In the majority of patients, the presence of a ventricular septal defect permits some blood flow into the right ventricular chamber. The inflow or sinus portion of the ventricle is absent, but the body or trabecular portion and the outflow or conus region are often quite well developed. The size of these portions of the ventricle varies, probably as a result of the size and position of the ventricular septal defect. The trabecular portion may be prominent, but when the ventricular septal defect is small at birth, only the conus is present. The ventricular septal defect may be of the perimembranous or malalignment types and occasionally is in the muscular septum (see Chapter 7). The defect varies in size from a large unrestrictive communication to a pinpoint opening. There is a tendency for the defect size to decrease postnatally, usually within the first 2–3 years after birth.

An atrial septal communication is necessary for both fetal and postnatal survival. The foramen ovale is usually of normal size or large and sometimes a fossa ovalis or ostium secundum type of defect is present. Prominent eustachian valves are also a common finding in individuals with tricuspid atresia. It has been suggested that these valves could possibly play a role in the etiology by modifying flow patterns during embryological development, but it is more likely that the alterations in flow during fetal life are responsible for their persistence.

Aortopulmonary transposition is commonly associated with tricuspid atresia, occurring in about one-quarter of all patients. The presence of transposition has formed the basis for one classification of tricuspid atresia.

Tricuspid atresia with normal aortopulmonary relationship

This group, also known as type 1, comprises 70–75% of patients. They may have no ventricular septal defect (type 1A), have a moderate-sized defect

Congenital Diseases of the Heart, 3rd edition. By A. Rudolph
 ISBN: 9781405162456

which is restrictive (type 1B), or have a large defect (type 1C). About half of all individuals with tricuspid atresia have the type 1B form. In the absence of a ventricular septal defect, a small amount of muscle tissue, sometimes with a small slit or area of fibrosis, just below the pulmonary valve may represent the right ventricle. The pulmonary valve and main pulmonary artery are small; pulmonary valvar stenosis is not uncommon, or there may be pulmonary atresia, but the left and right pulmonary arteries may be reasonably well developed. A patent ductus arteriosus is present; it may be small and often arises from the aorta at an acute inferior angle. The right atrium is large, with prominent pectinate muscles. The foramen ovale is patent and may be larger than normal. The left ventricle is slightly to moderately enlarged and hypertrophied and the aorta is dilated. The aortic isthmus is wider than normal in the infant, and coarctation of the aorta is not encountered.

When tricuspid atresia is associated with a ventricular septal defect that imposes no restriction between the ventricles, the right ventricle is usually fairly well developed. Although the inlet portion is absent, the trabecular and infundibular chambers may be almost normal in size. The pulmonary artery is large and this enlargement extends to the intrapulmonary vessels. The left atrium and ventricle are enlarged and the left ventricle is hypertrophied. The foramen ovale is open, but the orifice may be small. Pulmonary stenosis is not usually encountered when the ventricular septal defect is large. The ductus arteriosus is usually present postnatally but closes normally.

A small or medium-sized ventricular septal defect imposes some restriction between the ventricles. The degree of development of the right ventricle varies; the trabecular portion may be of reasonable size but is usually small. The conus is often normal, but may be small and narrow, with subvalvar stenosis, and the pulmonary valve may be stenosed. The pulmonary arteries are reasonably well developed and postnatally a normal ductus arteriosus is noted.

Tricuspid atresia with aortopulmonary transposition

Tricuspid atresia associated with transposition of the great arteries is known as type II; a ventricular septal defect is almost always present. Although it is possible that systemic blood flow could be supplied from the pulmonary artery through a ductus arteriosus, it appears that this is unusual, if it occurs at all. Therefore, a ventricular septal defect is necessary to provide systemic blood flow. The right ventricular infundibulum is usually quite well developed and leads to an aorta, which is anterior, with a valve that is quite cephalad in position. The ascending aorta is usually smaller than normal and there is a high incidence of aortic isthmus narrowing, often of severe degree, and aortic coarctation may be encountered. The pulmonary artery is placed posteriorly and the main branch vessels are large. The left atrium and ventricle show considerable enlargement and hypertrophy. Occasionally, patients with tricuspid atresia, ventricular septal defect, and aortopulmonary transposition also have subpulmonary stenosis.

Other anatomical disturbances may be associated with tricuspid atresia, such as truncus arteriosus communis. Mitral regurgitation may occur in association with left ventricular enlargement, usually when there is an associated ventricular septal defect. About 10–15% of patients with tricuspid atresia have a persistent left superior vena cava (SVC) that flows into the coronary sinus. This is an important consideration in performing an SVC to pulmonary artery anastomosis.

Infrequently, tricuspid atresia is associated with L-transposition or ventricular inversion and aortopulmonary transposition. In this condition the right atrium empties into the left ventricle through a mitral valve and this ventricle ejects into the pulmonary artery. The left atrium drains into the right ventricle through a tricuspid valve and the ventricle ejects into the aorta. Rarely, the tricuspid valve is atretic and induces functional disturbances similar to those of mitral atresia. This lesion is discussed in Chapter 11.

Embryological considerations

The embryological disturbances responsible for tricuspid atresia are not known, but possibly multiple mechanisms could be responsible. It was proposed that embryological development of pulmonary atresia could cause right ventricular hypoplasia, and tricuspid atresia resulted from diversion of flow away from the right side in early fetal life. This is unlikely because many individuals with tricuspid atresia and ventricular septal defect have a well-developed right ventricular infundibulum and pulmonary valve. Failure of ventricular alignment over the atrioventricular orifice could explain the development of tricuspid atresia. During cardiac development, the cardiac tube forms a rightward loop. The right ventricle develops from the bulbus cordis, which connects proximally with the left ventricle. The atrioventricular orifice leads into the left ventricle, but after looping, the ventricular septum migrates to the left and the atrioventricular orifice migrates to the right. This positions the right side of the atrioventricular orifice over the right ventricle to form the tricuspid valve. Failure of this migration could result in a double-inlet left ventricle if the common atrioventricular valve remains committed to the left ventricle. A similar disturbance in migration could affect positioning of the tricuspid valve over the right ventricle by a yet unexplained process. Another mechanism that has been suggested is that an *in utero* infection occurring very early in gestation could cause endocarditis of the valve, resulting in fusion of the leaflets; right ventricular hypoplasia is explained by absence of flow into the chamber.

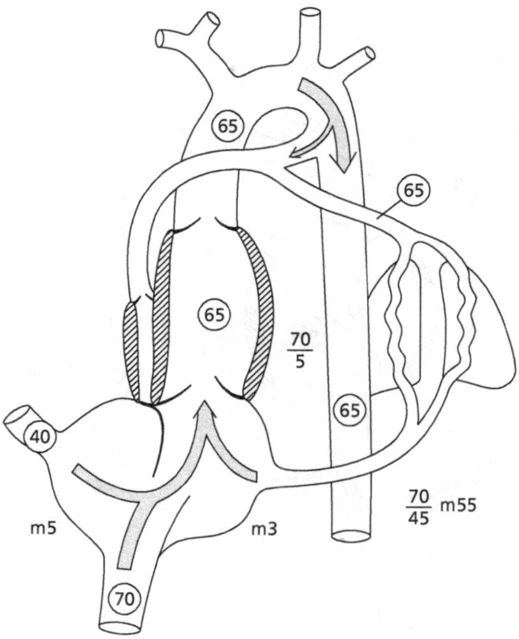

Figure 16.1 Tricuspid atresia with intact ventricular septum in a fetus: course of the circulation, oxygen saturations (circled), and pressures. m, mean pressure.

Hemodynamic considerations

Fetal circulation

Tricuspid atresia is compatible with survival and normal intrauterine development of the fetus, because the infant born with tricuspid atresia usually has no evidence of intrauterine distress or growth retardation. The total venous return from both the SVC and inferior vena cava (IVC) must pass through the foramen ovale. Thus, whereas normally only about 25% of combined ventricular output (CVO) traverses the foramen ovale (see Chapter 1), with tricuspid atresia the flow through the foramen ovale is four times greater and the foramen is considerably larger than normal. Blood from the SVC and IVC and pulmonary veins all flows into the left atrium and this results in complete admixture of all the systemic and umbilical venous blood returning to the heart in this chamber (Figure 16.1).

Assuming, as discussed in Chapter 1, that the CVO in the human fetus is about 450 mL/min per kg fetal body weight, that umbilical blood flow in the latter trimester is about 130 mL/min per kg, that umbilical venous oxygen saturation is about 85%, and that mixed systemic venous oxygen saturation is about 40%, then oxygen saturation of the mixed blood will be 52%. The usual difference in the oxygen saturations of blood distributed to the upper and lower parts of the fetal body is eliminated and saturation of blood distributed to the systemic and pulmonary circulations will be the same. The brain, which normally receives blood with an oxygen saturation of about 65%, will receive blood with a considerably lower oxygen saturation of 52%. It is unlikely that oxygen delivery to the brain is significantly reduced, because cerebral vasodilation in response to the hypoxemia can readily compensate to maintain oxygen supply. The oxygen saturation of blood delivered to the lungs will be slightly higher than normal, but the difference is probably not significant enough to materially alter pulmonary vascular resistance or pulmonary vascular development. In the fetus with tricuspid atresia and an intact ventricular septum, pulmonary blood flow is derived from the aorta

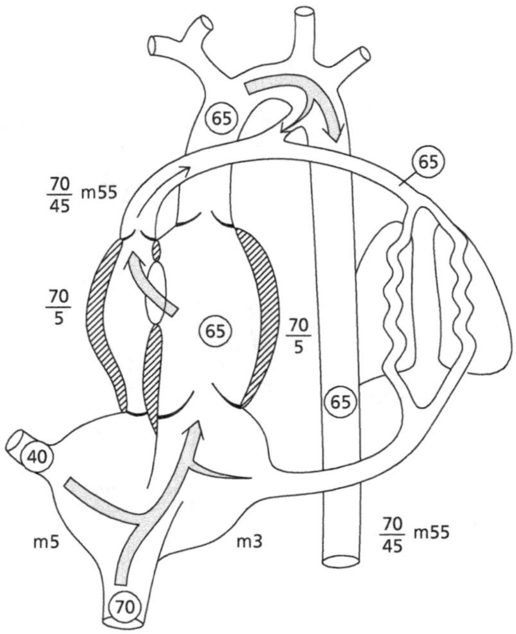

Figure 16.2 Tricuspid atresia with ventricular septal defect in a fetus: course of the circulation, oxygen saturations (circled), and pressures. m, mean pressure.

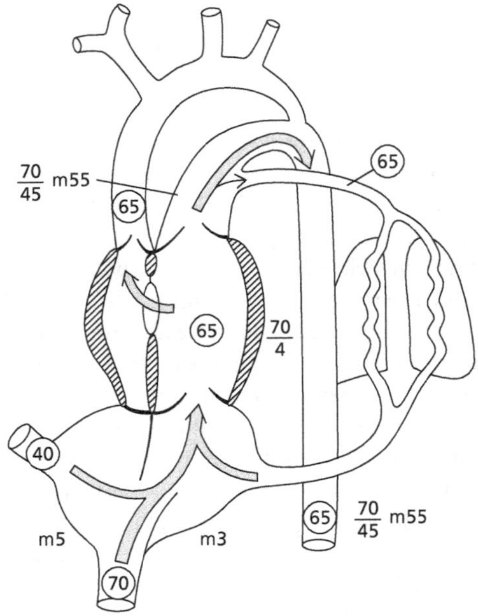

Figure 16.3 Tricuspid atresia associated with aortopulmonary transposition and a ventricular septal defect in a fetus: course of the circulation, oxygen saturations (circled), and pressures. m, mean pressure.

through the ductus arteriosus. When a ventricular septal defect is present, blood flow to the lungs may be provided either by flow of blood through the ductus arteriosus or by passage of blood from the left ventricle through the ventricular septal defect into the right ventricle and pulmonary artery (Figure 16.2). In either event, the Po_2 of blood perfusing the pulmonary circulation would be slightly higher than that in the normal fetal circulation. Possibly, it could result in some decrease in pulmonary vascular resistance and restrict development of pulmonary vascular smooth muscle (see Chapter 5). In view of the complete admixture of systemic and umbilical venous blood in the left atrium, there will also be no difference in the oxygen saturations of blood distributed to the various parts of the circulation in fetuses with tricuspid atresia with aortopulmonary transposition (Figure 16.3).

The slightly lower Po_2 and oxygen saturation of blood distributed to the heart and the brain do not appear to have any adverse effect on the fetus. Most fetuses with tricuspid atresia develop normally, but in a study of the outcome of 88 fetuses diagnosed with tricuspid atresia by ultrasound examination, four died *in utero* [1]. The cause of death was not apparent, but it has been suggested that constriction of the foramen ovale resulting in elevated venous pressure and hydrops could be responsible.

Tricuspid atresia with intact ventricular septum

When the ventricular septum is intact, total pulmonary blood flow is derived from the aorta through the ductus arteriosus. Whereas in the normal fetus a large proportion of passes across the ductus arteriosus from the pulmonary artery to the aorta, in the presence of tricuspid atresia with an intact ventricular septum only pulmonary blood flow traverses the ductus from the aorta to the pulmonary artery. The diameter of the ductus arteriosus may therefore be smaller than normal. Also, the ductus joins the descending aorta at an acute inferior angle compared with the normal oblique angle (see Chapter 6). Whether the ductus arteriosus responds in the usual manner to the stimuli that normally promote closure after birth has yet to be determined.

The aortic isthmus conducts about 10–15% of CVO in the normal fetus. In the fetus with tricuspid atresia and intact ventricular septum, the total cardiac output is ejected by the left ventricle into the ascending aorta, and the aortic isthmus carries the total blood flow to the descending aorta as well as pulmonary blood flow. This represents about 75% of CVO or about five to six times the normal flow. This probably accounts for the fact that the ascending aorta is large and the aortic isthmus has a wide diameter in the newborn infant with tricuspid atresia. The narrowed isthmus segment normally seen is not present in these infants; also, coarctation of the aorta has not been described in infants with tricuspid atresia and intact ventricular septum with normal origin of the aorta and pulmonary artery (see Chapter 12).

Tricuspid atresia with ventricular septal defect

Normal aortic and pulmonary artery relations

In the presence of a ventricular septal defect, it is difficult to predict the amount of blood that would flow through the defect into the right ventricle and pulmonary artery. Also, the amounts of blood that traverse the ductus arteriosus and the direction of flow could vary considerably. Blood from the left ventricle could pass through the right ventricle to the main pulmonary artery and be distributed either to the lungs, or through the ductus arteriosus to the descending aorta. This pattern of flow is likely to occur if the ventricular septal defect is large. However, if the defect is small, only a small volume of blood would pass to the right ventricle and pulmonary artery and it is then likely that blood would pass from the aorta through the ductus to the pulmonary circulation. It is difficult to predict which flow patterns prevail, but they are probably determined by the size of the ventricular septal defect and the degree of pulmonary stenosis (see Figure 16.2). It is not likely that aortic arch development would be affected.

With aortopulmonary transposition

When aortopulmonary transposition and a ventricular septal defect are present, blood is ejected from the left ventricle into the main pulmonary artery. The flow from the pulmonary artery through the ductus arteriosus to the descending aorta is probably similar to that which occurs normally in the fetus. However, if the ventricular septal defect is small and transmits little flow into the right ventricle and ascending aorta, a greater than normal flow must be carried by the ductus (see Figure 16.3).

In the fetus with tricuspid atresia and aortopulmonary transposition, the aorta arises from the hypoplastic right ventricle. Blood flow into the ascending aorta will be greatly affected by the size of the ventricular septal defect. If it is large, a reasonable amount of blood could enter the ascending aorta and it could be of normal size. Also, if aortic flow is not greatly reduced, flow across the isthmus could be adequate and the isthmus diameter could be normal. If the defect is smaller, flow into the ascending aorta would be limited and the ascending aorta would be hypoplastic; in addition aortic isthmus narrowing and aortic coarctation would be expected to be common (see Chapter 12). About 30–50% of patients with tricuspid atresia and transposition have aortic arch obstructions. If ascending aortic flow is restricted, an increased flow is carried by the ductus arteriosus to the descending aorta; if flow is severely limited, blood may flow retrogradely across the isthmus to provide some of the flow to the branches of the ascending aorta.

About one-third of individuals with tricuspid atresia and transposition have, in addition to the ventricular septal defect, some degree of pulmonary stenosis. If the stenosis is mild, it may not significantly influence the patterns of circulation. If it is more severe, it is necessary that the ventricular septal defect be large, because it will have to transmit the blood supply to the systemic circulation, umbilical circulation and, via the ductus arteriosus, most of the blood to the lungs.

Postnatal circulatory changes

The hemodynamic adjustments and consequent clinical features of tricuspid atresia after birth are influenced by the associated congenital anomalies, particularly the ventricular septal defect and aortopulmonary transposition. Three main hemodynamic complexes are discussed: tricuspid atresia with intact ventricular septum and hypoplastic right ventricle; tricuspid atresia with ventricular septal defect and normal origin of the great arteries; and tricuspid atresia with ventricular septal defect and aortopulmonary transposition.

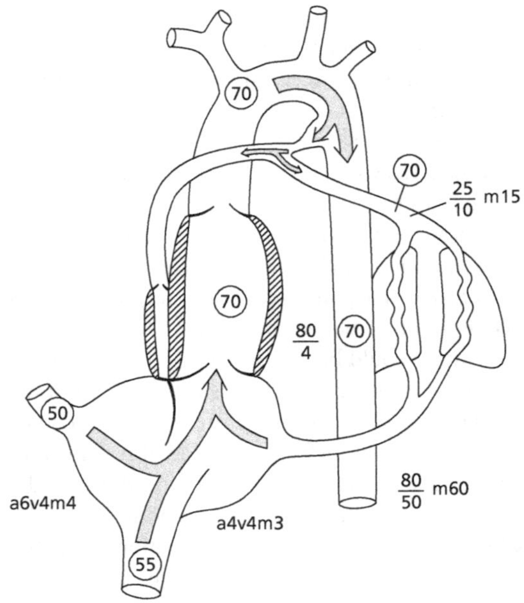

Figure 16.4 Tricuspid atresia with intact ventricular septum in a newborn infant: course of the circulation, oxygen saturations (circled), and pressures. Pulmonary blood flow is derived from the aorta through the ductus arteriosus. m, mean pressure.

Tricuspid atresia with intact ventricular septum

The course of the circulation after birth is essentially similar to that in the fetus, in that systemic and pulmonary venous admixture occurs at the left atrial level (Figure 16.4), but oxygen and carbon dioxide exchange must now take place in the lung instead of the placenta. The pulmonary vascular resistance may be expected to fall normally in response to an increase in alveolar oxygen levels associated with ventilation. If the medial muscle layer in pulmonary arterioles is not as well developed as in the normal infant, resistance could drop more rapidly than normal. Pulmonary blood flow is dependent on patency of the ductus arteriosus. As mentioned above, the ductus arteriosus tends to be small, because it transmits only blood flow to the lungs during fetal life. This is a relatively low flow compared with the postnatal requirements for pulmonary flow. The ductus may not be large enough to provide an adequate pulmonary flow.

Complete admixture of pulmonary and systemic venous returns occurs in the left atrium; the final oxygen saturation is therefore related to the pulmonary to systemic flow ratio (see Chapter 3). While the ductus is still open, a reasonably good pulmonary blood flow may be maintained. The infant will be cyanosed, but as long as pulmonary blood flow is adequate to provide oxygen uptake to satisfy tissue requirements, the infant will not demonstrate any clinical difficulties apart from the cyanosis. As the ductus arteriosus constricts, pulmonary blood flow falls. Systemic blood flow is usually well maintained, if not increased in response to the hypoxemia; with the decrease in pulmonary to systemic flow ratio, arterial oxygen saturation and Po_2 fall markedly. Eventually oxygen uptake falls below critical levels and anaerobic metabolism ensues, resulting in lactic acid accumulation and metabolic acidemia (see Chapter 3). The clinical manifestations in these infants are related to hypoxemia and acidemia rather than to cardiac failure. Hyperventilation occurs as a result of arterial and cerebral chemoreceptor stimulation by hypoxemia and acidemia, and even though pulmonary flow is low, adequate carbon dioxide elimination occurs, so that systemic arterial Pco_2 does not rise significantly.

The normal ductus arteriosus is relaxed when Po_2 falls to 35–45 mmHg. It is not known whether the ductus in infants with tricuspid atresia responds normally to Po_2, but if it does a drop in arterial Po_2 to below about 35 mmHg will tend to reopen the ductus, thus improving pulmonary blood flow. A balance may exist for some time after birth between the size of the ductus, pulmonary blood flow, and arterial Po_2. Eventually, the ductus tends to close even though Po_2 remains low, but the mechanisms responsible for the later closure are not known. The ductus arteriosus may close within a few days after birth, but its closure may be delayed for several weeks.

The size of the foramen ovale postnatally is important in infants with tricuspid atresia, because total systemic venous return must pass through it to the left atrium. The foramen ovale is invariably of adequate size and does not usually present any difficulties in the immediate postnatal period. During fetal life, except for pulmonary venous return, total venous return to the heart including umbilical–placental venous return passes through the foramen. After birth, the volume traversing the foramen ovale is considerably reduced by elimination of umbilical blood flow. Normally, a large increase in pulmonary blood flow occurs after birth; this results in elevation of left atrial pressure and functional closure of the foramen ovale. However, in infants with tricuspid atresia and intact ventricular septum, or with a ventricular septal defect and pulmonary stenosis, pulmonary blood flow is restricted after birth and the rise in left atrial pressure is limited. Passage of systemic venous blood through the foramen ovale is achieved with relatively small increases in right atrial pressure. Although inadequate size of the foramen ovale is not a significant concern in these infants, it may become a serious consideration after surgical introduction of an aortopulmonary shunt. The increased pulmonary venous return will elevate left atrial pressure and tend to close the valve of the foramen ovale; right atrial pressure will thus also have to be raised in order to maintain flow of systemic venous blood across the foramen ovale. A wide opening of the foramen may be indicated to reduce systemic venous pressure.

Tricuspid atresia with ventricular septal defect

Normal aortopulmonary relations

A wide spectrum of hemodynamic and clinical features may be associated with tricuspid atresia and ventricular septal defect depending on the size of the defect and the presence of right ventricular outflow tract stenosis. If the ventricular septal defect is very small or if there is marked right ventricular outflow obstruction, pulmonary blood flow will be restricted and the hemodynamic features will be similar to those described above for tricuspid atresia with intact ventricular septum.

The ventricular septal defect may be large enough so there is little or no restriction between the left and right ventricles. The pressures in the ventricles are similar and, in the absence of right ventricular outflow obstruction, systolic pressures in the aorta and pulmonary artery will be the same. With the fall in pulmonary vascular resistance after birth, pulmonary blood flow is readily established by flow through the ventricular septal defect into the right ventricular infundibulum and the pulmonary artery. Complete admixture of pulmonary and systemic venous returns occurs in the left atrium. The pulmonary to systemic flow ratio is determined by the relationship between systemic and pulmonary vascular resistances. During the first few days after birth, while pulmonary vascular resistance is still somewhat elevated, the increase in pulmonary blood flow is limited and systemic arterial oxygen saturation will be moderately reduced. With the subsequent fall in pulmonary vascular resistance, pulmonary blood flow increases markedly and, with the increase in pulmonary to systemic flow ratio to levels above 2.5, arterial oxygen saturation may reach levels as high as 88–92%. As mentioned above, it is possible that pulmonary vascular resistance may drop more rapidly than normal, so that a high pulmonary to systemic flow ratio could be achieved within a few days after birth. The high levels of pulmonary blood flow create an increased volume load on the left ventricle, and an increase in left ventricular end-diastolic and left atrial pressures. Left ventricular failure with pulmonary edema frequently ensues (Figure 16.5).

The increase in left atrial pressure will result in a corresponding increase in right atrial pressure to produce flow of systemic venous blood across the foramen. However, the elevation in left atrial

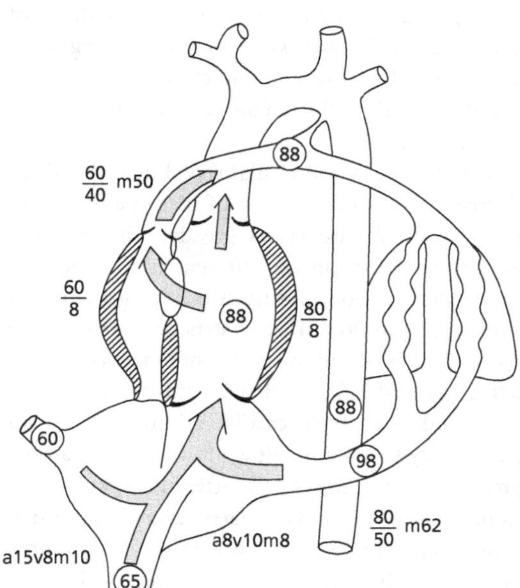

Figure 16.5 Tricuspid atresia with large ventricular septal defect in a newborn infant: course of the circulation, oxygen saturations (circled), and pressures. A large pulmonary blood flow has developed and cardiac failure often develops. m, mean pressure.

pressure also tends to close the foramen ovale, making the effective orifice smaller and thus causing a relatively greater increase in right atrial pressure, with systemic venous congestion. It is interesting to consider the phasic pressure relationships between the atria. Normally, the *v* wave in the left atrium is more prominent and the *a* wave in the right atrium is larger. An increase in pulmonary blood flow will increase the left atrial *v* wave, and thus tend to close the foramen ovale during this phase of the cardiac cycle. The flow of systemic venous blood across the foramen will occur predominantly in late diastole associated with atrial contraction and to a limited extent in early diastole. The right atrial *a* wave is increased and the main right-to-left atrial pressure difference is associated with atrial contraction.

Cardiac failure is often noted within 2–3 weeks after birth in these infants, whereas in ventricular septal defect without tricuspid atresia it tends to occur later (see Chapter 7 for discussion of cardiac failure). This could be related to a more rapid drop in pulmonary vascular resistance than occurs in the presence of ventricular septal defect alone. However, restriction of flow across the foramen ovale may be an important factor in the early manifestations of cardiac failure because systemic venous congestion will occur. Treatment of the cardiac failure may allow survival of the infant, and the subsequent course is variable.

The size of the ventricular septal defect tends to decrease with time in most of these patients, but the rate of closure varies greatly. This imposes an obstruction from the left ventricle to the pulmonary circulation, effectively behaving like a right ventricular outflow tract obstruction. Pulmonary blood flow falls, and this will result in a decrease in left atrial and left ventricular end-diastolic pressures and relief from cardiac failure. The fall in pulmonary to systemic flow ratio results in a progressive decrease in systemic arterial oxygen saturation, resulting in mild and later severe hypoxemia. This progression may begin within a few months after birth, but may be delayed for 3–4 years. Associated with the decrease in size of the ventricular septal defect, the pressure in the right ventricle falls progressively. A similar sequence of events may occur if there is hypertrophy, or lack of growth with age, of the infundibular region of the right ventricle. Right ventricular systolic pressure remains at left ventricular and aortic levels but pulmonary arterial pressure falls. This phenomenon is much less likely than ventricular septal defect closure. If the ventricular septal defect does not become smaller, and right ventricular and pulmonary arterial pressures remain high, there is a serious risk of pulmonary vascular disease. The increase in pulmonary vascular resistance also results in a decrease in pulmonary blood flow and pulmonary to systemic flow ratio, with a progressive decrease in arterial oxygen saturation.

About 50% of all infants born with tricuspid atresia have a moderately or severely restrictive ventricular septal defect and the hemodynamic features are related to the size of the defect. If the defect is severely restrictive, pulmonary blood flow will be low and hypoxemia will be the dominant feature, as in infants with an intact ventricular septum (see Chapter 16). If the defect is moderately large, the features will be similar to those described with nonrestrictive defects. However, the manifestations of cardiac failure are less evident and the infants have greater degrees of hypoxemia. Pulmonary blood flow is moderately increased, with pulmonary to systemic flow ratios of 1.5–2.5 and mild cyanosis is evident. The ventricular septal defect tends to become progressively smaller after birth, so that pulmonary blood flow falls and the degree of cyanosis increases.

With aortopulmonary transposition

When tricuspid atresia is associated with aortopulmonary transposition, the ventricular septal defect is usually large and there is no pressure difference between the left and right ventricles at birth. After birth, the course of the circulation is not very different from that in fetal life. However, after removal of the placental circulation and establishment of the postnatal pulmonary circulation there is reorientation of vascular resistances. Pulmonary blood flow is increased, and because all the pulmonary and systemic venous blood mixes in the left atrium, the final common arterial saturation is determined by the pulmonary to systemic flow ratio. In the immediate postnatal period, when pulmonary vascular resistance has not yet fallen markedly, pulmonary flow will not be very large and moderate arterial oxygen desaturation with moderate cyanosis may be evident. Later, pulmonary vascular resistance falls, perhaps more rapidly than usual. Pulmonary blood flow increases markedly, resulting in volume overload of the left ventricle and failure is common. Arterial oxygen saturation may be decreased to only 85–90% and thus mild cyanosis is noted.

Infants with tricuspid atresia and transposition often have associated aortic isthmus narrowing or aortic coarctation of moderate to severe degree. Blood flow to the descending aorta may, as in fetal life, be largely or wholly dependent on patency of the ductus arteriosus postnatally if aortic obstruction is severe. Only blood distributed to the coronary circulation and upper body would pass through the ventricular septal defect and into the ascending aorta. The ventricular septal defect would thus not have to be very large to accommodate this flow. This is an important consideration if it is planned to correct the aortic obstruction and close the ductus arteriosus, because total systemic flow to the upper and lower body would now have to traverse the ventricular septal defect. If it is too small to accommodate this increased blood flow, a pressure gradient will develop between the ventricles. The left ventricle may not be adequate to generate a pressure high enough to provide an adequate systemic blood flow, and systemic output will fall.

Flow to the descending aorta is maintained through the ductus arteriosus when aortic isthmus obstruction is severe. Descending aortic pressure depends on the size of the ductus arteriosus and on the relationship between pulmonary and systemic vascular resistances. While the ductus is widely dilated in the postnatal period, an adequate systemic blood flow and systemic arterial pressure can be maintained with pulmonary arterial pressure at normal postnatal systemic arterial pressures. The flow through the ductus arteriosus is lower than during fetal life, because umbilical–placental flow is eliminated. Therefore, it is possible that modest degrees of constriction of the ductus arteriosus could occur without a pressure gradient developing. Greater degrees of constriction will result in development of a pressure gradient, and if pulmonary arterial pressure is not maintained at adequate levels, systemic blood flow to the lower body will decrease, with a reduction in descending aortic pressure and inadequate tissue perfusion. A lack of oxygen supply to the tissues will result, with lactic acid accumulation and metabolic acidemia (see Chapter 3). Renal perfusion pressure and blood flow will fall and oliguria or anuria result. One of the factors inducing constriction of the ductus arteriosus is Po_2 of systemic arterial blood. Mixed arterial Po_2 is usually maintained at relatively high levels postnatally, so that the ductus may constrict, thus interfering with systemic blood flow to the lower body. In many lesions in which blood flow to the descending aorta is supplied by right-to-left shunting through the ductus arteriosus, oxygen saturations in the upper and lower body are different. However, with tricuspid atresia, because there is complete admixture of pulmonary and systemic venous blood in the left atrium, oxygen saturations in the aorta and pulmonary artery are the same, so no difference in saturation between the ascending and descending aortae is noted.

The patterns of blood flow are affected by many variables in infants with tricuspid atresia, ventricular septal defect, and aortopulmonary transposition (Figure 16.6). Flow of blood from the right to left atrium is affected by the size of the atrial communication. The distribution of blood flow from the left ventricle is determined by the relative resistances of the pulmonary circulation, the ventricular septal defect, and the right ventricular infundibulum. With aortic arch obstruction, the size of the ductus arteriosus and upper and lower body vascular resistances also influence blood flow distribution.

Since pulmonary vascular resistance tends to drop rapidly, pulmonary blood flow increases markedly in the first few days postnatally. This results in a high pulmonary to systemic flow ratio and therefore a relatively high mixed arterial oxygen saturation and Po_2. The left ventricle increases its stroke volume as a result of the increased pulmonary venous return to the left atrium, and left ventricular end-diastolic pressure increases. If the left ventricular output is not large enough to maintain adequate systemic blood flow, some increase in systemic vascular resistance will occur, with compromise of peripheral blood flow but maintenance of adequate perfusion pressure. The high mixed arterial oxygen saturation will tend to produce ductus arteriosus constriction, resulting in an increase

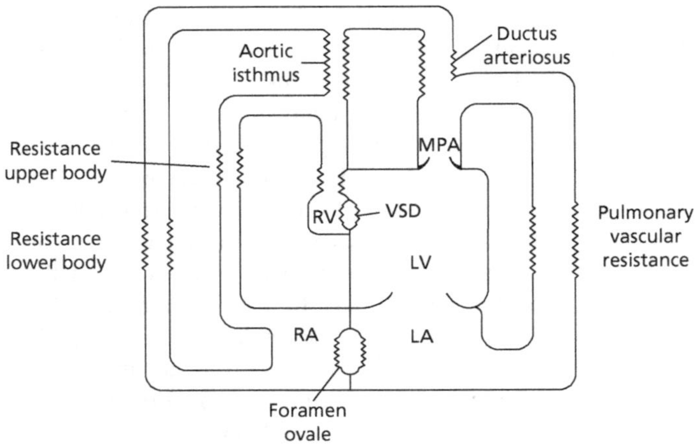

Figure 16.6 This circulation in a newborn infant with tricuspid atresia, aortopulmonary transposition, and a large ventricular septal defect. The circulatory distribution is influenced by the resistances at different sites in the circulation, as described in the text. LA, left atrium; LV, left ventricle; MPA, main pulmonary artery; RA, right atrium; RV, right ventricle; VSD, ventricular septal defect.

in outflow resistance to the lower body circulation. Left ventricular output would thus be directed preferentially, first to the pulmonary circulation, then to the ascending aorta, and last to the descending aorta. With increasing ductus arteriosus constriction, descending aortic pressure falls, with the consequences described above. Since systemic blood flow, especially that to the lower body, is reduced, total systemic venous return falls and this, with the high pulmonary blood flow, further increases the pulmonary to systemic flow ratio and mixed arterial oxygen saturation. Ductus constriction may be enhanced, aggravating the hemodynamic disturbance. Death results from a combination of left ventricular failure associated with the high pulmonary blood flow and metabolic acidemia due to tissue hypoxia associated with inadequate perfusion, particularly of the lower body.

The importance of the foramen ovale in this lesion is similar to that described above in the section on tricuspid atresia with ventricular septal defect and normal origin of the great arteries.

Clinical features

The associated lesions and the resulting hemodynamic disturbances determine the clinical features of tricuspid atresia.

Tricuspid atresia with intact ventricular septum

As a result of the inadequate pulmonary blood flow the main presenting feature is hypoxemia with cyanosis. The infant is usually cyanotic within a few hours after birth when the ductus arteriosus constricts, but cyanosis may be mild for several weeks after birth. Some infants present with severe cyanosis, hyperventilation, and acidemia within the first week after birth but others do quite well for several months, although it is rare for them to survive more than 3–4 months without treatment. The variability is almost certainly related to the diameter of the ductus arteriosus and the rate at which it closes. Occasionally, an infant who has been only mildly cyanotic may suddenly develop a marked increase in the degree of cyanosis and become progressively hypoxemic and acidemic, due to rapid closure of the ductus. When the infant becomes severely cyanotic, hyperventilation and peripheral pallor occur and unconsciousness follows; if resuscitative measures are not used, survival is unlikely. The episodic hypoxic spells noted in patients with pulmonary stenosis with ventricular septal defect are occasionally encountered in patients with tricuspid atresia.

On physical examination, cyanosis of varying degree is evident. Clubbing of the fingers and toes, common in older cyanosed children, is not usually noted before 3–4 months of age. Resting hyperventilation of moderate degree is common, but the lungs are clear on auscultation. In older children neck vein pulsation with a prominent *a* wave may be noted. The liver often is palpable 2–3 cm below the right costal margin and is not pulsatile; usually it is not enlarged but is displaced downward by the hyperinflated lungs. The peripheral pulses are usually prominent, particularly in the infant with marked cyanosis, probably due to increased cardiac output and stroke volume. The extremities are warm.

Examination of the heart is usually unremarkable. The most striking feature is the decreased impulse at the lower left sternal border related to lack of the right ventricle. This finding on palpation is particularly unusual in a newborn infant with cyanosis and is very suggestive of the diagnosis of tricuspid atresia. The cardiac impulse is predominantly apical but is not hyperactive in most infants and there is no clinical cardiomegaly. The first heart sound is accentuated; the second heart sound is invariably single and is often loud, particularly at the lower left sternal border, associated with aortic valve closure. In early infancy a grade 2–3/6 high-frequency continuous murmur may be heard at the upper left sternal border and under the left clavicle, resulting from flow through a small patent ductus arteriosus. It rarely has the rough quality of the murmur in patients with isolated patent ductus arteriosus because the ductus is narrow. In many infants with tricuspid atresia, no murmurs are audible. This may be related to the fact that the ductus is very small or that it has closed and pulmonary flow is provided by aortopulmonary collateral arteries.

Tricuspid atresia with ventricular septal defect

Normal aortopulmonary relations

As mentioned on p. 427, the size of the ventricular defect varies from a very small opening to a large hole with no restriction between the ventricles. If the defect is small, the features are similar to those with intact ventricular septum. However, a medium-frequency systolic murmur is audible at the lower left sternal border. The intensity and duration vary from grade 2/6 occupying only one-third of systole with a tiny defect, to grade 4/6 occupying most of systole with a somewhat larger defect. The cyanosis usually progresses rapidly within the first 3–4 months due to spontaneous closure of the defect and as this occurs, the murmur becomes softer and shorter.

Infants with unrestrictive ventricular septal defects often have moderate cyanosis in the immediate neonatal period but this usually becomes less prominent after the first week. By 2–3 weeks after birth, the arterial oxygen saturation is often 88–92%. Frequently there are no symptoms for 2–3 weeks after birth, but symptoms of cardiac failure, with dyspnea and tachypnea and excessive perspiration, soon become manifest. The peripheral pulses are initially normal but become weak when the infant is in failure. Often there is also pallor due to peripheral vasoconstriction. The liver is often enlarged considerably, to as much as 4–6 cm below the costal margin; occasionally the spleen may be slightly enlarged. Rales may be heard in the lungs. The heart is clinically enlarged and there is a hyperactive apical impulse associated with left ventricular volume overload. The first heart sound is well heard at the apex; the second sound may be of normal intensity but is often accentuated and may be well split. A loud, harsh, pansystolic murmur of grade 4–5/6 intensity is heard at the lower left sternal border and a low-frequency mid-diastolic murmur is often heard at the apex. These clinical features are very similar to those encountered in infants with a large isolated ventricular septal defect, apart from the cyanosis. However, because cyanosis is so mild, it may not be appreciated and the diagnosis of a large ventricular septal defect, not associated with other lesions, may be entertained (see Chapter 16). The cardiac failure may be severe and without medication or surgical treatment, the infant will succumb.

Diuretic and digitalis therapy may control cardiac failure and the subsequent course is variable, depending on whether the size of the ventricular septal defect decreases and whether right ventricular outflow obstruction or pulmonary vascular disease develops. All these changes will decrease pulmonary blood flow and result in similar changes in the clinical signs. The respiratory rate decreases and dyspnea improves, sweating is less prominent, and feeding improves. However, after a period of initial improvement the cyanosis increases, first becoming more prominent with exertion and then increasing progressively even at rest. This is associated with a progressive decrease in exercise tolerance. The heart size decreases and left ventricular hyperactivity becomes less apparent. The apical mid-diastolic murmur softens and later disappears. There is no consistent change in the systolic murmur, but it may become less harsh and shorter in duration as flow across the defect decreases. The second heart sound may be helpful in distinguishing between the fall in pulmonary blood flow resulting from an increase in pulmonary vascular resistance and that resulting from closure of the ventricular septal defect. Closure of the defect may decrease the intensity of the second sound, but it may become louder and narrower with increased pulmonary vascular resistance. The clinical course of patients with high pulmonary vascular resistance is discussed in Chapter 5. In older children, progressive clinical cardiomegaly occurs and a medium-frequency decrescendo systolic murmur is heard at the apex, radiating to the axilla, as a result of the development of mitral regurgitation.

With aortopulmonary transposition

In the more common form of this lesion there is no pulmonary or subpulmonary stenosis, so systolic pressure in the pulmonary artery is equal to that in the left ventricle. The clinical picture is variable and depends on the relationship of the resistances (see Figure 16.6). Most infants develop severe symptoms soon after birth. The main features are those of cardiac failure and of inadequate systemic blood flow; cyanosis is usually mild. When aortic isthmus obstruction is present, the femoral pulses may be normal after birth but are poorly felt or absent after the ductus arteriosus constricts. Differential cyanosis is not evident, as systemic and pulmonary venous returns are mixed completely in the left atrium and ventricle, so blood of similar oxygen saturation is distributed to the aorta and pulmonary artery. As pulmonary vascular resistance falls, evidence of left ventricular failure appears, with dyspnea, sweating, increasing cardiomegaly, and marked hyperactivity of the left ventricular impulse. If the ventricular septal defect is restrictive, the pulses in the upper extremities also become weak. The diagnosis of aortic isthmus obstruction may not be considered, because pulses may be weak in both the upper and lower extremities. If the ventricular septal defect is very restrictive at birth, systemic blood flow may be dependent on the ductus arteriosus and constriction of the ductus will result in a fall in systemic arterial pressure and blood flow.

The first heart sound is usually accentuated at the apex and the second sound is accentuated at the upper left sternal border and is usually only narrowly split. A medium-frequency pansystolic murmur of grade 3–4/6 intensity is heard at the mid and lower left sternal border. A low-frequency mid-diastolic murmur is often heard at the apex. Associated with the left ventricular failure and elevation in left atrial pressure, rales may be heard in both lungs. The liver becomes enlarged, often to 4–6 cm below the costal margin, because right atrial pressure becomes elevated considerably, and ascites and peripheral edema may occur. If systemic blood flow is markedly reduced, peripheral vasoconstriction with generalized pallor occurs, and severe metabolic acidemia may result due to inadequate oxygenation of the tissues. The clinical picture may be very similar to that of aortic atresia (see Chapter 11).

The current management in these infants is to correct the aortic arch obstruction surgically and to reduce pulmonary arterial pressure and blood flow by banding the pulmonary artery. This will result in improvement of cardiac failure, but will increase the degree of cyanosis. Postoperatively, a major concern is that progressive closure of the ventricular septal defect will induce functional subaortic stenosis with increasing pressure loading of the left ventricle. This is discussed in the section on management below.

Complications

The complications of most concern are those resulting from right-to-left shunt through the foramen ovale. Systemic arterial emboli may occur, the most serious of which is cerebral embolus. Cerebral abscess is most likely initiated by small septic emboli. Infective endocarditis is also a potential complication and the importance of prophylaxis must be stressed with parents and patients.

Investigations

Electrocardiography

The characteristic features of the electrocardiogram in patients with tricuspid atresia are right atrial hypertrophy, reflected by tall peaked P waves in standard leads II and III and the right precordial leads, left axis deviation, and left ventricular hypertrophy. Occasionally, atrioventricular conduction time is prolonged. These features are invariably present in patients with tricuspid atresia with intact ventricular septum and in the majority of those with ventricular septal defect and normal aortopulmonary position. The R wave is usually absent in the right precordial leads, but occasional individuals with an associated ventricular septal defect and a fairly well-developed right ventricle will have right precordial R waves evident. I have encountered several infants with ventricular septal defect and normal aortopulmonary position in whom the electrocardiogram showed pure R waves of 4–8 mm in V4R and V1 in addition to evidence of left ventricular hypertrophy. Some patients with tricuspid atresia, ventricular septal defect, and aortopulmonary transposition may have a frontal axis in the normal range and also demonstrate R waves in the right precordial leads.

Chest radiography

When pulmonary blood flow is reduced, the vascular markings in the lungs are poorly defined and the cardiac diameter is normal. The main pulmonary artery segment is not seen and the ascending aorta and aortic arch may be prominent. The right heart border may show a bulge at the lower edge, reflecting right atrial enlargement. The cardiac apex may be displaced downward and to the left, reflecting dominance of the left ventricle.

When pulmonary blood flow is increased, pulmonary vascular markings are increased; when cardiac failure occurs the vessel margins become hazy, particularly in the hilar regions, due to pulmonary edema. The heart is enlarged and frequently the apex is displaced downward to the left and posteriorly, reflecting left ventricular enlargement. The pulmonary artery segment may be normal in size or even prominent when there is normal aortopulmonary position; usually it is not well seen in the frontal projection when aortopulmonary transposition is present but the superior mediastinum may be widened in the lateral view. In older patients the heart nay be markedly enlarged and the left atrium is also very large as a result of the presence of mitral regurgitation.

Echocardiography

Ultrasound studies can usually define the morphological features of tricuspid atresia as well as the associated anomalies. The important features to evaluate include:

- size of the atrial septal communication;
- size of the right ventricle and pulmonary arteries;
- presence and severity of infundibular or pulmonary stenosis;
- presence and size of a ventricular septal defect;
- relationship of the aorta and pulmonary artery;
- presence and size of the ductus arteriosus;
- presence of aortic isthmus narrowing or coarctation;
- degree of mitral regurgitation and left ventricular function.

Following surgery, additional information should be obtained relating to further management (discussed below).

The atrial septal opening can be imaged, and with two-dimensional and color flow Doppler techniques the size of the communication can be determined. Bulging of the septum into the left atrium suggests that the atrial opening is restrictive. The position of the aorta and pulmonary artery should be assessed to determine whether they are normally related or transposed. Imaging of the right ventricle will show the cavity size and whether both outflow portions are present. It is important to detect the presence of right ventricular infundibular stenosis when the pulmonary artery arises from the right ventricle, but especially if there is transposition, because this creates subaortic stenosis. Although the pressure gradient can be estimated from peak velocity in Doppler flow studies, it may not be reliable, because the stenotic area may have some length. The size of the ventricular septal defect should be determined and the pressure gradient between the left and right ventricles estimated.

The aortic arch must be imaged carefully, particularly if there is aortopulmonary transposition, for the presence of aortic isthmus narrowing and aortic coarctation. The patency and size of the ductus arteriosus and pattern of flow in the ductus are examined by color flow Doppler. Left ventricular size in systole and diastole should be measured, and the presence and severity of mitral regurgitation and ventricular function assessed. This is most important if it is planned to perform cavopulmonary anastomosis.

Cardiac catheterization and angiocardiography

Cardiac catheterization was the mainstay of diagnosis of tricuspid atresia and the associated anomalies prior to the advent of ultrasonography. Since these techniques were introduced, cardiac catheterization is not often indicated in the initial evaluation of infants with tricuspid atresia. It is now mainly indicated prior to a procedure to bypass the return of venous blood from the right atrium to the pulmonary arteries directly. Cardiac catheterization and angiography are important in determining pulmonary arterial pressure and pulmonary vascular resistance, and the presence of constriction or kinking of pulmonary arteries. Left ventricular end-diastolic pressure is measured and the presence and degree of mitral regurgitation assessed. In some centers, balloon atrial septostomy is recommended in most infants with tricuspid atresia because of concerns that the foramen ovale may become restrictive (see Chapter 16).

From the groin approach the catheter can be readily passed across the foramen ovale to the left atrium and ventricle. From the left ventricle the catheter can also be manipulated into the aorta or, with transposition, into the pulmonary artery. Unless the ventricular septal defect is very small, the catheter can then be manipulated through the defect into the right ventricle and pulmonary artery or, with aortopulmonary transposition, into the aorta.

Oxygen saturation

The most important finding in tricuspid atresia is complete admixture of systemic and pulmonary venous return in the left atrium.

In patients with decreased pulmonary blood flow, systemic venous oxygen saturation is low. In infants with intact ventricular septum, it may be reduced to 20–30%. There is no significant difference in SVC, IVC, and right atrial blood samples. Left atrial oxygen saturation is reduced considerably, the amount of reduction depending on the pulmonary to systemic flow ratio. When pulmonary flow is markedly reduced, oxygen saturation levels as low as 30–40% may be recorded. Left ventricular and peripheral arterial oxygen saturations are similar to oxygen saturations in the left atrium, but commonly left atrial samples may be variable due to inadequate mixing of pulmonary venous and foramen ovale streams in the left atrium. Pulmonary venous blood is usually fully saturated with oxygen in these patients. Since there is hyperventilation relative to the decreased pulmonary blood flow, the Po_2 of pulmonary venous blood is often raised to above 100 mmHg while the infant is breathing air. Pulmonary venous Pco_2 may be decreased to 15–20 mmHg and pH increased to 7.42–7.48.

In patients with increased pulmonary blood flow, the oxygen saturations in the SVC, IVC, and right atrium are normal or only slightly reduced (50–70%). Left atrial, left ventricular, and systemic arterial oxygen saturations are usually slightly or moderately reduced, depending on the pulmonary to systemic flow ratio; levels of 75–92% may be recorded. The oxygen saturation data are similar when there is normal aortopulmonary position or aortopulmonary transposition, and also if aortic isthmus obstruction is present. Oxygen saturation in the pulmonary artery is identical to that in the systemic arteries. Pulmonary venous saturation may be normal, but when pulmonary congestion and edema are present, it may be reduced and oxygen saturation may vary in different pulmonary veins, depending on local alveolar ventilation–perfusion relationships.

Pressures

Infant with intact ventricular septum

Right atrial pressure exceeds left atrial pressure. Usually there are prominent *a* waves in the vena cava and right atrial pressure recordings, sometimes reaching 10–15 mmHg. The mean pressure difference between the right and left atria is usually not more than 3–5 mmHg in the newborn infant. The left atrial pressure level is usually normal, with a mean pressure of 2–5 mmHg, but the normal prominent *v* wave is usually not present when pulmonary blood flow is decreased; the *a* and *v* waves are of similar height. Left ventricular and aortic systolic pressures are usually normal, as is left ventricular end-diastolic pressure.

Ventricular septal defect and normal aortopulmonary position

Right atrial pressure is increased, with mean levels up to 15 mmHg, but it may be higher if left ventricular failure has developed. Left atrial mean pressure is also increased, and there may be a mean pressure difference of as much as 8–10 mmHg between the right and left atria. The right atrial *a* wave may be very tall and may reach 25–30 mmHg. The left atrial *v* wave is prominent, particularly when there is a large pulmonary venous return. Left ventricular end-diastolic pressure is increased, especially if there is cardiac failure. Left ventricular and aortic pressures are usually normal.

The pressures in the right ventricle and pulmonary artery are related to the degree of obstruction at the ventricular septal defect and the right ventricular infundibulum. It is unusual that the ventricular septal defect is unrestrictive. With large defects, pressures in the right ventricle and pulmonary artery are usually slightly lower than those on the left side in the young infant. Right ventricular and pulmonary arterial systolic pressures are often 40–60 mmHg, whereas left ventricular and aortic systolic levels are 80–90 mmHg. However, right and left ventricular pressures may be equal. A pressure difference may also be recorded between the right ventricle and the pulmonary artery. In older children pulmonary arterial pressure is usually considerably lower than systemic arterial pressure, because the ventricular septal defect becomes restrictive or outflow tract stenosis of the right ventricle develops.

Tricuspid atresia, ventricular septal defect, and aortopulmonary transposition

The atrial pressure relationships are similar to those in patients with normal aortopulmonary position. Systolic pressures in the left ventricle and the pulmonary artery are usually equal but there may be a pressure gradient of mild degree. Systolic pressure in the right ventricle and ascending aorta are usually equal to that in the left ventricle in the newborn infant; left ventricular pressure is normal. However, systolic pressure in the right ventricle and aorta may be 10–15 mmHg lower than that in the left ventricle in the presence of restriction of the ventricular septal defect or right ventricular infundibular stenosis. In children who undergo banding of the pulmonary artery, left ventricular systolic pressure may be markedly elevated and there is a large systolic gradient across the ventricular septal defect, which may increase progressively. In the presence of aortic isthmus obstruction, pressure in the descending aorta may be considerably lower than that in the pulmonary artery and pulse pressure be reduced. If the ductus arteriosus constricts markedly, descending aortic pressure may be reduced to 30–40 mmHg, with a very narrow pulse pressure.

Blood flows

In patients with tricuspid atresia, the pulmonary and systemic blood flows can be readily calculated if oxygen consumption is known, and pulmonary to systemic flow ratios can be determined easily. Systemic arterial and mixed systemic venous oxygen saturations can be measured to provide the systemic arteriovenous difference. Pulmonary venous blood can usually be sampled, but it may not be possible to obtain a pulmonary arterial sample. However, because systemic and pulmonary arterial saturations are identical, pulmonary arteriovenous difference can be calculated from the difference between pulmonary venous and systemic arterial oxygen content.

The equations for calculating flow are as follows:

$$\text{Systemic blood flow } (\dot{Q}\text{s}) = \frac{\dot{V}\text{o}_2}{C\text{sao}_2 - C\text{mvo}_2}$$

$$\text{Pulmonary blood flow } (\dot{Q}\text{p}) = \frac{\dot{V}\text{o}_2}{C\text{pvo}_2 - C\text{sao}_2}$$

Pulmonary to systemic flow ratio ($\dot{Q}$p/$\dot{Q}$s)

$$= \frac{C\text{sao}_2 - C\text{mvo}_2}{C\text{pvo}_2 - C\text{sao}_2}$$

where $\dot{V}\text{o}_2$ represents oxygen consumption, $C\text{sao}_2$ systemic arterial oxygen content, $C\text{mvo}_2$ mixed venous (right atrial) oxygen content, and $C\text{pvo}_2$ pulmonary venous oxygen content. Effective pulmonary flow ($\dot{Q}$ep) represents that portion of the mixed venous return that eventually reaches the lung for oxygenation and is calculated from the equation:

$$\dot{Q}\text{ep} = \frac{\dot{V}\text{o}_2}{C\text{pvo}_2 - C\text{mvo}_2}$$

Systemic blood flow is increased in children with marked systemic arterial hypoxemia but is decreased in those with large ventricular septal defects and cardiac failure. Pulmonary blood flow is decreased in patients with hypoxemia and increased in those with ventricular septal defects and relatively low pulmonary vascular resistance.

The presence of aortic isthmus narrowing or interruption usually interferes with the ability to calculate systemic blood flow when the descending aorta receives some of its blood supply from the pulmonary artery, because ascending and descending aortic oxygen content differs. This is *not* the case in patients with tricuspid atresia, because aortic and pulmonary arterial oxygen contents are the same.

The pulmonary to systemic flow ratio determines the systemic arterial oxygen saturation, because there is complete admixture of systemic and pulmonary venous bloods. The relationship between systemic arterial oxygen saturation and pulmonary to systemic flow ratio is discussed in Chapter 2.

Shunts

Calculation of shunts is complicated by the fact that there is admixture of pulmonary and systemic venous returns. Shunts cannot be calculated in the usual manner, because the actual amounts of blood passing from the systemic to the pulmonary and from the pulmonary to the systemic circulations are different from those that recirculate. Therefore, it is helpful to introduce the concept of anatomical and physiological shunts discussed in Chapter 4.

Because the total systemic venous return passes across the foramen ovale, the anatomical right-to-left shunt is equal to systemic blood flow. The physiological right-to-left shunt reflects that portion of the systemic venous return that does not pass to the lungs and is represented by the equation:

$$\text{Physiological right-to-left shunt} = \dot{Q}s - \dot{Q}ep$$

Anatomical left-to-right shunt is represented by the total pulmonary blood flow, because this is derived from flow to the right from the left ventricle, or to the pulmonary artery from the aorta through a patent ductus arteriosus. Physiological left-to-right shunt reflects the proportion of blood oxygenated in the lungs that recirculates to the lungs and can be calculated from the equation:

$$\text{Physiological left-to-right shunt} = \dot{Q}p - \dot{Q}ep$$

Angiocardiography

Angiography is an important part of the study of patients with tricuspid atresia. Most details of morphology are now usually clearly resolved by ultrasound studies. The most important information to be obtained by angiocardiography is the presence and degree of mitral regurgitation and the detailed morphology of the pulmonary arteries. This information is important if it is planned to refer the child for caval or atrial to pulmonary artery anastomosis (Fontan or modified Fontan procedure). Left ventricular injection of contrast material provides information about mitral valve insufficiency, as well as presence or absence of a ventricular septal defect and the size of the right ventricle. It also delineates the position of the great arteries and whether there is aortopulmonary transposition. The pulmonary arteries can be best visualized if an injection of contrast material is made directly into the arteries. Efforts should therefore be made to manipulate the catheter into the vessel. This may be done from the right atrium to left atrium and left ventricle and through the ventricular septal defect into the right ventricle and pulmonary artery. With aortopulmonary transposition, attempts should be made to enter the pulmonary artery from the left ventricle. If a systemic-to-pulmonary arterial shunt has been introduced, it may be possible to catheterize the pulmonary artery through the shunt from a retrograde arterial approach. Catheterization of the pulmonary artery is also important for measuring pressure. When aortopulmonary transposition is present, an angiogram into the ascending aorta will demonstrate aortic arch obstruction or coarctation.

Differential diagnosis

The differential diagnosis of tricuspid atresia may be considered with regard to the clinical presentations outlined above.

Infant with severe cyanosis

In the young infant, tricuspid atresia has to be differentiated from other lesions producing cyanosis with decreased pulmonary blood flow. The more important lesions to consider are pulmonary atresia with intact ventricular septum, severe pulmonary stenosis or atresia with ventricular septal defect, and single ventricle with severe pulmonary stenosis. The clinical features in these lesions are usually not helpful in distinguishing among these lesions. There may be a systolic ejection murmur when pulmonary stenosis rather than atresia is present but, apart from this, physical examination is similar in all the lesions. The radiograph is also not helpful, as it shows a heart of relatively normal size with decreased pulmonary vascular markings in all instances. The electrocardiogram is most helpful, as in tricuspid atresia there is left axis deviation and a left ventricular dominance pattern, whereas in severe pulmonary stenosis with or without a ventricular septal defect there is right ventricular hypertrophy.

The distinction between pulmonary atresia with intact ventricular septum and tricuspid atresia may be difficult when the tricuspid valve is very small and the right ventricle markedly hypoplastic in an infant with pulmonary atresia. The electrocardiogram may show absence of right ventricular forces but there is usually a normal or right frontal axis. The diagnosis is usually readily made by ultrasound studies.

Although aortopulmonary transposition is associated with a normal or increased pulmonary blood flow, it is a lesion that must be considered in the differential diagnosis in the immediate neonatal period, because the infant may also present with severe cyanosis and no significant cardiac murmurs. The electrocardiogram shows right rather than left ventricular dominance and the radiograph shows a narrow superior mediastinal shadow in the anteroposterior view in transposition and pulmonary vascular markings that are more prominent than in tricuspid atresia. The differentiation is obvious with ultrasound examination.

The lesion of double-inlet left ventricle and pulmonary stenosis may be very difficult to differentiate from tricuspid atresia. With hypoplastic right ventricle, the electrocardiogram may show dominant left ventricular forces. Even with ultrasound examination, the differential diagnosis may be difficult. As mentioned above, it has been proposed by some that tricuspid atresia represents one form of double-inlet left ventricle. It is not too important to make this differential, because the approach to management is similar.

Infant with cardiac failure

The infant with tricuspid atresia and a large ventricular septal defect usually presents in cardiac failure within the first few weeks after birth. The heart is hyperactive and there is a loud murmur typical of ventricular septal defect and an apical mid-diastolic flow rumble. Because these infants often have a high pulmonary to systemic flow ratio, arterial oxygen saturation may be as high as 88–92%. The usual initial clinical impression is that the infant has an isolated large ventricular septal defect. The left ventricular impulse is usually more prominent and the right ventricular impulse may not be increased in the infant with tricuspid atresia. The electrocardiogram shows right axis deviation and prominent right and left ventricular forces with a large ventricular defect. The diagnosis is differentiated readily by cardiac catheterization and angiography.

Tricuspid atresia with ventricular septal defect and aortopulmonary transposition also presents with cardiac failure in early infancy. It is difficult to differentiate this complex from tricuspid atresia with ventricular septal defect and normal aortopulmonary relationship. The clinical features are usually similar. Cyanosis is mild in both conditions and the physical findings of an active enlarged heart, with a loud pansystolic murmur and an apical mid-diastolic murmur, are similar to both complexes. The radiograph is quite similar, showing a large heart with increased pulmonary vascular markings. A narrow superior mediastinal shadow in the frontal view may be evident in aortopulmonary transposition. The electrocardiogram occasionally demonstrates a right axis shift with transposition, but usually shows a left axis with dominant left ventricular forces. Frequently infants with tricuspid atresia and transposition also have weak femoral pulses due to associated aortic arch obstructions. The diagnosis of tricuspid atresia is apparent from ultrasound studies.

Aortopulmonary transposition with a large ventricular septal defect without tricuspid atresia also presents with severe cardiac failure in infancy. Most of the clinical features are similar to those in infants who also have tricuspid atresia, but the electrocardiogram usually shows marked right axis deviation with prominent right ventricular forces on the precordial leads. In infants who have associated tricuspid atresia, the electrocardiogram usually shows dominant left ventricular forces and left axis deviation is more likely, although right axis deviation may be present. Aortic arch obstructions are also much more common in infants with associated tricuspid atresia.

Infants with double-outlet right ventricle of the Taussig–Bing type usually present with cardiac failure in early infancy. The presence of mild cyanosis and physical findings of increased precordial activity, prominent second heart sound, and precordial murmur are similar to those of tricuspid atresia with ventricular septal defect with either normal or transposed great vessels. Furthermore, aortic arch obstructions are not infrequently associated with Taussig–Bing anomaly. An additional finding that may make clinical differentiation difficult is the occasional finding of left axis deviation on the electrocardiogram in Taussig–Bing anomaly, although usually right ventricular forces are very prominent. The differentiation usually has to be made by ultrasound examination.

Principles of management

Currently, there is no means of providing an adequate replacement tricuspid valve and right ventricle, so all treatment must be considered palliative. Approaches to management depend on the presenting clinical features, including the following:

- increase pulmonary blood flow if it is markedly reduced;
- decrease pulmonary blood flow if it is markedly increased to manage cardiac failure and prevent pulmonary vascular obstruction;
- relieve aortic arch obstruction;
- provide an adequate atrial septal communication;
- reduce volume load on the left ventricle;
- maintain an adequate systemic blood flow;
- prevent complications of infective endocarditis and cerebral embolism.

Tricuspid atresia with intact ventricular septum and decreased pulmonary blood flow

In the infant, the immediate concern is to treat the hypoxemia and the resultant acidemia. The infant should be maintained at optimal environmental temperature to avoid increasing oxygen consumption by exposure. It was common practice to treat lactic acidemia resulting from hypoxia by administration of sodium bicarbonate or amine buffers. Many centers still recommend this therapy, but there is no convincing evidence to support this approach and it could in fact be harmful [2,3]. Although oxygen may be administered in high concentrations in inspired air, it may not provide much benefit in improving arterial oxygen saturation if pulmonary blood flow is greatly reduced (see Chapter 3). An intravenous infusion of prostaglandin (PG)E_1 should be started without delay to dilate or maintain patency of the ductus arteriosus in order to provide optimal pulmonary blood flow. Subsequent to this initial management, a surgical procedure is indicated to establish pulmonary blood flow. The early procedures all involved a connection between the systemic and pulmonary arterial circulation. The advantages and disadvantages of the Blalock–Taussig, Potts, and Waterston shunts are discussed in Chapter 14.

The particular concern with all systemic-to-pulmonary arterial shunts in tricuspid atresia is that the volume load on the single left ventricle is greatly increased, because it has to provide both systemic and pulmonary outputs. If the shunt volume is small, pulmonary blood flow will be low and arterial oxygen saturation will be relatively low. To maintain a higher oxygen saturation, the shunt flow would have to be considerably larger and left ventricular work would be greatly increased. There is increasing evidence to suggest that left ventricular myocardial function becomes impaired over time in patients with tricuspid atresia with systemic-to-pulmonary arterial shunts [4]. Furthermore, studies of left ventricular morphology have shown an increase in fibrous tissue in the myocardium in patients with tricuspid atresia [5,6]. The increased volume load on the ventricle induces enlargement and mitral valvar regurgitation may develop. Systemic-to-pulmonary arterial shunts may also have adverse effects with regard to plans for subsequent surgical procedures. The kinking and distortion of the right pulmonary artery resulting from a Waterston anastomosis may complicate the performance of a Fontan type of procedure (see Chapter 16). The left pulmonary artery may be distorted by the Potts shunt and disassembling the shunt involves extensive and often risky surgery. For these reasons, the shunt currently most favored is a modified Blalock–Taussig shunt, which involves interposing a conduit, such as a GoreTex tube, of appropriate diameter between a subclavian and a pulmonary artery. This has the advantages that the size of the conduit can be selected to avoid the risks of excessively increasing pulmonary arterial flow or pressure, and it can also be readily eliminated at the time of subsequent surgery without extensive dissection. It is recognized that the shunt will become restrictive as the child grows, but usually it is anticipated that a systemic venous to pulmonary arterial connection will be performed.

Systemic venous to right atrial communications have several advantages over arterial shunts. Pulmonary blood flow is provided by direct flow of venous blood into the pulmonary arteries. This reduces the volume load on the left ventricle. Also, because the systemic venous blood that passes directly into the pulmonary arteries is oxygenated in the lungs before it returns to the left ventricle, arterial oxygen saturation will increase. The following example demonstrates these issues.

> Assume an infant has a systemic blood flow of 1000 mL/min, that 40% returns to the SVC and 60% to the IVC, and that oxygen saturation is 60% in both SVC and IVC and 100% in the pulmonary vein. If SVC blood (400 mL/min) passes directly to the pulmonary artery, the final oxygen saturation of arterial blood will be 76%. The volume ejected by the left ventricle will be 1000 mL/min. If all systemic venous blood passes through the foramen ovale to the left ventricle and pulmonary flow is provided by an arterial shunt, pulmonary blood flow would have to be 700 mL/min and left ventricular output 1700 mL/min to provide an arterial oxygen saturation of 76%.

The first systemic venous to pulmonary arterial procedure developed was an SVC to pulmonary arterial anastomosis (Glenn procedure) performed by severing the SVC just above its connection with the right atrium. The SVC was anastomosed end to side to the right pulmonary artery. The right atrium at the SVC junction was sutured and the azygous vein and the right pulmonary artery proximal to the anastomosis ligated.

The Glenn shunt produced considerable improvement in arterial oxygen saturation, but it could be performed successfully in older children, usually above 3–4 years of age. Occasional success was achieved in younger infants but there was a high incidence of complications. It was generally assumed that the pulmonary vascular resistance, although not significantly increased above the normal range for infants, had not dropped adequately to accommodate the SVC flow at venous pressures, as compared with that achieved by right ventricular contraction. Following a venous shunt, blood flow to the right is markedly affected by respiratory patterns. It is thus markedly reduced by Valsalva forced expiration or prolonged crying. Also, pulmonary disease such as atelectasis or pneumonia may seriously affect oxygenation. Increasing pulmonary vascular resistance could cause a profound decrease in pulmonary blood flow. Recently, reduction in arterial oxygen saturation has been reported when patients ascend to altitudes above about 2450 m (8000 feet). Also, because most commercial flights are not pressurized to maintain altitudes equivalent to less than about 2450 m, consideration should be given to providing supplemental oxygen to these individuals during air travel. It is possible that this degree of hypoxemia could induce a mild increase in pulmonary vascular resistance that could interfere with lung perfusion by the pressure of the systemic veins.

Early complications of the Glenn procedure are related to elevation of SVC pressure resulting in suffusion and edema of the face and upper extremities. The concern is that these patients may develop cerebral congestion and edema, with the manifestations of benign intracranial hypertension. Usually the manifestations of SVC hypertension gradually subside. Later complications include the development of SVC to IVC collateral anastomoses and pulmonary arteriovenous fistulae. Collateral venous connections from the SVC to the IVC will decrease the blood flow to the right lung and also increase the return of blood with relatively low oxygen saturation to the left atrium and ventricle. This will result in a decrease in arterial oxygen saturation. In recent years the Glenn procedure has been modified so that the SVC is connected to the main pulmonary artery rather than the right pulmonary artery, the so-called bidirectional Glenn procedure. This has greatly reduced the likelihood for venous congestion in the upper body, presumably because the resistance to SVC flow is lower.

Pulmonary arteriovenous shunts frequently develop in the dependent portions of the right lung a few years after the Glenn procedure, but their presence may not be appreciated for 10–15 years. They result in increasing cyanosis and mounting limitation of exercise tolerance, because oxygen uptake in the lung is reduced. It is thought that the fistulae are due to exclusion of a factor released from the liver, which appears to protect against their development. This factor would have to have a very short half-life or be removed by passage of blood through the systemic circulation, because hepatic venous blood would eventually be distributed to the right lung through the SVC. The possibility that the liver removes a substance that induces arteriovenous fistulae has to be considered. This is unlikely because recent evidence indicates that inclusion of hepatic venous blood in perfusion of the lung reduces the likelihood for arteriovenous fistula formation and also appears to limit progression of fistulae that are already present. Little is known about the natural history of these shunts. Small fistulae may occur within a few months, particularly in younger patients, and they do appear to progress. Recently, it has been suggested that small shunts may be present in the lungs of some infants with atrial isomerism syndromes and congenital heart disease. The presence of aneurysms may be demonstrated by ultrasound techniques. A so-called contrast study is performed using saline solution that has been shaken with air and which therefore contains microbubbles. While injecting the saline into an arm vein, the rapid appearance of the microbubbles in the left atrium confirms the presence of rapid transit through fistulae. If the microbubbles all pass through the pulmonary microcirculation, they will be eliminated in the lung. It is important to appreciate that microbubbles may appear in the left atrium if there are SVC to IVC collateral veins. This is recognized by the fact that microbubbles will be seen in the IVC and cross the foramen ovale into the left atrium; their appearance may also be delayed.

Fontan and Baudet introduced the concept of complete redirection of systemic venous return to the pulmonary arteries directly. After performing a Glenn procedure, the right atrium was connected to the left pulmonary artery to direct IVC blood to the left lung. Subsequently the procedure was modified to connect the right atrium to the main pulmonary artery, which was obliterated proximal to the anastomosis. Some surgeons connected the right atrium to the right ventricle if the cavity was of reasonable size. More recently, the procedure has undergone further modifications. To bypass the right atrium, Kreutzer constructed an external tunnel along the lateral wall of the right atrium to direct IVC blood into the pulmonary artery. In the early experience with the Fontan procedure, the mortality was high, particularly in infants. It was therefore recommended that atriopulmonary or atrioventricular connections should not be performed below the age of 3–4 years. Other factors contributing to a high risk of serious complications and mortality are pulmonary vascular resistance greater than 4.0 units/m^2, pulmonary arterial mean pressure greater than 15 mmHg, significant mitral insufficiency, poor left ventricular function and elevated ventricular end-diastolic pressure, and small or distorted pulmonary arteries. The postoperative complications are related to elevated venous pressure; fluid retention with ascites and pleural effusion may persist for several months or longer. The most serious complication is protein-losing enteropathy, which may appear some time after the procedure and is associated with a high mortality. SVC pressure elevation may result in suffusion and edema of the face and upper extremities and benign intracranial hypertension. Experience has shown that if right atrial pressure is greater than 20 mmHg postoperatively, the outcome is usually poor, with a mortality of about 40%. Because the major postoperative concerns are related to the high venous pressure, the practice was developed of creating a fenestration either between the right and left atria or between the lateral tunnel and the left atrium to attempt to reduce venous pressures by permitting venous blood to enter the left side of the heart. This does cause mild postoperative cyanosis, but if venous pressure falls over time, the defect can usually be closed by interventional techniques.

Another important complication of the Fontan procedure is the development of atrial tachyarrhythmias. These may occur in the early postoperative period in about 20%, but may have a later onset in 15–20% of patients who have had an atriopulmonary connection. The incidence of serious arrhythmias has been reduced considerably by performing total cavopulmonary anastomosis. Atrial flutter following the procedure is often difficult to control. It may not respond to many of the drugs usually recommended and more drastic procedures such as radiofrequency ablation have been used, but success is variable.

A very important advantage of total diversion of systemic venous return to the pulmonary artery is the prevention of cerebral emboli and reduction in the risk for cerebral abscess. These are serious complications associated with right-to-left shunting through the foramen ovale and provide justification for proceeding with inferior cavopulmonary connection soon after the superior cavopulmonary anastomosis has been performed.

Current approach to management

The dilemma with these previous therapeutic techniques was that the venous anastomoses could not be performed until at least 2–3 years of age. Therefore arterial shunts were introduced. This placed an excessive volume load on the left ventricle and often left ventricular dysfunction or mitral insufficiency, or an increase in pulmonary vascular resistance had occurred by the time the venous shunt was contemplated. This greatly increased the risk of the procedure. In recent years, it has been recognized that a bidirectional superior cavopulmonary anastomosis is well tolerated in infancy. The SVC is anastomosed to the pulmonary artery to permit perfusion of both lungs. Arterial hypoxemia is greatly improved by this procedure and the child may do well for several years with the partial diversion of systemic venous blood directly to the pulmonary artery. Furthermore, the subsequent complete diversion can be accomplished with considerably lower risk than if the complete Fontan procedure is performed as a single operation. It is therefore now recommended that superior cavopulmonary anastomosis be performed in infancy in these patients. Although the procedure has been performed within 2–3 weeks after birth, it is generally believed that fewer postoperative problems develop if it is delayed until about 8–10 weeks after birth. Thus if it is possible to maintain the infant's arterial oxygen saturation above about 70% by PGE_1 infusion, it would be reasonable to delay until about 8 weeks before recommending cavopulmonary anastomosis. If arterial oxygen saturation cannot be maintained at that level, it is probably advisable to perform a modified Blalock–Taussig shunt initially and to consider a superior cavopulmonary diversion at about 6 months of age. One disadvantage of the use of PGE_1 is that by maintaining patency of the ductus, pulmonary blood flow could be too high and cause left ventricular volume overload and failure. Also, pulmonary arterial pressure could be maintained at relatively high levels and interfere with the maturation of pulmonary arterioles. However, as mentioned above, the ductus arteriosus is usually small in these patients and the likelihood of producing an excessive shunt or pulmonary hypertension is small. It is important to avoid introducing an excessively large left-to-right shunt by the use of a large tube for the Blalock–Taussig procedure or by maintaining wide patency of the ductus arteriosus. The patient should be monitored clinically and by ultrasound examination to ensure this is not occurring.

One concern with the superior cavopulmonary anastomosis is that pulmonary arteriovenous fistulae may develop in both lungs. It appears that when the diversion is done early in infancy, the fistulae may develop much sooner after surgery than in older individuals [7]. It is therefore important to monitor the patient for the presence of arteriovenous fistulae regularly after surgery by contrast ultrasound study. Should extensive fistulae be detected, completion of the total cavopulmonary diversion should be considered sooner than might otherwise be planned. As mentioned above, when hepatic venous blood is directed into the pulmonary circulation, it appears that progression of the fistulae is slowed and possible improvement may occur. It is usually recommended that the second stage be performed at 18–24 months of age.

In the past, many centers recommended that a balloon or blade atrial septostomy be performed routinely if an arterial shunt procedure was to be performed. It was thought that the increased pulmonary venous return would increase left atrial pressure and tend to close the foramen ovale. This would reduce systemic output and also result in systemic venous congestion. This was probably an important issue when the size of the shunt could not be carefully controlled. Currently, use of a graft of specific diameter as a modified Blalock–Taussig shunt limits the magnitude of pulmonary blood flow. Foramen ovale restriction is less likely to occur. If inadequate systemic cardiac output, or venous congestion, is evident after the procedure, the infant should be assessed by catheterization and an atrial septostomy can be performed if indicated.

Tricuspid atresia with ventricular septal defect

Decreased pulmonary blood flow

The infant who has tricuspid atresia with a ventricular septal defect and reduced pulmonary blood flow should be treated in the same manner as infants with intact ventricular septum. Many of these infants will maintain an adequate arterial oxygen saturation without PGE_1 infusion and the cavopulmonary anastomosis can be performed as the initial procedure after 2–3 months. The ventricular septal defect tends to close spontaneously.

Increased pulmonary blood flow

The main feature of this combination of lesions is increased pulmonary blood flow with cardiac failure in infancy. Immediate therapy is to treat cardiac failure. If the failure can be controlled by medical measures, it is probably advisable not to perform pulmonary artery banding, because in the majority of these infants the defect tends to become smaller and often closes spontaneously. The main concern is that, prior to the defect becoming small, pulmonary arterial hypertension may induce pulmonary vascular changes. The high pulmonary vascular resistance would preclude subsequent cavopulmonary anastomosis.

If the ventricular septal defect appears to be still fairly large by clinical examination and ultrasound study at about 3 months of age, cardiac catheterization should be performed to measure pulmonary arterial pressure and pulmonary vascular resistance. If the resistance exceeds 3–4 units, banding of the pulmonary artery should be performed to try to reduce the resistance in preparation for a cavopulmonary anastomosis at a later date.

Tricuspid atresia with ventricular septal defect and transposition with normal aortic isthmus

These patients present with severe cardiac failure as pulmonary resistance falls after birth. Cardiac failure should be treated with medical measures. If failure cannot be controlled, two approaches are possible. Banding of the pulmonary artery can be performed to reduce pulmonary arterial pressure and pulmonary blood flow. It has been noted that pulmonary arterial banding must be quite tight to avoid pulmonary vascular resistance reaching levels above 4 units/m^2. This is important with regard to the possibility of performing cavopulmonary anastomosis at a later date. Although there is a tendency for functional subaortic stenosis to develop spontaneously in these patients as a result of decrease in the size of the ventricular septal defect, it appears that banding tends to hasten the process. The subsequent procedure will have to be performed sooner than anticipated if this occurs. The combined increase in outflow resistance through the ventricular septal defect and outflow resistance into the banded pulmonary artery results in left ventricular pressure overload and enlargement and thus cardiac failure is likely to develop. The procedure requires that the outflow from the left ventricle into the aorta be relieved. Some success has been achieved by enlarging the ventricular septal defect surgically, but the procedure now being favored is bypass of the right ventricle by connecting the pulmonary artery, which is severed above the pulmonary valve, to the ascending aorta by an end-to-side anastomosis (Damus–Kaye–Stansel procedure). At the same procedure a superior cavopulmonary anastomosis is performed to the distal segment of pulmonary artery to provide pulmonary blood flow. The complete cavopulmonary connection is performed at a later date. The ability to accomplish this at one operation has prompted some centers to perform this procedure in infancy with no consideration of pulmonary artery banding. Considerable success has been achieved even in neonates, with mortality as low as about 10%.

Tricuspid atresia with ventricular septal defect and transposition with aortic isthmus obstruction or aortic coarctation

When this lesion is associated there is, in addition to the problem of cardiac failure due to high pulmonary blood flow, interference in blood flow to the descending aorta when ductus arteriosus constriction occurs. The initial therapy is to treat acidemia and cardiac failure. Infusion of PGE_1 should be started to maintain flow to the lower body. In the past surgical procedures were directed to relieving the aortic arch obstruction and decreasing pulmonary arterial blood flow by banding the pulmonary artery. A very high mortality was associated with this procedure, because in many individuals the ventricular septal defect was restrictive and systemic output was poor after surgery. Recently, an approach similar to that described above has been used. In a single procedure in the neonatal period, the aortic arch is repaired, a pulmonary arterial to aorta anastomosis (Damus–Kaye–Stansel) is performed, and then a bidirectional superior cavopulmonary connection is completed. Relatively few procedures of this type have been done, but the mortality is probably about 10–20%. A modification of the procedure consists of connecting the pulmonary artery to the descending aorta as an end-to-side anastomosis at the site of the aortic arch correction.

Long-term results

Systemic venous to pulmonary artery communication has greatly improved the outlook for individuals with tricuspid atresia. The 5-year survival following the Fontan procedure was about 80%, but with improvements in technique and the use of cavopulmonary anastomosis the outlook has improved further. Most patients have reasonably good exercise tolerance with regard to daily activities. However, their ability to perform is considerably less than the norm. Although the incidence of late-onset arrhythmias appears to have been reduced since the use of cavopulmonary anastomosis, serious arrhythmias are still a concern.

Protein-losing enteropathy is a serious complication following the Fontan atriopulmonary artery anastomosis; although the mechanism responsible has not been delineated, it appears to be associated with high systemic venous pressure. There is some evidence to suggest it occurs less frequently after anastomosis of the SVC and IVC to the pulmonary artery compared with the traditional Fontan procedure. Conversion of a traditional Fontan connection to a complete extracardiac cavopulmonary anastomosis has been successful in improving protein-losing enteropathy [8].

After initial improvement in exercise tolerance related to increased arterial oxygen saturation, patients who have had Fontan atriopulmonary connections show progressive decrease in performance. As discussed above the decreasing exercise capacity could be related to progressive left ventricular dysfunction, probably related to increasing left ventricular myocardial fibrosis. Left ventricular failure may become severe enough to require cardiac transplantation.

Although there is not as yet adequate long-term observation of individuals who have had total cavopulmonary anastomosis, there is some evidence to suggest that their prognosis is better than those who have had an atriopulmonary connection [9]. In a report of 261 patients who had either procedure, over a median period of 12.2 years about 30% had died and about 2% required cardiac transplantation [10].

An important complication is thromboembolism, which was considered to account for about 8% of deaths. The importance of providing antiplatelet or anticoagulant therapy to avoid this complication has been stressed [10].

It is apparent that although total cavopulmonary anastomosis is a procedure that can provide a reasonable lifestyle to patients with single ventricle physiology, the long-term outlook is not optimal and increasing numbers of these individuals are becoming candidates for cardiac transplantation.

References

1 Wald RM, Tham EB, McCrindle BW *et al.* Outcome after prenatal diagnosis of tricuspid atresia: a multicenter experience. Am Heart J 2007;153:772–778.

2 Forsythe SM, Schmidt GA. Sodium bicarbonate for the treatment of lactic acidosis. Chest 2000;117:260–267.

3 Weil MH, Tang W. Management of acidosis: the role of buffer agents. Crit Care 1997;1:51–52.

4 Baker EJ, Jones OD, Joseph MC, Maisey MN, Tynan MJ. Radionuclide measurement of left ventricular ejection fraction in tricuspid atresia. Br Heart J 1984;52: 572–574.

5 Ho SY, Jackson M, Kilpatrick L, Smith A, Gerlis LM. Fibrous matrix of ventricular myocardium in tricuspid atresia compared with normal heart. A quantitative analysis. Circulation 1996;94:1642–1646.

6 Binotto MA, Higuchi M de L, Aiello VD. Left ventricular remodeling in hearts with tricuspid atresia: morphologic observations and possible basis for ventricular dysfunction after surgery. J Thorac Cardiovasc Surg 2003;126: 1026–1032.

7 Bernstein HS, Brook MM, Silverman NH, Bristow J. Development of pulmonary arteriovenous fistulae in

children after cavopulmonary shunt. Circulation 1995;92(suppl II):309–314.

8 Marcelletti CF, Hanley FL, Mavroudis C *et al.* Revision of previous Fontan connections to total extracardiac cavopulmonary anastomosis: a multicenter experience. J Thorac Cardiovasc Surg 2000;119:340–346.

9 Giardini A, Hager A, Napoleone CP, Picchio FM. Natural history of exercise capacity after the Fontan operation: a longitudinal study. Ann Thorac Surg 2008;85:818–821.

10 Khairy P, Fernandes SM, Mayer JE Jr *et al.* Long-term survival, modes of death, and predictors of mortality in patients with Fontan surgery. Circulation 2008;117:85–92.

17

CHAPTER 17

Ebstein malformation of the tricuspid valve

Ebstein anomaly is a rare congenital abnormality of the tricuspid valve and the adjacent right ventricular wall. The physiological effects and clinical manifestations are extremely variable. The condition may result in death *in utero*, present with severe cyanosis in the newborn, or cause no symptoms until late adult life. The anomaly is also encountered with L-transposition (corrected transposition) and then involves the tricuspid valve, which is functioning as the mitral valve in the left atrioventricular sulcus.

Morphological and embryological features

Ebstein malformation is characterized by downward displacement of the attachments of the septal and posterior leaflets of the tricuspid valve away from the atrioventricular junction toward the trabecular portion of the right ventricle. The degree of displacement varies and the leaflets are usually adherent to the wall of the right ventricle, as well as being dysplastic. Normally, the septal leaflet of the tricuspid valve is attached to the ventricular septum slightly distal to the attachment of the septal leaflet of the mitral valve. In Ebstein anomaly, this separation is considerably increased. The morphological features of the leaflets that determine the functional disturbance, in addition to the degree of displacement, are the length of valve tissue that is not adherent, and the amount of thickening and dysplasia. When the leaflets are displaced, attached to the wall and thick and short, severe regurgitation is likely. The anterior leaflet has normal attachment to the atrioventricular annulus and is large and frequently redundant and has been described as sail-like. It is usually thickened, and muscular or fibrous bands may course through it. The anterior leaflet may also be abnormally attached distally to a muscular shelf at the junction of the inlet and trabecular portions of the right ventricle. The leaflet may be attached to produce complete obstruction between the inlet and trabecular portions of the ventricle, simulating tricuspid atresia. Occasionally one or more fenestrae are present in the anterior leaflet, allowing some passage of blood, but effectively causing tricuspid stenosis. When the anterior leaflet is very redundant, it may bulge into the outflow tract of the right ventricle, causing obstruction and making the functional size of the right ventricle exceedingly small. Displacement of the valve leaflets moves the orifice of the tricuspid valve distal to the atrioventricular sulcus to a varying degree. When the posterior and septal leaflets are markedly displaced and the anterosuperior leaflet bulges distally, the cavity of the right ventricle may be represented only by the outflow tract and it is unlikely to be capable of providing an adequate pulmonary blood flow. Atresia of the pulmonary valve is fairly frequent, occurring in almost 10% of infants with Ebstein anomaly [1].

The right ventricular wall is composed of two segments. The trabecular portion and the outflow, beyond the attachments of the tricuspid valve, have the appearance of normal right ventricular wall, but the wall of the ventricle between the atrioventricular junction and the displaced tricuspid valve leaflets is markedly thinned. This portion of the ventricle has been said to be atrialized and functionally is an extension of the right atrial cavity. The right atrium is enlarged by the distal displacement of the tricuspid valve, but may become

Congenital Diseases of the Heart, 3rd edition. By A. Rudolph
© 2009 Blackwell Publishing, ISBN: 9781405162456

extremely dilated as a result of severe tricuspid regurgitation.

The eustachian valve is often prominent in infants with Ebstein anomaly. In addition, abnormalities of the conduction system have been observed. The right bundle may be involved by fibrosis and, occasionally, accessory bundles have been noted in individuals with preexcitation syndrome. Atrial septal communications are present in about 90% of individuals with Ebstein anomaly; either a patent foramen ovale or a true fossa ovalis defect may be present. A small proportion of individuals has a ventricular septal defect, which is usually small. Rarely, Ebstein anomaly may be associated with atrioventricular septal defect.

Abnormalities of the left ventricle are commonly noted with Ebstein malformation. If the right ventricle and atrium are greatly enlarged, the ventricular septum may bulge to the left, reducing left ventricular cavity size. This may reduce ventricular filling and interfere with the ability of the ventricle to sustain an adequate output [2]. The left ventricular myocardium may also show variable degrees of fibrosis, usually beyond childhood.

Ebstein anomaly appears to arise fairly late in prenatal development. The tricuspid valve is formed from the endocardial surface of the right ventricle by a process known as delamination. The inner surface of the ventricle is undermined distal to the atrioventricular sulcus and the leaflets are lifted off the ventricular wall. The chordae tendineae are formed by the same process. Of interest is the fact that the anterosuperior leaflet is formed very early, but development of the septal and anteroinferior leaflets is delayed until the third to fourth month of gestational age. This wide interval separating the time at which the leaflets form helps to explain the discrepancy in their development. Although the exact cause of the anomaly is not known, Ebstein malformation has been observed in several infants born to mothers treated with lithium for psychiatric disorders early in pregnancy. It is not known whether the abnormality of the anterior leaflet is the primary abnormality and the involvement of the septal and posterior leaflets is secondary. Possibly abnormal development of the septal and posterior leaflets is the initial disturbance and this results in abnormal development of the already formed anterior leaflet. Perhaps development of all three leaflets is the result of a common underlying etiology.

Hemodynamic considerations

Fetal circulation

The majority of fetuses with Ebstein anomaly do not experience any difficulties *in utero*. Mild to moderate displacement of the tricuspid valve does not significantly alter the course of the circulation. However, severe forms of the anomaly may have serious adverse effects. Although there are several reports of Ebstein malformation in fetuses, little has been mentioned of the hemodynamic disturbances associated with the anomaly. The frequent association of right ventricular outflow obstruction has been noted [3,4]. This may occur if the anterosuperior leaflet is large and attached to the ventricular wall so that the right atrium is completely separated from the right ventricle. However, in most instances, the obstruction is due to pulmonary stenosis or atresia; although this could be a component of the embryological disturbance, it is very likely that it is the result of reduced right ventricular output. In the fetus, it is necessary for the right ventricle to develop a pressure as high as that in the systemic circulation to achieve flow across the pulmonary valve. Pulmonary vascular resistance is high in the fetus and the ductus arteriosus permits pressure in the pulmonary artery to be at systemic arterial levels. Decreased right ventricular output may be due to the fact that the functional portion of the right ventricle is so small that it cannot develop a pressure high enough to eject into the pulmonary artery. If the functional portion of the right ventricle is of reasonable size, the presence of severe tricuspid regurgitation may limit the volume of blood ejected across the right ventricular outflow into the pulmonary artery. With a very small functional ventricle or severe tricuspid regurgitation, the pulmonary valve would remain closed throughout the cardiac cycle and pulmonary blood flow would be provided by flow through the ductus arteriosus from the aorta. It is possible that persistent closure of the pulmonary valve for an extended period during fetal development may result in morphological atresia of the pulmonary valve.

If there is no flow across the pulmonary valve, the combined ventricular output of the heart will have to be achieved by the left ventricle. Venous return to the heart from systemic and umbilical veins must pass through the foramen ovale into the left atrium and ventricle to be distributed to the fetal body, lungs, and umbilical–placental circulation. Complete admixture of systemic and umbilical venous blood will occur and the oxygen saturation of mixed blood, based on assumptions of umbilical and systemic venous blood flows and oxygen saturations in human fetuses, will be about 55% (see Chapters 11 and 16). Thus the pulmonary circulation may receive blood of higher oxygen saturation than normal and this could lower pulmonary vascular resistance and limit pulmonary vascular smooth muscle development. Blood distributed to the ascending aorta and brain would have an oxygen saturation lower than the normal of about 65% and thus cerebral oxygen supply could be compromised under conditions of stress.

Several other factors could have important roles in affecting circulatory dynamics in fetuses with Ebstein malformation, including the severity of tricuspid regurgitation, left ventricular output, size of the foramen ovale, and the pulmonary circulation.

Tricuspid regurgitation

The magnitude of tricuspid regurgitation is probably dependent on the size of the functional right ventricle. If the ventricle is small, even if the tricuspid valve is quite incompetent, the volume of blood regurgitated will be small. Most of the blood will flow through the foramen ovale and the flow patterns will simulate those of tricuspid atresia (see Chapter 16). With a larger functional right ventricle the regurgitant volume can be large if the tricuspid valve is grossly incompetent. The more severe the regurgitation, the less likely that blood will be ejected into the pulmonary artery. If valvar regurgitation is marked, the right ventricle and right atrium will become markedly enlarged; right atrial and systemic and umbilical venous pressures will be increased. Tricuspid regurgitation may be associated with several consequences.

The turbulence in the right atrium and vena cavae could disrupt the preferential flow pattern of umbilical venous blood through the foramen ovale and of distal inferior vena cava and superior vena cava blood through the tricuspid valve. Thus, even if some right ventricular blood is ejected into the pulmonary artery, there would be a variable degree of mixing of the venous streams, so that the preferential flow of well-oxygenated blood from the ductus venosus through the foramen ovale would be disrupted. This could alter the oxygen saturations levels normally present in pulmonary arterial and ascending and descending aortic blood.

Severe tricuspid regurgitation will result in elevation of right atrial and venous pressures. If there is free access of blood across the foramen ovale into the left ventricle, the degree of increase in venous pressure will be limited, but if there is any interference with flow across the foramen, atrial and venous pressures could increase to a greater extent and result in fetal and placental edema (hydrops fetalis) and fetal demise [3,4].

The eustachian valve is often very prominent in fetuses with Ebstein malformation. It is not known whether this is a primary anomaly that is a component of Ebstein malformation or if it is the result of abnormal flow patterns. The latter concept seems more likely, because a large eustachian valve is commonly noted in the fetus with tricuspid atresia. It would be interesting to examine the relationship between the size of the eustachian valve and the dynamics of Ebstein malformation; it is possible that enlargement of the valve occurs in those fetuses with mild to moderate tricuspid regurgitation and significant outflow obstruction, simulating the hemodynamics of tricuspid atresia, whereas it may not be noted when tricuspid regurgitation is severe.

Left ventricular output

Marked enlargement of the right atrium and ventricle associated with regurgitation may cause ventricular septal displacement severe enough to reduce the size of the left ventricle during diastole and interfere with left ventricular filling. The reduced diastolic volume will restrict left ventricular stroke volume and left ventricular output could be severely compromised. This, combined with the reduced right ventricular flow into the pulmonary artery, will significantly reduce combined ventricular output. This reduction in combined ventricular output could result in redistribution of blood flow as occurs during fetal hypoxemia, with maintenance of flow to the brain and heart and reduction of flow to other tissues and the placenta (see Chapter 3).

Intrauterine growth retardation could result and it is of interest that infants with Ebstein malformation who die soon after birth and have the severest forms of the anomaly have birth weights about 30% less than those who survive.

Displacement of the ventricular septum to the left by a markedly enlarged right atrium and ventricle limits flow into the left ventricle and results in increased left ventricular end-diastolic and left atrial pressures. This will result in elevation of right atrial and systemic venous pressures and promote the development of fetal hydrops (see Chapter 1). Furthermore, the increased left atrial pressure will tend to move the atrial septum to the right and thus restrict the size of the foramen ovale.

Foramen ovale

The foramen ovale is usually of relatively normal size in fetuses with Ebstein malformation. In fetuses with Ebstein malformation and hydrops, it has been noted that the foramen may be restricted [5]. The size of the foramen ovale is probably related to the magnitude of tricuspid regurgitation and the degree of impingement on the left ventricular cavity. In those fetuses with minor amounts of regurgitation, either because the functional right ventricle is small or because tricuspid valve function is not grossly disturbed, the foramen ovale is probably of normal size. This would allow total systemic and pulmonary venous blood flow returning to the right atrium to pass across the foramen with only a minor increase in right atrial pressure. As mentioned above, restriction of the foramen ovale is probably the result of increased left atrial pressure associated with the reduction of left ventricular cavity size due to enlargement of the right ventricle and atrium caused by severe tricuspid regurgitation.

Restriction of the foramen ovale and elevation of left atrial pressure could possibly result in increased pulmonary venous and capillary pressures, with enhanced development of pulmonary vascular smooth muscle (see Chapter 5). Also, as mentioned above, foramen ovale restriction could contribute to the induction of fetal hydrops.

Pulmonary circulation and pulmonary vascular development

In fetuses with Ebstein malformation and severe or complete obstruction to right ventricular output, and in those with a small functional right ventricle with minimal flow across the pulmonary valve, complete admixture of systemic and umbilical venous blood will result in a higher than normal oxygen saturation of blood perfusing the lungs. This could result in a fall in pulmonary vascular resistance and lessen development of pulmonary vascular smooth muscle. This could be beneficial to the neonate, because pulmonary vascular resistance could fall rapidly after birth and this could help to reduce the degree of tricuspid regurgitation.

Adverse effects on pulmonary vascular development could result from two different mechanisms in fetuses with marked tricuspid regurgitation. As mentioned above, foramen ovale restriction could increase left atrial and pulmonary venous pressures and enhance pulmonary vascular smooth muscle development. In addition, the marked cardiomegaly that may result from tricuspid regurgitation often affects lung growth, with resultant pulmonary hypoplasia; this will be associated with reduced total pulmonary vascular cross-sectional area. A combination of these factors could have a major impact on establishment of an adequate pulmonary circulation after birth and thus elevated pulmonary arterial pressure will be maintained, and tricuspid regurgitation will be enhanced. This could explain the difficulty in resuscitating many infants with Ebstein malformation after birth and the high mortality in these infants.

Postnatal hemodynamics

Neonatal period

The physiological effects of Ebstein anomaly during the postnatal period are extremely variable, depending on the severity of the malformation and on the associated anomalies. If leaflet displacement is mild, the posterior and septal leaflets fairly well formed, and the anterior leaflet not too redundant, the postnatal circulation may be relatively normal. The right ventricle is of reasonable size and is capable of providing adequate pulmonary blood flow. Mild or insignificant tricuspid regurgitation may be present. If displacement of the septal and posterior leaflets is greater and the leaflets are short and dysplastic, tricuspid insufficiency may be more severe. During the immediate postnatal period, while pulmonary vascular resistance is still elevated, afterload on the right ventricle is high. The stroke volume ejected into the pulmonary artery is relatively low because afterload on the right ventricle is high. The high afterload tends to exaggerate the tricuspid regurgitation. Right atrial pressure is elevated and this favors right-to-left shunting through the atrial communication, resulting in varying degrees of systemic arterial hypoxemia. While the ductus arteriosus is still patent, adequate pulmonary blood flow may be maintained and the degree of cyanosis may be mild. Constriction of the ductus may reduce pulmonary blood flow and exaggerate the hypoxemia. As pulmonary vascular resistance begins to fall after birth, pulmonary blood flow from the right ventricular output increases and, as a result of the decrease in afterload, the degree of tricuspid regurgitation is reduced. Right atrial pressure falls and shunting through the atrial communication decreases or is abolished and cyanosis lessens or disappears.

The effect of the ductus arteriosus during the neonatal period is of considerable interest. If there is a significant degree of right ventricular outflow obstruction, the ductus may be very important in providing adequate pulmonary blood flow after birth. Also, right ventricular output may be restricted because the functional ventricle is small or if there is marked regurgitation. While pulmonary vascular resistance is still elevated after birth, the right ventricle may be incapable of providing adequate pulmonary blood flow. Under these circumstances, maintaining patency of the ductus may be crucial in providing adequate pulmonary blood flow.

The adverse effect of patency of the ductus arteriosus is that it elevates pulmonary arterial pressure; the resulting increased afterload on the right ventricle will tend to increase tricuspid regurgitation. As pulmonary vascular resistance falls, right ventricular output can increase and the degree of tricuspid regurgitation will diminish. As mentioned on p. 453, because there may be an increase in pulmonary arterial oxygen levels in the fetus, possibly pulmonary vascular resistance will be lower and pulmonary vascular smooth muscle development may be limited. This could permit a more rapid decline in pulmonary vascular resistance after birth compared with the normal infant. Thus there could be a fairly rapid increase in right ventricular output with reduction in tricuspid regurgitation. However, if the ductus arteriosus is patent, it may not only prevent the fall in pulmonary arterial pressure but also inhibit the fall in pulmonary vascular resistance. As discussed below in the section on management, the decision whether to maintain patency of the ductus or to permit or even induce closure is sometimes very difficult. There is evidence to indicate that if the ductus arteriosus is not required to maintain pulmonary blood flow, the survival of infants with Ebstein malformation is improved if the ductus is closed [6]. Because the fall in pulmonary vascular resistance after birth is so important in influencing the degree of tricuspid regurgitation, the possibility that treatment to reduce pulmonary vascular resistance would be beneficial should be seriously considered. Because introduction of an aortopulmonary shunt in those infants who have Ebstein malformation will have a similar effect to that of a patent ductus arteriosus, it would be preferable to avoid this procedure if possible. However, if it is decided to perform the procedure, it is very important to avoid introducing large shunts, because they would have the same adverse effects as a large patent ductus arteriosus.

Severe forms of the anomaly are characterized by marked displacement of the proximal attachments of the posteroinferior and particularly the septal leaflets, and abnormal distal attachment and often dysplasia of the leaflets. This results in severe tricuspid insufficiency. The atrialized portion of the right ventricular wall functions as part of the right atrium and the size of the functional portion of the right ventricle is greatly reduced. Right ventricular performance is thus greatly reduced. During the early postnatal period, while the ductus arteriosus is open and pulmonary vascular resistance is high, pressure in the pulmonary artery is maintained at systemic arterial levels. The right ventricle is not capable of generating a systolic pressure high enough to open the pulmonary valve and thus functional pulmonary atresia results. The total systemic venous return is routed through the atrial communication to the left atrium, where complete admixture of pulmonary and systemic venous return occurs. The systemic arterial oxygen saturation will be determined by the ratio of pulmonary to systemic blood flow (see Chapter 3). Right ventricular output will also be affected by the presence of even moderate degrees of pulmonary valvar or subpulmonary stenosis. In the presence of a ventricle that can eject only a small stroke volume, any increase in afterload induced by the obstruction would greatly restrict right ventricular stroke volume. Furthermore, if tricuspid insufficiency is severe, outflow obstruction of the ventricle would aggravate the regurgitation and output into the pulmonary artery would be greatly reduced. Thus infants with outflow obstruction have a high mortality.

The left ventricle is responsible for providing both pulmonary and systemic blood flows. If it is capable of increasing its output, it could provide adequate flows to both circulations. However, the greatly enlarged right atrium and ventricle may cause ventricular septal displacement that reduces left ventricular volume and limits inflow and thus outflow. If left ventricular output is restricted, it could interfere with either pulmonary blood flow or systemic flow or both. Reduction of pulmonary blood flow will result in increasing cyanosis. Decreased systemic flow will cause hypotension and poor peripheral perfusion; if this persists, anaerobic metabolism with metabolic acidemia will develop (see Chapter 3). This form of Ebstein malformation is associated with a high mortality in the neonate.

Within a few days improvement may occur. As pulmonary vascular resistance falls and the ductus arteriosus closes, pulmonary arterial pressure falls. Pressure generated by the right ventricle may now be adequate to open the pulmonary valve and provide adequate pulmonary blood flow for survival. The decrease in afterload on the right ventricle may reduce the degree of tricuspid regurgitation significantly and the magnitude of right-to-left shunt through the atrial communication will be greatly reduced. These infants may survive and present the features of Ebstein anomaly with moderately severe tricuspid regurgitation observed in older children (see Chapter 17).

In those infants in whom the distal portion of the anterior leaflet is tethered to the right ventricular wall to cause complete obstruction to flow into the right ventricle, the hemodynamic features are similar to those of infants with tricuspid atresia with intact ventricular septum (see Chapter 16). The complex of Ebstein anomaly associated with pulmonary atresia is discussed in Chapter 15.

Effect of arrhythmia

Although atrial tachyarrhythmias are not as frequent in the newborn period as at later ages, onset of tachycardia may have adverse effects. In the infant with cyanosis, tachycardia may further compromise output from the right ventricle and thus reduce pulmonary blood flow, as well as increase right atrial pressure. Thus right-to-left shunting through the atrial communication will increase and cyanosis will become more severe. In addition the altered phasic pressure relationships of the right and left atrium may enhance the right-to-left shunt and aggravate the degree of cyanosis. The tachyarrhythmia may also reduce left ventricular output and induce circulatory shock.

Hemodynamics beyond infancy

As in the infant, the hemodynamic disturbances and clinical manifestations of Ebstein anomaly are quite variable and are determined by:

- severity of obstruction of the tricuspid orifice;
- severity of tricuspid valve insufficiency, which is related to the degree of displacement of the valve leaflets and the extent of dysplasia of the leaflets;
- amount of functional right ventricle;
- presence of an atrial septal communication;
- cardiac rhythm disturbances.

Individuals with a minor degree of tricuspid valve displacement and fairly well formed leaflets will usually also have a right ventricle of almost normal size and have no obstruction and minimal valvar insufficiency. The atrial septal communication will be associated with left-to-right shunting, the magnitude of which will depend on the size of the defect. If a large left-to-right shunt is present, the hemodynamic features are the same as those in individuals with atrial septal defect (see Chapter 8). The malformation may only be recognized when the individual has an ultrasound study performed for suspected atrial septal defect, occurrence of tachyarrhythmias, or development of cyanosis with exertion or rhythm disturbance. Ebstein anomaly has been encountered as an incidental finding at autopsy in individuals dying at ages beyond 60 years.

Severe obstruction of the valve orifice is unusual beyond infancy. It may also be difficult to differentiate between orifice obstruction and limitation of right ventricular size, which may also interfere with ventricular filling from the atrium. The effect of both these abnormalities is to reduce right ventricular filling and raise right atrial pressure and induce greater right-to-left shunting through the atrial septal defect, with reduced systemic arterial oxygen saturation.

Tricuspid valve insufficiency occurs to varying degree in almost all patients with Ebstein anomaly. It is most severe with dysplastic, grossly displaced valve leaflets. When severe, it interferes with right ventricular output and is associated with increased right atrial pressure and atrial right-to-left shunting. Severe insufficiency is also likely to be associated with a small functioning right ventricular cavity. Thus it is apparent that whatever the specific morphological or functional abnormality of the valve, the hemodynamic effects are limitation of right ventricular output, raised right atrial and systemic venous pressures, and atrial right-to-left shunting. As in the neonatal period, marked enlargement of the right ventricle and atrium may displace the ventricular septum, reducing left ventricular cavity size and thus filling and stroke volume. The consequences of these disturbances are cyanosis, limitation of cardiac output, and right-sided cardiac failure. During the first year after birth, infants with marked tricuspid insufficiency present with right-sided cardiac failure and moderate cyanosis.

Effect of exercise

Many individuals with Ebstein anomaly are asymptomatic at rest and have minimal or no cyanosis. They may become more cyanosed and be markedly restricted in their tolerance of exercise. This could be related to the limitation in their ability to increase right ventricular output and thus raise cardiac output. The right-to-left shunt at the atrial level could provide some compensation. However, the increased venous return during exercise may exaggerate displacement of the ventricular septum and interfere with the ability of the left ventricle to increase its output. The decrease in systemic arterial oxygen saturation appears to be the more important factor in limitation of exercise. A number of individuals have shown marked improvement in physical performance after closure of the atrial communication. In other types of cyanotic congenital heart disease, although cyanosis increases with exercise, it may be better tolerated, because an increase in cardiac output may provide some increase in oxygen delivery to the tissues. However, this may not occur with Ebstein anomaly because left ventricular output is restricted.

Effect of arrhythmia

Arrhythmias are frequent, occurring in 20–30% of individuals with Ebstein malformation. Atrial tachyarrhythmias are most frequently encountered, and may be precipitated by exertion. The hemodynamic effects in the older individual are similar to those in the infant (see above) and to those associated with exercise. However, atrial right-to-left shunting may first become manifest in association with the onset of arrhythmia.

Effect of posture

Posture may have an important effect in determining the presence of cyanosis, particularly in adolescent and adult individuals. While sitting or standing, cyanosis may be minimal or absent, whereas cyanosis may appear when the individual is reclining. This is probably related to the fact that, during quiet standing, blood pools in lower body veins and venous return to the heart is reduced. The right ventricle is capable of ejecting the volume returning, so that right-to-left shunting through the atrial communication is minimal. On reclining, venous return increases and the right ventricle may not be capable of ejecting the larger volume, some of which shunts through the atrial communication. It is also possible that the increased velocity of inferior vena cava blood may result in streaming of venous blood across the atrial septal defect.

Clinical features

Ebstein malformation should be considered as a possible lesion in a fetus manifesting hydrops, tachyarrhythmia, or marked cardiomegaly. Any of these manifestations requires further study by ultrasound to confirm or exclude the diagnosis. In addition, a fetus in a mother who has been administered lithium during early pregnancy for treatment of bipolar disorder should be suspected as a possible candidate for the anomaly.

Neonatal presentation

The hemodynamic disturbances are variable, depending on the severity of the anomaly. In the presence of severe right ventricular outflow obstruction, the main concern is maintenance of pulmonary blood flow after birth. These infants show cyanosis, which becomes progressive as the ductus arteriosus constricts, resulting in severe hypoxemia progressing to hypoxia and metabolic acidemia. The presentation is similar to that of infants with severe pulmonary stenosis or pulmonary atresia with intact ventricular septum (see Chapter 15). These infants usually also have significant tricuspid regurgitation. The heart is thus usually enlarged clinically and the cardiac impulse is prominent at the lower left sternal border. The intensity of the first sound is usually decreased and the second sound is single and also soft. A decrescendo systolic murmur of variable intensity is heard at the lower left sternal border and it may radiate to the right of the sternum.

The infant with little or no outflow obstruction but with severe tricuspid regurgitation also presents with cyanosis. Severe intrauterine cardiomegaly may have resulted in pulmonary hypoplasia and expansion of the lungs may not be achieved, even with ventilatory assistance. Little or no blood may be ejected by the right ventricle into the pulmonary artery and pulmonary blood flow may be provided exclusively by the ductus arteriosus. As mentioned above, functional closure of the pulmonary valve may result from the high pulmonary arterial pressure. In the early neonatal period, the cyanosis may progress rapidly if the ductus arteriosus constricts. During this period, administration of prostaglandin (PG)E_1 may improve or prevent progression of the cyanosis by increasing pulmonary perfusion through the ductus arteriosus. However, it could potentially have an adverse effect by increasing the degree of tricuspid regurgitation and right ventricular failure (see above). In addition to the cyanosis, the infant has a markedly enlarged heart; the impulse may be prominent at the lower sternal region. Auscultatory findings are similar to those in the infant with obstructed right ventricular outflow. Hepatomegaly of mild to moderate degree is usually noted. The mortality of infants with Ebstein malformation who present with significant symptoms at birth is very high [7].

With less severe anomalies, the infant is cyanosed at birth but within a few days, associated with the decrease in pulmonary vascular resistance, cyanosis begins to lessen and the infant's condition improves as the degree of tricuspid regurgitation also decreases. Mild to moderate hepatomegaly is present. Perfusion is poor and blood pressure is reduced. The heart is markedly enlarged. Precordial pulsation is not significantly increased but some increase in cardiac pulsation over the lower sternum may be appreciated. The first heart sound is usually split with prominence of the second component. The tricuspid closure sound may be very prominent because the anterior leaflet is often large and redundant; closure may generate the so-called "slatting sail" sound. The second sound is frequently widely split due to the presence of right ventricular conduction delay. A third sound is also frequently audible. A systolic murmur of grade 2–4/6 is usually heard most prominently over the lower sternal region. A short, low-frequency, mid-diastolic murmur may also be heard over the lower sternal region. A number of infants die during the first year as a result of cardiac failure and hypoxemia.

Presentation in the child and adolescent

The mildest forms of Ebstein malformation may cause no symptoms and may not be recognized clinically. If tricuspid insufficiency is mild to moderate, symptoms may not be noted at rest, but cyanosis and limitation may be noted with exertion. Most individuals have decreased exercise tolerance. With increasing age, the tendency is for cyanosis and cardiac failure to become more severe, but the rate of progression is variable. Palpitations may be experienced in young children, but are more common in adolescents and adults. The sudden onset of fluttering in the chest with weakness, dyspnea, and increased cyanosis may occur with tachyarrhythmia. Sudden death may occur, probably as a result of ventricular tachycardia.

Physical examination usually shows normal physical and intellectual development. Although cyanosis may not be present at rest, patients often have a flushed or ruddy complexion. The pulse volume may be decreased in patients with severe tricuspid insufficiency, and pulse pressure is reduced. The precordial activity is usually not increased but the heart may be markedly enlarged. The auscultatory findings are similar to those described above for the infant. The first sound is split, with a loud late tricuspid component. The second sound is widely split and the split does not vary with respiration. A third sound is often present and a fourth sound may be heard. A medium-frequency systolic murmur of grade 2–4/6 starting with the first sound and extending through about two-thirds or all of systole is heard at the lower sternal region. A short, low-frequency, mid-diastolic murmur is often present at the lower left sternal border.

Investigations

Electrocardiography

The common findings on the electrocardiogram are tall peaked P waves, prolonged atrioventricular conduction, and right bundle-branch block. In infants the changes are often relatively mild; the P waves are only moderately prominent and right ventricular conduction delay is present, but complete bundle-branch block is not usual. With advancing age, the typical changes become manifest. The voltage of the QRS complexes in the right precordial leads is usually low. Preexcitation or Wolff–Parkinson–White (WPW) syndrome is common, occurring in up to about 25% of individuals. Usually the B type of WPW syndrome is found with Ebstein malformation, with a pattern of left axis deviation and QRS complexes suggesting left bundle-branch block. The preexcitation is intermittent and between the episodes the electrocardiogram shows the usual pattern of Ebstein anomaly.

Arrhythmias occur commonly and, as mentioned above, their frequency increases with advancing age. It has been reported that almost 80% of individuals with Ebstein anomaly will experience arrhythmia. In adolescents and adults, arrhythmia is the presenting feature in almost half of the patients [7]. Atrial and ventricular ectopic beats are common. Paroxysmal supraventricular tachycardia, atrial flutter, or atrial fibrillation are the usual arrhythmias, but unsustained ventricular tachycardia may also occur.

Chest radiography

The heart size varies from almost normal to marked enlargement. It is not uncommon for the heart size to be normal in the neonate with no or mild symptoms. However, infants with marked cyanosis and tricuspid regurgitation usually have very large hearts. On the anteroposterior view, the heart has a somewhat globular shape, with the right atrium bulging into the right chest; on the lateral view the right atrium fills the retrosternal space. The pulmonary artery segment is not prominent and pulmonary vascular markings are usually decreased in the infant with marked cyanosis.

Beyond infancy, the heart size is largely determined by the degree of tricuspid insufficiency. In individuals with mild leaflet displacement, the heart is often only slightly enlarged, but the right atrium may be prominent. The pulmonary artery is usually not enlarged and the pulmonary vasculature is normal. Occasionally, with mild tricuspid valve involvement, a large left-to-right shunt through the atrial septal communication is associated with enlargement of the main pulmonary artery and prominent pulmonary vessels in the lung fields. Severe tricuspid insufficiency is associated with marked cardiomegaly, with massive right atrial enlargement.

Echocardiography

Ultrasound has become the mainstay in diagnosis and assessment of severity of Ebstein malformation. The morphology and motion of the tricuspid valve leaflets is delineated more clearly than with angiocardiography. M-mode echocardiography was not very reliable in diagnosing the anomaly; delayed closure of the tricuspid valve relative to the mitral valve was considered a criterion for the diagnosis. However, two-dimensional echocardiography has greatly facilitated the diagnosis. Characteristically, the proximal attachment of the septal leaflet of the valve is displaced inferiorly toward the apex. Normally the septal leaflet attaches slightly distal to the septal attachment of the mitral valve. This separation is accentuated in Ebstein anomaly; a distance between the attachments greater than 8 mm/m^2 body surface area is considered diagnostic. Other criteria that have been suggested are a separation of more than 15 mm in children or more than 20 mm in adults. The displacement of the posterior leaflet can also be observed. The septal and posterior leaflets should be examined to assess the extent of tethering to the adjacent myocardium and the degree of dysplasia, because these features have important surgical implications. The anterosuperior leaflet is seen to be large and billowing; the distal attachments of the leaflet should be defined to assess whether the tricuspid orifice into the functional portion of the right ventricle is obstructed. The atrial septum should be examined to assess the size of the defect. The ventricular septum may be displaced into the ventricular cavity to a varying degree. The size of the left ventricle and its function should be assessed. Doppler flow studies are useful in determining the magnitude of tricuspid regurgitation and the direction and extent of shunting through the atrial septal communication.

Cardiac catheterization

The advent of two-dimensional echocardiography has largely eliminated the need for cardiac catheterization or angiography for diagnosis of Ebstein malformation. The main indication for transvenous procedures is to undertake electrophysiological studies and possibly perform ablation procedures for arrhythmias. In the early experience with catheterization, there was a high risk, usually as a result of the induction of serious arrhythmia. However, with improved monitoring, more careful catheter manipulation, and ability to terminate arrhythmia, the risks have been greatly reduced.

From the groin approach the catheter is readily passed through the inferior vena cava. The diagnosis may be suspected if the catheter forms a wide loop in a greatly enlarged right atrium. Some difficulty may be experienced in manipulating the catheter across the tricuspid orifice into the right ventricle because the large billowing anterior leaflet may create obstruction. If the right ventricle is catheterized, considerable difficulty may be experienced in entering the pulmonary artery, because the course of the catheter may be distorted by the tricuspid valve. From the right atrium, the catheter can usually be passed readily across the atrial septal communication into the left atrium and ventricle. Occasionally, however, the atrial enlargement results in marked displacement of the atrial septum and it may be difficult to locate the atrial septal defect.

Oxygen saturation data

In the cyanosed newborn infant, mixed venous oxygen saturation is usually decreased as a result of arterial hypoxemia as well as reduced cardiac output. In the infant with severe cyanosis, metabolic acidemia may develop. In the older child with mild tricuspid valve abnormalities, a left-to-right shunt at the atrial level may result in an increase in right atrial and right ventricular oxygen saturation. Systemic arterial oxygen saturation is reduced when an atrial right-to-left shunt is present. In the neonate, oxygen saturation may be markedly decreased to 40–50%. In older children and adults, arterial saturation is usually in the range 80–90%, but it may be lower.

Pressures

Pressures in the vena cava and right atrium may be normal, but with significant tricuspid regurgitation the mean atrial pressure may be increased to 10–15 mmHg and the *v* wave is prominent. The pressure in the atrialized portion of the ventricle is identical to that in the atrium. Right ventricular systolic pressure is usually normal but may be increased mildly to about 35–40 mmHg. Rarely, in association with marked subvalvar or valvar obstruction of the pulmonary valve, right ventricular systolic pressure may be elevated to near systemic arterial levels. End-diastolic pressure in the right ventricle may be elevated, particularly when tricuspid regurgitation is severe. Systemic arterial pressure, as well as pulse pressure, may be reduced in infants with reduced cardiac output, but in older individuals arterial pressure is usually normal. However, it may fall if severe cardiac failure develops.

Prior to the use of ultrasound techniques for diagnosing Ebstein anomaly, it was difficult, even after catheterization, to be sure of the diagnosis. A very useful technique is to correlate the pressure contour with the intracardiac electrocardiogram. A catheter with a built-in electrode adjacent to the hole at the tip is maneuvered, with continuous pressure monitoring, through the tricuspid orifice into the right ventricle. Both the pressure and intracardiac electrocardiogram are recorded simultaneously while the catheter is withdrawn. In the ventricle, the typical ventricular pressure and electrocardiogram are noted. In the patient with Ebstein malformation, with gradual withdrawal of the catheter, an area can be identified where the pressure contour is characteristic of the atrial chamber but the electrocardiogram is typical of that in the right ventricle. On further withdrawal, the pressure and electrocardiogram are characteristic of the right atrium.

Blood flows and vascular resistances

Pulmonary blood flow is often greatly reduced in the newborn infant with severe cyanosis. Systemic flow is often also decreased in the infant with severe symptoms. In the early neonatal period, pulmonary vascular resistance is still elevated, not having undergone the normal postnatal decline. Within a few days, pulmonary vascular resistance falls and pulmonary blood flow increases. As the infant improves, systemic blood flow increases to normal levels. In the older child, blood flows are in the normal range, unless cyanosis or cardiac failure occurs. Pulmonary blood flow may exceed systemic flow if there is a left-to-right shunt. The pulmonary to systemic flow ratio is rarely greater than about 1.7–2:1. Systemic flow is higher than pulmonary flow if a significant right-to-left shunt is present. Systemic vascular resistance is usually normal but may be increased in the presence of severe tricuspid insufficiency.

Angiocardiography

An injection of contrast medium into the right atrium reveals the enlarged chamber, consisting of the atrium itself and the atrialized portion of the right ventricle. An indentation on the diaphragmatic margin of the chamber may designate the site of the atrioventricular annulus. The large billowing anterior valve leaflet may be seen extending well to the left of the spine. Contrast medium may also be observed passing through the atrial septal communication into the left atrium. An injection into the right ventricle may show a chamber of almost normal size, but usually the functioning right ventricular chamber is small. In severe malformations, particularly in infants, only the outlet chamber of the ventricle is evident. In the neonate, the pulmonary valve may not open and differentiation between morphological and functional pulmonary atresia is difficult. With the right ventricular injection, contrast material usually fills the right atrium. Although this is usually due to valvar insufficiency, it may be difficult to assess the degree of tricuspid regurgitation because the catheter may distort the abnormal valve. Frequently the tip of the catheter withdraws proximal to the tricuspid valve due to the small size of the ventricle. The main and branch pulmonary arteries are usually small in infants with significant cyanosis. In older individuals, the diameter of the arteries is sometimes decreased. In relation to the greatly enlarged atrium and ventricular shadow, they have an appearance of being very small. The intrapulmonary vessels are poorly filled in infants with severe cyanosis, but in older individuals are usually normal. A left ventricular angiogram may show the chamber to be relatively small due to encroachment by displacement of the ventricular septum.

Differential diagnosis

In the newborn infant with severe cyanosis, the differential diagnosis between Ebstein malformation and other lesions may be difficult. On auscultation, splitting of the first and second sound, a prominent third sound, and possibly a fourth sound suggest the diagnosis. Although the heart may be of normal size in a cyanosed infant with Ebstein anomaly, this is quite unusual; the presence of marked cardiomegaly should make one suspect the diagnosis. Electrocardiographic features suggesting Ebstein anomaly are right bundle-branch block and type B WPW syndrome. However, these are not common in infants. The absence of prominent right ventricular forces in the precordial leads, with right ventricular conduction delay and the presence of tall peaked P waves, suggest a diagnosis of Ebstein anomaly or tricuspid atresia. With tricuspid atresia there is usually left axis deviation. The diagnosis is apparent with ultrasound study.

In older individuals, the association of cyanosis and tachyarrhythmia should strongly suggest the possibility of Ebstein anomaly. Other clinical phenomena that should lead to consideration of the anomaly are exercise limitation and appearance of cyanosis on exertion, and postural cyanosis on reclining. In individuals with Ebstein malformation with mild abnormality of the valve and only a small left-to-right shunt through the atrial septal communication, the diagnosis of atrial septal defect of the secundum type may be entertained. The wide splitting of the second sound and short mid-diastolic murmur at the lower left sternal border are findings common to both lesions. The differential diagnosis may be difficult on clinical examination, because the electrocardiogram may not be helpful, showing right ventricular conduction delay with only mildly prominent right forces. The chest radiograph may also be unhelpful, but marked prominence of the right atrium makes the diagnosis of Ebstein malformation more likely. The diagnosis may not be appreciated until an ultrasound study is performed.

Principles of management

The spectrum of morphological abnormalities and functional disturbance is so varied that treatment plans for patients must be individualized. Individuals with a mild tricuspid valve anomaly may never experience symptoms and require no therapy. The therapeutic options include various forms of surgery to modify the morphology and management of arrhythmias with drugs or ablation procedures. In the sections below I discuss the treatment options for the following clinical presentations:

- cardiac failure or arrhythmia in the fetus;
- severe cyanosis in the neonate;
- severe tricuspid regurgitation with cardiac failure;
- cyanosis with severe exercise limitation;
- paradoxical embolism;
- supraventricular or ventricular tachycardia.

Some centers have also suggested that marked cardiomegaly, or moderate cyanosis without severe limitation, are indications for surgery.

Ebstein anomaly in the fetus

The mortality is high in fetuses in whom the diagnosis has been established [3–5]. Generally, little can be offered. However, in one report, improvement of cardiac failure, manifested by hydrops, has been achieved by administering digoxin directly to the fetus [8]. Digoxin therapy should probably be considered for these fetuses, but the likelihood of improvement is small. Furthermore, infants in whom the diagnosis of Ebstein anomaly had been made *in utero* have a very high mortality during the newborn period. If fetal arrhythmia is detected, treatment should be instituted by administering drugs to the mother. Many drugs have been recommended. Digoxin has occasionally terminated supraventricular tachycardia but is not likely to be effective in Ebstein anomaly. Currently, class II antiarrhythmic (β-adrenoceptor blocking) agents are favored. Sotalol, a drug with class III as well as class II effects, has been used in some patients.

Newborn infant with severe cyanosis

The infant should receive oxygen and other measures for management of hypoxemia (see Chapter 14). In the early postnatal period, while pulmonary vascular resistance is still relatively high, PGE_1 should be administered by intravenous infusion to maintain ductus arteriosus patency in order to provide adequate pulmonary blood flow. If severe right ventricular outflow obstruction is present, it will be necessary to maintain ductus patency with PGE_1 until a decision is made about subsequent therapy. If there is little or no right ventricular outflow obstruction, as pulmonary vascular resistance falls after birth, the decrease in pulmonary arterial pressure and afterload on the right ventricle will reduce the degree of tricuspid regurgitation and manifestations of cardiac failure. At this stage, maintaining patency of the ductus arteriosus may interfere with the fall in pulmonary arterial pressure and prevent the reduction in severity of tricuspid regurgitation. Infusion of PGE_1 should be gradually reduced or terminated while the infant's oxygen saturation, Po_2 and pH are carefully monitored. If arterial oxygen saturation or Po_2 falls significantly, or if pH falls, the PGE_1 infusion should be restarted immediately. If the infant does not tolerate cessation of PGE_1, subsequent attempts to stop the infusion can be made after several days. Administration of pulmonary vasodilators such as sildenafil or nitric oxide prior to stopping the prostaglandin infusion may allow adequate pulmonary perfusion.

If adequate pulmonary blood flow cannot be maintained without PGE_1, an aortopulmonary shunt is recommended. In the early experience with aortopulmonary shunts, results were very disappointing and mortality was high. This was probably related to the inability of the left ventricle to increase its output to provide both pulmonary blood flow and adequate systemic blood flow, because of infringement of its cavity by septal displacement. Currently, in addition to performing a modified Blalock–Taussig shunt, the tricuspid valve is closed, either by suturing the large anterior leaflet to the ventricular wall or by inserting a pericardial patch in the orifice. This eliminates tricuspid regurgitation and reduces septal displacement, and improves left ventricular performance [9]. It has also been recommended that if significant pulmonary valvar insufficiency is evident, the pulmonary valve orifice should be sealed. Considerable success has been achieved with this approach. This procedure commits the patient to surviving with a single ventricle. Subsequently, a superior cavopulmonary anastomosis is established after about 6–8 months. Completion of the Fontan-type operation can be accomplished later (see Chapter 16).

Ebstein anomaly with severe tricuspid insufficiency

The need for surgery for tricuspid insufficiency may arise during infancy, but may not be necessary until later in childhood or even until adulthood. Because of technical difficulties in small infants, it is preferable to delay the procedure until an older age if possible. Several different approaches have been used and techniques have improved progressively. Early attempts at reconstruction of the valve did not achieve great success, so prosthetic valve replacement was recommended. Although some successes were reported, the results were not uniformly encouraging. However, with advances in technique, reconstruction has been considerably improved and almost 80% of patients requiring surgery are amenable to some type of reconstruction. Various techniques are still used, but usually the atrialized portion of the right ventricle is plicated, a posterior tricuspid annuloplasty is performed, and an attempt is made to improve leaflet function. Techniques that have been used to achieve this include use of the large anterior leaflet to create a monocusp, and freeing the posterior and septal leaflets from their attachment to the ventricular wall to provide more mobility. Recently, the use of special suture to attempt to reconstitute chordae tendineae, and to replace shortened chordae and thus improve valve motility to create better closure, has been successful in some children [10].

If right atrial enlargement is severe and right ventricular function very poor, it may not be possible to achieve a significant reduction of tricuspid regurgitation and provide an adequate right ventricular output. Under this circumstance, introduction of a bidirectional superior cavopulmonary shunt has, in many instances, resulted in considerable improvement by reducing the volume load on the right ventricle [11,12].

Atrial septal defect closure

Occasionally, older children or adults with Ebstein anomaly develop increasing limitation associated with cyanosis. The heart may not be markedly enlarged and tricuspid insufficiency may not be severe. In some of these individuals, closure of the atrial septal defect has been successful in relieving both the cyanosis and symptoms. Although this has been accomplished surgically, currently closure of the defect by interventional cardiac catheterization techniques would be the recommended approach (see Chapter 8).

Arrhythmia

Supraventricular tachycardias are often very resistant to drug therapy in individuals with Ebstein malformation. Drugs may be very effective, but because of the considerable incidence of one or more accessory pathways in these patients, it is recommended that if they manifest arrhythmia, an electrophysiological procedure be performed. Abnormal conducting pathways should be ablated by radiofrequency. The success rate of ablation procedures is not as high in patients with Ebstein anomaly as in those with hearts with normal morphology, because multiple pathways are often present. For this reason, recurrence of tachycardia after initial success may occur.

References

1 Stellin G, Santini F, Thiene G *et al.* Pulmonary atresia, intact ventricular septum, and Ebstein anomaly of the tricuspid valve. Anatomic and surgical considerations. J Thorac Cardiovasc Surg 1993;106:255–261.

2 Inamura N, Taketazu M, Smallhorn JF, Hornberger LK. Left ventricular myocardial performance in the fetus with severe tricuspid valve disease and tricuspid insufficiency. Am J Perinatol 2005;22:91–97.

3 Hornberger LK, Sahn DJ, Kleinman CS, Copel JA, Reed KL. Tricuspid valve disease with significant tricuspid insufficiency in the fetus: diagnosis and outcome. J Am Coll Cardiol 1991;17:167–173.

4 Sharland GK, Chita SK, Allan LD. Tricuspid valve dysplasia or displacement in intrauterine life. J Am Coll Cardiol 1991;17:944–949.

5 Pavlova M, Fouron JC, Drblik SP *et al.* Factors affecting the prognosis of Ebstein's anomaly during fetal life. Am Heart J 1998;135:1081–1085.

6 Wald RM, Adatia I, Van Arsdell GS, Hornberger LK. Relation of limiting ductal patency to survival in neonatal Ebstein's anomaly. Am J Cardiol 2005;96:851–856.

7 Celermajer DS, Bull C, Till JA *et al.* Ebstein's anomaly: presentation and outcome from fetus to adult. J Am Coll Cardiol 1994;23:170–176.

8 Hsieh YY, Lee CC, Chang CC, Tsai HD, Yeh LS, Tsai CH. Successful prenatal digoxin therapy for Ebstein's anomaly with hydrops fetalis. A case report. J Reprod Med 1998;43:710–712.

9 Reemtsen BL, Fagan BT, Wells WJ, Starnes VA. Current surgical therapy for Ebstein anomaly in neonates. J Thorac Cardiovasc Surg 2006;32:1285–1290.

10 Reddy VM, McElhinney DB, Brook MM, Silverman NH, Stanger P, Hanley FL. Repair of congenital tricuspid valve abnormalities with artificial chordae tendineae. Ann Thorac Surg 1998;66:172–176.

11 Quinonez LG, Dearani JA, Puga FJ *et al.* Results of the 1.5-ventricle repair for Ebstein anomaly and the failing right ventricle. J Thorac Cardiovasc Surg 2007;133: 1303–1310.

12 Marianeschi SM, McElhinney DB, Reddy VM, Silverman NH, Hanley FL. Alternative approach to the repair of Ebstein's malformation: intracardiac repair with ventricular unloading. Ann Thorac Surg 1998;66:1546–1550.

18

CHAPTER 18

Aortopulmonary transposition

Aortopulmonary transposition, or transposition of the great arteries, is a congenital heart lesion characterized by abnormal origin of the aorta and pulmonary artery from the ventricular complex. The atria and the ventricles are normally related or concordant; the right atrium connects through a tricuspid valve to a ventricle with the morphological features of a normal right ventricle; the left atrium leads through a mitral valve into a morphological left ventricle. However, the ventricular–arterial relationships are discordant, with the aorta arising from the right ventricle and the pulmonary artery from the left ventricle. The spatial relationships of the great arteries are also often abnormal. Normally, the pulmonary artery is placed anteriorly and to the right in the superior mediastinum. The aorta arises posteriorly and to the left and the valve is also caudal to the pulmonary valve. In aortopulmonary transposition, the aorta is placed anteriorly at its origin from the right ventricle and the pulmonary artery is posterior, arising from the left ventricle. The aortic valve is also positioned cephalad to the pulmonary valve. However, the relationships of the aorta and pulmonary artery may vary considerably; the diagnosis should be based on the presence of ventricular–arterial discordance rather than the spatial relationships of the aorta and pulmonary artery.

Transposition of the aorta and pulmonary artery is frequently associated with other congenital cardiac lesions, such as ventricular septal defect (present in about 50% of individuals) and left ventricular outflow tract obstruction, which functionally is pulmonary stenosis. In addition, atrioventricular septal defect, tricuspid atresia, and various types of single ventricle may be associated with transposition. Tricuspid atresia with transposition is discussed in Chapter 16. Congenitally corrected transposition is a condition in which the spatial relationships of the aorta and pulmonary artery are abnormal but the ventricles are inverted, so that there is atrioventricular discordance as well as ventricular–arterial discordance. The right atrium leads through a mitral valve into a morphological left ventricle, which gives rise to a pulmonary artery. The left atrium connects via a tricuspid valve to a morphological right ventricle from which arises the aorta. Because there is both atrioventricular and ventricular–arterial discordance, the circulatory dynamics are normal. In this chapter, I discuss aortopulmonary transposition with normal ventricular alignment.

Morphological considerations

Although aortopulmonary transposition is now defined as ventricular–arterial discordance, in the past it was characterized by the anterior position of the aorta in relation to the pulmonary artery. The aortic valve is abnormally anterior, superior, and to the right. There is a well-developed conus or infundibulum in the subaortic region of the right ventricle, and this is the most anterior portion of the heart. The right ventricular muscle mass is usually normal postnatally, but its growth rate is not reduced as in the normal heart after birth and within a few weeks it is clearly hypertrophied compared with the normal. There is wide separation between the septal leaflet of the tricuspid valve and the aortic valve. In the early postnatal period, the thickness of the left ventricular wall is similar to that of the right left ventricle. In the absence of an associated large ventricular septal defect, the growth rate of the right ventricle decreases and

Congenital Diseases of the Heart, 3rd edition. By A. Rudolph
 ISBN: 9781405162456

within a few weeks after birth the thickness of the left ventricular wall is comparable to that of the right ventricular wall in a normal heart. The pulmonary valve is posterior to the aortic valve and is also displaced more inferiorly and toward the right than usual. There is no ventricular muscle tissue between the mitral and pulmonary valves, resulting in contiguity of the septal leaflet of the mitral valve with the pulmonary valve. The superior vena cava (SVC) and inferior vena cava (IVC), the pulmonary veins, and the atria are usually normal. During the postnatal period the ductus arteriosus usually becomes quickly constricted, with only a small lumen, and the foramen ovale shows a normal orifice. In the absence of other lesions, the ascending aorta is often quite large in diameter and the isthmus frequently is as wide as the descending aorta, suggesting that there has been greater than normal flow across the isthmus in fetal life (see Chapter 12). Aortic isthmus obstruction or coarctation may occur but is not common.

Associated lesions are quite common with aortopulmonary transposition. Ventricular septal defects, ranging from small to very large, are frequently encountered and are important in determining the hemodynamic and clinical manifestations. The defects may be located in any portion of the ventricular septum (see Chapter 7), but quite frequently involve the outlet septum. When the defect is located in the subpulmonary region of the septum, it may be difficult to distinguish between aortopulmonary transposition with a ventricular septal defect and double-outlet right ventricle of the Taussig–Bing type. In the latter condition, the aorta arises anteriorly and the pulmonary artery, which is posterior, overrides the ventricular septal defect. The outlet septum may be displaced toward the right, creating narrowing of the subaortic region; this gives the impression that the pulmonary artery arises largely from the left ventricle, suggesting the diagnosis of transposition. Functionally, the two complexes behave similarly and management is similar. Although a conus beneath both semilunar valves is characteristic of double-outlet right ventricle, it would be expected that there would be separation between the mitral and pulmonary valves; this may be poorly defined, so that differentiation may be difficult. The presence of subaortic stenosis, which is also commonly associated with aortic coarctation and narrow aortic isthmus, strongly supports the diagnosis of Taussig–Bing anomaly.

Large atrial septal defects of the fossa ovalis or ostium secundum type may occur, but they are not as common as ventricular septal defects. Frequently, systemic systolic pressure in the right ventricle displaces the ventricular septum into the left ventricular outflow tract and causes subvalvar pulmonary stenosis. Less commonly, more severe degrees of stenosis may be related to a fibrous shelf below the pulmonary valve and occasionally abnormal attachment of the mitral valve may encroach on the outflow tract of the left ventricle. The pulmonary valve orifice itself may be small and sometimes the valve is stenotic. When transposition is associated with a ventricular septal defect, subvalvar pulmonary stenosis may be due to displacement of the outlet septum into the left ventricular outflow. The main pulmonary trunk tends to be shorter than normal and frequently the trunk is oriented toward the right. With this orientation the right pulmonary artery is often considerably larger than the left, which may appear to be hypoplastic.

Changes in the pulmonary vasculature after birth vary, depending on the associated lesions. When a large ventricular septal defect is present, the pulmonary arteriolar vessels retain their thick muscular medial layer, and there is usually appearance of intimal proliferation and fibrosis within the first year of life. The pulmonary vascular obstructive changes appear to occur earlier than when a ventricular septal defect is not associated with transposition and, not infrequently, infants of 3–6 months of age have well-developed pulmonary vascular changes. In the absence of a large ventricular septal defect, the vessels tend to show normal maturational changes, but intimal proliferation with thrombosis and fibrosis occurs in a small number of infants, as early as a few months after birth. The occurrence of increased pulmonary vascular smooth muscle development with high pulmonary vascular resistance in both the fetus and neonate with aortopulmonary transposition has been recognized [1]. This association is discussed on p. 471.

Lesions of the tricuspid valve, with associated underdevelopment of the right ventricle, are sometimes associated with aortopulmonary transposition.

The association of ventricular septal defect, underdeveloped right ventricle, and small tricuspid valve with functional stenosis and aortopulmonary transposition is occasionally observed. When this complex is present, there is also a high incidence of aortic isthmus narrowing or aortic coarctation and persistent patent ductus arteriosus. A more severe form with tricuspid atresia may also occur, with a smaller right ventricle and a ventricular septal defect; aortic isthmus narrowing is commonly associated (see Chapter 16).

The coronary arteries both originate from the aorta. Both coronary arteries arise from the aortic sinuses adjacent to the pulmonary artery. Whereas normally the noncoronary sinus is the right posterior sinus, in aortopulmonary transposition the right anterior sinus does not give rise to a coronary artery. Unlike in normal individuals, the right coronary artery tends to be larger than the left; the left circumflex artery arises from the right coronary in about 20% of individuals. A single coronary artery occurs in about 10% of patients with transposition.

Apart from the manifestations of hypoxia and, if present, cardiac failure, there are no other generalized pathological findings in aortopulmonary transposition. Other congenital anomalies are not common. One interesting finding in some newborn infants with transposition is the presence of islet hypertrophy in the pancreas. Whether this is a true association or coincidental is questionable.

Embryological considerations

The disturbances in embryological development of the heart responsible for aortopulmonary transposition are not yet fully defined. One hypothesis suggests that it is based on lack of spiraling of the septum that grows in the primitive truncus arteriosus communis to separate it into the aortic and pulmonary trunks. The introduction of new models of embryological development of the conotruncal region by Keith, Lev, and van Praagh has resulted in a much broader concept of transposition. These hypotheses stress the importance of the development of the conus region, whether it preferentially develops on the left or right side or bilaterally, and its ultimate position in relation to the aorta and the pulmonary artery. The discussion that follows refers to transposition, in which there is normal position of the atria and ventricles with atrioventricular concordance, so-called D-transposition. Keith has maintained that the abnormal relationships of the aorta and pulmonary artery to the respective ventricles are due to alterations in resorption of conal tissue in the subaortic and subpulmonary regions. During development of the conotruncal region, the pulmonary artery is related to the left conus and the aorta to the right conus. It was suggested that normally the right conus is resorbed, bringing the aorta over the left ventricle. Aortopulmonary transposition was claimed to be due to resorption of the left rather than the right conus and this placed the pulmonary artery over the left ventricle. Van Praagh has presented a hypothesis of an abnormality of conal development based on differential rates of conal growth rather than on resorption of conal tissue. He stresses the fact that in typical aortopulmonary transposition there is always well-developed conus related to the aorta and absent conal tissue in relation to the pulmonary artery. This results in separation of the aortic and tricuspid cusps and also in contiguity of the mitral and pulmonary valve cusps. Therefore, he has proposed that there is differential growth of the left and right coni. Normally, preferential growth of the left conus, which is subpulmonary in location, displaces the pulmonary valve anteriorly and to the left, so that the aortic valve is pushed posteriorly and to the right; because right conus growth is significantly less, the aortic valve is contiguous with the mitral valve. Aortopulmonary transposition, it is claimed, is caused by preferential growth of the right-sided conal tissue, which brings the developing aorta anteriorly and to the right in relation to the right ventricle. The left conus does not grow and thus the pulmonary artery overlies the left ventricle and is contiguous with the mitral valve. Whether abnormalities in either differential conus resorption or growth are responsible for transposition is yet to be resolved.

The hypothesis that aortopulmonary transposition is due to abnormal growth of the spiral septum has lost support in recent years. It has been claimed that the normal spiral relationships of the proximal portion of the aorta and pulmonary artery are due to growth of endocardial cushions that develop in a spiral arrangement in the ventral aorta connected to the bulbus cordis. It has been proposed that if growth of the septum is straight rather than spiral, the anterior portion of the aorta will connect with the right ventricle and the posterior portion, from which the pulmonary artery develops, with the left ventricle. A modified version of this concept proposes that a disturbance in the hemodynamic patterns of flow in the developing embryonic heart explains the lack of spiraling of the septum. This, it is suggested, results in disappearance of the normal separate streams of blood entering the ventral aorta; the lack of these streams interferes with normal molding and allows the septum to develop in a single straight plane. Van Praagh has criticized the theory that abnormal development of the spiral septum is responsible for transposition, because alterations in the positions of the coronary arteries and of the semilunar valve cusp alignment would be expected. Thus if the septum did not develop appropriately, the left coronary artery would be expected to arise from the pulmonary artery. It has been proposed that spiraling of the septum is related to differential conus growth or resorption.

Aortopulmonary transposition has generally not been associated with genetic syndromes and its occurrence was assumed to be sporadic. However, a report from Italy indicates that congenital cardiovascular malformations were encountered in 10% of families with a child with transposition; also the most common lesion that occurred was transposition [2]. Recently, variants of the *CFC1* gene have been noted to occur in individuals with laterality defects, who also develop congenital cardiovascular malformations [3]. *CFC1* mutations have also been identified in patients with heterotaxy syndrome, some of whom had aortopulmonary transposition [4].

Hemodynamic considerations

The presence and extent of the associated lesions determine the circulatory dynamics in individuals with aortopulmonary transposition. The lesions that commonly affect the hemodynamic and clinical features are ventricular septal defect, pulmonary stenosis, and atrial septal defect. The size of the defects and severity of the stenosis are important in determining the manifestations. Five groups are considered.

1 Aortopulmonary transposition with inadequate communication between the pulmonary and systemic circulation.
2 Aortopulmonary transposition with a large communication between the pulmonary and systemic circulation:
   (a) Ventricular septal defect
   (b) Atrial septal defect.
3 Aortopulmonary transposition with ventricular septal defect and pulmonary stenosis.
4 Aortopulmonary transposition with ventricular septal defect and hypoplastic right ventricle.
5 Aortopulmonary transposition with ventricular septal defect and tricuspid atresia (see Chapter 16).

Fetal circulation

Aortopulmonary transposition is compatible with fetal survival and normal body growth and development. There is no evidence that there is a significantly high incidence of aortopulmonary transposition in stillbirths. The gestational development of the fetus also appears to be normal in most cases; in fact, there is a tendency for these infants to be rather large and heavy at birth. This relatively normal development of the fetus is related to the presence of the foramen ovale and the ductus arteriosus.

Aortopulmonary transposition with no related cardiac lesions

Although no measurements of oxygen saturation in the fetus with aortopulmonary transposition are available, it may be assumed that the oxygen content of blood ejected by the left and right ventricles is different from that in the normal fetus. Figure 18.1 shows the oxygen saturations that might be expected in various vessels and cardiac chambers in the normal fetus. Figure 18.2 shows the values for oxygen saturation that I have speculated might be observed in a fetus with aortopulmonary transposition and intact ventricular septum [5]. The patterns of venous return to the heart are probably not altered significantly in the fetus with transposition, although, as discussed below, it is possible that some minor alterations may result from the changes in afterload on the left and right ventricles.

The patterns of blood flow in the normal fetus are discussed in Chapter 1. SVC blood, which has an oxygen saturation of 35–40%, returns to the

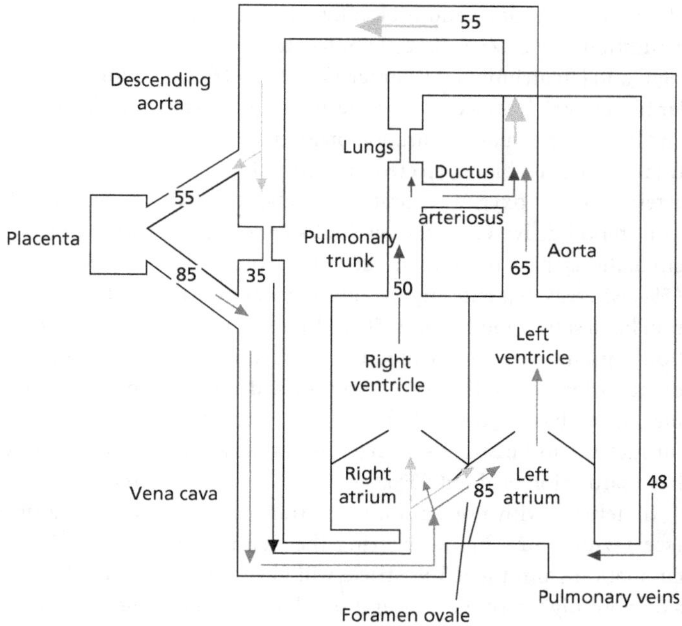

Figure 18.1 Circulation in the normal fetal lamb showing the patterns of blood flow and oxygen saturations in the cardiac chambers and vessels. Oxygen saturation is higher in the ascending aorta than the descending aorta. Pulmonary arterial oxygen saturation is quite low. For a detailed description see the text. From Rudolph [5] with permission. (See color plate 18.1).

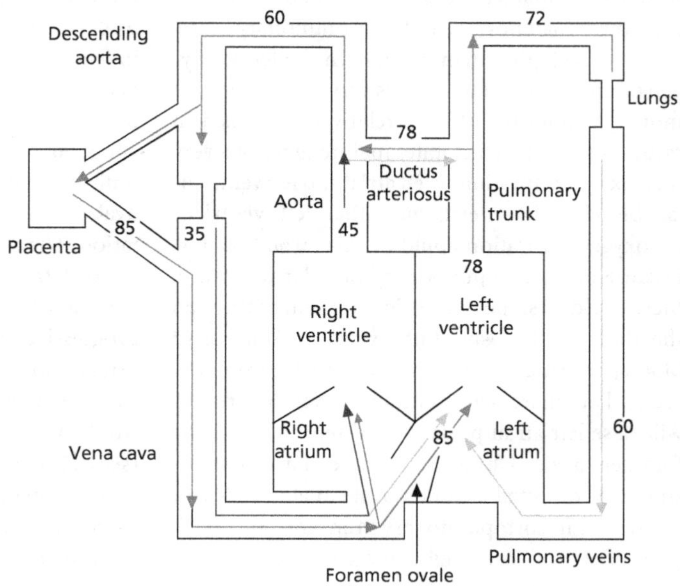

Figure 18.2 Patterns of blood flow and oxygen saturations in cardiac chambers and vessels in the fetus with aortopulmonary transposition. Assumptions of volumes of blood flow were used in calculating oxygen saturations in the main vessels. The pulmonary artery arises from the left ventricle; pulmonary arterial oxygen saturation is considerably greater than normal. The aorta arises from the right ventricle and oxygen saturation in the ascending aorta is less than normal. Descending aortic blood oxygen saturation is similar to that in the normal fetus. From Rudolph [5] with permission. (See color plate 18.2).

right atrium and is largely directed through the tricuspid valve to the right ventricle. Distal IVC blood has a similar oxygen saturation and is also predominantly directed through the tricuspid valve. An average of about 50% of umbilical venous blood, with an oxygen saturation of about 85%, is distributed to the portal circulation and the remainder passes through the ductus venosus. However, the proportion of umbilical venous return passing through the ductus venosus varies in individual fetuses from 20 to 80%. Ductus venosus blood is preferentially directed through the foramen ovale into the left atrium where it is joined by pulmonary venous blood, which has an oxygen saturation of about 48%. Hepatic venous blood, with an oxygen saturation of 65–75%, is distributed to both the right and left atrium (see Chapter 1). Left ventricular blood, which is ejected into the ascending aorta and its branches, has a saturation of about 65% and right ventricular blood, ejected into the pulmonary artery, has an oxygen saturation of about 50%. Thus blood delivered to the cerebral and coronary circulations has an oxygen saturation of about 65%, whereas that entering the pulmonary circulation has a saturation of about 50%. A large proportion of pulmonary arterial blood passes through the ductus arteriosus to the descending aorta; descending aortic blood, derived from the ductus and through the aortic isthmus from the ascending aorta, has a saturation of about 55%.

In fetuses with aortopulmonary transposition (see Figure 18.2), blood entering the pulmonary circulation from the left ventricle will have a considerably higher oxygen saturation than normal. The pulmonary vascular resistance, which is very sensitive to small changes in Po_2, will be considerably lower than normal and thus pulmonary blood flow will be higher than normal. In the fetus, oxygen consumption of the lung is very low, so the pulmonary venous blood has a relatively high oxygen saturation and this facilitates maintenance of a very high oxygen saturation of left atrial and left ventricular blood. I have estimated that left ventricular oxygen saturation could be 75–80%. Possibly, because of the low pulmonary vascular resistance, there could be some bidirectional shunting through the ductus arteriosus, but oxygen saturation of blood perfusing the lung will still be extraordinarily high. The increased pulmonary venous return will raise left atrial pressure and tend to close the foramen ovale. Ultrasound studies have demonstrated a restricted foramen ovale in about 20% of fetuses with aortopulmonary transposition [6,7]. The effect of the high oxygen saturation of pulmonary arterial blood on the small pulmonary blood vessels could be to reduce the development of pulmonary smooth muscle and thus make the pulmonary vessels less reactive to vasoactive stimuli. However, the relative effects of the high pulmonary arterial oxygen saturation and the effects of increased pulmonary arterial pressure could determine pulmonary vascular smooth muscle development.

In addition to the effect of the high oxygen saturation of pulmonary arterial blood on the pulmonary circulation, it could also have an effect on the ductus arteriosus. Pulmonary arterial blood passes through the ductus to the descending aorta and thus the ductus, which is normally exposed to blood with an oxygen saturation of about 50%, would be subjected to an an oxygen saturation of 75–80%; this could induce constriction. As shown in fetal lambs, constriction of the ductus results in pulmonary arterial hypertension and, as discussed in Chapter 5, this could induce increased development of pulmonary arteriolar smooth muscle and result in high pulmonary vascular resistance after birth. Ultrasound examination has demonstrated the presence of ductus arteriosus constriction and abnormal shunting in some fetuses with transposition [6,7], and persistent pulmonary hypertension of the newborn has been observed in some neonates with aortopulmonary transposition.

The vasodilator effects of increased oxygen saturation on the pulmonary circulation are more likely to occur in late gestation. The pulmonary vessels in fetal lambs are poorly reactive to changes in Po_2 before about 100 days' gestation and in human fetuses they are relatively unresponsive before about 30 weeks' gestation (see Chapter 5). It is thus unlikely that significant changes in the foramen ovale would be evident before about 30 weeks' gestation. The constrictor effect of oxygen on the ductus of fetal lambs is insignificant below about 90 days' gestation and the response to Po_2 increases progressively to term. The response of the ductus to Po_2 has not been defined in relation to human fetal gestational age, but it is unlikely that constriction would be prominent before 25–30 weeks' gestation (see Chapter 6).

It is apparent that many factors could interact to influence flow patterns in the fetus with aortopulmonary transposition. Thus an increase in pulmonary blood flow will increase pulmonary venous return and elevate left atrial pressure, tending to close the foramen ovale. This could reduce the flow of ductus venosus blood across the foramen ovale and reduce the oxygen saturation of left ventricular and pulmonary arterial blood, thus countering the fall in pulmonary vascular resistance. Although the fall in pulmonary vascular resistance resulting from exposure to high oxygen saturation could reduce pulmonary vascular smooth muscle development, the rise in pulmonary arterial pressure associated with ductus constriction could enhance smooth muscle development. It remains to be determined what the roles of these various influences are in the responses of the pulmonary circulation, the ductus arteriosus, and the foramen ovale.

It has now been recognized that detection of foramen ovale or ductus arteriosus constriction in the fetus with aortopulmonary transposition by ultrasound examination predicts that postnatal adaptation is likely to be difficult. The neonate usually has severe hypoxemia, does not usually show improvement with prostaglandin (PG)E_1 infusion, and may succumb within a few hours without drastic intervention [7]. Also persistent pulmonary hypertension of the newborn may be a prominent feature, which also presents difficult management problems. These features are discussed below.

The alterations of blood flow patterns in transposition will also affect the oxygen saturation and Po_2 of blood distributed to various parts of the fetal body. Normally, in lamb fetuses near term the oxygen saturation of blood in the ascending aorta is about 65% and Po_2 is 25–28 mmHg. However, in the fetus with transposition, the blood distributed to the ascending aorta from the right ventricle will have an oxygen saturation of about 45% (see Figure 18.2), similar to that in the pulmonary artery of the normal fetal lamb. Coronary blood flow would have to be about 1.5 times higher than normal to provide the same oxygen delivery as in the normal fetus. Similarly, cerebral blood flow would have to increase by 150% to provide the same oxygen delivery. The cerebral circulation in fetal lambs responds to hypoxemia by vasodilation with an increase in blood flow; thus cerebral oxygen delivery and oxygen consumption are maintained (see Chapter 1). There is evidence from ultrasound studies that cerebral vascular resistance is decreased in fetuses with aortopulmonary transposition, as shown by the reduced pulsatility index in Doppler flow velocity waveforms in the middle cerebral artery [8]. This should allow for adequate oxygen supply to the brain during fetal development. However, head circumference was significantly lower in neonates with aortopulmonary transposition compared with normal infants [9,10]. Whether this is related to a lower oxygen content in the blood supplying the brain or to associated genetic factors is not known. It is possible that although increased blood flow may usually be able to compensate for the low oxygen saturation, oxygen supply to the brain may be compromised at times of stress.

Blood from the ascending aorta that crosses the isthmus to the descending aorta will be joined by blood with higher Po_2 from the pulmonary artery that traverses the ductus arteriosus. The Po_2 of descending aortic blood will therefore be somewhat higher than that of ascending aortic blood and also higher than normal. This difference will depend on volume of flow from the pulmonary artery to the descending aorta; if the ductus arteriosus is constricted, this flow may be quite low.

The proportions of blood ejected by the left and right ventricles, and passing through vessels and shunts, could be significantly affected by the presence of aortopulmonary transposition. The output of the fetal ventricles is very sensitive to changes in afterload. In the normal fetus, a large proportion of the blood ejected by the right ventricle passes through the ductus arteriosus to the relatively low-resistance umbilical–placental circulation. However, in the fetus with transposition, if the ductus arteriosus is constricted, flow to the placenta will be derived from the right ventricle across the aortic arch and isthmus to the descending aorta. This could explain the fact that in newborn infants with transposition, the aortic isthmus shows less narrowing than normal (see Chapter 12). In the fetus with transposition, the left ventricle ejects into the pulmonary trunk, which connects with the ductus arteriosus and gives rise to the pulmonary arteries. The afterload is therefore determined by the pulmonary vascular resistance and, through the ductus arteriosus, by the low-resistance placental circulation. The afterloads on the ventricles will affect their emptying and therefore could influence the relative proportion of IVC blood distributed to the right ventricle and, through the foramen ovale, into the left ventricle.

It is difficult to explain the fact that abnormalities of the foramen ovale and ductus arteriosus are detected in only about 20% of fetuses with aortopulmonary transposition. This could possibly be explained by the amount of well-oxygenated umbilical venous blood that passes across the foramen ovale, with the resultant increase in pulmonary arterial oxygen saturation. As mentioned in Chapter 1, 20–80% of umbilical venous blood may bypass the liver through the ductus venosus, and ductus venosus blood is preferentially directed across the foramen ovale into the left atrium. Thus if a large proportion of umbilical venous return passes through the ductus venosus, it might be expected that pulmonary arterial oxygen saturation will be very high in the fetus with transposition and affect the pulmonary circulation and ductus arteriosus. However, if the major proportion of umbilical venous blood is distributed through the hepatic circulation, only a small volume would be preferentially directed across the foramen ovale and oxygen saturations in the two ventricles would be closer.

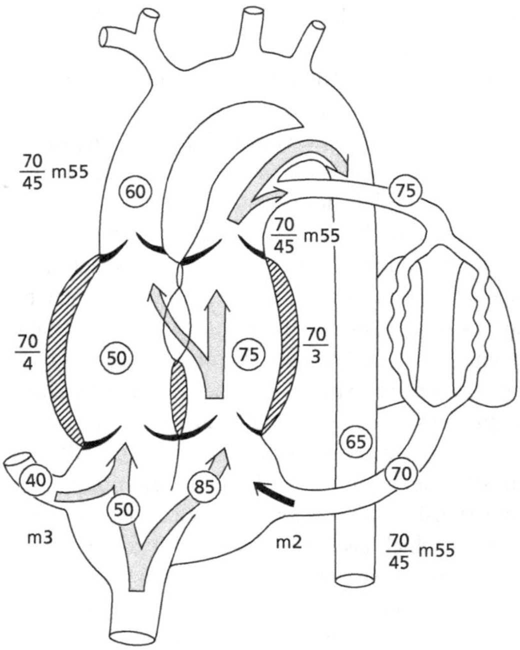

Figure 18.3 Aortopulmonary transposition with ventricular septal defect in a fetus: course of the circulation, oxygen saturations (circled), and pressures. m, mean pressure.

Aortopulmonary transposition with ventricular septal defect

When a large ventricular septal defect is present, the course of the circulation may be modified. Depending on the afterload on each ventricle, some shunting could occur in either direction, and it is possible that bidirectional shunting could occur. The high oxygen saturation of pulmonary arterial blood will decrease pulmonary vascular resistance, and during systole blood will probably shunt from the right to the left ventricle. This will result in some decrease in Po_2 of blood distributed to the lungs as well as through the ductus arteriosus. During diastole, a large volume will return from the pulmonary veins to the left atrium and ventricle and thus a shunt from the left to the right ventricle is likely to occur. This will add blood with a higher Po_2 to the ascending aortic stream and thus tend to limit the abnormal decrease in upper body Po_2 (Figure 18.3). The presence of a large ventricular septal defect will tend to allow some bidirectional shunting and limit the large changes in oxygen saturation that probably occur in the presence of an intact septum.

Aortopulmonary transposition with ventricular septal defect and pulmonary stenosis

If pulmonary stenosis is severe, blood entering the left ventricle will be largely ejected through the ventricular septal defect into the right ventricle. This would result in almost complete admixture of SVC and IVC streams, so that the Po_2 of ascending and descending aortic and pulmonary arterial blood would be similar. Blood supply to the lungs would be provided by flow from the aorta to the pulmonary artery beyond the stenosis through the ductus arteriosus. The blood distributed to the lungs would therefore have a lower Po_2 than that in transposition with no associated defects and there would be a lesser reduction in pulmonary vascular resistance (Figure 18.4). Ascending and descending aortic blood will have a similar Po_2 and this will be higher than that in transposition without other lesions.

Aortopulmonary transposition with ventricular septal defect and hypoplastic right ventricle

Inflow into the right ventricle is impeded and IVC blood will pass preferentially across the foramen to the left atrium. If right ventricular hypoplasia is severe and the tricuspid valve is small, even SVC blood may be directed across the foramen ovale. The right ventricle may receive only a small

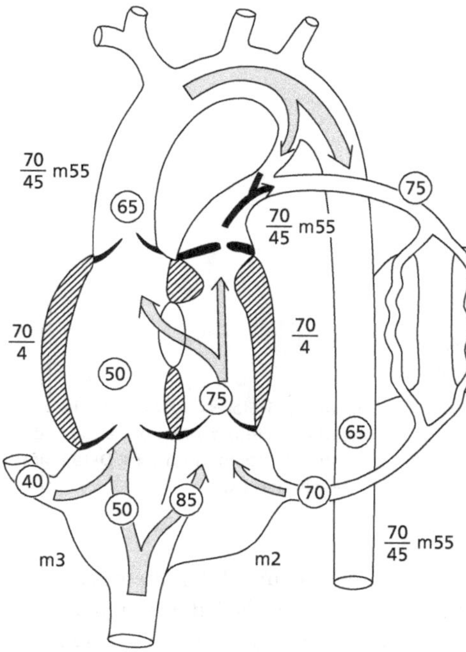

Figure 18.4 Aortopulmonary transposition with ventricular septal defect and pulmonary stenosis in a fetus: course of the circulation, oxygen saturations (circled), and pressures. m, mean pressure.

proportion of blood through the tricuspid valve and be supplied from the left ventricle through the ventricular septal defect. Because the volume of blood ejected by the right ventricle will be limited, the ascending aorta may be poorly developed and carry only the blood flow to the coronary circulation, the upper extremities, and the head. Aortic isthmus flow will be markedly reduced, and this could account for the fact that aortic isthmus narrowing or tubular hypoplasia of the aortic isthmus is encountered frequently in this complex (see Chapter 12). Left ventricular blood will be ejected into the pulmonary trunk and a large proportion will pass through the ductus to the descending aorta. Depending on the degree of reduction in aortic isthmus flow, a greater proportion of descending aortic flow will be derived from the ductus arteriosus, which therefore could be wider than normal. As in other aortopulmonary transposition complexes, the normal Po_2 relationships between the ascending and descending aortae would be reversed. However, if the right ventricle receives most of its blood from the left ventricle, the difference in Po_2 between the ascending and descending aortae will be small.

Postnatal circulation

General considerations

For the function of gas exchange to be assumed by the lung after birth, it is necessary not only for ventilation to occur but also for an effective pulmonary circulation to be established. Pulmonary blood flow must be increased and oxygenated blood must also be distributed to the systemic circulation. If the normal separation of the left and right sides of the heart by closure of the ductus arteriosus and foramen ovale ensued after birth in the infant with aortopulmonary transposition, oxygen supply to the tissues would not be possible. Systemic venous blood returning from the SVC and IVC to the right atrium will be ejected by the right ventricle into the aorta and thus would be recirculated. Pulmonary venous blood returning to the left atrium will be ejected by the left ventricle into the pulmonary artery, thus recirculating oxygenated blood through the pulmonary circulation. It is essential that there be some means for systemic venous blood to enter the pulmonary circulation to be oxygenated and also for pulmonary venous blood to pass into the systemic arterial system to supply oxygen to the tissues. This bidirectional shunting after birth may occur through persistent patency of fetal channels, the foramen ovale and the ductus arteriosus, or through abnormal channels, such as ventricular or atrial septal defects.

The general principles outlined in the following three sections will then be applied to postnatal circulatory adjustments in infants with aortopulmonary transposition and various associated defects.

Shunting and effective flows

There has been considerable confusion regarding the interpretation of left-to-right and right-to-left shunts in patients with aortopulmonary transposition. A left-to-right shunt represents the volume of blood passing from the left atrium or ventricle, or the aorta, directly into the right side of the heart. In most congenital cardiac lesions, it reflects the volume of pulmonary venous or oxygenated blood that recirculates through the lungs. However, in aortopulmonary transposition the pulmonary venous blood shunted from the left to the right side of the

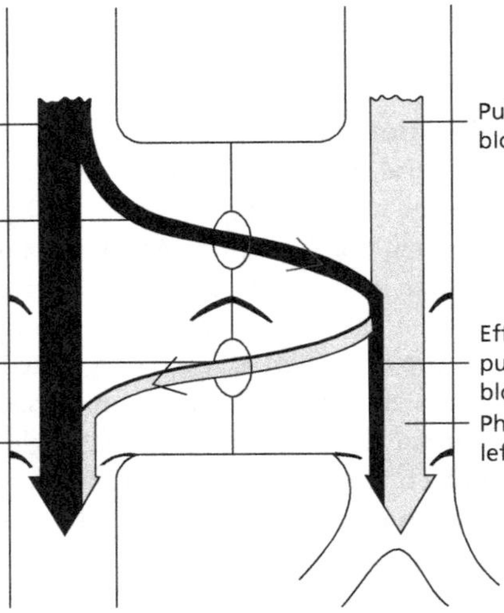

Figure 18.5 Flows and shunts in the heart of an infant with both atrial and ventricular communications. Details are given in the text.

heart enters the systemic circulation and does not recirculate to the lungs. The pulmonary venous blood returning to the left atrium and ventricle that is not shunted is ejected into the pulmonary artery and does recirculate.

To avoid confusion, it is convenient to introduce the concept of anatomical and physiological shunting (see Chapter 4). The anatomical left-to-right shunt represents the volume of blood actually passing from the left to the right side of the heart. The physiological left-to-right shunt reflects the volume of pulmonary venous blood that is recirculated through the lungs. Similarly, the anatomical right-to-left shunt is a measure of the actual amount of blood shunted from the right atrium or ventricle, or from the aorta, to the left atrium and ventricle or the pulmonary artery. The physiological right-to-left shunt represents the volume of systemic venous blood that reenters the systemic arteries without passing through the lung.

From the functional point of view, the amount of oxygen that can be taken up in the lungs is dependent on the volume of systemic venous blood that reaches the lungs; this is termed the *effective pulmonary blood flow*. In aortopulmonary transposition, the maximal amount of systemic venous blood that can reach the lungs is the anatomical right-to-left shunt. However, it cannot be assumed that the anatomical right-to-left shunt equals the effective pulmonary blood flow when there is bidirectional shunting. This is best explained in a model in which it is assumed that there is a shunt from the right atrium to the left atrium and from the left ventricle to the right ventricle (Figure 18.5). Some of the systemic venous blood shunted into the left atrium may be shunted back to the right ventricle without reaching the lungs and thus the effective pulmonary blood flow would be somewhat smaller than the anatomical right-to-left shunt. If the anatomical shunt is small in proportion to the total systemic or pulmonary blood flow, the error involved in calculations in which it is assumed that anatomical right-to-left shunt equals effective pulmonary flow will be quite small. However, if the anatomical shunt is a large percentage of systemic or pulmonary flow, the error may be quite large.

The anatomical left-to-right shunt must be identical to the anatomical right-to-left shunt in aortopulmonary transposition. Temporary small differences in the actual shunts may occur, but any prolonged difference would result in depletion of the blood volume in one circulation, with overloading of the other. The methods and difficulties involved in calculation of shunts in patients with aortopulmonary transposition are described in Chapter 4.

Pulmonary and systemic blood flow and arterial oxygen concentration

In most congenital heart lesions with right-to-left shunting of blood, the most important single factor that determines the level of arterial oxygen saturation is the magnitude of pulmonary blood flow. This is exemplified in tetralogy of Fallot (see Chapter 14). In aortopulmonary transposition, the most important factor is the amount of mixing between the pulmonary and systemic circulations, as represented by the physiological right-to-left and left-to-right shunts. However, when there is very effective mixing, due usually to a large ventricular or atrial septal defect, the magnitude of pulmonary blood flow and the ratio of pulmonary to systemic flow will influence the arterial oxygen saturation. In the absence of a large communication, pulmonary blood flow may be increased markedly, yet arterial oxygen saturation may be greatly reduced. As mentioned on p. 474, when there is poor mixing, the calculated effective pulmonary blood flow provides a reliable measure of actual anatomical left-to-right and right-to-left shunts. In these instances, knowledge of actual pulmonary blood flow is not important in relation to arterial Po_2, but may be important with regard to left ventricular dynamics and assessment of pulmonary vascular resistance.

Although systemic blood flow is important in providing oxygen to the tissues, the total available oxygen supply is provided by the oxygenated blood that passes from the left to the right side of the heart, namely the physiological left-to-right shunt. If systemic blood flow is large, the oxygen saturation of arterial blood will be low; if it is decreased, oxygen saturation will be higher.

Therefore the main concerns in the postnatal adjustment of infants with aortopulmonary transposition without adequate mixing are the magnitude of the shunts, the size of effective pulmonary blood flow, and the total oxygen uptake for delivery to the tissues.

Pulmonary and systemic blood flow and effective mixing

When there is effective mixing of pulmonary and systemic venous returns in patients with aortopulmonary transposition, the level of arterial oxygen saturation is influenced by the pulmonary to systemic flow ratio. A large pulmonary to systemic flow ratio will result in a relatively high systemic arterial oxygen concentration and tissue hypoxia will not occur; the physiological disturbances will be related to the ability of the ventricles to maintain the high pulmonary blood flow. If the ventricles are not able to do so, cardiac failure supervenes. If there is effective mixing but pulmonary flow is reduced by the presence of pulmonary stenosis or increased pulmonary vascular resistance, the pulmonary to systemic flow ratio will be decreased and arterial oxygen saturation will be lower. If the ratio is markedly reduced, hypoxemia with resultant hypoxia may result.

Aortopulmonary transposition with inadequate pulmonary–systemic communication

Elimination of the low-resistance umbilical–placental circulation at birth results in a marked increase in systemic vascular resistance. In the presence of aortopulmonary transposition, the right ventricle, which ejects into the aorta, is confronted with a greater afterload and initially its stroke volume will fall. End-diastolic volume and pressure will be elevated to raise stroke volume and the right atrial *a* wave will increase. The decrease in pulmonary vascular resistance associated with ventilation will reduce the afterload on the left ventricle, allowing a greater stroke volume into the pulmonary artery. If the ductus arteriosus remains open, the fetal flow pattern will be reversed and blood will flow from the aorta to the pulmonary artery, the quantity of flow being determined by the size of the ductus and the pulmonary arterial and aortic pressures (Figure 18.6). If the ductus is widely patent and pulmonary arterial and aortic pressures are the same, the flow will be determined by relative resistance in the pulmonary and systemic circulations. In the early postnatal period, while pulmonary vascular resistance is still relatively high, pulmonary blood flow as well as the ductus shunt are not very large, but with further maturation of the pulmonary vasculature, an increasing pulmonary blood flow will develop.

We do not know whether the decline in pulmonary vascular resistance after birth follows the normal pattern in infants with aortopulmonary transposition. If, as mentioned on p. 470, the pulmonary arterioles have poorly developed medial smooth muscle, it might be expected that the decrease in pulmonary vascular resistance after birth would be more rapid than normal. However, if pulmonary vascular smooth muscle development

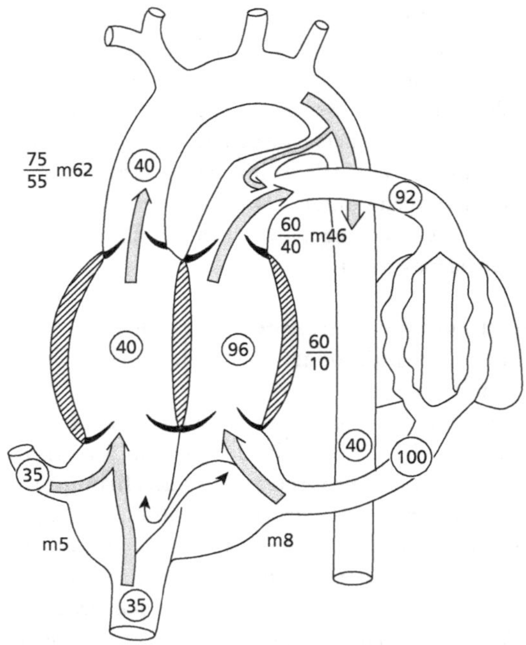

Figure 18.6 Aortopulmonary transposition with no associated defects in a newborn infant: course of the circulation, oxygen saturations (circled), and pressures demonstrate the important roles of the ductus arteriosus and the foramen ovale. m, mean pressure.

has been enhanced by prenatal ductus arteriosus constriction (see Chapter 18), pulmonary vascular resistance may be high and fall only slowly after birth. In this circumstance, pulmonary blood flow will be low and thus cyanosis may be severe.

Another factor that must be considered is whether systemic arterial hypoxemia may affect the postnatal changes in the pulmonary circulation. Early studies in fetal lambs suggested that a reduction in systemic arterial Po_2 and pH might induce pulmonary vasoconstriction through chemoreflex mechanisms. If this occurred in infants after birth, the low systemic arterial Po_2 often encountered in infants with aortopulmonary transposition may cause reflex vasoconstriction of the pulmonary circulation and delay the postnatal decrease in pulmonary vascular resistance. However, current evidence suggests that the pulmonary arterioles are primarily affected by local Po_2 and pH levels in the lung and that reflex effects of systemic arterial hypoxemia are of minor importance (see Chapter 5). It is of interest that blood flow to the right lung is greater than that to the left in about half the individuals with aortopulmonary transposition. This could be related to the orientation of the pulmonary outflow and main pulmonary artery toward the right; it could explain the frequent observation that the right is often larger than the left pulmonary artery.

The increase in pulmonary blood flow after birth results in an increase in venous return to the left atrium, which is associated with an elevation of pressure, particularly of the *v* wave. Blood flow from the aorta to the pulmonary artery through the ductus arteriosus results in an even further increase in venous return to the left atrium, left ventricle, and pulmonary circulation. The increase in left atrial and left ventricular diastolic pressures will increase the output of the left ventricle and thus large pulmonary flows are established. If an adequate communication exists between the left and right atria, the increased left atrial pressure will result in shunting to the right atrium, with a balancing of volumes in the pulmonary and systemic circulations; also, left atrial pressure will not reach very high levels. However, with a normal foramen ovale, the increase in left atrial pressure tends to close the foramen ovale flap, as it does in the normal infant, thus permitting a progressive increase in left atrial pressure. The higher the left atrial pressure, the more effectively the foramen ovale is sealed.

If the foramen ovale is the sole channel by which blood can pass from the left to the right side of the heart, there will be interference with passage of pulmonary venous blood to the systemic circulation. Distension of the left atrium and atrial septum may stretch the foramen ovale and allow some flow during certain phases of the cardiac cycle. Also, the elevated pulmonary venous and left atrial pressures could promote flow of pulmonary venous blood through bronchial venous connections into the azygous vein and thus into the systemic circulation. In adult dogs the flow of blood through bronchial veins is related to pressure relationships between the pulmonary and systemic veins [11]. When systemic venous pressure is higher than pulmonary venous pressure, systemic venous blood flows into the pulmonary veins, but when pulmonary venous pressure is higher, flow occurs into the systemic veins. The prolonged survival of those infants in whom no apparent communication exists between the pulmonary and systemic circulations is probably related to bronchial arterial and venous flows.

Role of the ductus arteriosus

During the immediate postnatal period, while pulmonary vascular resistance is relatively high and the ductus widely patent, bidirectional shunting through the ductus may occur. This has been observed by color flow Doppler studies and during selective right and left ventricular angiography within the first day or two after birth. During systole, if pulmonary arterial and aortic pressures are similar, shunting from the pulmonary artery to the aorta may occur. This is probably related to the dynamics of flow in the ductus region; the high velocity of blood ejected into the pulmonary artery during systole carries blood through the ductus to the descending aorta. During diastole, however, blood flows from the aorta to the pulmonary artery because pulmonary vascular resistance is lower than systemic vascular resistance. This pattern of shunting through the ductus arteriosus will result in a reduced oxygen saturation in the lower compared with the upper extremities (see Chapter 3). While the ductus arteriosus is widely patent, pulmonary arterial pressure remains elevated; this may delay the rate of decline in pulmonary vascular resistance and prevent a rapid increase in pulmonary blood flow and left atrial pressure, thereby avoiding sealing of the foramen ovale. These mechanisms may allow a reasonable amount of bidirectional shunt through both the foramen ovale and ductus arteriosus, adequate to prevent severe hypoxemia.

When the ductus arteriosus begins to constrict, associated with the drop in pulmonary vascular resistance, pulmonary arterial pressure falls and shunting from the pulmonary artery to the aorta is eliminated. Aortic to pulmonary arterial shunting continues while the ductus is patent; pulmonary blood flow is increased and the volume of blood in the pulmonary circulation is increased. If the foramen ovale does not permit an adequate shunt from the left to the right atrium, pulmonary blood volume will increase progressively, resulting in a rise in pulmonary arterial and left atrial pressures. Pulmonary edema will ensue. The increase in pulmonary arterial pressure will limit the magnitude of the aortic to pulmonary arterial shunt through the ductus, but only when left atrial and pulmonary venous pressures are markedly increased.

It is not known whether the ductus arteriosus in infants with aortopulmonary transposition responds to the same influences that affect the normal ductus. If it does, the sensitivity and time course of these responses are yet to be determined. As mentioned on p. 471, the ductus may be constricted prenatally and this will affect postnatal blood flow patterns.

Atrial dynamics and foramen ovale shunting

The behavior of the foramen ovale after birth is crucial in determining the clinical features of infants with aortopulmonary transposition. The hemodynamic changes tending to close the foramen ovale have been mentioned above. As discussed in Chapter 8, the degree of competency of the foramen ovale varies greatly. If the valve effectively seals the foramen, severe symptoms are likely within a few hours or the first day or two after birth. If the valve of the foramen ovale is somewhat short, the orifice may not be sealed completely, and a small opening may exist between the edge of the crista dividens and the upper margin of the valve. Although this may permit only a small shunt in the normal circulation, a much larger shunt may occur if left atrial pressure is greatly increased, particularly if the foramen is stretched. This variation in normal anatomy of the foramen ovale could explain differences in the amount of atrial left-to-right shunting and hence in onset of symptoms in infants with aortopulmonary transposition. It is important to recognize that if prenatal restriction of the foramen ovale is noted by ultrasound examination, it is highly likely that foramen ovale shunting will be very limited and the infant may develop severe hypoxia soon after birth.

Even if the foramen ovale is incompetent, it is difficult to conceive that any right-to-left shunt can occur when mean pressure in the left atrium significantly exceeds that in the right atrium. It was proposed that shunting could occur intermittently; flow first occurred in one direction and then, after several minutes or longer, shunting was reversed. However, it is not necessary to invoke this hypothesis, because bidirectional shunting can be explained on the basis of variations in pressure differences between the two atria during different phases of the

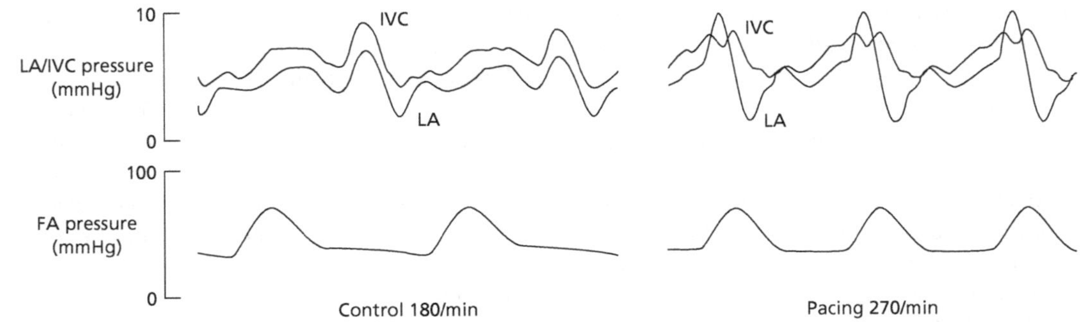

Figure 18.7 Left and right atrial pressure contours showing change in pressure differences resulting from atrial arrhythmia. LA, left atrium; IVC, inferior vena cava; FA, femoral arterial.

cardiac and respiratory cycles. Normally, the pressure pulse in the right atrium shows a dominant *a* wave and a smaller *v* wave; the left atrial pressure tracing has a small *a* wave and a prominent *v* wave. It is evident that the dominant *v* wave in the left atrial pressure pulse is related to pulmonary venous drainage and not to its communication with the left ventricle. In patients with anomalous pulmonary venous drainage to the right atrium, the pulmonary venous pressure shows a dominant *v* wave in its intrapulmonary portion, but for a short distance proximal to its connection with the right atrium there is a dominant *a* wave. Also, the left atrial pressure does not show a tall *v* wave in patients with total anomalous pulmonary venous connection.

With aortopulmonary transposition, the fact that the atrial communications are reversed, in that the right atrium connects with the systemic, or right, ventricle and the left atrium with the pulmonary, or left, ventricle, does not alter their normal *a* and *v* wave contours. The right atrial *a* wave is usually higher than normal, because the right ventricle is the systemic ventricle and end-diastolic pressure is similar to that of the normal left ventricle after birth. Thus during atrial systole, blood shunts from the right to left atrium through the foramen ovale. During the rapid-filling phase of the atria, the height of the left atrial *v* wave exceeds that of the right atrial *v* wave, tending to produce left-to-right atrial shunting. However, the left-to-right atrial shunt will depend on the competency of the foramen ovale. The phasic pressure relationships between the atria are influenced by respiration. During inspiration, the increased venous return to the right atrium and decreased pulmonary venous flow would favor shunting from the right atrium to the left atrium, whereas expiration would tend to promote increased left-to-right shunting. The marked increase in cyanosis that occurs during crying in infants with aortopulmonary transposition could well be related to changes in atrial shunting. Arrhythmias can produce serious deleterious effects in infants with aortopulmonary transposition; this could be due to interference with atrial shunting associated with changes in atrial pressure pulses (Figure 18.7).

Blood gases and hydrogen ion concentration

If mixing between the pulmonary and systemic circulations is inadequate, systemic arterial Po_2 will fall markedly, not uncommonly to 20–25 mmHg. This level of hypoxemia usually results in tissue hypoxia, with an increase in anaerobic glycolysis, production of lactic acid, and development of severe metabolic acidemia (see Chapter 3). The systemic arterial hypoxemia and acidemia may stimulate the carotid and cerebral chemoreceptors, causing an increase in respiration. However, the carotid chemoreceptor is relatively insensitive to hypoxemia in the first few days after birth (see Chapter 3). Pulmonary blood flow is increased within a few days after birth, so that actual ventilation–perfusion relationships may be normal or decreased. However, because much of the pulmonary blood recirculates through the lungs, the Pco_2 of pulmonary venous blood is reduced and pulmonary venous pH rises. When only a small volume of pulmonary venous blood is shunted into the systemic circulation, although Pco_2 is low, it does not result in a low systemic arterial Pco_2; the level in the systemic artery is usually normal or slightly reduced or increased. If hypoxia is severe, anaerobic glycolysis is increased and carbon dioxide production is reduced, because lactic acid is not metabolized (see Chapter 3).

Effects of oxygen administration

When a newborn infant is noted to be cyanotic, it is customary to administer high oxygen concentrations in inspired air in an attempt to raise systemic arterial Po_2. In infants with aortopulmonary transposition, the effect of increasing inspired oxygen is related to the amount of systemic–pulmonary mixing. In infants with very poor mixing, little increase in systemic arterial Po_2 will result, because the increase is related to the effective rather than the total pulmonary blood flow.

Pulmonary venous blood is usually fully saturated with oxygen, and administration of 100% oxygen will raise the oxygen content by a maximum of about 1.5 mL/dL by increasing the dissolved oxygen in plasma (see Chapter 3). This represents an increase of about 10% in the amount of oxygen either attached to hemoglobin or dissolved in plasma. In most infants with low effective pulmonary flow, administration of 100% oxygen, even by assisted ventilation, produces an increase of less than 5–10 mmHg. in systemic arterial blood Po_2. However, this small increase could provide enough elevation in oxygen supply to retard the progression of acidemia. This finding is quite helpful in distinguishing between transposition and primary lung disease in the newborn infant; the infant with lung disease on assisted ventilation with high-oxygen gas mixtures usually shows a considerable increase in systemic arterial Po_2. Oxygen administration could have potentially undesirable effects in some infants with aortopulmonary transposition. An increase in inspired oxygen could hasten the decrease in pulmonary vascular resistance, and reduce pulmonary arterial pressure. If the ductus arteriosus is still open, the shunt from the aorta to the pulmonary circulation could increase and, if the foramen ovale is small, left atrial hypertension and pulmonary edema may develop (see Chapter 18).

Metabolism

Environmental temperature is very important in infants with aortopulmonary transposition. Because they have difficulty in maintaining an adequate oxygen supply, every attempt should be made to avoid increasing oxygen demands. If they are not maintained in a neutral thermal environment, oxygen requirements are increased; because oxygen uptake and supply are limited, cooling may exaggerate tissue hypoxia and metabolic acidemia (see Chapter 3).

An additional problem encountered in the newborn infant with aortopulmonary transposition is hypoglycemia. Anaerobic glycolysis increases with severe hypoxia; for the same amount of energy production, more glucose has to be metabolized, because complete glycolysis is halted at the lactate level during oxygen lack. Another factor that may play a role in some newborn infants with aortopulmonary transposition is hyperinsulinism. As mentioned above, many infants with transposition are large for gestational age and pancreatic islet hypertrophy has been reported.

Effects of PGE_1

Although the ductus arteriosus is often smaller than normal in infants with aortopulmonary transposition, administration of PGE_1 produces dilatation in the postnatal period. In the infant with only a small foramen ovale, PGE_1 may have a considerable beneficial effect in the first few days after birth. While pulmonary arterial pressure is still elevated, dilatation of the ductus may enhance bidirectional shunting and thus facilitate mixing between the systemic and pulmonary circulations. Within a few days after birth, when pulmonary arterial pressure has fallen, shunting from the pulmonary artery to the aorta will not occur and blood will shunt only from the aorta to the pulmonary artery. If the foramen ovale is patent and permits shunting of the blood added to the pulmonary circulation and left atrium to the right atrium, mixing between the two circulations will be enhanced and arterial oxygen saturation will increase. However, if the valve of the foramen ovale is competent, the volume of blood shunted into the pulmonary circulation will exceed that passing across the foramen and left atrial pressure will increase markedly resulting in pulmonary edema. Also, arterial oxygen saturation will not increase significantly. Although this is not a common event associated with PGE_1 administration, it can occur and should be recognized.

Course in infancy and childhood

Infants with aortopulmonary transposition with inadequate systemic–pulmonary communication do not usually survive more than a few months. As mentioned above, a few may survive beyond a year and this could be due to a modest atrial communication or possibly, as mentioned on p. 476, by developing a large bronchial circulation. If they do survive, there is a considerable risk of early pulmonary vascular obstructive disease. This is discussed below.

Presence of a small ventricular septal defect

A small ventricular septal defect is commonly present in infants with aortopulmonary transposition. The hemodynamic changes with a small defect will be similar to those described for the ductus arteriosus. In the early postnatal period, while pulmonary vascular resistance is still elevated, only a small shunt will occur from the right to the left ventricle. As pulmonary vascular resistance falls, right-to-left ventricular shunting will increase, raising pulmonary blood flow and left atrial as well as left ventricular diastolic pressure. Left-to-right atrial flow of blood is necessary to establish bidirectional shunting. Although some left-to-right ventricular shunt will develop as left ventricular diastolic pressure increases, it is limited because at the low pressures in diastole, only a small shunt will occur through the small defect. As described above for the ductus arteriosus (p. 477), if the foramen ovale does not permit adequate flow from the left to the right atrium, left atrial and pulmonary venous pressures will increase and pulmonary edema may develop. The tendency is for the size of the ventricular septal defect to decrease over time, and this will result in a fall in arterial oxygen saturation.

A ventricular septal defect of moderate size may permit somewhat greater bidirectional mixing, with less hypoxemia. A spectrum thus exists between the infants with very small or insignificant ventricular septal defects and those with very large ventricular defects, as described in the following section.

Aortopulmonary transposition with large pulmonary–systemic communication

Although a widely patent ductus arteriosus may be present in infants with aortopulmonary transposition, it is unusual for ductus patency to persist for more than a few weeks after birth. The large communications usually encountered are ventricular septal defects, but occasionally a large atrial septal defect is encountered.

Large ventricular septal defect

When a large ventricular septal defect is present, shunting between the pulmonary and systemic circulation may be so effective that only minimal systemic arterial hypoxemia occurs, but severe cardiac failure is often encountered. The development of cardiac failure is primarily dependent on the relationship of pulmonary and systemic vascular resistances.

Effects of changes in pulmonary and systemic vascular resistances

Elimination of the placental circulation results in an immediate increase in systemic vascular resistance and right ventricular afterload. The fall in pulmonary vascular resistance after birth associated with ventilation permits an increase in pulmonary blood flow. Blood from the right ventricle will be directed through the ventricular septal defect to the lower-resistance pulmonary circulation (Figure 18.8). Pulmonary blood flow will be increased, with a resultant increase in pulmonary venous return and elevation in left atrial pressure. The foramen ovale will be closed and, unless it is incompetent, no shunting of blood will occur in either direction. If it is incompetent, however, blood may flow from the left to the right, particularly when left atrial pressure is markedly increased. The increased pulmonary blood flow will thus pass almost entirely through the mitral valve into the left ventricle, which is now confronted with a large volume overload. If the ventricular septal defect is large, i.e., if its diameter is equal to or greater than that of the aortic valve orifice, pressures in the two ventricles will remain equal. During systole, blood would flow preferentially to the lower-resistance pulmonary circulation, and thus systemic venous blood will pass from the right to the left ventricle and then to the pulmonary circulation to be oxygenated. During ventricular diastole, the increased venous return to the left atrium and the left ventricle will elevate left ventricular pressure above right ventricular pressure, thus favoring shunting of oxygenated blood to the right ventricle, with an increase in systemic arterial oxygen saturation.

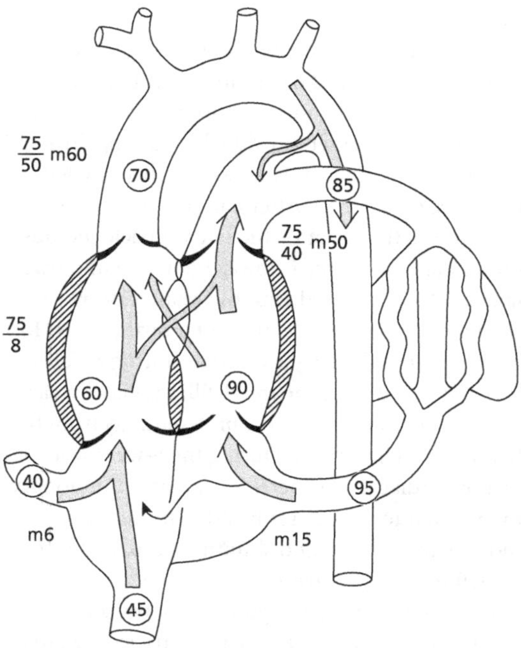

Figure 18.8 Aortopulmonary transposition with a large ventricular septal defect in a newborn infant: course of the circulation, oxygen saturations (circled), and pressures. A large pulmonary flow and left ventricular failure have developed. m, mean pressure.

The ratio of pulmonary to systemic vascular resistance is very important in determining the amount of mixing and the symptomatology in these patients. In the immediate postnatal period, while pulmonary vascular resistance is still relatively high, little right-to-left ventricular shunting will occur in systole and pulmonary blood flow will be only slightly greater than normal. Because the volume of blood returning to the left side is not increased, little shunting would occur from the left to the right ventricle. With a relatively small degree of mixing, systemic arterial Po_2 will be significantly reduced and moderate cyanosis will be evident. The volume load on the heart is not greatly increased, so cardiac failure does not occur. As pulmonary vascular resistance falls, pulmonary blood flow rises and bidirectional shunting is enhanced. This results in a higher systemic arterial Po_2 and oxygen saturation. It is not unusual for Po_2 to be above 60 mmHg and arterial oxygen saturation to be 85–88%. The increased pulmonary blood flow and pulmonary venous return introduce a large volume overload on the left ventricle. Increased cardiac activity and cardiac enlargement result and, if the left ventricle is not capable of maintaining the large flow, cardiac failure develops (see Chapter 7 for a description of the mechanisms causing cardiac failure).

The presence of a large ventricular septal defect will maintain left ventricular and pulmonary arterial systolic pressures at systemic levels. This will delay the postnatal fall in pulmonary vascular resistance and the child will be subject to the risk of developing a subsequent increase in pulmonary vascular resistance with permanent pulmonary vascular obstructive changes (see Chapter 5). The increase in pulmonary vascular resistance causes a decrease in pulmonary blood flow and relief from cardiac failure but also a decrease in arterial oxygen saturation. Progressive increase in pulmonary vascular resistance usually develops at a much younger age than in individuals with ventricular septal defect alone. Not infrequently, pulmonary vascular changes are already present by 3–4 months of age and significant changes are almost always present by 1 year of age. The reason for the earlier onset of pulmonary vascular obstruction in infants with transposition and a large ventricular septal defect is not known. One possible explanation is that the main pulmonary artery is short and the kinetic forces of left ventricular ejection may be more readily transmitted to the peripheral vessels, creating greater shear forces. As mentioned above, flow to the right lung is often greater than that to the left; it would be interesting to observe whether there are differences in pulmonary vascular pathology in the two lungs.

Effect of foramen ovale and atrial shunting

The size of the foramen ovale and the competence of the valve may affect circulatory dynamics in these infants. In the early postnatal period, while pulmonary vascular resistance is still relatively high and pulmonary blood flow has not increased markedly, right atrial pressure may exceed left atrial pressure. During atrial systole, right-to-left shunting may occur. When pulmonary vascular resistance falls and pulmonary flow increases, left atrial pressure rises. If the foramen ovale is competent, left atrial pressure may increase markedly. This will raise left ventricular diastolic pressures and increase shunting from the left to right ventricle in diastole, facilitating mixing. The elevated left atrial and pulmonary venous pressure may result in pulmonary edema. If the foramen ovale is incompetent, blood will flow from the left to the right atrium, particularly during the *v* wave of the cycle; this provides pulmonary venous blood to the systemic circulation and aids in mixing. Right-to-left shunting of blood would occur across the ventricular septal defect, providing systemic venous blood to the pulmonary circulation to be oxygenated. An incompetent foramen ovale will not allow marked increases in left atrial and pulmonary venous pressures.

Intact ventricular septum with large atrial septal defect

A large atrial septal defect is not a common association with aortopulmonary transposition but it is the most desirable lesion with regard to prognosis. Bidirectional shunting allows good systemic–pulmonary mixing so that cyanosis is usually mild. The left ventricle handles a large volume of blood, but at a relatively low pressure, so cardiac failure is not a major concern. In the immediate postnatal period, while pulmonary vascular resistance is relatively high, pulmonary blood flow may be increased only slightly. If the ductus arteriosus is patent, bidirectional shunting may occur through this vessel. As pulmonary vascular resistance falls, aortic to pulmonary flow will occur through the ductus arteriosus, thus aiding in mixing, and pulmonary blood flow will increase.

After the ductus arteriosus closes, left ventricular and pulmonary arterial pressures fall as pulmonary vascular resistance decreases. Pulmonary blood flow will be increased, but because the left ventricle ejects a large volume at low pressure, cardiac failure is not likely to occur. With the fall in pulmonary vascular resistance, the left ventricle is faced with a lower afterload and stroke volume will increase. This will result in greater emptying with a smaller residual volume. During atrial systole and in the rapid-filling phase of ventricular diastole, blood will flow preferentially from the right to the left atrium, and the volume entering the left ventricle will be greater than that entering the right ventricle. During the *v*-wave component, blood will flow mainly from the left atrium to the right atrium.

Atrial shunting patterns

It is of interest to compare the shunting patterns in these patients with those in individuals with atrial septal defects with normal aortopulmonary relationships. In the latter individuals, shunting through the atrial septal defect is almost exclusively left to right (see Chapter 8). Afterload of the right ventricle is lower than that of the left ventricle, because pulmonary resistance is lower than systemic resistance. This, associated with the relative decrease in right ventricular muscle mass after birth, allows for greater filling of the right ventricle during atrial systole and also during the rapid-filling phase in early diastole, so that flow occurs preferentially from the left to the right atrium. During the *v*-wave portion of the cardiac cycle there is a greater pulmonary than systemic venous return, due to the large pulmonary blood flow, and shunting occurs also from the left to the right atrium.

In patients with aortopulmonary transposition, the aorta arises from the right ventricle; the afterload of the right ventricle is greater than that of the left. The left ventricle will therefore empty more than the right ventricle when pulmonary vascular resistance has fallen. Thus, during atrial systole and the rapid-filling phase, blood will preferentially enter the left ventricle and flow will occur from the right atrium to the left atrium. However, during the *v*-wave portion of the cycle, when pulmonary venous return is greater than systemic, blood will tend to flow into the right atrium from the left atrium, and this creates a bidirectional shunt pattern (Figure 18.9).

The atrial shunting will be subject to changes in pulmonary and systemic vascular resistances, as in patients with isolated atrial septal defects. Thus, a decrease in systemic vascular resistance could decrease right-to-left atrial shunting and increase the shunt from the left to the right atrium. Similarly, an increase in left ventricular outflow resistance, due to either increased pulmonary vascular resistance or pulmonary stenosis, could increase left-to-right and decrease right-to-left atrial shunting. Either of these changes could interfere with adequacy of mixing and result in a decrease in systemic arterial oxygen saturation.

Atrial arrhythmias could seriously interfere with atrial shunting patterns. Not only will rapid rates reduce the time period over which a pressure

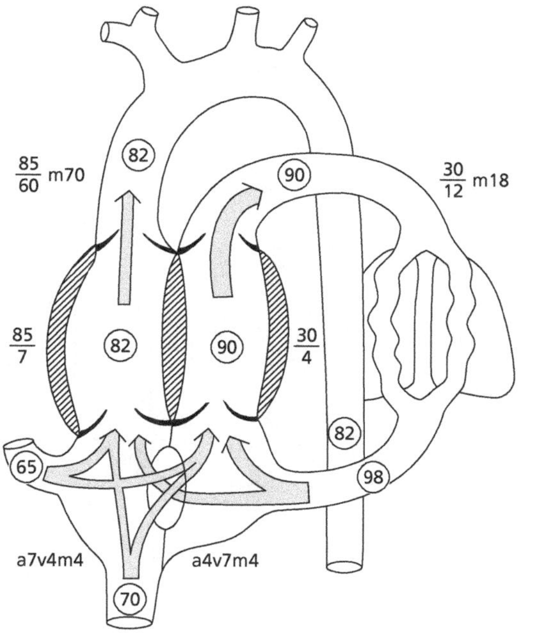

Figure 18.9 Aortopulmonary transposition with a large atrial septal communication and intact ventricular septum: course of the circulation, oxygen saturations (circled), and pressures. m, mean pressure.

difference will be present, but also the normal atrial pressure contour will be altered. Atrial arrhythmias are therefore poorly tolerated in infants with transposition.

The course of infants in whom an atrial communication is created by balloon atrial septostomy or surgery is similar to that of those with naturally occurring atrial septal defects. The mixing may be so effective that systemic arterial oxygen saturation may reach 80–85%. Usually, in the first week or two after birth, the arterial oxygen saturation is lower, but a gradual improvement occurs, presumably associated with a decrease in pulmonary vascular resistance. The patients may be asymptomatic for several years, with no evidence of cardiac failure and only moderate hypoxemia.

Development of the bronchial circulation

Some children with aortopulmonary transposition and an atrial septal communication have been noted to develop a prominent bronchial arterial circulation. The reason for this is not known. My impression is that it is related to the degree of systemic arterial hypoxemia. Infants in whom an atrial septal defect has been created and who maintain systemic arterial oxygen saturation of 80–85% appear to have small bronchial arteries, whereas those with saturations of only 65–70% appear to have a well-developed bronchial arterial circulation. It is possible that systemic arterial hypoxemia is a stimulus to the development of a bronchial to pulmonary arterial collateral circulation.

Development of the pulmonary circulation

The postnatal hemodynamic pattern in children with aortopulmonary transposition and a large atrial septal defect is similar to that in the individuals with an isolated atrial septal defect. Pulmonary arterial pressure falls after birth and pulmonary vascular smooth muscle regresses. In individuals with atrial septal defect with normal aortopulmonary relationship, pulmonary vascular obstructive changes are unusual; if they do develop, it is rare before the age of 15–20 years. Individuals with aortopulmonary transposition with an atrial communication appear to be more likely to develop pulmonary vascular obstruction and at a much earlier age. The reason for the different behavior of the pulmonary circulation is not known. My impression is that early pulmonary vascular changes are more frequent in patients in whom systemic arterial oxygen saturation has been below about 70% during the first 6–12 months after birth. The reduced systemic arterial oxygen saturation cannot have a direct effect because the pulmonary vessels are exposed to normal alveolar oxygen and high oxygen saturation levels in pulmonary arterial and pulmonary venous blood. One mechanism that should be considered is an increased hematocrit, with increased blood viscosity. The lower the systemic arterial oxygen saturation, the higher the hematocrit. The high hematocrit will increase the shear on the small pulmonary vessels and this, associated with the increased shear related to the high pulmonary blood flow, may result in early intimal proliferation and luminal obstruction. Another possibility that should be considered is that the increased bronchial arterial collateral circulation directs blood with a low arterial oxygen saturation through the pulmonary vessels and may contribute to the development of pulmonary vascular obstruction. The increase in pulmonary vascular resistance will result in an increase in pulmonary arterial and left ventricular pressures and a decrease in systemic–pulmonary mixing, with a further reduction in systemic arterial oxygen saturation. A progressive increase in pulmonary vascular resistance and systemic hypoxemia will occur. Later, progressive cardiac failure develops.

Development of left ventricular outflow obstruction

It has been noted that many infants with aortopulmonary transposition, in whom atrial septal defects have been created, develop obstruction of the left ventricular outflow during the first 3–24 months after birth. The obstruction is below the level of the pulmonary valve and is usually associated with displacement of the ventricular septum into the subvalvar area. This is probably related to the systemic pressure in the right ventricle. The obstruction is usually not severe and the pressure gradient across the left ventricular outflow tract is not usually more than 30–40 mmHg. In some patients more severe stenosis may result from a fibromuscular shelf on the septal side of the outflow tract. Obstruction has also been noted to result from abnormal attachment of the anterior leaflet of the mitral valve that projects across the outflow tract during systole. Pulmonary valvar stenosis has also been encountered, but is not common.

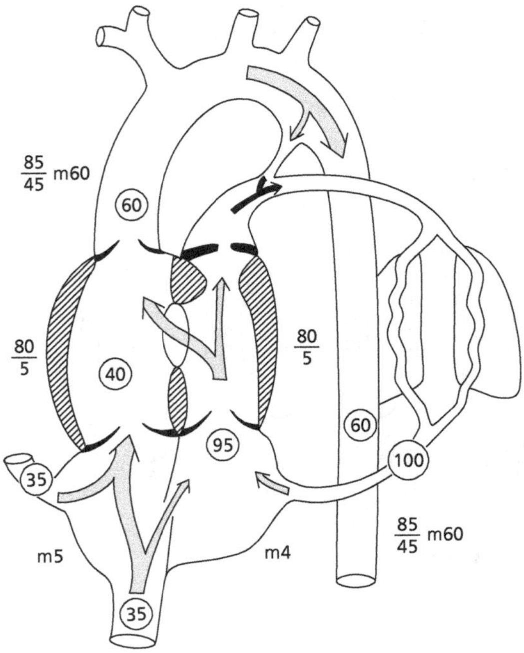

Figure 18.10 Aortopulmonary transposition with severe pulmonary stenosis and ventricular septal defect in a newborn infant: course of the circulation, oxygen saturations (circled), and pressures. m, mean pressure.

Aortopulmonary transposition with ventricular septal defect and pulmonary stenosis

The hemodynamic disturbances and symptomatology of this complex vary considerably after birth and depend on the size of the ventricular septal defect and the degree of pulmonary stenosis. The more common condition encountered in aortopulmonary transposition is a large ventricular septal defect with severe pulmonary stenosis. It is also possible that left ventricular outflow obstruction may develop or increase in severity with advancing age. In the immediate postnatal period, with severe pulmonary stenosis, blood will flow preferentially into the systemic circulation (Figure 18.10). Thus, a left-to-right ventricular shunt will be present, carrying pulmonary venous blood through the ventricular septal defect into the systemic circulation. If the foramen ovale is patent, systemic venous blood may be shunted through the foramen into the left atrium during atrial systole, but the shunt may be small because the left atrial *a* wave may be prominent as a result of the pulmonary stenosis. With a large ventricular septal defect bidirectional shunting may be present, but flow across the defect during diastole may be limited by low compliance of a hypertrophied left ventricle. It is of interest that even though the oxygen saturation of pulmonary arterial blood is high, because it is derived from the left ventricle, the important factor in determining the level of oxygen saturation of systemic arterial blood is the adequacy of pulmonary blood flow. This determines the total uptake of oxygen (see Chapter 3).

Blood flow to the lungs has to be provided by a communication from the aorta to the pulmonary artery beyond the stenosis. The ductus arteriosus is important in the postnatal course of these infants. In the immediate postnatal period, while it still is patent, aortic to pulmonary arterial flow will increase as pulmonary vascular resistance falls, and pulmonary blood flow will increase. While pulmonary flow is maintained, adequate oxygen uptake occurs and, in view of the good mixing, oxygen supply to the tissues is provided to permit aerobic glycolysis. The systemic arterial Po_2 may be reduced to 35–50 mmHg, but it is unlikely that acidemia will be present. In infants with this lesion, the ductus appears to remain open for a longer period after birth than normal. It is usually smaller than normal and it is possible that because it does not carry the usual flows in fetal life, it does not develop normally and may not possess the usual postnatal responsiveness. However, the ductus usually constricts within a few days and pulmonary blood flow falls, resulting in systemic arterial hypoxemia. The hemodynamic effects of aortopulmonary transposition with ventricular septal defect and pulmonary stenosis are similar to those of infants with ventricular septal defect and severe pulmonary stenosis or tetralogy of Fallot (see Chapter 14). However, there is an added disadvantage. With tetralogy of Fallot, pulmonary venous blood all returns to the left ventricle and is ejected into the aorta. With aortopulmonary transposition, some of the pulmonary venous blood returning to the left ventricle is ejected into the pulmonary artery and does not traverse the ventricular septal defect to the systemic arterial circulation. Therefore, to provide a similar amount of oxygen to the systemic circulation, a larger pulmonary blood flow is required. In view of the fact that pulmonary blood flow is not increased, the ventricles do not eject a large volume. Cardiac enlargement is not usually present and cardiac failure does not usually occur. If pulmonary flow and bronchial flow are adequate to prevent severe hypoxemia, these patients may tolerate the lesion well and may survive for many years without treatment.

Aortopulmonary transposition with ventricular septal defect and hypoplastic right ventricle

The postnatal adaptations in this lesion depend on the severity of right ventricular hypoplasia. If the right ventricle is fairly well developed, the hemodynamic disturbances are similar to those in aortopulmonary transposition with ventricular septal defect. However, if the ventricle is very small, the manifestations are similar to those of tricuspid atresia with ventricular septal defect and aortopulmonary transposition (see Chapter 16).

Neurological complications of aortopulmonary transposition

Survival beyond infancy is associated with a high incidence of neurological complications in patients with aortopulmonary transposition who have not undergone surgery to separate the pulmonary and systemic circulations. A relationship exists between the severity of systemic arterial hypoxemia and the incidence of neurological complications. However, severe neurological deficits have occurred in infants after atrial septostomy, who have arterial oxygen saturations of about 85%. The neurological disturbances are the result of severe hypoxemia, cerebral emboli, or venous thrombosis. Cerebral abscesses are also encountered, but this is unusual in early infancy and occurs most commonly after the first year.

Clinical features

The symptoms and signs of aortopulmonary transposition are determined by the presence of the associated lesions. The clinical manifestations are presented for the groups mentioned above.

Aortopulmonary transposition with inadequate systemic–pulmonary communication

Infants with this anomaly are usually cyanotic at birth or within a few hours after birth. However, there are usually no immediate postnatal symptoms; respiration is normal and, commonly, the infants appear robust and tend to be heavier than usual. Characteristically, attention is first directed to the infant by the nurse, who comments on the presence of cyanosis in the otherwise apparently healthy infant. Examination at this time is not helpful. The peripheral pulses are usually readily palpable and are equal in the upper and lower extremities. There is no hepatomegaly and no clinical cardiomegaly. A parasternal cardiac impulse, indicating prominent right ventricular activity, is felt but this is not noticeably different from the normal infant. The first heart sound is prominent at the lower left sternal border and the second heart sound is loud and narrowly split. It is often heard better at the lower rather than the upper left sternal border. Murmurs are not usually heard, but a short grade 2–3/6 systolic murmur may be audible at the mid-left sternal border. These findings would correspond to the phase, described in the section on postnatal circulatory adjustments, when the ductus arteriosus and foramen ovale are widely open and adequate mixing is present.

The electrocardiogram is not helpful, as it shows right ventricular hypertrophy of a degree that is normal for a newborn infant. However, it is of interest that, unusually, the electrocardiogram shows dominant left ventricular forces. In two infants in whom I observed this, they developed severe hypoxia soon after birth. My assumption is that they had prenatal constriction of the ductus arteriosus with pulmonary hypertension that placed a large pressure load on the left ventricle.

Chest radiography may or may not be helpful. The heart is usually normal in size and the pulmonary vascular markings are normal in appearance. The radiographic picture so often described, of a large heart with increased pulmonary vascularity, is not at all typical of aortopulmonary transposition with poor mixing in the newborn infant. It is representative of aortopulmonary transposition with a large ventricular septal defect. Because the pulmonary artery usually lies directly behind the aorta, the superior mediastinum is narrow in the frontal plane but is wide in the lateral view. The thymic shadow is usually small or not observed, and this is rather unusual in a robust infant. The reason for the small thymus shadow is not clear. Arterial blood gases vary, depending on the degree of mixing between the pulmonary and systemic circulations. While the ductus arteriosus is still open, the $P\text{o}_2$ may be reduced to only 35–40 mmHg. $P\text{co}_2$ and pH are usually normal. A small difference in arterial oxygen saturation between the upper and lower body may be recorded by oximetry, with a slightly higher saturation in the lower body. This is the result of shunting of pulmonary arterial blood through the ductus arteriosus to the descending aorta. Administration of 100% oxygen results in a small increase in arterial $P\text{o}_2$ and oxygen saturation.

Although symptoms may progress rapidly, frequently clinical deterioration is delayed for 2–4 days after birth. Cyanosis becomes more severe and respiratory rate and depth increase, but there is usually no chest retraction and no grunting. The chest may appear expanded due to the increased respiratory effort. As a result of this hyperventilation, the diaphragm and liver may be displaced downward and the liver margin may be palpable 2–3 cm below the right costal margin, suggesting that there is hepatomegaly. In the early phase, the heart rate is usually normal but tachycardia to 140–160/min soon develops. With progressive severe hypoxemia and acidemia, heart rate may slow to 80–100/min. The pulses are usually easily palpated and blood pressure is normal. The heart is usually slightly enlarged; other features are similar to those described above. A systolic murmur of grade 2–3/6 intensity may be heard at the upper left sternal border. The electrocardiogram does not show any further changes, but the presence of upright T waves in the right precordial leads suggests that there is abnormal right ventricular hypertrophy.

The chest radiograph usually shows no significant cardiomegaly in the early stages of severe hypoxemia and acidemia, but progressive cardiomegaly develops. However, no specific chamber enlargement is characteristic. The pulmonary vascular markings also increase in prominence but do not achieve the prominence noted in large left-to-right shunt lesions. When hyperventilation is present, pulmonary vascularity may not be prominent if the film is taken in marked inspiration. The narrow superior mediastinal shadow in the anteroposterior view, with no evidence of a main pulmonary artery segment but prominence of pulmonary vascular markings, are characteristic features of aortopulmonary transposition.

Systemic arterial blood gases show severe hypoxemia, with $P\text{o}_2$ of 18–25 mmHg, acidemia, and pH of 7.1–7.25. $P\text{co}_2$ is usually normal or only slightly increased to 40–45 mmHg. $P\text{o}_2$ usually rises by only 5–10 mmHg with 100% oxygen inhalation, even with assisted ventilation. Progressive and often rapid deterioration occurs, with increasing hyperpnea, increasing cyanosis and, later, pallor of the skin develops. Pulse rate slows and it becomes weaker, and body temperature falls. The systemic arterial pH drops rapidly to below 7.0 and if pH has been this low for an hour or more, survival is questionable.

Aortopulmonary transposition with large ventricular septal defect

In the immediate postnatal period, these infants usually do not demonstrate any signs of heart disease. Mild cyanosis, which increases during crying, may be present. Physical examination at this time is not remarkable. The heart is not enlarged and cardiac activity is normal. The first heart sound is normal and the second sound is usually accentuated and narrowly split and best heard over the mid-sternal region. A systolic murmur of grade 2–3/6 intensity is usually present at the lower left sternal border, but no murmurs may be audible. The electrocardiogram usually shows right ventricular hypertrophy of a degree not abnormal for a newborn infant. An upright T wave in the right precordial leads may persist after the first few days, suggesting abnormal right ventricular hypertrophy. The chest radiograph may show slight cardiomegaly. Pulmonary vascularity usually appears normal but may be slightly increased. The typical narrow superior mediastinal shadow in the frontal view and wide shadow on the lateral view is frequently observed. Systemic arterial blood gases show a Po_2 that is moderately reduced, usually to 40–50 mmHg, but pH and Pco_2 are normal.

As pulmonary vascular resistance falls, a progressive increase in symptoms occurs. The time period after birth at which clinical deterioration occurs is variable, but usually cardiac failure develops within 1–3 weeks. Symptoms tend to develop somewhat sooner than is usually noted in infants with ventricular septal defect and normal origin of the great arteries. This may be partly related to a more rapid decrease in pulmonary vascular resistance.

The usual features of predominant left ventricular failure are evident. Increasing dyspnea and tachypnea are early findings. The infant tires with feeding, is irritable, and perspires excessively. Rales may be heard in the lungs and the liver enlarges. In view of the good systemic–pulmonary mixing, the infant usually has only mild cyanosis. The heart rate is increased to 160–180/min and the pulse volume is weak. The heart is clinically enlarged and on palpation there is increased cardiac activity with a prominent right as well as left ventricular impulse. The first sound is usually accentuated at the lower left sternal border. The second sound is split and is heard best at the mid-sternal region. A third heart sound and low-frequency mid-diastolic flow murmur are often heard at the apex. A prominent grade 3–4/6 harsh pansystolic murmur is heard maximally at the lower left sternal border, radiating to the whole precordium. The electrocardiogram now may show right and left atrial hypertrophy. There is almost always evidence of right ventricular hypertrophy, as indicated by tall R waves in the right precordial leads, and there are usually also prominent R waves in the left precordial leads. The electrical axis is usually +75° to +150°. The chest radiograph at this stage shows cardiomegaly, often of a marked degree, involving both ventricles. The contour is quite characteristic; there is a narrow superior mediastinal shadow with absence of the main pulmonary artery segment. The left and right pulmonary artery shadows are often well seen through the heart shadow and there is a marked increase in pulmonary vascular markings. When the infant is in cardiac failure, often there is also a haziness of the lung fields, particularly in the hilar regions, indicating the presence of pulmonary edema. Blood gases still show only mild to moderate decreases in Po_2, usually to 40–50 mmHg. However, with the development of pulmonary edema there is often mild respiratory acidemia, with Pco_2 elevated to 45–50 mmHg and pH reduced to 7.30–7.35. If treatment is not instituted, progressive pulmonary edema and decreased systemic blood flow ensue and the infant succumbs.

If the infant survives the period of acute left ventricular failure, chronic cardiac failure usually persists, with moderate degrees of tachypnea and dyspnea, hepatomegaly, excessive perspiration, and poor weight gain. Episodes of more acute failure may occur, frequently in association with respiratory infections, and the infant may die during one of these. The symptoms usually continue throughout the first year, but improvement in symptoms may occur in association with progressive increase in pulmonary vascular resistance. A gradual decrease in the severity of symptoms of failure is associated with a decrease in hepatomegaly and heart size. Cardiac activity becomes less prominent and the apical mid-diastolic murmur may disappear due to decreased pulmonary venous return and mitral orifice flow. Cyanosis increases in severity. As mentioned above, pulmonary vascular disease develops more rapidly in infants with ventricular septal defect and transposition than in those with normal aortopulmonary relationships. Although it is often advanced within 1–2 years, the course is variable. The severity of cyanosis increases, and the complications of pulmonary vascular disease, such as increasing dyspnea, cardiac failure, and hemoptysis develop (see Chapter 5). The chest radiograph shows a decrease in heart size and pulmonary vascular markings, particularly in the peripheral areas of the lung. The enlarged main pulmonary artery segment is not well visualized because it is within the cardiac shadow, but the right and left pulmonary arteries may enlarge markedly and become prominent in the hilar regions.

Aortopulmonary transposition with large atrial septal defect

This complex does not commonly occur naturally, but was frequently encountered in patients with aortopulmonary transposition who had balloon atrial septostomy or septectomy in the postnatal period to create a large atrial septal communication. Mild to moderate cyanosis is present in the postnatal period but, after a few days, cyanosis lessens, although it increases with crying. The heart is not enlarged soon after birth but increases moderately in size over a few weeks. Mild symptoms of cardiac failure may be present, but it is usually readily controlled. The cardiac impulse increases in activity but is not as prominent as when a large ventricular septal defect is present. The first heart sound is accentuated at the lower left sternal border. The second sound is loud and heard best at the mid-sternal region; the sound is created by the aortic valve, which is anterior. A medium-frequency ejection systolic murmur of grade 2–3/6 intensity is present at the mid-left sternal border and a short grade 2/6 low-frequency mid-diastolic murmur is often heard near the apex. The electrocardiogram shows evidence of right ventricular hypertrophy and on the chest radiograph the heart is moderately enlarged and the pulmonary vascular markings are quite prominent.

These infants usually grow quite well and are relatively asymptomatic, except for mild to moderate cyanosis, which increases on exertion. After a variable period, pulmonary vascular disease may develop, with the same sequence as described in the section on aortopulmonary transposition with large ventricular septal defect. There is a decrease in peripheral lung vascular markings, enlargement of the central pulmonary arteries, progressive cardiac enlargement, increasing cyanosis, and cardiac failure.

Aortopulmonary transposition with ventricular septal defect and pulmonary stenosis

The symptoms and signs of this complex are quite similar to those encountered in patients with ventricular septal defect and severe pulmonary stenosis with normal aortopulmonary relationship (tetralogy of Fallot), and clinical differentiation may be impossible. The baby is usually cyanotic soon after birth but otherwise is in no distress. If pulmonary stenosis is severe, cyanosis increases rapidly as the ductus arteriosus constricts; if pulmonary flow is markedly reduced, severe hypoxemia and acidemia ensue, with the consequences outlined in the section on aortopulmonary transposition with inadequate systemic–pulmonary communication. On physical examination, the pulses are well felt and there is no significant hepatomegaly. The heart is not enlarged; there is a right ventricular impulse at the lower left sternal border but it is not hyperactive. The first heart sound is best heard at the lower left sternal border. The second sound is single and loud at the mid-sternal region. A harsh stenotic systolic murmur of grade 3–4/6 intensity is heard at the mid-left sternal border, radiating to the upper right and left sternal borders and often to both lungs. If pulmonary atresia is present, a systolic murmur is usually not heard. A soft continuous murmur may be heard inferior to the clavicle due to flow through the ductus arteriosus. The development of symptoms and signs is similar to that seen in patients with ventricular septal defect and severe pulmonary stenosis with normal aortopulmonary relationship. If the infant does not develop severe hypoxemia in early infancy, cyanosis gradually increases and by 3–4 months of age, hypoxic spells may occur. Later, squatting may be noted, as with tetralogy of Fallot (see Chapter 14).

Aortopulmonary transposition with ventricular septal defect and hypoplastic right ventricle

The symptoms and signs in this complex are similar to those seen in patients with aortopulmonary transposition and a large ventricular septal defect. The most important clinical feature, which sometimes helps to indicate the presence of a hypoplastic right ventricle, is the electrocardiographic finding of a decrease in or absence of right ventricular forces on the precordial leads and sometimes left axis deviation.

Neurological complications

Neurological complications may manifest with a variety of symptoms. In infancy, the most common presentation is drowsiness, often with convulsions, which may be focal. Hemiplegia often develops within a few hours. The infant may recover rapidly and be left with persistent hemiplegia or weakness of only one arm. The development of a cerebral abscess may be difficult to recognize clinically. The symptoms and signs that should make one seriously consider the diagnosis of cerebral abscess are unexplained fever, change in behavior, such as drowsiness, irritability, failure to recognize the parents, and convulsions.

Investigations

Echocardiography

The introduction of two-dimensional and Doppler flow techniques has made it possible to diagnose the presence of aortopulmonary transposition, detect the presence of associated lesions, and obtain information relevant to surgical correction. Furthermore, it is possible to perform balloon atrial septostomy under echocardiographic guidance should it be deemed necessary. The diagnosis can be made during fetal life with reasonable assurance by 18 weeks' gestation and often earlier. The crucial feature to detect is the presence of ventriculoarterial discordance, with normal atrioventricular relationship. In addition to these features, other important information to obtain includes:

- presence of associated lesions, such as the atrial communication, ductus arteriosus, ventricular septal defect, and outflow tract stenosis of the left ventricle;
- origin and course of the coronary arteries;
- patterns of blood flow.

If the diagnosis of aortopulmonary transposition is made during fetal life, it is crucial to assess the foramen ovale and ductus arteriosus for evidence of restriction; repeated observation for these findings should be made. Preparation should be made to provide urgent therapy immediately after birth, because severe hypoxia, which may not respond to usual therapy, is likely to ensue (see Chapter 18).

The pulmonary artery originates from the posterior left ventricle and is recognized by branching into the left and right pulmonary arteries a short distance from the valve. The aorta, which arises from the anterior right ventricle, is directed cephalad and the first branches are some distance from the valve. The aorta is usually anterior and to the right of the pulmonary artery, but may be directly anterior or slightly to the left. Because spiraling of the great arteries does not develop, the aorta and pulmonary artery are parallel to one another. The aortic valve is clearly separated from the tricuspid valve and the subaortic infundibulum is well developed. However, the pulmonary valve is contiguous with the mitral valve and mitral–pulmonary contiguity is considered an important feature of aortopulmonary transposition. The presence of a ventricular septal defect should be explored. The defect may be in any of the locations in the septum described in Chapter 7. The size of the defect should be assessed and the patterns of blood flow through the defect defined by color Doppler flow studies. Differentiation between aortopulmonary transposition with a large ventricular septal defect and double-outlet right ventricle of the Taussig–Bing variety associated with a subpulmonary ventricular septal defect may be difficult. In both conditions the aorta arises from the anterior right ventricle; the pulmonary artery is posterior and arises from the left ventricle in transposition, whereas in Taussig–Bing anomaly it overrides the ventricle. The presence of the ventricular septal defect may make it difficult to distinguish the position of the pulmonary artery in relation to the ventricle. An important differentiation is that in Taussig–Bing anomaly there is supposedly a separation between the mitral and pulmonary valves. If there is a substantial separation, the diagnosis is not in doubt, but often the separation is questionable and the issue cannot be resolved. The aortic arch should be carefully imaged to detect either isthmus narrowing or coarctation. The presence of aortic obstruction strongly suggests the presence of Taussig–Bing anomaly, but does not completely exclude the possibility of transposition.

The atrial septum should be examined to determine the size of the foramen ovale or the presence of a fossa ovalis defect. The direction of blood flow through the foramen should be assessed by color flow Doppler study. The degree of patency of the ductus arteriosus should also be assessed and the direction of flow studied. When the ductus is large, shunting from the aorta to the pulmonary artery will be noted during diastole and shunting from the pulmonary artery to the aorta during systole. When the ductus has constricted and pulmonary vascular resistance has fallen, shunting will be exclusively from the aorta to the pulmonary artery. The outflow tract of the left ventricle should be examined for obstruction. If present, it is most commonly subvalvar in location. The most common form of obstruction is mild encroachment on the outflow by displacement of the upper portion of the ventricular septum by the relatively high pressure in the right ventricle. In this event, the magnitude of the pressure gradient cannot be assessed accurately from peak velocity. More severe stenosis may be due to a fibromuscular ring in the subvalvar region.

Particularly since the introduction of the arterial switch operation, it has become extremely important to identify the origin and course of the coronary arteries, because they have to be relocated during surgery. Abnormalities such as origin of the left circumflex from the right coronary artery (a common anomaly) and single right or, less commonly, single left coronary artery should be recognized. It is particularly important to identify whether a large coronary artery courses between the aorta and pulmonary artery or is closely applied to the wall of one of these vessels.

If the child has already had an atrial septostomy, the ultrasound study should define the size of the atrial communication and the patterns of shunting. If an atrial baffle procedure has been performed, the presence of vena cava compression and pulmonary venous obstruction should be excluded. If an arterial switch procedure has been done, particular attention should be directed to assessing the presence of peripheral pulmonary stenosis.

Cardiac catheterization and angiography

General considerations

Since the advent of ultrasound techniques, cardiac catheterization is rarely performed in infants with transposition. In addition to the use of catheterization for diagnostic purposes, balloon atrial septostomy was the most important therapeutic procedure; however, in recent years this procedure can be performed using two-dimensional echocardiography for guidance. Cardiac catheterization is indicated in the rare infant in whom the foramen ovale is almost closed and creation of an atrial communication is urgent. If a rapid attempt to perform balloon atrial septostomy under ultrasound guidance is not successful, catheterization is indicated to create an atrial communication by either balloon or blade septostomy. If the procedure is planned, the infant should be kept warm, hypoglycemia should be corrected, oxygen administered, and systemic arterial blood gases monitored repeatedly to assess progression of metabolic acidemia; acidemia should be corrected while preparations are being made. Intravenous PGE_1 should be administered to attempt to maintain ductus arteriosus patency (see below). If the procedure is performed, the diagnosis can be rapidly confirmed by angiography from the right and left ventricles.

If oxygen consumption is not measured directly, it may be unreliable to assume oxygen consumption based on body weight or surface area and age, particularly in the very cyanotic newborn infant. Oxygen consumption tends to be lower than normal in infants with severe hypoxia; it is usually slightly reduced but may be as low as 90–100 mL/min per m^2 it may also be altered by changes in environmental and body temperature. However, it is possible to calculate the relative flow relationships even if actual flows cannot be measured.

Blood flows and shunts

Table 18.1 shows an example of how to calculate flows and shunts in a newborn infant with an intact ventricular septum and small shunts across the foramen ovale and ductus arteriosus, as shown in Figure 18.6.

Systemic blood flow ($\dot{Q}s$) can be calculated in the usual manner from the equation:

Table 18.1 Calculation of flows and shunts.

	Oxygen saturation (%)	*Oxygen content (mL/L)*
Superior vena cava	35	70.0
Aorta	40	80.0
Pulmonary vein	100	200.0
Pulmonary artery	92	184.0
Oxygen capacity 200 mL/L		
Oxygen consumption 120 mL/min/m^2		

Flows

Pulmonary blood flow ($\dot{Q}p$) = 120/(200 − 184) = 7.5 L/min/m^2

Systemic blood flow ($\dot{Q}s$) = 120/(80 − 70) = 12.0 L/min/m^2

Effective pulmonary blood flow ($\dot{Q}ep$) = 120/(200 − 70) = 0.9 L/min/m^2

Shunts

Anatomical right-to-left shunt = $\dot{Q}ep$ = 0.9 L/min/m^2

Anatomical left-to-right shunt = Anatomical right-to-left shunt = 0.9 L/min/m^2

Physiological right-to-left shunt = $\dot{Q}s - \dot{Q}ep$ = 11.1 L/min/m^2

Physiological left-to-right shunt = $\dot{Q}p - \dot{Q}ep$ = 6.6 L/min/m^2

$$\dot{Q}s = \frac{\dot{V}O_2}{\text{Systemic arterial oxygen content} - \text{Systemic mixed venous oxygen content}}$$

Oxygen saturations of systemic arterial and venous blood are often very low. At low levels of saturation oximetry is not very accurate, so that there may be considerable error in calculation of systemic blood flow. Also, because an atrial left-to-right shunt is often present, a true mixed venous sample cannot be obtained, and SVC or IVC oxygen content has to be used in the calculation.

Pulmonary blood flow ($\dot{Q}p$) is calculated from the equation:

$$\dot{Q}p = \frac{\dot{V}O_2}{\text{Pulmonary venous oxygen content} - \text{Pulmonary arterial oxygen content}}$$

In patients with aortopulmonary transposition, pulmonary arterial oxygen content is usually very high; the arteriovenous oxygen difference is therefore low, so that small variations in measurement of oxygen saturation will result in major errors in calculation of flow (see Chapter 4). Another concern is that a mixed pulmonary venous sample cannot be obtained because not all pulmonary veins can be sampled. Using oxygen content from one pulmonary vein may not be representative of mixed pulmonary venous blood, particularly if pulmonary edema is present.

Some individuals with aortopulmonary transposition, particularly those who have marked cyanosis, have a large bronchial arterial collateral circulation, which provides systemic arterial blood to precapillary pulmonary vessels. With transposition, the oxygen saturation of bronchial arterial blood may be markedly reduced. If it makes a major contribution to total pulmonary capillary flow, use of pulmonary arterial oxygen content in the calculation could greatly underestimate pulmonary blood flow.

Effective pulmonary blood flow ($\dot{Q}ep$) is determined by the following equation:

$$\dot{Q}ep = \frac{\dot{V}O_2}{\text{Pulmonary venous oxygen content} - \text{Mixed systemic venous oxygen content}}$$

Although calculation of systemic and pulmonary blood flows is subject to considerable error, estimation of effective pulmonary blood flow is not likely to be quite as inaccurate. There is usually a large difference in oxygen content of pulmonary venous and systemic venous blood, so that small errors in measurement do not produce great alterations in the estimated effective pulmonary blood flow.

Shunt calculations

The terms "anatomical" and "physiological" shunting have been introduced to help understand the hemodynamic changes associated with aortopulmonary transposition (see Chapter 4).

1 *Anatomical shunts.* In individuals with aortopulmonary transposition, anatomical right-to-left shunt reflects the volume of blood flowing from the right atrium or ventricle to the left atrium or ventricle or from the pulmonary artery to the aorta. Anatomical left-to-right shunt represents flow from the left atrium or ventricle to the right atrium or ventricle or from the aorta to the pulmonary artery. Apart from temporary small variations, anatomical left-to-right and right-to-left shunts must be equal (see Chapter 4). Effective pulmonary

flow reflects the volume of systemic venous blood that passes to the pulmonary circulation to be oxygenated. It may be equated with anatomical right-to-left shunt minus the blood which has been shunted from the left atrium and ventricle and pulmonary artery to the right side, but which passes back to the left side of the heart.

2 *Physiological shunts.* Physiological right-to-left shunt represents the portion of the systemic venous blood that enters the systemic arterial circulation without being oxygenated. It may be calculated by subtracting effective pulmonary flow from systemic blood flow. Physiological left-to-right shunt is the portion of blood that has been oxygenated and recirculates through the lungs. It is calculated by subtracting effective pulmonary blood flow from total pulmonary blood flow.

Bronchial arterial collateral blood flow

The presence of a bronchial collateral circulation can be demonstrated but not quantified by measuring oxygen saturation or Po_2 in a pulmonary arterial wedge blood sample. If there is little or no bronchial arterial collateral flow, the oxygen saturation and Po_2 of the wedge sample will be higher than that of pulmonary arterial blood and similar to that of pulmonary venous blood, i.e., almost 100% saturation and Po_2 90–100 mmHg. If a large bronchial flow is present, the wedge sample oxygen saturation and Po_2 will be lower than in pulmonary arterial blood, and closer to those of aortic blood.

Aortopulmonary transposition with inadequate communication

Oxygen saturations and blood gases

The oxygen saturation in SVC and IVC blood is low; in infants with severe hypoxia, it may be reduced to as low as 20–25%. Usually there is only a small increase in saturation of 8–10% in the right atrium or ventricle, and oxygen saturation in the ascending aorta is similar to that in the right ventricle; descending aortic saturation may be 5–15% higher due to shunting from the pulmonary artery through the ductus arteriosus. Pulmonary venous oxygen saturation is usually normal and decreases by 5–10% in the left atrium or ventricle. Oxygen saturation in the pulmonary artery may be somewhat lower than that in the left ventricle if a patent ductus arteriosus is present.

The systemic arterial Po_2 is markedly reduced. Even when the infant is not clinically symptomatic, it is rarely above 35 mmHg and in the severely hypoxemic infant it may be 20–25 mmHg. In most instances, the systemic arterial Pco_2 is in the normal range but may be increased slightly to about 45 mmHg. Systemic arterial pH may be normal, but with severe hypoxia, pH falls to as low as 7.0 or less. The contrast between systemic arterial and pulmonary venous blood gases is striking. Pulmonary venous blood reflects the hyperventilation that occurs as a result of systemic arterial hypoxemia and acidemia. While breathing air, pulmonary venous Po_2 may be increased to 110–115 mmHg, Pco_2 reduced to 15–20 mmHg, and pH increased to 7.45–7.48. Administration of 100% oxygen increases pulmonary venous Po_2 to above 400 mmHg but may have little effect on systemic arterial Po_2, especially if effective pulmonary blood flow is very low.

Pressures

Right and left atrial pressures are usually mildly elevated. The right atrial *a* wave is dominant and may be increased to 15 mmHg; the *v* wave is prominent in the left atrial tracing. Usually, mean pressure in the left atrium is slightly higher than that in the right atrium, or the mean pressures may be similar. Right ventricular systolic pressure is at normal systemic arterial levels. Left ventricular and pulmonary arterial pressures vary, depending on postnatal age and patency of the ductus arteriosus. If the ductus arteriosus is still widely patent, systolic pressures may be at systemic arterial levels, but if the ductus is constricted or closed the systolic pressures in the left ventricle and the pulmonary artery are reduced to 40–60 mmHg within 1–2 weeks after birth and fall to 30–35 mmHg within 4–6 weeks. Systemic vascular resistance is slightly decreased and pulmonary vascular resistance is variable. Pulmonary arterial pressure and pulmonary vascular resistance tend to fall within 2–3 weeks after birth, unless the ductus arteriosus remains patent. Ductus arteriosus patency may delay or prevent the usual decline in pulmonary vascular resistance.

Angiocardiography

Angiocardiography was the most important method of diagnosis prior to the use of ultrasound techniques. Right ventricular injection of contrast material shows a normally positioned anterior ventricle with a normal tricuspid valve. The aorta arises anteriorly and the aortic valve is more cephalad than normal. A well-developed subaortic infundibulum is evident and there is considerable separation between the aortic and tricuspid valves. Whereas in the normal heart the posterior right aortic cusp is the noncoronary cusp, in aortopulmonary transposition the noncoronary cusp is anterior and to the right. Not infrequently, the left circumflex coronary branch arises from the right coronary artery on the posterior surface of the heart. If the aorta is not well visualized from the right ventricular injection, a direct aortic injection may be necessary. The diameter of the aorta is usually moderately increased, and a patent ductus arteriosus with shunting to the pulmonary artery may be visualized. Large bronchial arteries arising from the descending aorta and filling the pulmonary circulation may be seen.

The left ventricular injection shows a normal smooth-walled ventricle, placed posteriorly and ejecting into a posteriorly placed pulmonary artery. The pulmonary valve is more caudal than normal, and there is contiguity of the mitral and pulmonary valves. Shunting from the pulmonary artery to the descending aorta through the ductus arteriosus may be observed in the early postnatal period.

Aortopulmonary transposition with large ventricular septal defect in infancy

Oxygen saturations and blood gases

Mixed venous saturation is either normal or slightly reduced. An increase in oxygen saturation at the atrial level of 8–10% is quite common, due either to shunting from the left atrium to the right atrium or to tricuspid regurgitation. A large increase in oxygen saturation to 80–90% is noted in the right ventricle; aortic saturation is the same or slightly higher. Pulmonary venous and left atrial oxygen saturation is often reduced to 90–94%, in association with the pulmonary edema resulting from heart failure. Oxygen saturation in the left ventricle or the pulmonary artery may be slightly lower than that in the left atrium due to right-to-left shunting through the ventricular septal defect or ductus arteriosus. Oxygen saturation in the pulmonary artery is usually 5–10% higher than that in the aorta, but with good mixing, saturations may be similar. Systemic arterial oxygen saturation is usually 80–90%.

Systemic arterial Po_2 is usually moderately reduced to 55–70 mmHg, but may be slightly higher. Pco_2 is often increased to about 45 mmHg, and pH may be normal or slightly reduced (7.30–7.35), reflecting a mild respiratory acidemia and hypoxemia associated with pulmonary edema.

Pressures

The right atrial pressure is increased, the level depending on the degree of cardiac failure, but it may reach a mean of 12–15 mmHg; the *a* wave is dominant. The left atrial pressure is usually higher and in severe failure may reach a mean of 15–20 mmHg; the *v* wave is prominent. Left and right ventricular systolic pressures are almost identical. The pulmonary arterial and aortic systolic pressures are identical, but pulmonary arterial diastolic pressure may be considerably lower and pulmonary arterial mean pressure may be 10–15 mmHg lower than aortic mean pressure. Pulmonary blood flow is markedly increased and systemic blood flow is either normal or moderately reduced.

Angiocardiography

Many of the anatomical features are similar to those described above. However, from both the right and left ventricular injections there is almost simultaneous filling of the aorta and pulmonary artery due to the excellent mixing across the ventricular septum. Contrast injection into the aorta may demonstrate a patent ductus arteriosus in addition to the ventricular septal defect. It will also demonstrate the presence of aortic isthmus narrowing or coarctation. A marked increase in pulmonary blood flow and prominent main and peripheral pulmonary arteries are evident. The left atrium may be considerably enlarged and the left ventricle is usually also large, with a large ejection fraction.

Ventricular septal defect in childhood

If the infant survives the period of severe cardiac failure, during the first year there is a serious risk of pulmonary vascular disease. Associated with the increased pulmonary vascular resistance there is a reduction in pulmonary blood flow. The systemic arterial oxygen saturation decreases and there is only a smaller increase in oxygen saturation from the right atrium to the right ventricle. Pulmonary arterial pressure shows an increase in diastolic and mean pressures to equal systemic arterial levels. Left atrial mean pressure falls and the *v* wave becomes less prominent.

Aortopulmonary transposition with large atrial septal defect

The presence of a large atrial septal defect as the sole lesion associated with aortopulmonary transposition is unusual as a spontaneous occurrence. However, it was common as a result of the creation of a large atrial communication by balloon atrial septostomy or surgery.

Oxygen saturations

There is a large increase of 10–20% in oxygen saturation at the right atrial level, and often a further small increase in the right ventricle due to streaming, but oxygen saturation in the aorta and systemic arterial equals that in the right ventricle. Depending on the degree of mixing, systemic arterial oxygen saturation varies, but with a very large defect it may be as high as 85–90%. The pulmonary venous oxygen saturation is normal, but with a large defect it may be slightly reduced to 92–95%. Saturation in the left atrium is lower than that in pulmonary veins due to atrial right-to-left shunting and there may be a further small fall in the left ventricle due to streaming. In early infancy, if the ductus arteriosus is patent, oxygen saturation in the pulmonary artery may be lower than that in the left ventricle due to aortopulmonary shunting.

Pressures

When the atrial communication is very large, the right and left atrial mean pressures are similar and there is also almost complete equalization during all phases of the cardiac cycle. Usually the atrial septum is somewhat restrictive, so there may be similar and normal mean pressures, but the *a* wave is dominant in the right atrium and the *v* wave in the left atrium. Right ventricular end-diastolic pressure is in the normal range and right ventricular systolic pressure is increased to systemic arterial levels. In the immediate neonatal period and while the ductus arteriosus is widely patent, left ventricular and pulmonary arterial pressures are similar to systemic arterial pressures. After a few weeks, the left ventricular pressure falls to systolic levels of 25–40 mmHg and the pulmonary arterial pressure to 25–40/10–20 mmHg, with a mean of 15–30 mmHg. Frequently, a systolic pressure gradient of 30–40 mmHg develops across the subvalvar region of the left ventricular outflow tract within a few months after birth. As mentioned above, this subvalvar pulmonary stenosis is mild and is due to displacement of the ventricular septum with bulging into the outflow tract. If pulmonary vascular obstruction develops, calculated pulmonary vascular resistance increases, and pulmonary arterial and left ventricular pressures rise to systemic arterial levels or higher. Pulmonary blood flow falls and there is a decrease in systemic arterial oxygen saturation.

Angiocardiography

Apart from the fact that a large amount of contrast medium crosses the atrial septum in either left-sided or right-sided injections into the heart, the findings are similar to those described above. If pulmonary vascular obstruction develops, the pulmonary arteries become markedly dilated and the central pulmonary vessels are large and tortuous, but peripheral pulmonary vessels are poorly filled and pulmonary arterial emptying of contrast medium is slow.

Aortopulmonary transposition with ventricular septal defect and pulmonary stenosis

The findings at cardiac catheterization will depend on the size of the ventricular septal defect and the severity of pulmonary outflow obstruction. The following findings represent those found with a large ventricular defect and severe pulmonary stenosis.

Oxygen saturations

A small increase in oxygen saturation may be noted at the right atrial level, particularly in young infants. Oxygen saturation in the right ventricle increases by 5–10%, and a further small increase may be noted in the aorta due to streaming from the left ventricle through the ventricular septal defect. Systemic arterial oxygen saturation may be reduced to 35–45%, with a Po_2 of 20–25 mmHg; pH may be markedly reduced due to metabolic acidemia. The pulmonary venous oxygen saturation is normal and oxygen saturation in the left atrium may be slightly lower due to shunting through the foramen ovale from the right atrium.

Pressures

The right and left atrial mean pressures are usually similar, but the right atrial *a* wave is prominent, as is seen normally. The left atrial *v* wave may be less evident than usual, especially if pulmonary blood flow is very low. Left and right ventricular systolic pressures are equal and at systemic arterial levels. If the pulmonary artery can be catheterized, it is found to have a mean pressure at or slightly below its usual normal level but with decreased systolic and diastolic excursion and narrowed pulse pressure. However, the pulmonary arterial pressure may be slightly higher if the ductus arteriosus is still patent.

Angiocardiography

Identification of the positions of the great vessels differentiates between tetralogy of Fallot and aortopulmonary transposition with pulmonary stenosis. The aorta is seen to be anterior, arising from the infundibulum of the right ventricle. The pulmonary artery arises posterior to the ventricular septum from the left ventricle. The pulmonary stenosis is most commonly subvalvar, with a narrow ring beneath the valve. The valve may be thickened and have poor motion and the diameter of the main pulmonary artery is usually decreased. An aortic injection of contrast material may show a patent ductus arteriosus or possibly prominent large bronchial vessels arising from the descending aorta, with filling of the pulmonary circulation peripherally.

Aortopulmonary transposition with ventricular septal defect and hypoplastic right ventricle

The cardiac catheterization findings are similar to those described for aortopulmonary transposition and ventricular septal defect (see Chapter 16). The lesion is diagnosed by the right ventricular angiogram, which demonstrates a right ventricle with a small cavity. The ventricle is sometimes smooth-walled, suggesting that there is subendocardial fibroelastosis, but it may show normal trabeculation. The diameter of the tricuspid orifice is also decreased. The outflow region of the ventricle, including the subaortic infundibulum, may be of adequate size, but the ascending aorta may be small.

Differential diagnosis

The lesions with which aortopulmonary transposition may be confused, depending on the particular symptom complexes that may be encountered, are related to the associated lesions.

Aortopulmonary transposition with inadequate systemic–pulmonary communication

This has to be distinguished from other conditions that produce severe cyanosis in the newborn period. The clinical presentation of an infant with hyperventilation, marked cyanosis, and insignificant or no cardiac murmurs is characteristic of aortopulmonary transposition. Sometimes it is rather difficult to exclude the diagnosis of primary pulmonary disease. Idiopathic respiratory distress is much more common in premature infants, whereas babies with aortopulmonary transposition tend to be large and overweight. The pattern of breathing in respiratory disorders is usually one of markedly increased effort often with sternal retractions, whereas in aortopulmonary transposition there is increased depth and rate of breathing but usually it is not labored. Chest radiography is usually helpful, because in lung disease there is evidence of diffuse lung infiltration, areas of atelectasis, or the diffuse granular density of respiratory distress syndrome. In aortopulmonary transposition there may be some prominence of pulmonary vascular markings, but otherwise the lungs are clear; also, the typical cardiac contour of aortopulmonary transposition may be evident. Blood gas measurements are usually helpful in distinguishing these conditions. Arterial $P\text{CO}_2$ is usually normal or decreased in infants with transposition, whereas high $P\text{CO}_2$ levels are common in primary lung disease. $P\text{O}_2$ may be very low in both conditions, but administration of 100% oxygen usually causes a significant increase in $P\text{O}_2$ of at least 10–15 mmHg in infants with lung disease, whereas usually only a small rise of 5–8 mmHg results with transposition.

The differential diagnosis of aortopulmonary transposition from cyanotic congenital heart lesions with markedly decreased pulmonary blood flow may be difficult. The clinical features of infants with pulmonary atresia with or without a ventricular septal defect or with tricuspid atresia may be similar to those of infants with aortopulmonary transposition. Severe hypoxia and acidemia are associated with hyperventilation. Usually the second sound is loud and narrow or single in all these conditions and murmurs may be absent. The electrocardiogram may be helpful. Left axis deviation and an absence of right ventricular forces in the precordial leads supports the diagnosis of tricuspid atresia. In pulmonary atresia with ventricular septal defect, the electrocardiogram is similar to that in aortopulmonary transposition, showing prominent right ventricular forces. In pulmonary atresia with intact ventricular septum there is usually right ventricular hypertrophy, although if the right ventricle is very hypoplastic, left ventricular forces may be dominant.

Chest radiography may also be helpful. In tricuspid or pulmonary atresia, the heart is normal in size, there is absence of the main pulmonary artery segment, and pulmonary vascular markings are deficient. In aortopulmonary transposition, the heart size is often slightly or moderately increased. The superior mediastinum is narrow in the anteroposterior view but broad in the lateral view. The pulmonary vascular markings are normal or slightly increased. The differentiation is readily made by ultrasound studies.

Aortopulmonary transposition with large ventricular septal defect in infancy

During infancy, the main clinical features are those of cardiac failure with mild cyanosis, so many lesions that produce this picture have to be excluded. The conditions most likely to be confused with transposition with ventricular septal defect are mentioned.

Double-outlet right ventricle (Taussig–Bing anomaly)

This is perhaps one of the most difficult differential diagnoses that may be encountered. The clinical features are similar, and the onset of failure may occur at similar periods after birth. The electrocardiogram occasionally shows left axis deviation with double-outlet right ventricle but not with transposition with ventricular septal defect. As mentioned above, even with ultrasound study it may be difficult to distinguish between the two lesions. The important differentiating feature is contiguity of the mitral and pulmonary valves in transposition with ventricular septal defect. In Taussig–Bing anomaly, there is a subpulmonary infundibulum, with separation of the valves. However, the degree of separation may be inconspicuous, so that differentiation may not be reliable. Aortic arch obstruction is frequently associated with Taussig–Bing anomaly, but is unusual with transposition. If it is present, the assumption can be made that the diagnosis is Taussig–Bing anomaly, unless the evidence for aortopulmonary transposition is clear.

Tricuspid atresia with ventricular septal defect

This lesion may produce heart failure with minimal cyanosis soon after birth, either when the lesions are present alone or in association with aortopulmonary transposition. Physical examination may be quite similar to that in aortopulmonary transposition with ventricular septal defect but the right ventricular impulse may be less prominent. The electrocardiogram is helpful in that it usually shows left axis deviation and absent or small right ventricular forces in the precordial leads. The diagnosis is made readily by ultrasound examination.

Double-inlet left ventricle with aortopulmonary transposition

This lesion presents with mild cyanosis and cardiac failure soon after birth. Its presentation is very similar to that of tricuspid atresia with ventricular septal defect and aortopulmonary transposition. The electrocardiogram shows either left or right axis deviation. The lesion is recognized by ultrasound examination, which shows both atrioventricular valves connecting with the left ventricle and there is a rudimentary outlet chamber from which the aorta arises.

Atrioventricular canal defect

This lesion often presents with cardiac failure soon after birth. Cyanosis is not usual in these infants, but may occur if the defect is large. The second sound is loud and well split in this lesion and a loud systolic murmur is heard at the lower left sternal border and often also at the apex. The electrocardiogram shows left axis deviation as compared with the right axis deviation of transposition. The chest radiograph shows a very prominent main pulmonary artery segment in atrioventricular septal defect. Occasionally, aortic arch obstruction is associated with atrioventricular septal defect. Ultrasound study differentiates the lesions.

Truncus arteriosus communis

There are many features common to this lesion and aortopulmonary transposition with ventricular septal defect. Cardiac failure often appears early and cyanosis is usually mild. The pulse pressure may be wide with truncus arteriosus, but this is not a constant feature in the infant with cardiac failure. The second sound is loud and single but may be similar with transposition. A prominent systolic ejection click is common with truncus arteriosus. Chest radiography may show deficiency of the pulmonary artery segment in both lesions, and the electrocardiogram is similar. Ultrasound examination will distinguish the lesions.

Total anomalous pulmonary venous return

In those infants in whom there is no major obstruction to pulmonary venous return, the presenting feature is cardiac failure with mild cyanosis. Usually cardiac failure tends to occur 3–4 weeks after birth rather than after 1–3 weeks as with aortopulmonary transposition with ventricular septal defect. The second sound is widely split without marked accentuation. The pulmonary artery is enlarged on the chest radiograph and the electrocardiogram shows right axis deviation with deficiency in left ventricular forces; there is usually also complete reversal of RS progression in the precordial leads. The diagnosis is made by ultrasound study.

Aortopulmonary transposition with large atrial communication

These patients may show few symptoms, usually manifesting cyanosis that is mild at rest and increases with exercise. The more important lesions to be considered in the differential diagnosis are Ebstein anomaly, total anomalous pulmonary venous return, abnormal drainage of a systemic vein to the left atrium, and atrial septal defect with pulmonary arterial hypertension.

Ebstein anomaly

The onset of cyanosis in Ebstein anomaly may be delayed for several years but often appears in early infancy. The softness and wide splitting of the second sound and the frequent presence of triple or quadruple rhythm help to distinguish this lesion from aortopulmonary transposition. The chest radiograph shows sparse pulmonary vascular markings and the heart is considerably enlarged when Ebstein anomaly presents in infancy. The electrocardiogram is often helpful; with Ebstein malformation, the P wave is peaked and usually ventricular conduction delay with low precordial voltages is noted, as compared with prominent right forces in aortopulmonary transposition. Wolff–Parkinson–White syndrome, with right or left conduction delay, may be seen with Ebstein anomaly. The diagnosis of displacement of the tricuspid valve and the normal origin of the great arteries in Ebstein anomaly is readily made by ultrasound examination.

Total anomalous pulmonary venous return

Total anomalous pulmonary venous return without obstruction of the pulmonary veins may be readily confused. As mentioned above, the clinical examination and chest radiograph are helpful. The differential diagnosis of this, as well as the other lesions mentioned, is readily made by ultrasound study.

Aortopulmonary transposition with ventricular septal defect and pulmonary stenosis

This complex should be differentiated from those lesions that produce the clinical picture of marked cyanosis with decreased pulmonary blood flow. The more important lesions to be considered are ventricular septal defect with pulmonary stenosis and normal aortopulmonary relations (tetralogy of Fallot), double-outlet right ventricle with pulmonary stenosis, pulmonary atresia with intact ventricular septum, atrioventricular septal defect with pulmonary stenosis, and tricuspid atresia and single ventricle with pulmonary stenosis. The clinical examination may be similar in all these lesions. The chest radiograph may not be helpful, because the pulmonary artery segment may be absent or deficient and the cardiac contour similar, although with tricuspid atresia the right atrium may be prominent. The electrocardiogram is helpful, because left axis deviation is present with atrioventricular septal defect and tricuspid atresia. Differentiation is made by ultrasound study.

Aortopulmonary transposition with ventricular septal defect and hypoplastic right ventricle

The most important lesion with which this may be confused is tricuspid atresia with ventricular septal defect. The details of differential diagnosis are discussed in the section on tricuspid atresia (see Chapter 15); ultrasound study makes the distinction.

Principles of management

The management of patients with aortopulmonary transposition is determined by the associated lesions and the physiological disturbances.

Aortopulmonary transposition with inadequate systemic–pulmonary communication

Initial management

If the diagnosis of aortopulmonary transposition has been made prenatally, the infant should be delivered at an institution with facilities for caring for newborns with severe cardiac lesions; it is particularly important that the ability to perform balloon atrial septostomy urgently, if necessary, is available. This is particularly likely if restriction of the foramen ovale or constriction of the ductus arteriosus has been detected *in utero*. These infants often have severe hypoxemia and acidemia when first referred for treatment. In a report by Jouannic *et al.* [7], more than half of the fetuses with aortopulmonary transposition and abnormal foramen ovale or ductus arteriosus required immediate resuscitation, including ballon atrial septostomy within 30 min after birth; two died despite urgent treatment. Another important consideration is the possible association of persistent pulmonary hypertension of the newborn. I believe that this condition is probably related to prenatal constriction of the ductus arteriosus. It is associated with a very high neonatal mortality. Roofthooft *et al.* [1] reported that 12.5% of 112 patients with aortopulmonary transposition presented with this association and four of these infants died despite intensive therapy. If the diagnosis has not been made during fetal life and the infant does not show rapid response to usual resuscitative measures, the possibility that urgent balloon atrial septostomy will be indicated should be seriously considered.

Administration of high-oxygen gas mixtures does not usually raise the arterial Po_2 by more than 5–8 mmHg, but 100% oxygen should be given because it may have some beneficial effect. Arterial blood gases and pH should be measured promptly, either from an umbilical arterial catheter or by arterial puncture. It should be appreciated that the Po_2 of ascending aortic blood may be several mmHg lower than that measured from an umbilical arterial sample, because of ductus arteriosus shunting from the pulmonary artery to the descending aorta. It was, and still is in some centers, common practice to administer sodium bicarbonate or amine buffer if the infant with severe hypoxia develops acidemia. Although this is somewhat controversial, there is no convincing evidence that this is beneficial and in fact could be harmful [12,13]. Blood glucose concentration should be measured; hypoglycemia is common in these infants (see Chapter 18). Glucose should be administered as necessary to maintain normal blood glucose levels. PGE_1 should be administered to maintain ductus arteriosus patency. If the infant is not already on assisted ventilation, it is advisable to intubate the trachea to be prepared to assist ventilation should apnea result from PGE_1 infusion. The main concern with administration of PGE_1 in infants with aortopulmonary transposition is that if the ductus arteriosus does not remain widely patent and pulmonary vascular resistance and pulmonary arterial pressure fall, shunting through the ductus will be exclusively from the aorta to the pulmonary artery. This could result in pulmonary edema if the foramen ovale is effectively closed. This is most unlikely to occur in infants during the first 2–3 weeks postnatally, so there should be no hesitation in infusing prostaglandin. Beyond this time, when pulmonary vascular resistance may have dropped significantly and pulmonary arterial pressure is low, it is important to carefully observe arterial Po_2 and any increased respiratory effort or requirement for higher inspiratory ventilatory pressures. This will require that PGE_1 be stopped and further procedures considered immediately. Usually urgent balloon atrial septostomy is indicated, unless a surgical procedure can be done promptly.

Procedures

A number of procedures have been developed for treatment of transposition with intact ventricular septum: creation of an atrial communication; correction of pulmonary and systemic flows by atrial baffle; and correction of flows by arterial switch.

Creation of an atrial communication

This is a palliative procedure designed to provide better mixing between the systemic and pulmonary circulations. It was first performed surgically by the Blalock and Hanlon technique, but was associated with a high mortality. Balloon atrial septostomy, developed by Rashkind, dramatically improved the outlook of infants with transposition. Prior to the availability of PGE_1 the procedure was done urgently soon after birth. However, PGE_1 usually improves oxygenation in newborn infants with transposition and the indications for the procedure are currently being modified.

Balloon atrial septostomy was first performed with fluoroscopic guidance of the catheter from an IVC approach across the foramen ovale into the left atrium [14]. The balloon is inflated in the left atrium and rapidly withdrawn across the foramen to tear the membranous inferior margin to create a larger opening. Although this procedure usually increases arterial oxygen saturation to 70–85%, it is not effective in some infants; in some, after initial improvement, oxygen saturation again falls. Several factors may account for this: the foramen ovale may be stretched, but not torn; the valve of the foramen may herniate into the right atrium but not be torn; the tissue may be too tough to be torn by the balloon. In some of these infants, as well as in older infants in whom the tissues are tough, an opening may be made by blade septotomy, followed by balloon septostomy. In the blade technique, developed by Park *et al.* [15], a catheter that has a retractable blade at its tip is manipulated into the left atrium. The blade is then opened and slowly withdrawn across the septum; this is repeated several times and followed by balloon septostomy. In recent years balloon atrial septostomy has been performed with echocardiographic guidance of the catheter. This has the advantage that the procedure can be performed in the intensive care nursery. In addition, the adequacy of tearing of the septum can usually be appreciated.

If arterial oxygen saturation does not improve following balloon atrial septostomy, and an effective tear of the septum has been accomplished, consideration should be given to the possibility that pulmonary vascular resistance is high and is interfering with bidirectional shunting through the defect. Lack of improvement could also be related to lung disease. If pulmonary vascular resistance is elevated, use of pulmonary vasodilator agents such as sidenafil or inhaled nitric oxide should be considered (see Chapter 5).

Balloon atrial septostomy was for many years performed in all infants with transposition with inadequate mixing. Surgery to create an atrial baffle by the Mustard procedure (see below) was usually not recommended before 2–3 years, because mortality in infancy was very high. Although infants usually survived after balloon atrial septostomy, many complications occurred. These included cerebral vascular occlusions due to emboli, cerebral abscess, infective endocarditis, and pulmonary vascular obstruction. In addition, many infants continued to have moderately severe hypoxemia and there have been concerns about neurological and intellectual development. Recently, the arterial switch procedure is being performed in early infancy, and some controversy exists about the use of balloon atrial septostomy. Some centers still perform atrial septostomy first and then the arterial switch procedure a few weeks after birth. Others recommend that the definitive surgery of arterial switch be performed within a few days, in which case there is no need to perform atrial septostomy. If PGE_1 infusion permits the infant to maintain adequate oxygenation, there appears to be little indication to perform balloon atrial septostomy prior to performing the arterial switch. However, in some centers, there is concern that prolonged PGE_1 infusion causes the great vessels to become friable due to edema of the walls; it is maintained that this increases the risk of postoperative bleeding. It is recommended that PGE_1 be stopped for 2–3 days prior to surgery. Others do not feel that PGE_1 causes a significant problem with the surgery.

Atrial baffle procedures

The Mustard procedure has been used extensively with great success [16]. With cardiopulmonary bypass, the right atrium is opened widely and the atrial septum excised. A baffle, which in the original procedures was formed of pericardium, is sewed into the atrium to direct all pulmonary venous blood to the tricuspid valve and all SVC and IVC blood to the mitral valve. This allows all systemic venous blood to enter the left ventricle and pulmonary circulation and pulmonary venous blood to enter the right ventricle and aorta. Subsequently, the baffle was created with woven material such as Dacron. The Senning technique accomplished the same redirection of pulmonary and systemic venous return, but involved use of the atrial septum and reorientation of the walls of the atria [17]. An important advantage is that no foreign material is required for this procedure. The Senning procedure was associated with a high mortality in early experience and was abandoned. Subsequently, Senning modified the technique and it became the favored procedure. Both procedures were associated with a high mortality in infants, and many suffered the complications of atrial septostomy mentioned above while awaiting surgery. However, the survival with surgery in infancy improved and in the most recent experience, mortality was less than 5% even in infancy. The Senning procedure was favored in infants.

These procedures have been extremely effective in producing physiological correction of pulmonary and systemic flow patterns. Many individuals have been followed for 30 years or more and continue to lead normal lives [18]. In several studies it has been demonstrated that the long-term results, for both survival and performance, are better following the Senning than the Mustard procedure. However, numerous complications, both short term and long term have been noted, including obstruction of systemic or pulmonary venous return, atrial arrhythmias, poor exercise tolerance, right ventricular failure, and unexplained sudden death.

With experience and improvement in technique, the incidence of venous channel obstruction has decreased greatly. The most common obstruction of systemic venous return involves the SVC. It results in suffusion and edema of the face and upper extremities and, on occasion, benign intracranial hypertension. If symptoms are not severe, treatment is not indicated, and the symptoms improve due to development of collateral circulation to IVC channels. Surgical relief of obstruction entailed considerable risk, but the obstruction can now usually be relieved by dilation of the obstructed site by interventional techniques, with little risk. Obstruction of pulmonary venous return is more serious, because it results in pulmonary edema with dyspnea. The increase in pulmonary venous pressure may also induce an increase in pulmonary vascular resistance. The obstruction should be relieved by interventional techniques or, if necessary, by surgery.

Atrial arrhythmias are common after atrial baffle procedures. In the original series of patients where the Mustard procedure was used, more than two-thirds had experienced atrial arrhythmias by 20 years after the procedure. It is thought the high incidence is related to damage to the sinus node either directly or by severing the sinus node artery, and to severing internodal preferential conducting pathways in the atrial walls or septum. Sinus node dysfunction may result in bradycardia and is frequently associated with atrial ectopic tachycardia, flutter, or fibrillation. Although the bradycardia is not usually a serious problem, as many as 10–15% of these individuals may at some time require pacemaker insertion. The atrial flutter often occurs at an atrial rate lower than that typically encountered with spontaneous atrial flutter. With flutter rates of 150–250/min and one-to-one atrioventricular conduction, the presence of flutter may not be appreciated. It is therefore important to consider the diagnosis in these individuals if heart rates are rapid. The supraventricular tachycardias in these patients are notoriously difficult to treat with antiarrhythmic drugs. The drugs should be used with caution because of potential adverse effects in the presence of sinus node dysfunction. Modifications of technique have resulted in some reduction in the incidence of serious atrial rhythm disturbances, but they are still a serious early and late concern.

Almost 90% of those surviving the procedure live a reasonably normal life for up to 20 or more years and consider that their activities are normal. However, studies of exercise tolerance have shown that more than half of the individuals have limitations in exercise capacity. This is associated with both a reduction in cardiac output response and a limited heart rate response to exercise. The cause of the limitation in heart rate response is unclear, but the reduced cardiac output response could be related to the fact that the right ventricle is not capable of providing an adequate stroke volume with exercise.

The ability of the right ventricle to function as the systemic ventricle has been a major concern. In the more than 20 years of follow-up of patients who have had atrial baffle procedures, the incidence of right ventricular failure has not been high, but it is not known whether the ventricle will continue to perform adequately with further observation. Two important factors that contribute to the likelihood of failure are tricuspid valve insufficiency and persistent atrial tachycardia, particularly atrial flutter. Abnormalities of the tricuspid valve are not common and it has been suggested that many instances of tricuspid insufficiency are related to minor damage resulting from closure of a ventricular septal defect through the valve at the time of surgery. When right ventricular failure is associated with tricuspid insufficiency, ventricular enlargement may dilate the annulus, aggravating the insufficiency. Right ventricular failure is poorly tolerated because pulmonary venous pressures become elevated and pulmonary edema ensues. If arrhythmia is associated and can be controlled by antiarrhythmic therapy, improvement may result. If right ventricular failure cannot be controlled by medical measures, thought can be given to preparing the patient for an arterial switch procedure (see below) or cardiac transplantation. Recently, promising results have been achieved with the β-adrenoceptor blocker carvedilol in treating right ventricular dysfunction in patients with aortopulmonary transposition who have had atrial inflow corrective procedures. Considerable improvement in exercise tolerance was noted after 4 months of therapy [19]. It remains to be seen if this improvement persists.

Sudden death has occurred at various times after surgery. It has been noted after both Mustard and Senning procedures, and may occur many years after surgery in an individual who is otherwise doing well. It has occurred in individuals who have no apparent arrhythmia. The cause of death in these individuals is as yet unexplained, but is most probably related to arrhythmia.

In view of concerns about the long-term outlook for the right ventricle to perform effectively as the systemic ventricle, and the frequency of postoperative arrhythmias, the atrial baffle procedure is no longer considered the procedure of choice. Rather, it is performed in unusual circumstances, such as when coronary arterial abnormalities are present. The procedure currently favored is the arterial switch.

Arterial switch procedure

This procedure, developed by Jatene *et al.* [20], involves redirection of the aorta and pulmonary artery, so that each is connected to provide a concordant relationship between the ventricles and the great arteries. The aorta and pulmonary artery are separated just distal to the sinuses of the respective valves and then anastomosed so that the aorta arises above the pulmonary valve connected to the left ventricle and the pulmonary artery is connected to the aortic valve over the right ventricle. In early experience, the right pulmonary artery was frequently compressed, but this has been overcome by positioning the distal segment of the aorta behind the pulmonary arterial bifurcation. The reorientation of the aorta and pulmonary artery also requires that the coronary arteries be transposed. If they were not moved, coronary blood flow would be inadequate, because they would be perfused by the low pressure of the pulmonary artery. Each coronary artery is removed from the aortic sinus with a large cuff of aortic wall. They are then transposed to the segment of pulmonary artery just above the sinuses. It is particularly important that undue stretching, distortion, or kinking of the arteries be avoided. If a coronary artery is closely applied to the wall of the aorta or pulmonary artery in its course, the transfer may be difficult or impossible. The arterial switch operation can now be performed during the neonatal period in many centers, with a mortality of 5% or less. Most patients have few problems after successful repair. The main concerns are supravalvar pulmonary stenosis, innervation of the heart and coronary vessels, coronary arterial abnormalities, and function of the pulmonary valve in the aortic position.

Stenosis of the right pulmonary artery was common before the procedure was modified to position the distal aortic segment behind the branching of the pulmonary artery when it was anastomosed to the pulmonary stump. The current concern is that in the process of removing the coronary arteries with the cuffs of aortic wall, the lumen of the new pulmonary artery just above the valves may be narrowed in the repair process. Patches of pericardium or other material are introduced to try to avoid encroachment on the lumen. However, a mild degree of supravalvar stenosis is common following surgery. Systolic pressure gradients of 30–50 mmHg are usually of no concern, but larger gradients may require attention. Transvenous balloon dilatation has been performed successfully in some of these individuals, but there is some concern that coronary arterial damage could be produced by the procedure. The stenosis may progress with time and in some instances has required surgical relief.

The nerve supply to the heart courses along the great arteries and coronary vessels. Sectioning of the aorta and pulmonary artery will also cut the nerves supplying the heart. A study with meta-iodobenzylguanidine (MIBG) imaging before and after the arterial switch procedure has confirmed the interference with sympathetic nerve innervation [21]. Soon after surgery no evidence of MIBG uptake was observed. However, within a few weeks after surgery, uptake was again observed, indicating that sympathetic innervation had been restored. However, this test is relatively insensitive, and it is possible that normal innervation was not achieved. This raises the possibility that the myocardium may not respond normally during exercise and that disturbances of innervation could be responsible for the decreased coronary perfusion reserve that has been observed in some individuals after the procedure (see below).

Coronary artery abnormalities are the predominant cause of early mortality or morbidity after the arterial switch procedure. Interference with coronary perfusion may result from torsion or kinking of the artery, or from stenosis of the ostium at the site of insertion into the pulmonary stump. The left ventricle may not perform adequately to maintain perfusion and the electrocardiogram will show ST- and T-wave changes indicating coronary insufficiency. In the few years of observation of patients who have had successful arterial switch procedures in infancy, few late coronary arterial complications have been recognized. However, instances of late-onset ostial stenosis and of reduced perfusion of one coronary artery are beginning to be recognized. The left is often smaller than the right coronary artery in patients with aortopulmonary transposition and it is usually responsible for diminished perfusion. Studies using positron emission tomography of the response to coronary vasodilators have provided some evidence indicating that coronary blood flow reserve is limited. It has been suggested that vasomotor responses of the coronary circulation are impaired. It is possible that although the nerve supply does regenerate after the arterial switch procedure, normal innervation of the vessels may not be reestablished. It is important to follow these patients carefully and routine exercise testing should be instituted as soon as the child is cooperative. Should any evidence of coronary insufficiency be evident by symptomatology or routine electrocardiography, studies of myocardial perfusion and coronary angiography are indicated. There is concern that as these patients are followed for longer periods after surgery, an increasing incidence of coronary insufficiency may be observed. A recent report noted a 5% incidence of coronary lesions following the arterial switch procedure, associated with coronary perfusion disturbance. Most could be treated successfully by coronary angioplasty, but mammary bypass was required in some [22].

Although there is no evidence that the pulmonary artery will not perform adequately as the aortic valve after the arterial switch procedure, there is still some concern that it may show dysfunction over years of observation. Mild degrees of insufficiency have been noted in some children, but the fate of the pulmonary valve when functioning as an aortic valve has not been defined. Recently, Bove *et al.* [23] reported that 10% of patients with intact ventricular septum developed significant neoaortic valve regurgitation within 4.8 ± 3.9 years after the arterial switch procedure; in patients with aortopulmonary transpositon with ventricular septal defect, it occurred in almost 25% of patients.

The arterial switch procedure requires that the left ventricle be capable of generating enough force to maintain adequate cardiac output at systemic arterial pressures. In the early postnatal period, although pulmonary arterial and left ventricular pressures fall in infants with aortopulmonary transposition with intact ventricular septum, left ventricular mass is adequate to provide the output at systemic arterial pressure. Beyond 6–8 weeks after birth, however, the likelihood that left ventricular muscle is able to perform adequately decreases progressively. It is generally considered that the arterial switch procedure can be performed prior to 8 weeks postnatally, with a good chance that cardiac output will be maintained after surgery. If the procedure is planned beyond this period, it is necessary to attempt to increase left ventricular muscle mass to make it capable of generating the force necessary to provide an adequate cardiac output. This has been accomplished by banding the pulmonary artery to increase left ventricular pressure and so induce hypertrophy of the muscle. The procedure is quite successful in infants in whom the arterial switch procedure has been delayed, for various reasons, beyond the age of 2 months. However, the older the patient, the more difficult it is to achieve adequate left ventricular hypertrophy. It is difficult to gauge the degree of pulmonary stenosis that will produce hypertrophy without inducing cardiac failure. It may be necessary to perform increasing degrees of stenosis with two or three procedures over several years to develop adequate hypertrophy. The arterial switch procedure has been recommended in patients who have developed tricuspid insufficiency or right ventricular failure after an atrial baffle procedure. It is always necessary to induce left ventricular hypertrophy to accomplish this. Although it has been performed successfully in a number of individuals, there is serious concern whether the hypertrophied left ventricle will maintain adequate function over time. Postnatal hypertrophy is accomplished largely by increase in myocyte size and capillary growth does not match the increase in myocyte mass. There is thus less coronary reserve, and this may be further compromised by coronary arterial complications associated with the arterial switch procedure (see Chapter 18).

Aortopulmonary transposition with large ventricular septal defect

The main concern in these infants is the development of severe cardiac failure. Treatment includes administration of diuretic agents and digitalis. Prior to the development of the arterial switch procedure, the approach consisted of performing a pulmonary arterial banding procedure to reduce pulmonary blood flow and improve cardiac failure, as well as reduce the risk for increasing pulmonary vascular resistance with pulmonary vascular obstruction. Subsequently, at the age of 2–3 years, the ventricular septal defect was closed and an atrial baffle procedure performed. The mortality was greater than with the baffle procedure alone, but good long-term results were achieved. Currently, the approach is to close the ventricular septal defect and perform an arterial switch procedure. The surgical risks of this procedure are somewhat higher than with the arterial switch procedure alone, but current experience is that about 90% of these infants are alive after 5 years. The complications associated with the switch procedure are similar to those described on p. 502.

Aortopulmonary transposition with ventricular septal defect and pulmonary stenosis

In the neonatal period, the procedures described above for treating infants with severe cyanosis should be instituted (see Chapter 18). PGE_1 should be administered to maintain patency of the ductus arteriosus. Because the procedures currently available for redirecting blood flow have a high mortality when performed in early infancy, most centers recommend that a modified Blalock–Taussig procedure be performed, with introduction of an interposition graft between a subclavian and pulmonary artery.

When the stenosis involves the subvalvar region and is not severe, it may be possible to excise a localized fibrous narrowing, close the ventricular septal defect, and perform an arterial switch procedure. This complex procedure is attended by a very high mortality in early infancy, but has been performed successfully in older infants and children. There is no concern about whether the left ventricle can maintain an adequate systemic blood flow after the procedure, because pressure in the ventricle has been maintained at systemic levels by the ventricular communication and pulmonary stenosis. When the stenosis is severe or involves the valve, it would be inappropriate to perform an arterial switch

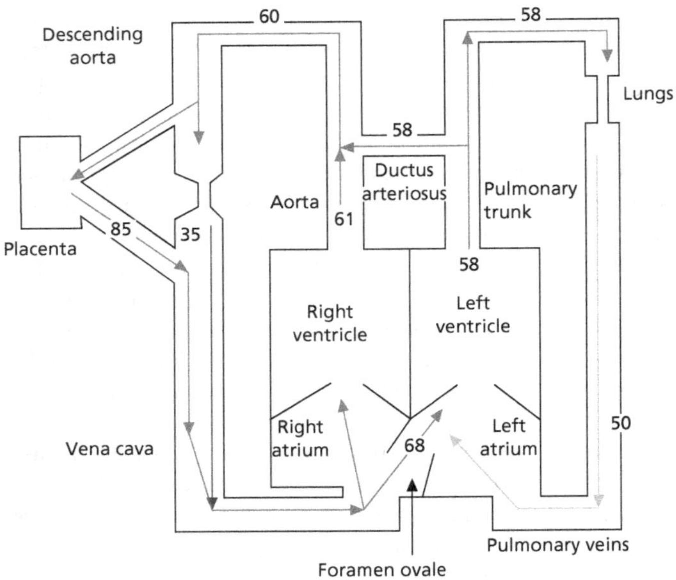

Figure 18.11 Patterns of blood flow and predicted oxygen saturations in cardiac chambers and vessels in the fetus with aortopulmonary transposition after closure of the ductus venosus. Assumptions of volumes of blood flow were used in calculating oxygen saturations in the main vessels. The pulmonary artery arises from the left ventricle. Compared with Figure 18.2, the oxygen saturation of blood perfusing the lungs and ductus arteriosus is reduced considerably and ascending aortic blood oxygen saturation is increased. From Rudolph [5] with permission. (See color plate 18.11).

procedure because of concerns for stenosis or insufficiency of the aortic outflow. The procedure currently recommended is to place a baffle to close the ventricular septal defect and direct the left ventricular outflow through the defect into the aorta arising from the right ventricle. The pulmonary artery is divided above the valve and the stump above the valve is sutured closed. A valved conduit, such as a pulmonary or aortic homograft, is inserted from the right ventricle to the distal segment of the pulmonary artery. This operation, known as the Rastelli procedure [24], still has a relatively high risk in most centers if performed during infancy. For this reason in most centers it is recommended that a modified Blalock–Taussig shunt be inserted in infancy as a temporary maneuver. The Rastelli procedure is then performed at about 12–18 months of age. Although the results with this procedure are very good, the graft will require replacement within several years due to the development of stenosis or insufficiency of the valve. Early and more frequent replacement of the conduit is necessary if the procedure is done before the age of 4 years [25]. It is important to maintain these patients on aspirin anticoagulant therapy and to provide antibiotic prophylaxis for infective endocarditis.

Aortopulmonary transposition with ventricular septal defect and hypoplastic right ventricle

If the right ventricle is only slightly reduced in size, it is possible to treat the patient in the same manner as transposition with a large ventricular septal defect. If the ventricle is severely hypoplastic, the approach should be the same as that for tricuspid atresia with ventricular septal defect and transposition (see Chapter 16).

Aortopulmonary transposition with restricted foramen ovale or constricted ductus arteriosus in the fetus

As mentioned above, detection of these abnormalities in the fetus herald early onset of severe hypoxemia with possible early mortality in the neonate. Even with urgent balloon atrial septostomy, the infant may not survive. This could be related to the presence of high pulmonary vascular resistance, probably related to prenatal ductus arteriosus constriction with pulmonary arterial hypertension. I have speculated whether intervention in the fetus with a narrow ductus arteriosus could possibly relieve the constriction and thus avoid the early postnatal stress. I have suggested that because the constriction is probably the result of exposure to pulmonary arterial blood resulting from preferential flow of ductus venosus blood across the foramen ovale, closure of the ductus venosus in the fetus could possibly induce relaxation of the ductus [5]. Figure 18.11 shows the predicted effect of closing the ductus venosus on oxygen saturations in the cardiac chambers and major vessels.

References

1 Roofthooft MT, Bergman KA, Waterbolk TW, Ebels T, Bartelds B, Berger RM. Persistent pulmonary hypertension of the newborn with transposition of the great arteries. Ann Thorac Surg 2007;83:1446–1450.

2 Digilio MC, Casey B, Toscano A *et al.* Complete transposition of the great arteries. Patterns of congenital heart disease in familial precurrence. Circulation 2001;104: 2809–2814.

3 Selamet Tierney ES, Marans Z, Rutkin MB, Chung WK. Variants of the CFC1 gene in patients with laterality defects associated with congenital cardiac disease. Cardiol Young 2007;17:268–274.

4 Goldmuntz E, Bamford R, Karkera JD, dela Cruz J, Roessler E, Muenke M. CFC1 mutations in patients with transposition of the great arteries and double-outlet right ventricle. Am J Hum Genet 2002;70:776–780.

5 Rudolph AM. Aortopulmonary transposition in the fetus. Speculation on pathophysiology and therapy. Pediatr Res 2007;61:375–380.

6 Maeno YV, Kamenir SA, Sinclair B, van der Velde ME, Smallhorn JF, Hornberger LK. Prenatal features of ductus arteriosus constriction and restrictive foramen ovale in D-transposition of the great arteries. Circulation 1999;99:1209–1214.

7 Jouannic JM, Gavard L, Fermont L *et al.* Sensitivity and specificity of prenatal features of physiological shunts to predict neonatal clinical status in transposition of the great arteries. Circulation 2004;110:1743–1746.

8 Jouannic JM, Benachi A, Bonnet D *et al.* Middle cerebral artery Doppler in fetuses with transposition of the great arteries. Ultrasound Obstet Gynecol 2002;20: 122–124.

9 Rosenthal GL. Patterns of prenatal growth among infants with cardiovascular malformations: possible fetal hemodynamic effects. Am J Epidemiol 1996;143:505–513.

10 Manzar S, Nair AK, Pal MG, Al-Khusaiby SM. Head size at birth in neonates with transposition of great arteries and hypoplastic left heart syndrome. Saudi Med J 2005;26:453–456.

11 Auld PA, Rudolph AM, Golinko RJ. Factors affecting bronchial collateral flow in the dog. Am J Physiol 1959;197:617–623.

12 Forsythe SM, Schmidt GA. Sodium bicarbonate for the treatment of lactic acidosis. Chest 2000;117:260–267.

13 Weil MH, Tang W. Management of acidosis: the role of buffer agents. Crit Care 1997;1:51–52.

14 Rashkind WJ, Miller WW. Creation of an atrial septal defect without thoracotomy. A palliative approach to complete transposition of the great arteries. JAMA 1966; 196:991–992.

15 Park SC, Zuberbuhler JR, Neches WH, Lenox CC, Zoltun RA. A new atrial septostomy technique. Cathet Cardiovasc Diagn 1975;1:195–201.

16 Mustard WT, Keith JD, Trusler GA, Fowler R, Kidd L. The surgical management of transposition of the great vessels. J Thorac Cardiovasc Surg 1964;48:953–958.

17 Senning A. Correction of the transposition of the great arteries. Ann Surg 1975;182:287–292.

18 Hörer J, Herrmann F, Schreiber C *et al.* How well are patients doing up to 30 years after a Mustard operation? Thorac Cardiovasc Surg 2007;55:359–364.

19 Doughan AR, McMonnell ME, Book WM. Effect of beta blockers (carvedilol or metoprolol XL) in patients with transposition of great arteries and dysfunction of the systemic right ventricle. Am J Cardiol 2007;99:704–706.

20 Jatene AD, Fontes VF, Souza LC, Paulista PP, Neto CA, Sousa JE. Anatomic correction of transposition of the great arteries. J Thorac Cardiovasc Surg 1982;83:20–26.

21 Kondo C, Nakazawa M, Momma K, Kusakabe K. Sympathetic denervation and reinnervation after arterial switch operation for complete transposition. Circulation 1998;97:2414–2419

22 Raisky O, Bergoend E, Agnoletti G *et al.* Late coronary artery lesions after neonatal arterial switch operation: results of surgical coronary revascularization. Eur J Cardiothorac Surg 2007;31:894–898.

23 Bove T, De Meulder F, Vandenplas G *et al.* Midterm assessment of the reconstructed arteries after the arterial switch operation. Ann Thorac Surg 2008;85:823–830.

24 Rastelli GC, Wallace RB, Ongley PA. Complete repair of tranposition of the great arteries with pulmonary stenosis. A review and report of a case corrected by using a new surgical technique. Circulation 1969;39:83–95.

25 Horer J, Schreiber C, Dworak E *et al.* Long-term results after the Rastelli repair for transposition of the great arteries. Ann Thorac Surg 2007;83:2169–2175.

CHAPTER 19

Truncus arteriosus communis

Lesions classified as truncus arteriosus, persistent truncus arteriosus, or truncus arteriosus communis comprise about 2% of congenital cardiac anomalies in various autopsy series; they are an important cause of death in infancy. The complex is characterized by the presence of a single semilunar valve and annulus with a single great vessel, usually termed the common trunk, arising from the ventricles. The condition is to be distinguished from those lesions in which a single arterial trunk connects with the ventricles but which are associated with atresia of either the aortic or pulmonary valve with small or atretic vessels.

Morphological and embryological considerations

Morphology

Several classifications have been described for truncus arteriosus complexes. The one most commonly used is that of Collett and Edwards, who described four main groups.

- Type I: a short common pulmonary artery segment arises on the right side of the common trunk just above the truncal valve and this gives rise to a separate left and right pulmonary artery; the ascending aorta arises from the left side of the common trunk.
- Type II: the common trunk continues up as the ascending aorta; the pulmonary arteries arise a short distance above the truncal valve from the posterior surface of the trunk as separate left and right pulmonary arteries from two orifices, very close to one another. Since the original description, a variant of this type has been noted in which the two pulmonary arteries arise from a single orifice on the posterior surface of the truncus. Some have alluded to this as a type I $^1/_2$ truncus.
- Type III: this is similar to type II but the pulmonary arteries arise more laterally and somewhat more distant from the semilunar valves.
- Type IV is characterized by an absence of any vestige of a pulmonary artery or pulmonary arterial branches. Blood supply to the lungs is derived entirely from major aortopulmonary collateral arteries (MAPCAs). Whether this type is a true truncus arteriosus has been questioned. It has been suggested that it represents an extreme form of tetralogy of Fallot with pulmonary atresia, in which there is no vestige of pulmonary arteries and the term *pseudotruncus* has been applied.

Van Praagh has suggested a different classification, in which truncus lesions are divided into types A and B. Type A is associated with a ventricular septal defect; van Praagh types A1 and A2 are comparable to the same types in the other classification. In type A3, one pulmonary artery is absent and in type A4 there is associated aortic isthmus atresia or hypoplasia. Type B has an intact ventricular septum, but it is a rarity. Since the conotruncal septum completes the closure of the ventricular septum, these patients almost always have a ventricular septal defect, usually of large size, just beneath the truncus valve. Usually, the position of the truncus in relation to the ventricular septal defect is such that it straddles the left and right ventricles evenly in about half the patients. In others it may be placed preferentially over one or other ventricle to a varying extent.

The truncal semilunar valve usually consists of three cusps; about 25% of patients have four cusps and about 10% have a bicuspid valve. Rarely, five or even six cusps are present. The cusps are often thickened and dysplastic and have limited mobility.

Congenital Diseases of the Heart, 3rd edition. By A. Rudolph
© 2009 Blackwell Publishing, ISBN: 9781405162456

Insufficiency of this valve is common, occurring in about 50% of patients. It varies in degree, but as many as 25% of patients are considered to have moderate to severe insufficiency. Stenosis of the truncal valve has been observed in about 25% of patients, but is usually of mild degree and rarely does the valve appear to be severely obstructed morphologically. However, because flow through the valve is large, the stenosis may be very significant functionally. Coronary artery anomalies are also common, occurring in about 25% of patients. In about half, there is a single coronary artery; in others two coronary arteries are present but they arise from a single ostium in the truncal root. Other coronary artery anomalies have been noted.

Aortic arch anomalies are commonly associated with truncus arteriosus. A right aortic arch is present in about 25% of patients and interruption of the arch is noted in about 10%. In infants with an interrupted arch, there is frequently a large chamber above the truncal valve, which leads primarily to a large ductus arteriosus. The small ascending aorta and the pulmonary arteries also arise from this chamber. This morphology is confusing and the presence of aortic arch interruption is frequently overlooked, because the ductus arteriosus is thought to be the arch. The ductus arteriosus is usually small, or even absent when the aortic arch is normally developed, but occasionally a normal ductus may be present when the arch is normal.

The morphology of the pulmonary arteries varies considerably in individuals with truncus arteriosus. As mentioned, in type I the left and right arteries arise from a short common trunk. In types II and $I^1/_2$, the pulmonary arteries are usually large, but occasionally stenosis is evident at the origins of the left and right pulmonary arteries; this stenosis may not be present at birth but may develop later in life. In type III, the pulmonary arteries originate more distally; their size varies, but generally they are smaller than in types I and II. Only one pulmonary artery may originate from the truncus; the other artery may be present, is usually hypoplastic, and is supplied by a ductus arteriosus. One or both pulmonary arteries may be absent and lung flow is provided from MAPCAs (see Chapter 14). The peripheral pulmonary arteries are usually normally developed in types I and II truncus arteriosus. However, following birth, the vessels tend to retain a greater amount of medial smooth muscle and, if the lesion is not corrected, there is a serious risk of development of pulmonary vascular obstructive changes with progressive increase in pulmonary vascular resistance (see Chapter 5). In type III, there is a high incidence of stenosis of the pulmonary arteries, either at the ostium or along the length of the vessel; this provides some protection to the pulmonary arterioles and limits the risk for obstructive changes. In type IV, pulmonary blood flow is provided by MAPCAs (discussed in Chapter 14).

A related lesion is the so-called hemitruncus, in which one pulmonary artery, most commonly the right, is connected to the ascending aorta, whereas the left pulmonary artery arises from the right ventricle and there is a separate pulmonary annulus and valve. This condition cannot be considered to be a truncus arteriosus communis and is not discussed.

Embryology

The concept has been presented that persistent truncus arteriosus is related to failure of development of the spiral septum in the conotruncus. This septum was described in the chick embryo to be formed from two ridges, one arising from the left anterior side and the other from the right posterior; these grow toward each other, join, and separate the conotruncus into the aorta and pulmonary artery. The concept that truncus arteriosus is exclusively due to failure of development of the spiral septum has been challenged. It has been pointed out that the main pulmonary trunk is not formed entirely by separation of the truncus, but also by fusion of the proximal portions of the two sixth branchial arches, which extend into the left and right pulmonary arteries and, on the left, into the ductus arteriosus. When viewed from above, the ventral aorta rotates clockwise just above the ventricular conus, and the right sixth arch migrates with it, meeting the left sixth arch at its origin. The fusion of these two arches at their origin, with dissolution of the intervening membrane, produces a common channel from which the right pulmonary artery arises and which continues into the ductus arteriosus and the left pulmonary artery. This rotation of the truncus is considered very important in the normal morphological development of the relationships between the aorta and the pulmonary artery. If the spiral ridges do not develop completely, there is lack of separation of the truncus from the pulmonary trunk formed from the sixth branchial arches. The failure of spiral ridges to develop will also result in abnormal formation of the semilunar valve, and instead of the total of six leaflets that normally develop (three in the aorta and three in the pulmonary artery) usually only two, three, or four cusps form. Also, since the spiral septum contributes to the closure of the uppermost portion of the ventricular septum, a defect will persist between the ventricles just beneath the common semilunar valve. The embryological development of this region may be even more primitive; if there is lack of adequate rotation of the ventral aorta, the left and right sixth arches will not join. This, associated with failure of spiral ridges to develop, will result in a single vessel arising from the ventricles, with the pulmonary arteries arising either posteriorly, close to each other, from the large trunk or separately from each other from the lateral sides of the trunk.

The actual cause of the embryological disturbance that results in the development of truncus arteriosus lesions is not known. One concept that has been considered is that flow of blood returning to the heart follows certain patterns and that there is spiraling of superior vena cava (SVC) and inferior vena cava (IVC) returns in the heart when it is still in the bilocular form. It has been suggested that these flow patterns could be important in molding the developing heart and in producing various types of rotation. Perhaps, alterations in blood flow patterns at an early stage of development contribute to the formation of a truncus arteriosus lesion.

Recently, it has been shown in the avian embryo that neural crest cells in the occipital region of the embryo migrate to the third, fourth, and sixth branchial arches, as well as to the aortic sac and the aortopulmonary outflow [1]. These cardiac neural crest cells are important in development of the walls of the great arteries and the aortopulmonary septum. It has been suggested that when the number of these cells falls below a critical level, the septum separating the conotruncus into the aorta and pulmonary artery does not develop. Ablation of the cardiac neural crest region in the chick embryo results in a high incidence of persistent truncus arteriosus. The lack of these cells may also alter flow patterns in the branchial arches and this could contribute to the disturbances in alignment. The cardiac neural crest cells express the *PAX3* gene and it has been postulated that mutations of this gene could be important in causing cardiac defects such as truncus arteriosus. This does not explain the different types of truncus arteriosus, unless one postulates that the number of neural crest cells involved determines the degree of maturational defect. Studies in the mouse embryo have indicated that a mutation of *Wnt5a* may be responsible for persistent truncus arteriosus [2]. *Wnt5a* is expressed in pharyngeal mesoderm adjacent to cardiac neural crest cells and in the conotruncus at the time the septum between the aorta and pulmonary artery begins to be formed.

The occurrence of truncus arteriosus in individuals with chromosome 22q11 deletions has also pointed to genetic associations. In different series 20–33% of patients with persistent truncus arteriosus have 22q11 deletions [3]. There is also a high incidence of DiGeorge syndrome in patients with truncus arteriosus. No information is currently available regarding the incidence of 22q11 deletions in those instances where aortic arch obstruction is associated with truncus arteriosus, but it is likely to be very high.

Hemodynamic considerations

Fetal circulation

The main effect of truncus arteriosus is to produce a variable degree of mixing of left and right ventricular blood just above the semilunar valve. SVC and IVC blood returning to the heart probably follow their normal course into the left and right atria and into the ventricles. Normally, blood in the fetal left ventricle has a higher oxygen saturation than that in the right ventricle (see Chapter 1). Based on estimates of systemic venous and umbilical venous blood flows and on oxygen saturations of systemic and umbilical venous blood, if blood from the two ventricles mixes completely, the oxygen saturation of the mixed blood will be about 55% (see Chapter 1). Thus blood distributed from the ascending aorta will have a lower oxygen saturation compared with the normal of about 65%. Blood distributed to the lungs and to the descending aorta will be slightly higher than the normal of about 50%. The degree of mixing will be related to the morphology. In type I truncus arteriosus, in which there is a common pulmonary trunk, right ventricular blood may be directed preferentially to the pulmonary trunk; only a relatively small amount of left ventricular blood enters the pulmonary artery, so that oxygen saturation will be only minimally higher than normal. However, in types II, III and IV, right and left ventricular blood will probably mix more effectively and therefore blood distributed to the ascending and descending aortae, as well as the pulmonary artery, will have similar oxygen saturations. The higher Po_2 of blood distributed to the lungs may lower pulmonary vascular resistance and possibly retard the degree of development of pulmonary vascular smooth muscle as compared with the normal fetus (see Chapter 5).

The patterns of blood flow and blood oxygen saturations and pressures that might be expected are shown in Figure 19.1. The size of the ductus arteriosus will also be important in determining patterns of flow. The ductus is usually small or absent in truncus arteriosus; therefore, during fetal life a large proportion of blood flow to the descending aorta will traverse the aortic arch and isthmus, so that the isthmus diameter may be greater than normal. If the ductus arteriosus is large in a fetus with type I truncus, flow could pass preferentially through the ductus to the descending aorta. Flow into the ascending aorta will be reduced and this may result in narrowing of the aortic isthmus and possibly contribute to the development of interruption of the aorta at this site. However, it is likely that the association of aortic arch interruption with persistent truncus is primarily due to an embryological disturbance rather than abnormal flow patterns, because both lesions are commonly associated with 22q11 deletions. When aortic arch interruption is associated with truncus arteriosus, the ductus is large and provides all blood flow to the lower body of the fetus and to the placenta.

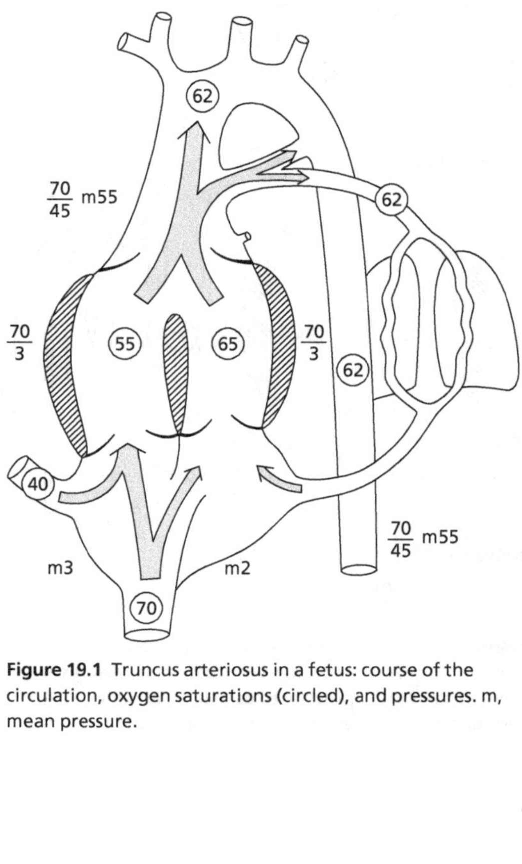

Figure 19.1 Truncus arteriosus in a fetus: course of the circulation, oxygen saturations (circled), and pressures. m, mean pressure.

Circulatory changes after birth

The origin of the pulmonary arteries and the aorta from a single trunk provides equal perfusion pressure in these vessels beyond the semilunar valve. Blood flows to the lungs and the systemic circulation are therefore determined by the relative resistances in these circulations. After birth, systemic vascular resistance is increased by removal of the low-resistance umbilical–placental circulation as well as by hormonal influences (see Chapter 2). Ventilation of the lungs with air reduces pulmonary vascular resistance rapidly initially and then more gradually due to postnatal maturation of the small pulmonary vessels (see Chapter 5). The pulmonary vasodilatation results in an increase in pulmonary blood flow; as pulmonary vascular resistance progressively decreases and systemic vascular resistance progressively increases after birth, an increasing pulmonary blood flow and pulmonary to systemic flow ratio results. The factors that affect pulmonary blood flow are pulmonary vascular, or arteriolar, resistance and the size of the pulmonary arteries.

The pulmonary to systemic flow ratio determines systemic arterial oxygen saturation and Po_2 after birth. If it is assumed that there is complete or almost complete admixture of pulmonary and systemic venous blood at the high ventricular or truncus level, the greater the pulmonary to systemic flow ratio, the higher the systemic arterial oxygen saturation (see Chapter 3).

In the infant with truncus arteriosus who has large pulmonary arteries with no orifice stenosis, the decreased pulmonary vascular resistance after birth will produce a modest increase in pulmonary blood flow, and systemic arterial oxygen saturation will increase immediately to about 75–80%. The pulmonary blood flow returning to the left atrium results in an increase in left atrial pressure; this, associated with a decrease in IVC return by elimination of umbilical venous return, closes the foramen ovale. Left ventricular end-diastolic pressure also increases slightly, but the ventricle is capable of ejecting the volume of blood presented. In the early postnatal period the arterial oxygen saturation and Po_2 are moderately reduced, but there are no other hemodynamic disturbances. The course of the circulation in the neonatal period is shown in Figure 19.2. The continuing decrease in pulmonary vascular resistance after birth results in a progressive increase in pulmonary blood flow. Systemic arterial oxygen saturation increases due to the increase in pulmonary to systemic flow ratio and may reach 88–90%. The increased pulmonary venous return to the left atrium and ventricle produces a progressive elevation of left atrial and left ventricular end-diastolic pressures and an increase in left ventricular stroke volume. The large increase in pulmonary blood flow will result in left ventricular failure if the volume load is presented rapidly to the ventricle so that there is inadequate time for compensatory left ventricular hypertrophy. Usually, the decrease in pulmonary vascular resistance occurs over a 2–3 week period, but many infants with truncus arteriosus develop cardiac failure within the first week after birth. This early onset of failure is usually due to the presence of associated truncal valve insufficiency. However, lack of normal development of pulmonary vascular smooth muscle before birth may result in a more rapid postnatal decline of pulmonary vascular resistance (see above). The early manifestations of cardiac failure are associated with left ventricular failure and pulmonary edema, but right ventricular failure also develops (Figure 19.3). Other factors contributing to the development of cardiac failure are discussed in detail in Chapter 7.

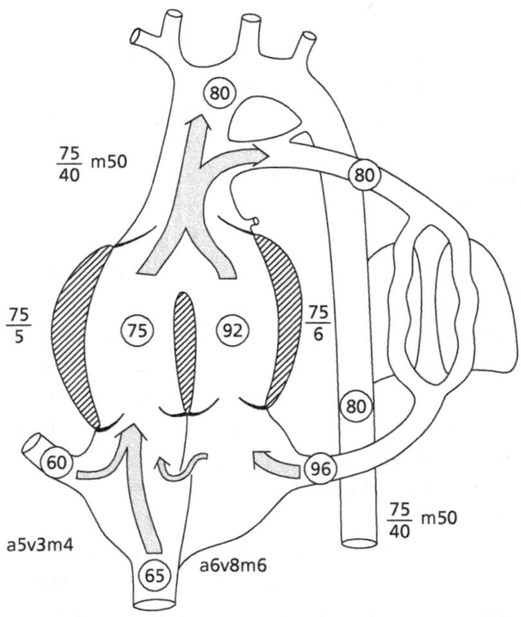

Figure 19.2 Truncus arteriosus in a newborn infant: course of the circulation, oxygen saturations (circled), and pressures. The pulmonary ostia are not stenosed and the pulmonary vascular resistance has dropped moderately. m, mean pressure.

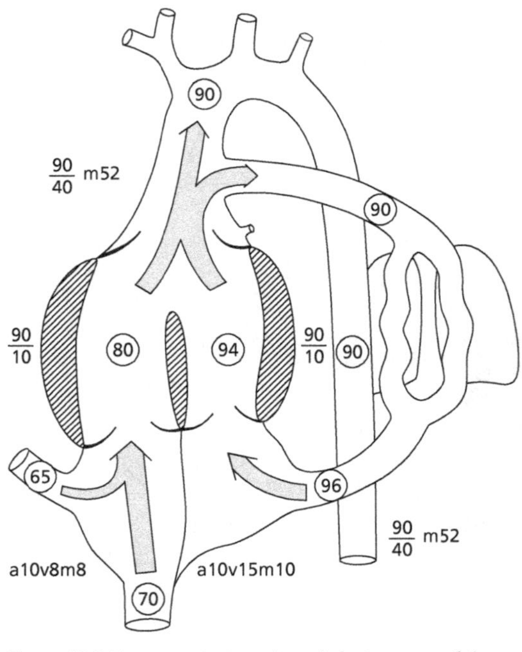

Figure 19.3 Truncus arteriosus in an infant: course of the circulation, oxygen saturations (circled), and pressures. Pulmonary vascular resistance has fallen markedly, resulting in cardiac failure. m, mean pressure.

Because the low pulmonary vascular resistance produces a rapid runoff from the truncus into the pulmonary circulation, a low diastolic pressure and wide pulse pressure might be expected in the truncus and the aorta and its branches. This accounts for the prominent pulses noted in these infants. Although this is noted in some infants with truncus arteriosus with high pulmonary to systemic flow ratios, arterial pulses are not always prominent. This could be due to the fact that, when pulmonary vascular resistance is very low, a large proportion of blood ejected during systole passes from the truncus into the pulmonary circulation during systole. The amount entering the aorta and the systemic circulation is small and therefore systolic pressure is rather low and the pulse pressure is not increased. In these infants the pulmonary blood flow is very high and cardiac failure is common. When pulmonary blood flow is not markedly increased, as in those infants who have mild to moderate pulmonary artery stenosis, arterial systolic pressure is higher and pulse pressure is increased. Reduction in pulmonary blood flow by either progressive pulmonary artery stenosis or development of pulmonary vascular disease will decrease diastolic runoff and pulse pressure will approximate normal.

Many infants succumb from heart failure in early infancy; if this can be controlled, the pulmonary vessels develop the secondary changes related to persistent pulmonary hypertension and increased blood flow (see Chapter 5). Severe intimal proliferation and occlusive pulmonary vascular disease may occur within the first year, but sometimes the process is slower and may take many years before marked vascular obstructive changes develop. As pulmonary vascular resistance increases, pulmonary blood flow decreases and left ventricular failure improves because the volume overloading is reduced. Associated with the decreased pulmonary to systemic flow ratio, the arterial oxygen saturation falls progressively.

In infants who have moderate degrees of stenosis or diffuse narrowing of the pulmonary arteries, a finding more common in type II and especially type III truncus, pulmonary blood flow does not increase greatly after birth. Associated with the decrease in pulmonary vascular resistance, arterial oxygen saturation will be increased to a limited extent. When the pulmonary arteries are reasonably well developed, the flow may be adequate to maintain an arterial saturation of 75–85%, but not large enough to cause left ventricular failure. These patients may have a more favorable course, with only moderate cyanosis; however, the stenosis tends to become progressively more severe with advancing age. This could be due to lack of growth of the orifice appropriate for age, but usually appears to be associated with an intimal proliferative process. The time course for this process varies greatly; it may develop during the first year, but may be slower, so that the child may have mild cyanosis with no other symptoms for several years. The stenosis of the pulmonary ostia creates a pressure drop between the truncus and the pulmonary arteries and thus protects the pulmonary arterioles against the development of pulmonary vascular disease. Some patients have stenosis of the ostium of one pulmonary artery, with a free opening in the other. This usually results in a moderately large total pulmonary blood flow, which maintains arterial oxygen saturation in the range 75–85%, but cardiac failure is not common. The arterioles in the lung supplied by the artery with a narrow ostium are protected from the development of vascular obstruction, but progressive disease occurs in the other lung, and increasing cyanosis will develop. In type IV truncus arteriosus, also referred to as pseudotruncus, pulmonary arteries are absent and pulmonary blood flow is provided by MAPCAs. The circulatory dynamics are similar to those in tetralogy of Fallot with pulmonary atresia and are presented in Chapter 14.

In all patients with truncus arteriosus, the relationship between pulmonary and systemic vascular resistances determines the pulmonary to systemic flow ratio. A decrease in systemic vascular resistance not associated with any change in pulmonary vascular resistance will result in preferential flow into the systemic circulation and the proportion of ventricular output distributed to the lung will decrease. Thus pulmonary to systemic flow ratio is reduced, resulting in a fall in arterial oxygen saturation. The fall in pressure in the aorta and the truncus will result in reduction in pulmonary blood flow and a fall in total oxygen uptake in the lung, which will further contribute to the decrease in arterial oxygen saturation. These mechanisms are similar to those occurring in tetralogy of Fallot and are discussed in detail in Chapter 14. A fall in systemic vascular resistance, which often occurs with sedation or during anesthesia, will result in a decrease in arterial oxygen saturation. Similarly, the fall in systemic vascular resistance associated with exercise will result in a fall in pulmonary to systemic flow ratio, but the fall in arterial oxygen saturation is greater because oxygen consumption is increased.

Truncal valve anomalies

Truncal valve insufficiency

This association is common, occurring in about half of all individuals with persistent truncus. About half of these patients have moderate to severe insufficiency, which has a major influence on the circulatory dynamics, as well as on the clinical presentation and prognosis. The fetal heart may be enlarged because of the large volume load resulting from the valvar insufficiency *in utero*. The afterload presented by the pulmonary circulation is high *in utero*, but decreases rapidly postnatally as a result of the pulmonary vasodilatation associated with ventilation. However, resistance in the aortic distribution increases after birth because the relatively low-resistance umbilical circulation is eliminated. Thus the total afterload on the truncus is probably not changed significantly. However, pulmonary blood flow increases as pulmonary vascular resistance falls, and this results in a greater volume of blood returning to the left atrium and ventricle and an increase in total cardiac output. Truncal regurgitation will thus increase after birth; the combination of increased pulmonary blood flow and truncal regurgitation places a huge volume load on the ventricle and cardiac failure is very likely to result.

After repair of the truncus arteriosus by connecting the pulmonary arteries to the right ventricle, the volume of blood passing through the truncal valve, which now functions as the aortic valve, is only the systemic blood flow. The output across the valve is thus greatly reduced and the amount of regurgitation may decrease considerably.

Truncal valve stenosis

This is not as common as insufficiency. Severe stenosis is unusual, and is not well tolerated because it presents an increased afterload on both ventricles. After pulmonary vascular resistance has fallen, a large proportion of the volume traversing the valve is delivered to the pulmonary circulation. Severe stenosis will restrict the combined output and systemic blood flow could be markedly compromised.

Milder degrees of stenosis, with systolic pressure gradients of up to about 60 mmHg, are encountered. The magnitude of the pressure gradient does not have the same implications as in isolated aortic stenosis, because a large volume traverses the valve. After correction of the truncus, the output across the valve is greatly reduced, because only systemic blood flow now passes through it and the gradient will be reduced significantly.

Aortic arch anomalies

As mentioned above, about 10% of patients with truncus arteriosus have aortic arch interruption. In the early postnatal period, the arterial oxygen saturation is moderately reduced, but as pulmonary vascular resistance falls and pulmonary blood flow increases, it increases to as high as 85–90%. Mixing of left and right ventricular blood in the truncus is usually almost complete, although oxygen saturation in the pulmonary artery may be slightly lower than that in the ascending aorta. Blood flow to the descending aorta is derived exclusively through the ductus arteriosus, so that if there is some degree of preferential flow of right ventricular blood into the pulmonary artery, there may be a somewhat lower oxygen saturation in descending as compared with ascending aortic blood. The difference is not usually more than about 5%. While the ductus arteriosus is widely patent, pressure and blood flow in the descending aorta are well maintained, but the flow is also determined by pulmonary vascular resistance. If resistance is low, blood will be preferentially distributed to the lungs and the volume passing to the descending aorta will be limited. To maintain normal flow to the descending aorta, the ventricles would have to increase their output, but pulmonary blood flow would be greatly increased, resulting in left atrial and left ventricular enlargement. The predominant features are those of cardiac failure. Constriction of the ductus arteriosus will reduce blood flow into the descending aorta, resulting in poor perfusion of the lower body. It will also tend to further increase pulmonary blood flow and thus exaggerate the cardiac failure. Factors responsible for the manifestations of cardiac failure are discussed in Chapter 7. Because pulmonary blood flow is high and systemic blood flow is normal or, especially when ductus arteriosus constriction occurs, reduced, the arterial oxygen saturation and Po_2 are maintained at high levels. If ductus arteriosus constriction results in marked reduction in flow to the lower body, oxygen delivery to the lower body will occur despite relatively high oxygen saturation; tissue hypoxia may result and metabolic acidemia develop (see Chapter 3).

Without surgical treatment, the majority of infants with truncus arteriosus types I or II succumb during the first year as a result of cardiac failure. If cardiac failure can be controlled, some patients survive to adolescence and even adult life. Pulmonary vascular changes usually begin to develop within the first year and may progress rapidly. This is associated with a reduction in pulmonary blood flow and progressive fall in arterial oxygen saturation. The consequences of pulmonary vascular obstructive disease are discussed in Chapter 5.

Infants with type III truncus arteriosus may not develop severe cardiac failure, because some degree of stenosis of the pulmonary arteries is common. Pulmonary blood flow is therefore not increased markedly when pulmonary vascular resistance falls. As a result of the lower pulmonary to systemic flow ratio, arterial oxygen saturation is considerably reduced. Also, there is frequently progressive stenosis of the pulmonary arteries with a progressive fall in arterial oxygen saturation. Patients with type IV truncus are similar to those with tetralogy of Fallot and pulmonary atresia (see Chapter 14).

Clinical features

Although many clinical features are common to all types of persistent truncus arteriosus, there are some differences in presentation, largely related to the pulmonary to systemic flow ratio. The different types are therefore presented separately.

Truncus arteriosus types I and II

In the immediate postnatal period mild cyanosis is noted, usually with no other symptoms. Cyanosis then decreases as pulmonary blood flow increases, but large increases in flow usually result in cardiac failure, manifested by increased respiratory effort, excessive perspiration, and hepatomegaly. This usually develops within about 2–4 weeks, but may appear during the first week if there is insufficiency of the truncal valve. The upper and lower extremity pulses may be well felt, but usually when the infant is in cardiac failure the pulses are not very prominent. If cardiac failure improves, as the infant develops, the pulse pressure may increase and the pulses will have a bounding character. If truncus arteriosus is complicated by aortic arch interruption, the upper and lower extremity pulses may both be normal or somewhat reduced during the first few days after birth, but as the ductus arteriosus constricts, the lower extremity pulses become progressively weaker. Blood pressure measurements often show a narrow pulse pressure in the infant in cardiac failure, but it widens with increasing age. The lower extremity blood pressure falls when the ductus arteriosus constricts if aortic arch interruption complicates the persistent truncus.

The heart becomes clinically enlarged, with a diffuse impulse; usually activity at the lower left sternal border predominates, but with truncal valve insufficiency the apical impulse is often hyperactive. The first sound is accentuated and is loud at the mid-left sternal border; usually the sound is single, but it may be narrowly split. It is difficult to explain this observation, as one would expect to hear a single second sound when only one semilunar valve is present. It is possible that because the valve cusps are frequently thickened, they do not all close simultaneously. A prominent systolic ejection click is frequently heard at the lower or mid-left sternal border; if present in an infant in cardiac failure, the diagnosis of truncus arteriosus should be considered. A third heart sound may be present at the apex.

In infants with cardiac failure there is usually a medium-frequency systolic ejection murmur at the upper left sternal border, radiating to both lungs. A low-frequency mid-diastolic murmur is often heard at the apex. An early decrescendo diastolic murmur may be audible along the left sternal border, associated with truncal valve insufficiency. When pulmonary vascular disease develops, cyanosis increases but the manifestations of cardiac failure improve; also, precordial activity decreases, the systolic murmur becomes softer, and the mid-diastolic murmur disappears.

Truncus arteriosus type III

The clinical features are determined by the size of the pulmonary arteries and the severity of stenosis of the pulmonary ostia. If the pulmonary arteries are large and there is minimal stenosis, pulmonary blood flow will be large and the features are similar to those of types I and II. Usually there is some restriction to pulmonary blood flow; the symptoms of cardiac failure are not usually severe and a moderate degree of cyanosis is evident. The pulses are usually prominent in both upper and lower extremities and the blood pressure shows a wide pulse pressure. Precordial activity is increased at the lower left sternal border but the cardiac impulse is not very hyperactive. The heart sounds are similar to those described above, but continuous murmurs may be heard at the upper left or right sternal border or in the back; these murmurs may radiate to the chest. They are due to flow across the stenotic ostia of the pulmonary arteries. In the early postnatal period, the features are related to moderate increases in pulmonary blood flow, because the ostial stenosis is usually not evident or is mild. Within weeks to months, the stenosis progresses and cyanosis increases and the continuous murmurs become more common. Progressive occlusion of the pulmonary arteries results in disappearance of murmurs and severe cyanosis. One pulmonary artery may be connected with the truncus, but receives its blood flow through a ductus arteriosus. Closure of the ductus will result in an increase in cyanosis.

Truncus arteriosus type IV

The clinical features are described in the section on tetralogy of Fallot with pulmonary atresia in Chapter 14.

Investigations

Electrocardiography

The electrocardiogram varies greatly. Most patients have a normal axis or right axis deviation of varying degree. Right ventricular forces are almost always increased and usually there is combined ventricular hypertrophy. Occasionally, left ventricular forces may be dominant.

Chest radiography

The heart size is increased within a few days after birth in types I and II truncus arteriosus; this is related to the increase in pulmonary blood flow. When significant truncal valve insufficiency is present, cardiomegaly may be noted at birth. The enlargement usually involves both ventricles, but often left ventricular enlargement dominates, particularly if aortic insufficiency is associated. The pulmonary vascularity is increased within a few days after birth, showing initially prominent pulmonary arteries extending to the periphery of the lung fields. When cardiac failure ensues, pulmonary edema may produce haziness of the markings, particularly in the hilar regions. The characteristic feature of persistent truncus arteriosus is a narrow superior mediastinum due to absence of the main pulmonary artery. However, although this finding is common, it may not be evident in type I truncus because the presence of a pulmonary trunk may create a shadow in the pulmonary artery region. The aortic arch is right-sided in about 25% of patients with truncus arteriosus; it has been suggested that the presence of a right aortic arch associated with increased pulmonary vascular markings should create a high degree of suspicion for the diagnosis of persistent truncus. In types III and IV truncus, the heart is not usually as large and the pulmonary arterial markings are not as prominent. The superior mediastinum is usually narrow and the pulmonary arterial segment is not evident. Significant stenosis of one or both pulmonary arteries is associated with a decrease in pulmonary arterial markings. When pulmonary vascular obstructive disease develops, the heart size decreases; the central pulmonary arterial markings are very prominent, but there is a paucity of peripheral arterial markings in the lungs.

Echocardiography

Two-dimensional imaging and color flow Doppler studies have made it possible to obtain most of the information necessary for diagnosis and therapeutic considerations in patients with persistent truncus arteriosus. The single large trunk exiting the heart can be defined. The truncus overrides the ventricular septum to variable degrees. Usually it is positioned fairly evenly over both ventricles, but it may be displaced to lie predominantly over either the left or right ventricle. The ventricular septal defect can be defined; it is usually large and in the outlet septum, but occasionally extends to the membranous septum. The truncal semilunar valve should be carefully examined; it is contiguous to the mitral valve. Most commonly, the valve is tricuspid, but may be quadricuspid or bicuspid. Rarely one or five cusps are present. The vale leaflets are often thickened and may not move freely. Truncal valve insufficiency is common, but it is difficult to gauge the severity of the regurgitation accurately. With color flow Doppler studies, the duration of regurgitation during diastole, the degree to which the ventricles fill, and the breadth of the regurgitant jet have been used as indications of severity. The presence of stenosis of the valve is demonstrated by assessing the velocity of flow beyond the truncal valve. The flow velocities to the pulmonary arteries and aorta may be different, so that it may be difficult to assess the degree of stenosis accurately. However, significant degrees of stenosis are unusual.

Defining the origin of the pulmonary arteries is one of the most important aspects of the examination. The presence of a partial aortopulmonary septum characterizes type I truncus; the origin of both the left and right pulmonary arteries from the common pulmonary trunk segment confirms the diagnosis. In type II truncus, the pulmonary arteries can be seen to originate from the posterior aspect of the truncus a short distance above the valve. In this type it is important to identify the relationship of the coronary artery ostia to the pulmonary artery origins, because damage to coronary arteries could result from surgery to separate the pulmonary arteries from the trunk. Pulmonary arteries may be difficult to identify in type III truncus because they arise some distance from the truncal valve and are frequently small. It is important to attempt to locate the origin of the pulmonary arteries to distinguish the lesion from tetralogy of Fallot with pulmonary atresia, in which only a single arterial trunk (the aorta) exits the heart. The size of the pulmonary arteries should be measured and the presence of stenosis assessed by Doppler flow examination.

Coronary artery anomalies should be defined. As mentioned above, a common origin of both coronary arteries from a single ostium or origin of both coronary arteries from ostia in the same sinus of Valsalva occur in about 25% of patients with truncus arteriosus. The anomalies are not usually important in surgical repair.

The presence of interruption of the aorta may be difficult to identify by ultrasound examination. The large ductus arteriosus may readily be mistaken as the arch of the aorta. It is therefore important to search for the origin of the innominate and carotid and subclavian arteries. A feature that strongly suggests the presence of interruption is the smooth continuous curve of the left side of the ascending aorta image into the left carotid artery. Other features readily identified by ultrasound examination are the presence of a right aortic arch, which is found in 25–30% of patients, and persistent left superior vena cava draining into the coronary sinus (10–15% of individuals with persistent truncus).

Cardiac catheterization and angiocardiography

General considerations

Prior to the introduction of ultrasound examination, cardiac catheterization and angiocardiography were usually necessary to make a definite diagnosis of truncus arteriosus. The procedure is now not usually necessary, because most of the morphological features can be defined by ultrasound examination. Occasionally, it may not be possible to identify the precise origin of pulmonary arteries by ultrasound studies and catheterization is necessary. Other indications for catheterization include definition of the presence and severity of obstruction at the pulmonary artery ostia and along the course of the pulmonary arteries. Although delineation of the presence of coronary artery anomalies is not as important as it was previously, it is still potentially important if surgery is being considered. Another important indication for catheterization is to estimate pulmonary vascular resistance to decide whether it is too greatly elevated to consider surgery. This issue is usually raised in infants or children who have survived the infancy period and have developed pulmonary vascular changes.

Approach and catheter manipulation

It is usually easy to pass the catheter into the truncus from the right ventricle; it then may pass into the ascending aorta and to the innominate artery or around the arch to the descending aorta. In type I truncus the catheter may enter the pulmonary trunk and then the left or right pulmonary artery. The course is such that it may not be recognized that the catheter has passed through the truncus to reach the pulmonary arteries, and it may be considered to be normal. The exact course of the catheter may be even more difficult to resolve when it enters the truncus and passes to the descending aorta through the ductus arteriosus. It is commonly not appreciated that the infant has an interruption of the aortic arch, because the ductus is close to the arch. It may therefore be difficult to distinguish passage across a normal arch from passage across the ductus to the descending aorta. Another lesion that must be differentiated from truncus arteriosus is aortopulmonary fenestration; in this lesion, the catheter may be passed from the pulmonary artery through the fenestration into the ascending aorta and then around the arch to the descending aorta. It is difficult, from the course of the catheter alone, to distinguish these conditions.

To assess the presence of pulmonary ostial or pulmonary arterial stenosis, it is important to attempt to catheterize each pulmonary artery and to measure pressure along the course of the artery and across the ostium. Catheterization of the pulmonary arteries is often more readily achieved from a retrograde arterial approach.

Oxygen saturation and blood gases

Superior and inferior vena caval oxygen saturations are usually normal but may be reduced if cardiac failure is present or if there is a marked decrease in systemic arterial saturation. In infants with a large pulmonary blood flow, an increase in right atrial oxygen saturation may be noted, due to left-to-right shunting across the foramen ovale; the increase is usually only 5–8% but may be as high as 15–20%. Right ventricular oxygen saturation is sometimes increased compared with right atrial levels, due to left-to-right shunting through the ventricular septal defect or to truncal valve insufficiency. This is variable, and samples obtained in the body or apex of the ventricle frequently show only a small increase in saturation. The fact that both left and right ventricular blood is ejected into the truncus during systole and that little blood from the left ventricle crosses the ventricular septal defect to enter the body of the right ventricle probably explains these findings. However, a sample taken in the right ventricle just below the semilunar valve does demonstrate the increase in oxygen saturation. Pulmonary venous oxygen saturation may be reduced to 85–90% in infants with pulmonary edema; $P\text{O}_2$ may be as low as 40–50 mmHg and $P\text{CO}_2$ increased to 40–45 mmHg.

When pulmonary blood flow is markedly reduced, usually in type III or IV truncus, pulmonary venous $P\text{O}_2$ may be raised to 110–115 mmHg, $P\text{CO}_2$ reduced to 15–20 mmHg, and pH increased to 7.45–7.48 due to an increase in the ventilation–perfusion ratio. Oxygen saturation in the left atrium is often lower than that in the pulmonary vein due to right-to-left shunting across the foramen ovale. Oxygen saturations in the left ventricle are often similar to those described for the right ventricle; the inflow and apical regions have oxygen saturations similar to those in the left atrium, but the outflow region may have a lower saturation, because the right ventricular stream may produce shunting at this site.

Although it is usually assumed that mixing of left and right ventricular blood is fairly complete in truncus arteriosus, there may be considerable differences in oxygen saturations in the pulmonary and systemic arteries. This is particularly likely in type I truncus, but may also be observed in type II. Oxygen saturation in the pulmonary artery may be as much as 8–10% lower than that in the systemic arteries in type I truncus, but the difference is less in type II. In patients in whom the pulmonary arteries arise from the posterior or lateral portions of the truncus or from the aorta, the oxygen saturations in systemic and pulmonary arterial blood are usually identical. The actual levels of oxygen saturation and $P\text{O}_2$ are related to the pulmonary to systemic flow ratio; with large pulmonary blood flow, levels of 85–90% are usual. In the infant with type IV truncus, the systemic arterial oxygen saturation may be as low as 25–30% with a $P\text{O}_2$ of 20–25 mmHg, and pH may be markedly reduced.

The effects of oxygen administration on systemic arterial oxygen saturation and $P\text{O}_2$ are also related to the magnitude of pulmonary blood flow; 100% oxygen administration can increase the amount of dissolved oxygen by about 1.5 mL/dL in pulmonary venous blood. If pulmonary blood flow is large, this can constitute a major contribution of oxygen to the total mixture of pulmonary and systemic venous return. Oxygen saturation may increase to 100% and Po_2 to 150–250 mmHg. However, if pulmonary blood flow is very low, the amount of additional oxygen provided in dissolved form is relatively small and there is only a small rise in oxygen saturation and Po_2 of systemic arterial blood (see Chapter 3).

The changes in arterial oxygen saturation may be very useful in evaluating the responsiveness of the pulmonary circulation to vasodilator agents. This is discussed in detail below in the section on vascular resistances.

Blood flows and shunts

Systemic blood flow is reduced in infants in cardiac failure, but it may be increased in patients who have a markedly decreased arterial oxygen saturation. Pulmonary blood flow varies greatly, from very high levels in patients with no pulmonary arterial stenosis and relatively low pulmonary vascular resistance to low levels in patients with pulmonary stenosis, high pulmonary vascular resistance or absent pulmonary arteries.

Calculation of shunts is not very reliable because, in many instances, there is bidirectional shunting and the shunts may occur at different levels. Thus, blood shunted left to right at the atrial level may then be shunted right to left through the ventricular septal defect or into the truncus and then to the aorta. Therefore, it is not feasible to estimate the magnitude of the true or anatomical shunt. An estimate of the total volume of pulmonary venous blood that recirculates through the lungs (physiological left-to-right shunt) and the systemic venous blood that enters the systemic arteries without entering the lungs (physiological right-to-left shunt) can be made from the following equations:

$$\text{Physiological left-to-right shunt} = \dot{Q}p - \dot{Q}ep$$

$$\text{Physiological right-to-left shunt} = \dot{Q}s - \dot{Q}ep$$

where $\dot{Q}p$ is pulmonary blood flow, $\dot{Q}s$ systemic blood flow, and $\dot{Q}ep$ effective pulmonary blood flow. The physiological left-to-right shunt is large in patients with large pulmonary blood flows and the physiological right-to-left shunt is large in those with marked cyanosis. Pulmonary to systemic flow ratios may be as high as 3.5–4.0 when pulmonary flow is high, or reduced to 0.5 when pulmonary flow is low.

Pressures

Right atrial pressure may show a slightly increased *a* wave to levels of 8–10 mmHg but mean pressure is normal, although it may be raised in infants in cardiac failure. Right ventricular end-diastolic pressure may be increased to 8–10 mmHg and systolic pressure is at systemic arterial levels. The systemic arterial and truncus pressures vary considerably. Infants with a huge pulmonary blood flow usually have cardiac failure and systolic and diastolic pressures are reduced. In patients with normal or reduced pulmonary flows, systemic arterial pressures are usually normal. In older infants and children, in whom pulmonary blood flow is moderately increased, there is often a low diastolic pressure and wide pulse pressure. The left atrial mean pressure is increased in patients with large pulmonary blood flows and the *v* wave is large and may reach 15–20 mmHg, but left ventricular end-diastolic pressure is usually only moderately increased to about 10–15 mmHg. When pulmonary flow is reduced, mean pressure in the left atrium may be 2–3 mmHg lower than, or equal to, that in the right atrium; the *a* wave is lower and the *v* wave may be equal to the *a* wave. Pressure in the pulmonary artery is identical to that in the truncus and the ascending aorta in the absence of ostial stenosis. However, when marked stenosis is present, it may be reduced to low levels, with mean pressures of only 10–15 mmHg. When pulmonary blood flow is derived from a MAPCA arising from the descending aorta, pressure in it may vary from systemic arterial levels to very low levels if the orifice is stenosed.

Pulmonary and systemic vascular resistances

Systemic vascular resistance is usually normal when arterial oxygen saturation is above about 65%, but may be increased when saturation is reduced as a result of cardiac failure. Pulmonary vascular resistance, representing the resistance across the pulmonary vascular bed, is high, in the range 8–10 units/m^2 in the immediate postnatal period. In infants with no pulmonary arterial ostial stenosis, the pulmonary vascular resistance falls to 3–5 units/m^2 within the first few weeks after birth but it does not reach normal levels. In some patients, pulmonary vascular resistance may rise quite rapidly again within the first year, but occasionally may not reach levels above 8 units/m^2 for several years, although there is invariably a progressive increase in resistance. In patients with pulmonary stenosis, pulmonary vascular resistance is low.

Estimation of pulmonary vascular resistance in each lung is difficult; this is important in patients who have stenosis of the pulmonary artery to one lung, with systemic pressure in the other pulmonary artery. It is not possible to calculate the magnitude of pulmonary flow to each lung by the Fick method, unless it is feasible to measure oxygen uptake in each lung. A reasonable indication of the magnitude of flow to each lung can be obtained by radioisotope injection, with scanning of both lungs or by computed tomography or magnetic resonance imaging.

For decisions regarding possible surgery in older infants and children who have developed an increased pulmonary vascular resistance, it is important to know whether the pulmonary vessels are still reactive. The response to pulmonary vasodilator agents has been used to assess this, but pressure measurements are not helpful because the pulmonary arterial and aortic pressures both fall if either pulmonary or systemic vasodilatation occurs. An estimate of the effect of vasodilator drugs can be obtained by measuring systemic arterial and mixed venous oxygen saturations before and after administration of a pulmonary vasodilator agent (see Chapter 5). The study is most reliable if the mixing of pulmonary and systemic venous return is fairly complete, but is useful even if mixing is not complete. If the pharmacological agent produces a greater reduction in pulmonary than systemic vascular resistance, there will be a relative increase in pulmonary blood flow, since perfusion pressures are the same, and the mixed systemic arterial oxygen saturation will increase. However, if there is little effect on pulmonary vascular resistance, the oxygen saturation will either fall slightly or not change. It is important to measure mixed venous oxygen saturation to be sure that it does not change significantly after administration of the drug.

Angiocardiography

Injections of contrast medium into the left or right ventricle may show the truncus and the sites of origin of the pulmonary arteries, but these features are usually more clearly demonstrated with a direct injection into the truncus. Both left and right ventricular injections define the ventricular septal defect, because the injection results in passage of contrast material across the defect. With the right ventricular injection, the pulmonary arteries may fill preferentially in type I truncus. If the injection in the truncus is made through a catheter passed progradely through the truncal valve, it may be difficult to accurately assess the degree of truncal valve insufficiency. This is more reliably evaluated by injecting into a catheter passed retrogradely from a peripheral artery. This injection demonstrates the presence of one semilunar valve and it may be possible to determine the number of cusps. Also the presence of a right aortic arch will be identified. When a common pulmonary segment is present, it is located on the left posterior aspect of the wide common truncus just above the valve and the left and right pulmonary arteries arise from it. When the pulmonary arteries arise from the truncus directly, the presence of ostial stenosis should be assessed and the diameter of each vessel noted. The coronary arteries should be examined to determine whether there is any anomaly. However, in those individuals with large pulmonary blood flows, the contrast medium may be so diluted that coronary arteries are not well visualized. If the artery to the lung arises some distance from the truncal valve or from the descending aorta, it may be advisable to inject contrast medium into the aorta just proximal to the vessel to give better visualization than can be obtained from a supravalvar injection. If a catheter can be manipulated into the artery, an injection can be made directly to assess its size and possible distal stenosis. When pulmonary arterial ostial stenosis is marked, blood flow to the lung may be decreased and the vessels are narrow. In the absence of stenosis, the pattern of the pulmonary vessels may give some indication of the level of pulmonary vascular resistance. When it is not greatly increased there is rapid flow of contrast medium into the lung, with filling of the small vessels and pulmonary capillaries, and venous filling appears early and the veins are clearly visualized. When pulmonary vascular resistance is high, the central pulmonary arteries are dilated and often tortuous but there is poor filling of smaller vessels, deficient capillary filling, and a poorly visualized venous phase.

As with ultrasound examination, the diagnosis of aortic arch interruption may be difficult by angiography. The truncus is seen as a large chamber above the valve; the pulmonary arteries usually originate from the lateral sides of the truncus and a small ascending aorta arises from the upper portion. The ductus passes posteriorly and to the left. The large ductus arteriosus leading from the truncus to the descending aorta can readily be mistaken for the aortic arch and the ascending aorta is thought to be the innominate artery. The appearance of the left carotid artery, as described in the ultrasound section above, is often helpful in diagnosing the interruption.

Differential diagnosis

In infants in failure, truncus arteriosus must be distinguished from other lesions that cause cardiac failure and are associated with mild cyanosis. Lesions such as aortopulmonary transposition with ventricular septal defect, double-outlet right ventricle, tricuspid atresia with ventricular septal defect with or without aortopulmonary transposition, single ventricle and total anomalous pulmonary venous drainage are the more important lesions to consider. The left axis deviation and dominant left ventricular forces in the electrocardiogram noted with tricuspid atresia and the paucity of left ventricular forces in patients with total anomalous pulmonary venous drainage are helpful differentiating points. The absent or small pulmonary artery segment on the radiograph suggests either truncus arteriosus or aortopulmonary transposition but, as mentioned above, the pulmonary arterial shadow may be present in some instances. Ultrasound examination readily differentiates the various lesions.

In older infants and children, the presence of a continuous murmur with evidence of a large left-to-right shunt may create confusion with aortopulmonary fenestration or patent ductus arteriosus. The patient with truncus arteriosus is cyanotic, but this may be so mild that it may not be appreciated; also, if cardiac failure is present, cyanosis may occur due to pulmonary edema associated with any of the lesions. The radiograph may be helpful if the pulmonary artery segment is deficient. Ultrasound studies usually readily provide the correct diagnosis.

In patients with markedly decreased pulmonary blood flow, the differentiation must be made from other causes of marked cyanosis with reduced pulmonary flow. These include pulmonary atresia with intact ventricular septum, tricuspid atresia, atrioventricular septal defect with pulmonary stenosis, double-outlet right ventricle with pulmonary stenosis, and tetralogy of Fallot with severe pulmonary stenosis or pulmonary atresia. The differential diagnosis of these lesions is discussed in Chapters 14, 15 and 16.

Principles of management

Without treatment, most patients with truncus arteriosus die within 6–12 months after birth, usually due to severe cardiac failure. Within the past 15–20 years the management has changed dramatically. Surgical repair can now be accomplished with a relatively low mortality, even in small infants. The principle of the operation is to close the ventricular septal defect so that the left ventricle communicates with the aorta. A valved or nonvalved conduit is placed between the right ventricle and the pulmonary arteries.

Prior to the development of this approach, the only palliative procedure that was available was pulmonary arterial banding. If there was a common pulmonary artery segment, it was sometimes possible to band the short common segment with good results, but when the pulmonary arteries arise directly from the truncus it was necessary to band each vessel separately. This was an extensive procedure and it was very difficult to estimate how much constriction should be produced in each artery. The procedure had a high mortality, and inadequate or excessive narrowing of one or both vessels at the site of banding was common after the surgery.

In early experience with surgical repair, the mortality in infants was high, and it was preferred in most centers to delay the procedure for 2–3 years. Cardiac failure was treated with digitalis and diuretic agents. If a good response was obtained, the infant was followed and assessed repeatedly with regard to the possible development of increasing pulmonary vascular resistance. If it was noted that precordial activity became less prominent, that cardiac failure improved, that the apical mid-diastolic flow murmur disappeared, and that cyanosis increased, it was likely that pulmonary vascular resistance was increasing and surgery was performed.

Recently it has been recommended that surgery be performed in early infancy. This eliminates the risks for persistent cardiac failure and the development of pulmonary vascular disease. In most centers, a valved aortic or pulmonary arterial homograft is used as the conduit between the right ventricle and the pulmonary arteries. In type I truncus, the common pulmonary trunk segment is separated from the truncus and this is attached to the homograft. In types II and III truncus, the individual pulmonary arteries are detached and some reconstruction is required to make the connection. In type IV truncus, a unifocalization procedure is performed, as described for tetralogy of Fallot with pulmonary atresia (see Chapter 14).

If truncal valve insufficiency is either not present or is mild, surgical results are excellent. In a series of 65 patients in whom surgery was performed within the first postnatal month, 23% had moderate to severe truncal valve insufficiency and 12% had an interrupted aortic arch. A valved aortic or pulmonary allograft was used for right ventricular outflow reconstruction and the aortic valve was repaired or replaced to relieve the insufficiency. Surgical mortality was only 5% [4]. These excellent results are not achieved in all centers. Although these exceptional results are achievable in the first postnatal month, many consider that outcomes are somewhat improved if surgery is delayed until the second to third month. The practice at these centers is to routinely perform the surgery at 2–3 months, unless the infant has uncontrollable cardiac failure or has an associated interruption of the aortic arch.

The presence of moderate to severe truncal valve insufficiency dramatically influences survival. Whether detected before or after surgical repair, in early experience the mortality was about 33% soon after surgery, with another 20% succumbing within 10 years. Mechanical or homograft replacement was attended by a high operative mortality and did not achieve good results. Recently, several centers have reported encouraging results with direct repair of truncal valves with marked insufficiency [4]. It remains to be seen whether this approach will be successful.

The association of interrupted aortic arch considerably increases the mortality with repair of truncus arteriosus, and it was suggested that the repair be performed in two procedures. However, recently, excellent results have been achieved with complete repair of both lesions during the first month after birth [4].

The conduit placed between the right ventricle and the pulmonary artery in the earliest procedures on patients with truncus arteriosus were nonvalved tubes. They were quite effective, but it was important to use narrow tubes to avoid development of marked pulmonary insufficiency. The second approach was to use a woven tube graft with a porcine valve (Hancock valve). Subsequently, aortic or pulmonary allografts, which included the semilunar valve, have been used. Most recently, bovine jugular vein grafts with a tricuspid bovine venous valve have been used. These bovine conduits appear to be as effective as aortic homografts [5].

The insertion of a conduit between the right ventricle and the pulmonary arteries during early infancy usually requires that it be replaced at some later period. The period after which replacement is necessary varies greatly, but in various centers the median is 5–6 years. Replacement is necessary because the conduit may become too small with age and right ventricular pressure increases. Also the homograft valve may become thickened and stenosed resulting in right ventricular hypertension. Another concern is the development of homograft valve regurgitation. The indications for replacement are reviewed in Chapter 14.

In types II and III truncus, relief of obstruction at the orifice, or more distally in the pulmonary arteries, is frequently necessary. Surgical attempts were often not successful and were often associated with restenosis. Transcatheter balloon dilation of the obstructed area, often with the insertion of a stent, has been quite successful in relieving these stenoses.

References

1 Restivo A, Piacentini G, Placidi S *et al.* Cardiac outflow tract: a review of some embryogenetic aspects of the conotruncal region of the heart. Anat Rec A Discov Mol Cell Evol Biol 2006;288:936–943.

2 Schleiffarth JR, Person AD, Martinsen BJ *et al.* Wnt5a is required for cardiac outflow tract septation in mice. Pediatr Res 2007;61:386–391.

3 Momma K, Ando M, Matsuoka R. Truncus arteriosus communis associated with chromosome 22q11 deletion. J Am Coll Cardiol 1997;30:1067–1071.

4 Thompson LD, McElhinney DB, Reddy M, Petrossian E, Silverman NH, Hanley FL. Neonatal repair of truncus arteriosus: continuing improvement in outcomes. Ann Thorac Surg 2001;72:391–395.

5 Sierra J, Christenson JT, Lahlaidi NH, Beghetti M, Kalangos A. Right ventricular outflow tract reconstruction: what conduit to use? Homograft or Contegra? Ann Thorac Surg 2007;84:606–610.

Index

Note: page numbers in *italics* refer to figures, those in **bold** refer to tables

The manufacturer's authorised representative in the EU for product safety is Oxford University Press España S.A. of El Parque Empresarial San Fernando de Henares, Avenida de Castilla, 2 – 28830 Madrid (www.oup.es/en or product.safety@oup.com). OUP España S.A. also acts as importer into Spain of products made by the manufacturer.

Printed in the USA/Agawam, MA
March 10, 2025

884105.029